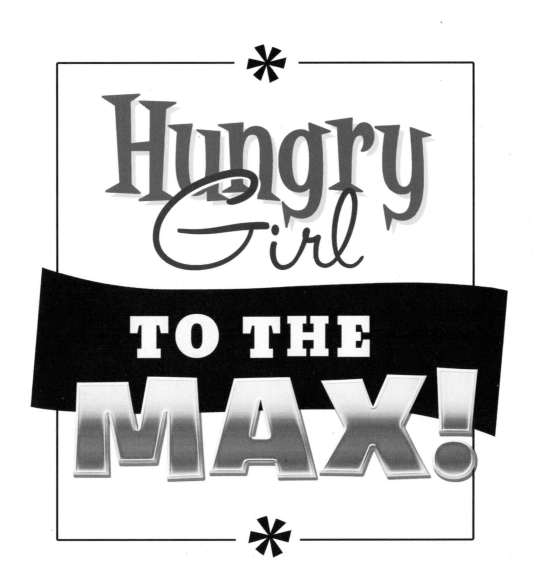

DISCARD

ALSO BY LISA LILLIEN

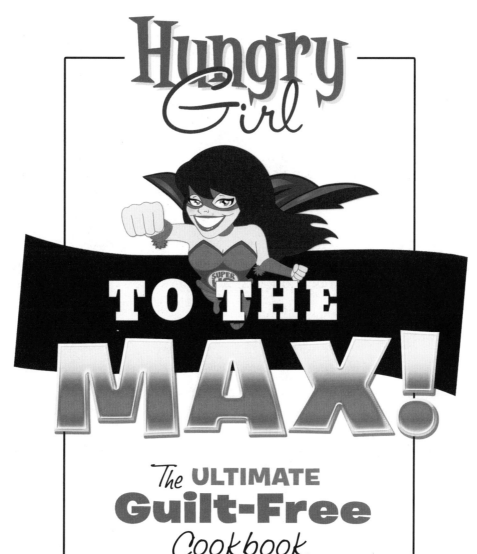

Hungry Girl
TO THE MAX!

The ULTIMATE Guilt-Free Cookbook

LISA LILLIEN

Greenwood Public Library
PO Box 839 Mill St.
Greenwood, DE 19950

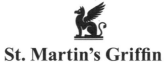

St. Martin's Griffin
New York

The author's references to various brand-name products and services are for informational purposes only and are not intended to suggest endorsement or sponsorship of the author or her book by any company, organization, or owner of any brand.

HUNGRY GIRL TO THE MAX! THE ULTIMATE GUILT-FREE COOKBOOK. Copyright © 2012 by Hungry Girl, Inc. All rights reserved. Printed in the United States of America. For information, address St. Martin's Press, 175 Fifth Avenue, New York, N.Y. 10010.

www.stmartins.com

Cover design and book design by Elizabeth Hodson

Illustrations by Jack Pullan

Food styling and photography by General Mills Photography Studios

      Photographer: Val Bourassa

      Food Stylists: Nancy Johnson and Carol Grones

      Photography Assistant: Dusty Hoskovec

ISBN 978-0-312-67678-0

First Edition: October 2012

10 9 8 7 6 5 4 3 2 1

CONTENTS

CHAPTER 3
PARFAITS

CHAPTER 4
PANCAKES AND FRENCH TOAST

CHAPTER 5
FAUX-FRYS: POPPERS, ONION RINGS, CHICKEN NUGGETS & MORE 90

CHAPTER 6
SWAPPUCCINOS & SHAKES   120

CHAPTER 9
PASTA

CHAPTER 12
BURGERS & FRIES   268

CHAPTER 15
PARTY FOODS, COCKTAILS & HOLIDAY 356

Recipe Guide by Category

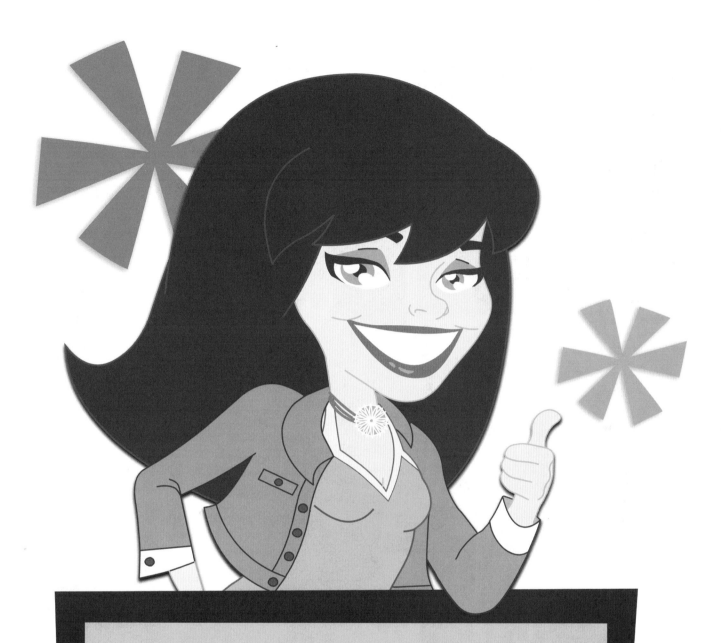

ACKNOWLEDGMENTS
(thankyouthankyouthankyou!!!)

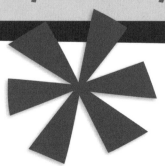

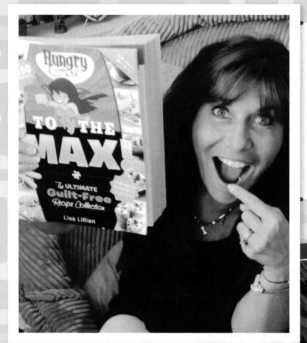

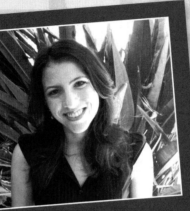

These people deserve
HUGE thanks
(and I figured you'd wanna see
what they look like) . . .

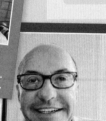

Bill Stankey
My manager's awesome . . .
and ALWAYS on the phone.

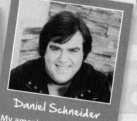

Daniel Schneider
My amazing husband & the
creator of Dan-Good Chili!
(LOVE YOU!)

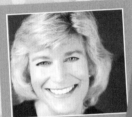

Amanda Pisani
Proofreading PRO. (Hope there
are no typos on this page!)

Jamie Goldberg
Managing Editor/Superwoman who
sacrificed many nights of sleep for this
book! (Hug her if you see her!)

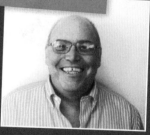

John Murphy
PR KING at St. Martin's Press . . .
Everyone loves John!

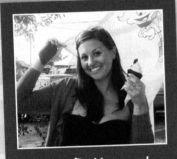

Lynn Bettencourt
Worked her butt off on this book . . .
from thousands of miles away!

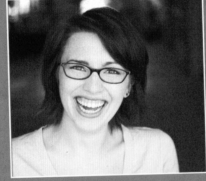

Dana DeRuyck
Editor, recipe developer . . . What CAN'T
Dana accomplish? I can answer that:
NOTHING!

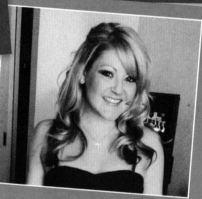

Callie Pegadiotes
Food-stylist/photographer extraordinaire
& SO much more. (She snaps ALL the
recipe pics in HG emails!)

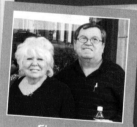

**Florence &
Maurice Lillien**
My crazy-cute parents. (My
mom's amazing stuffed cabbage
is featured in this book!) XOXO

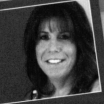

Meri Lillien
My sis . . . who seeks out
new guilt-free foods like
it's her JOB!

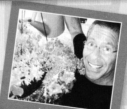

Jay Lillien
My bro . . . He doesn't
work on HG books, but
he deserves thanks
nonetheless!

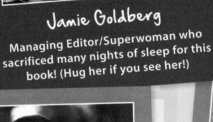

Melissa Klotz
Daily-email designer &
production wizard!

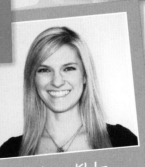

Matthew Shear
Publishing head honcho at
St. Martin's Press! (And he's
ALWAYS smiling!)

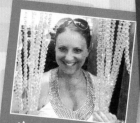

Michelle Weintraub

Marketing & analyst guru and newest HG full-timer!

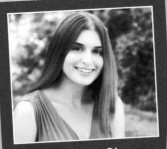

Samantha Oliver

Editorial brainiac. (She's read this book cover to cover several times!)

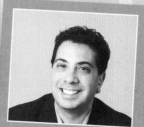

John Vaccaro

Voice of reason/ BFF/Hungry Boy!

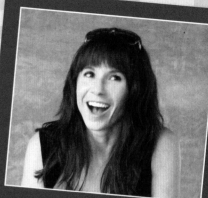

Elizabeth Hodson

HG's DESIGN QUEEN! She's designed ALL 7 GORGEOUS HG books (this page included)!

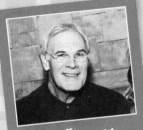

Tom Fineman

The world's BEST attorney (and my very close friend!)

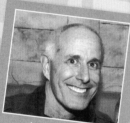

Jeff Becker

My cuddly business manager (and the FUNNIEST CPA in history)!

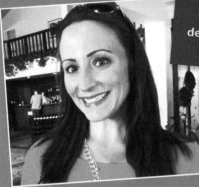

Lisa Friedman

Jill of all trades! (The HG HQ does not run without her!)

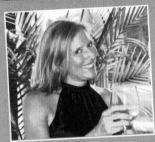

Alison Kreuch

Advertising & Marketing VP/LIFESAVER!!!

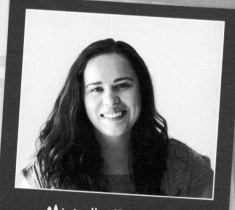

Michelle Ferrand

Kitchen genius (she's made EVERY recipe in this book more than once!).

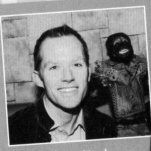

John Karle

Has done PR for all 7 HG books … and we STILL love each other!

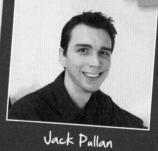

Jack Pullan

HG artist. He sure knows his way around a pencil … He draws all the HG character art!

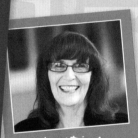

Nanci Dixon

Manages the photo studio at General Mills (where our book photos are shot!). Yay, Nanci!

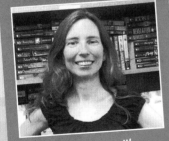

Anne Marie Tallberg

St. Martin's Press Marketing MAVEN. (Please get the word out about this book, Anne Marie!)

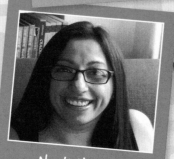

Neeti Madan

Without her super-agent skills, you wouldn't be holding this book!

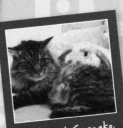

Jackson & Cupcake

My furry babybooboos!!!

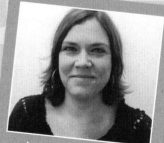

Jennifer Enderlin

Editorial mastermind at St. Martin's Press … JEN ROCKS!

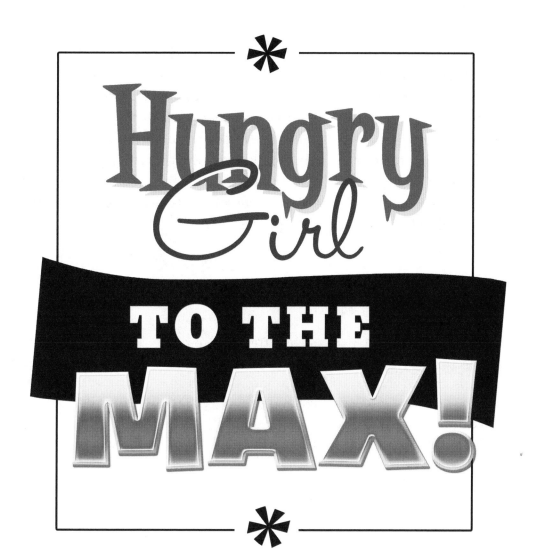

INTRODUCTION

Welcome to *HUNGRY GIRL TO THE MAX! The Ultimate Guilt-Free Cookbook*, a.k.a. your HUNGRY GIRL BIBLE. This is the most MASSIVE and complete Hungry Girl book in existence—a must-have for anyone who craves decadent food without the high-calorie price tag. What's inside? A whopping 650 guilt-free recipes for any and every food you crave. We've taken HG classics—egg mugs, faux-frys, oversized oatmeal bowls, crock-pot recipes, foil packs, fast-food swaps, and more—and put them in one tremendous must-own collection. Then we developed hundreds more of these favorites just for YOU. Love our Lord of the Onion Rings? There are EIGHT versions to enjoy. Is Hungry Girlfredo your favorite? TEN terrific variations to chomp on. New to HG, or just wanna know more? Keep reading . . .

HUNGRY GIRL IN A HUNDRED WORDS OR LESS

Hungry Girl is a lifestyle brand that started as a free daily email service about guilt-free eating. The emails (read by over a million people a day) feature news, food finds, recipes, and real-world tips and survival strategies. Hungry Girl was started by me, Lisa Lillien. I'm not a doctor or nutrition professional; I'm just hungry! Back in 2004, I decided I wanted to share my love and knowledge of guilt-free eating with the world, so Hungry Girl was born. To sign up for the daily emails or to see what you've missed since the beginning, go to hungry-girl.com.

GUILT-FREE EATING 101

The Hungry Girl way of eating is a bridge between the average American junk-food-packed diet and the idealistic way of eating perfectly healthy foods at all times. It's a realistic approach to better-for-you eating that people can actually live with and feel good about. HG recipes fulfill real-world cravings for EVERYTHING—including fattening things like fried food, pizza, and mac 'n cheese—without containing a tremendous amount of calories and fat. These recipes can help you to achieve and maintain a healthy weight without feeling deprived.

INSIDE THE HG RECIPE LAB . . .

When creating HG recipes, the goal is to make them taste delicious while keeping them low in fat and calories. We also aim for high fiber and protein counts to help you feel full and satisfied. Nutritional information is also provided for sodium, carbs, sugars, etc., so you can look at a recipe and decide if it works for you. You can, of course, make substitutions for products and ingredients, but the taste and nutritional info will vary accordingly. It's that simple . . .

THE 411 ON CLASSIC RECIPES REVISITED

This book contains many classic HG recipes, and some of 'em have been updated. For example, we've SUPER-SIZED our very first oatmeal bowls. The ingredients called for in this book are also easier to find than ingredients in past books. When a recipe's nutritionals differ slightly from those in a previous HG cookbook, it's because the recipe has been revamped a bit. The nutritional stats for each version of the recipe are 100 percent accurate—the recipes themselves are just slightly different.

BEHIND THE NUTRITIONALS: HOW WE DO IT

The stats for each recipe are carefully calculated by doing extensive research—using extremely reliable nutritional databases and countless product labels. When recipes call for generic ingredients (like tortillas or burger patties), we calculate averages based on a wide variety of national brands. Also taken into account are the small amounts of calories and fat in many so-called no-calorie and fat-free ingredients. We work extremely hard to determine the most accurate nutritional information possible for our recipes—not only because we care about you, but because the Hungry Girl staff and I make and eat them too!

NAVIGATING TO THE MAX

With more than 600 recipes, we knew we had to make it super-easy to find what you're looking for. In addition to the table of contents and the recipes listed at the start of each chapter, we've added symbols throughout the book to help you quickly spot what you're after . . .

15 Minutes or Less
This symbol lets you know a recipe should take you no more than fifteen minutes from start to finish! That includes prep and cook time.

30 Minutes or Less
Just like the 15-minute version, this one points out recipes that take 30 minutes or less to whip up.

Meatless
You guessed it—no meat here! That includes beef, poultry, and fish. Some recipes give the option of a meatless ingredient. If you want your meal without meat, go with the meatless choice.

Single Serving
Pretty straightforward. These are recipes for one.

5 Ingredients or Less
Fans of HG know that we like to keep things simple. And these recipes contain just five ingredients or less!

Photos
These recipes can be seen in one of the book's photo inserts. The number in the symbol tells you which insert. Find photos of all the recipes at hungry-girl.com/books!

Flip to the back of the book for **COMPLETE LISTS of every recipe in each of these categories**. And for more helpful assistance, check out our **super-deluxe index**!

SPLENDA & SUGAR SWAPPIN'!

Many HG desserts call for Splenda No Calorie Sweetener (granulated) because it has around 90 percent fewer calories than sugar. We use real sugar in recipes when not much sweetener is needed or when the taste of real sugar makes a big difference.

Some people prefer one or the other across the board, so we've provided recipe stats if made with the alternative for every recipe! The few exceptions are recipes in which the nutritional difference is negligible; in those cases, the ingredients are listed interchangeably.

GET THE PHOTOS AND POINTSPLUS® VALUES FOR ALL 650 RECIPES!

Not every single recipe is lucky enough to have a photo here, so we've captured each and every one for your online viewing pleasure!

Also, we're big fans of Weight Watchers, and we know many of you are too. For your convenience, we've provided the Weight Watchers *PointsPlus*® value* for each and every recipe in *HUNGRY GIRL TO THE MAX!* online.

Visit **hungry-girl.com/books** for the photos and values!

*The PointsPlus® values for these recipes were calculated by Hungry Girl and are not an endorsement or approval of the recipe or developer by Weight Watchers International, Inc., the owner of the PointsPlus® registered trademark.

RECOMMENDED PRODUCTS

PANTRY

No-calorie sweetener packets
Splenda
Truvia

Hot cocoa mix packets with 20 to 25 calories each
Swiss Miss Diet
Nestlé Fat Free

Baked tortilla chips
Guiltless Gourmet
Baked! Tostitos Scoops!

Canned pure pumpkin
Libby's

Thick teriyaki marinade or sauce
Newman's Own
Lawry's

Creamy tomato soup with 4g fat or less per serving
Amy's Chunky Tomato Bisque

Moist-style cake mix
Betty Crocker
Pillsbury

Sugar-free French vanilla powdered creamer
Coffee-mate Sugar Free French Vanilla

BREAD PRODUCTS

Light bread
Sara Lee Delightful
Nature's Own 40 Calories

100-calorie flat sandwich buns
Arnold Select/Brownberry/Oroweat Sandwich Thins
Pepperidge Farm Deli Flats
Nature's Own Sandwich Rounds

Medium-large high-fiber flour tortillas with 110 calories or less each
La Tortilla Factory Smart & Delicious
 Low Carb High Fiber and 100 Calorie
Mission Carb Balance
Tumaro's Healthy and Low in Carbs
Flatout Light Wraps

Light English muffins
Thomas' Light Multi-Grain
Weight Watchers

Corn taco shells
Old El Paso Stand 'N Stuff
Taco Bell
Ortega

Corn tortillas
Mission 6-inch tortillas
Mission Super Size (medium-large tortillas)

Light buns
Sara Lee Delightful
Wonder 80 Calorie

FRIDGE

Fat-free liquid egg substitute
Egg Beaters Original
Better'n Eggs

Light whipped butter or light buttery spread
Brummel & Brown
Land O' Lakes Whipped Light Butter

Light vanilla soymilk
8th Continent Light
Silk Light

Fat-free yogurt
Yoplait Light
Fiber One
Weight Watchers

Fat-free Greek yogurt
Fage Total 0%
Chobani 0%

Sugar-free pancake syrup
Log Cabin Sugar Free
Mrs. Butterworth's Sugar Free
Cary's
Joseph's

Sugar-free and low-sugar fruit preserves, jelly, and jam
Smucker's Sugar Free and Low Sugar Preserves, Jelly, and Jam
Polaner Sugar Free Preserves with Fiber

Sugar-free pudding snacks with 60 calories or less each
Jell-O Sugar Free
Handi-Snacks Sugar Free
Snack Pack Sugar Free

Fat-free or light caramel dip (often found in the produce section)
Marzetti Fat Free and Light Caramel Dip
Litehouse Low Fat and Original

Hot dogs with about 40 calories and 1g fat or less each
Hebrew National 97% Fat Free Beef Franks
Hoffy Extra Lean Beef Franks
Veggie Patch Veggie Dogs

Center-cut bacon and turkey bacon
Oscar Mayer
Hormel
Jennie-O
Applegate

Precooked real crumbled bacon
Oscar Mayer
Hormel

Turkey pepperoni
Hormel

Light/low-fat salad dressing
Newman's Own Lite
Litehouse (low-fat varieties)

FREEZER

Meatless hamburger-style patties with 100 calories or less each
Boca Original Vegan Meatless Burgers
Amy's Bistro Burgers
MorningStar Farms Grillers Vegan

Ground-beef-style soy crumbles
Boca Meatless Ground Crumbles
MorningStar Farms Meal Starters Grillers Recipe Crumbles

Meatless or turkey sausage patties with 80 calories or less each
MorningStar Farms Original Sausage Patties
Jimmy Dean Turkey Sausage Patties

Low-fat waffles
Eggo Nutri-Grain Low Fat Whole Wheat
Van's Lite Totally Natural

Fat-free ice cream
Breyers Fat Free
Dreyer's/Edy's Slow Churned Light (not fat-free but fantastic, and it'll barely affect a recipe's stats!)

HOW TO HG-IFY YOUR KITCHEN

Stock up on basic kitchen equipment, HG-style.
Here's what you'll need ...

Stovetop cookware:
a basic skillet, a wok or large skillet, and small and large nonstick pots

Baking needs:
a couple of baking sheets, an 8-inch by 8-inch pan, a 9-inch by 13-inch pan, and a 12-cup muffin pan

Microwave-safe essentials:
large mugs, bowls, and plates

Measuring must-haves:
spoons, cups, and a kitchen scale

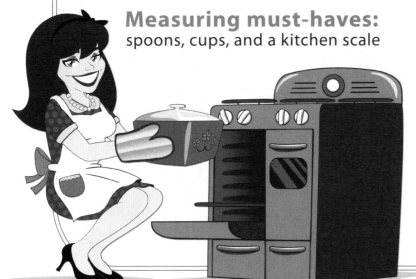

Countertop tools:
a crock pot/slow cooker, a good blender, a Magic Bullet or other small food processor (optional), a meat mallet (optional), a strainer, and kitchen shears (optional, but helpful!)

Now you know everything. Nothin' left to do but start whipping up delicious guilt-free recipes. ENJOY!

CHAPTER 1

EGG MUGS AND EGG BAKES

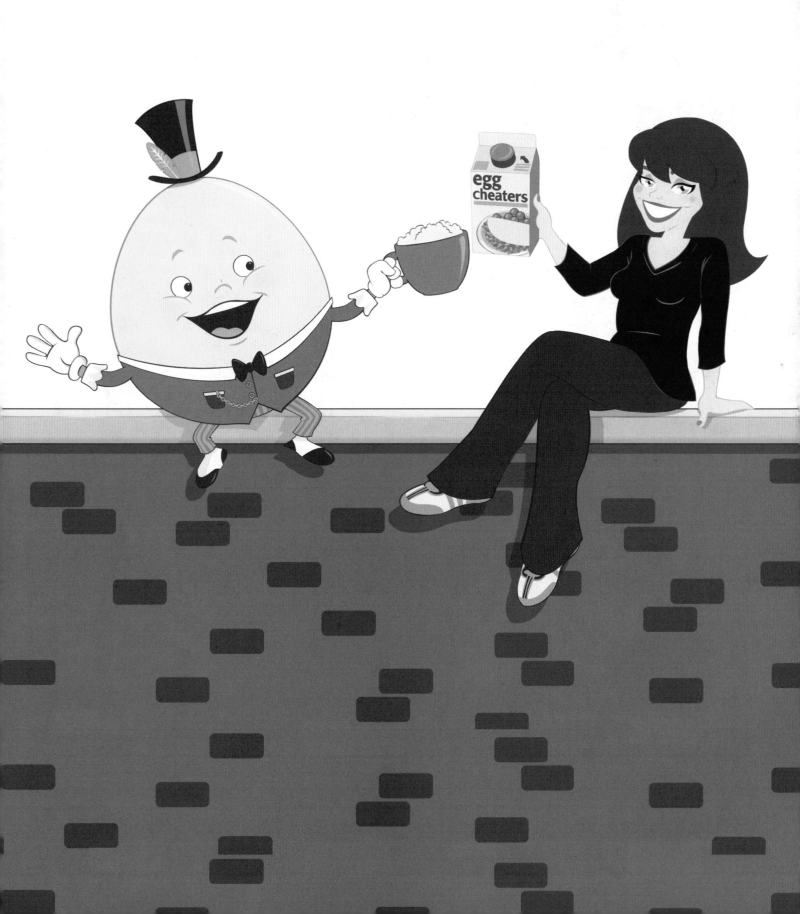

EGG MUGS AND EGG BAKES

EGG MUGS

The Egg Mug Classic
Mug Foo Young
Bean 'n Cheesy Soft Taco in an Egg Mug
Eggs Bene-chick Mug
Egg Mug Neptune
California Love Mug
BTA (Bacon, Tomato, Avocado) Egg Mug
Chicken Fajita Scramble Mug
Buffalo Chicken Egg Mug
Crunchy Beefy Taco Egg Mug
Denver Omelette in a Mug
Pizza! Pizza! Egg Mug
Say Cheese! Egg Mug
Mexi-licious Egg Mug
Egg Mug Lorraine
The HG Special Egg Mug
It's All Greek to Me Egg Mug
Egg Mug Burger-rama
All-American Egg Mug
Bacon-Cheddar Egg Mug
Meat Lover's Egg Mug
Egg Mug Florentine
Chili Cheese Egg Mug
Thanksgiving in an Egg Mug
Hawaiian Scramble in a Mug
Veggie Eggs-plosion Mug
Cheesy Chicken & Broccoli Egg Mug
Cheesy Jalapeño Egg Mug
Chicken Teriyaki Egg Mug

EGG BAKES

The Original Ginormous Egg Bake
Egg Bake Olé
Totally Fly Thai-Style Egg Bake
El Ginormo Southwest Egg Bake
Cheesy-Onion Egg Bake
The Breakfast Club Egg Bake
Cheesy Bacon-Apple-Bella Egg Bake
Good Morning Mega Quiche
Cheesy Sausage 'n Hash Egg Bake
Caramelized Onion 'n Spinach Egg Bake
Ham-It-Up Egg Bake
Sweet Treat a la Soufflé

Eggs are underrated as far as we're concerned. This section will prove this quite clearly. Enjoy . . .

MUG IT UP!

* When choosing a mug, the bigger, the better. The egg mixture will puff and rise as it cooks. Your best bet is a tall, wide mug with a 16-ounce capacity. Don't own any oversized mugs? Use a microwave-safe BOWL. We won't tell . . .

* Some microwaves are more powerful than others. You may need to adjust cook times for your specific appliance.

* After you're finished eating, SOAK YOUR MUG in warm, soapy water. That egg sticks! (Consider yourself warned.)

ABOUT YOUR EGG BAKE . . .

* Cool it! Literally. Let your oven-baked dish cool for 5 to 10 minutes before digging in. The omelette will pull away from the edges a bit, making it easier to cut and serve.

* Your egg bake may deflate a little once it has cooled. Worry not; it'll still be huge.

* Use a big spatula to remove a serving . . . It's the right utensil for the job!

A QUICK GUIDE TO SYMBOLS:

15 Minutes or Less

This symbol lets you know a recipe should take you no more than fifteen minutes from start to finish! That includes prep and cook time.

30 Minutes or Less

Just like the 15-minute version, this one points out recipes that take 30 minutes or less to whip up.

Meatless

You guessed it—no meat here! That includes beef, poultry, and fish. Some recipes give the option of a meatless ingredient. If you want your meal without meat, go with the meatless choice.

Single Serving

Pretty straightforward. These are recipes for one.

5 Ingredients or Less

Fans of HG know that we like to keep things simple. And these recipes contain just five ingredients or less!

Photos

These recipes can be seen in one of the book's photo inserts. The number in the symbol tells you which insert. Find photos of all the recipes at hungry-girl.com/books!

EGG MUGS

Discovered by sheer accidental laziness, egg mugs have become a staple in the world of Hungry Girl. No pots or pans required for these piping-hot, super-simple, protein-packed breakfasts. We've got a SLEW of 'em right here and now, for your chewing pleasure . . . ENJOY!!!

THE EGG MUG CLASSIC

125 calories

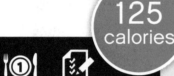

You'll Need: large microwave-safe mug, nonstick spray
Prep: 5 minutes
Cook: 5 minutes

Entire recipe: 125 calories, 1.5g fat, 547mg sodium, 3.5g carbs, 0g fiber, 2.5g sugars, 20g protein

INGREDIENTS

¾ cup fat-free liquid egg substitute
1 wedge The Laughing Cow Light Creamy Swiss cheese

DIRECTIONS

In a large microwave-safe mug sprayed with nonstick spray, microwave egg substitute for 1½ minutes.

Mix in cheese wedge, breaking it into pieces. Microwave for 1 minute, or until set. Stir and enjoy!

MAKES 1 SERVING

MUG FOO YOUNG

150 calories

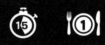

You'll Need: large microwave-safe mug, nonstick spray
Prep: 5 minutes
Cook: 5 minutes

Entire recipe: 150 calories, 0.5g fat, 629mg sodium, 8g carbs, 1g fiber, 3g sugars, 27g protein

INGREDIENTS

¼ cup roughly chopped bean sprouts
¼ cup chopped mushrooms
¾ cup fat-free liquid egg substitute
1 ounce cooked and chopped skinless chicken breast
1 tablespoon chopped scallions
½ teaspoon reduced-sodium/lite soy sauce
½ teaspoon dried minced onion
⅛ teaspoon garlic powder
2 tablespoons fat-free chicken gravy

DIRECTIONS

In a large microwave-safe mug sprayed with nonstick spray, microwave sprouts and mushrooms for 30 seconds, or until slightly softened.

Blot away excess moisture. Add all remaining ingredients *except* gravy. Stir and microwave for 1½ minutes.

Stir and microwave for 1 minute, or until set.

Stir, top with gravy, and microwave for 10 seconds, or until gravy is warm. Dig in!

MAKES 1 SERVING

BEAN 'N CHEESY SOFT TACO IN AN EGG MUG

190 calories

You'll Need: small bowl, large microwave-safe mug, nonstick spray
Prep: 5 minutes
Cook: 5 minutes

Entire recipe: 190 calories, 0.25g fat, 835mg sodium, 20g carbs, 4g fiber, 2.5g sugars, 25g protein

INGREDIENTS

¼ cup fat-free refried beans
¼ teaspoon taco seasoning mix
¾ cup fat-free liquid egg substitute
½ of a 6-inch corn tortilla
1 tablespoon shredded fat-free cheddar cheese
1 tablespoon salsa

DIRECTIONS

In a small bowl, mix beans with taco seasoning.

In a large microwave-safe mug sprayed with nonstick spray, microwave egg substitute for 1½ minutes.

Tear tortilla half into bite-sized pieces and add to the mug. Stir in seasoned beans and cheese.

Microwave for 1 minute, or until set. Top with salsa and dig in!

MAKES 1 SERVING

EGGS BENE-CHICK MUG

153 calories

You'll Need: large microwave-safe mug, nonstick spray, small microwave-safe bowl
Prep: 5 minutes
Cook: 5 minutes

Entire recipe: 153 calories, 1.75g fat, 831mg sodium, 15.5g carbs, 3g fiber, 2.5g sugars, 20g protein

INGREDIENTS

½ cup fat-free liquid egg substitute
½ light English muffin, lightly toasted
1 ounce sliced 97% to 98% fat-free ham (about 2 slices), roughly chopped
2 teaspoons fat-free mayonnaise
1 teaspoon Dijon mustard
1 drop lemon juice

DIRECTIONS

In a large microwave-safe mug sprayed with nonstick spray, microwave egg substitute for 1 minute.

Tear muffin half into bite-sized pieces and add to the mug. Add ham and stir. Microwave for 1 minute, or until set, and stir.

In a small microwave-safe bowl, thoroughly mix mayo, mustard, and lemon juice. Microwave for 15 seconds, or until warm. Pour over your egg mug, stir, and dig in!

MAKES 1 SERVING

HG SODIUM TIP:
Shave about 140mg of sodium off the stats by using reduced-sodium ham.

For more recipes, tips & tricks, sign up for FREE daily emails at **hungry-girl.com**!

EGG MUG NEPTUNE

188 calories

You'll Need: small microwave-safe bowl, large microwave-safe mug, nonstick spray
Prep: 5 minutes
Cook: 5 minutes

Entire recipe: 188 calories, 2g fat, 802mg sodium, 22.5g carbs, 3g fiber, 3.5g sugars, 22g protein

INGREDIENTS

½ teaspoon light whipped butter or light buttery spread
½ tablespoon fat-free mayonnaise
½ teaspoon Best Foods/Hellmann's Dijonnaise
½ teaspoon lemon yogurt (or plain yogurt with a drop of lemon juice)
⅔ cup fat-free liquid egg substitute
½ light English muffin, lightly toasted
1½ ounces (about ¼ cup) roughly chopped imitation crabmeat

DIRECTIONS

Microwave butter in a small microwave-safe bowl for 10 seconds, or until melted. Add mayo, Dijonnaise, and yogurt. Mix well.

In a large microwave-safe mug sprayed with nonstick spray, microwave egg substitute for 1½ minutes.

Tear muffin half into bite-sized pieces and add to the mug. Add crab and stir. Microwave for 45 to 50 seconds, until set, and stir.

If you like, microwave mayo mixture for 10 seconds, or until warm. Pour over egg mug and dig in!

MAKES 1 SERVING

CALIFORNIA LOVE MUG

140 calories

You'll Need: large microwave-safe mug, nonstick spray
Prep: 5 minutes
Cook: 5 minutes

Entire recipe: 140 calories, 4.5g fat, 456mg sodium, 7g carbs, 2g fiber, 3g sugars, 16g protein

INGREDIENTS

½ cup chopped spinach leaves
½ cup sliced mushrooms
½ cup fat-free liquid egg substitute
2 tablespoons diced tomato
1 wedge The Laughing Cow Light Creamy Swiss cheese
1 ounce (about 2 tablespoons) diced avocado

DIRECTIONS

In a large microwave-safe mug sprayed with nonstick spray, microwave spinach and mushrooms for 1½ minutes, or until softened.

Blot away excess moisture. Add egg substitute, stir, and microwave for 1 minute.

Mix in tomato and cheese wedge, breaking the wedge into pieces. Microwave for 1 minute, or until set. Top with avocado and enjoy!

MAKES 1 SERVING

BTA (BACON, TOMATO, AVOCADO) EGG MUG

175 calories

You'll Need: large microwave-safe mug, nonstick spray | **Prep:** 5 minutes | **Cook:** 5 minutes

Entire recipe:
175 calories, 7.25g fat, 813mg sodium, 8.5g carbs, 3g fiber, 3.5g sugars, 19.5g protein

INGREDIENTS

½ cup fat-free liquid egg substitute
⅓ cup chopped tomato, patted dry
2 tablespoons precooked real crumbled bacon
1 ounce (about 2 tablespoons) diced avocado
2 tablespoons salsa

Optional seasonings: salt and black pepper

DIRECTIONS

In a large microwave-safe mug sprayed with nonstick spray, microwave egg substitute for 1 minute.

Stir in tomato and bacon. Microwave for 1 minute, or until set. Top with avocado and salsa. Eat up!

MAKES 1 SERVING

CHICKEN FAJITA SCRAMBLE MUG

163 calories

You'll Need: large microwave-safe mug, nonstick spray | **Prep:** 5 minutes | **Cook:** 5 minutes

Entire recipe:
163 calories, 0.75g fat, 583mg sodium, 12g carbs, 1.25g fiber, 5.5g sugars, 26g protein

INGREDIENTS

¼ cup chopped red bell pepper
¼ cup chopped onion
1 ounce cooked and chopped skinless chicken breast
1 teaspoon fajita seasoning mix
½ cup fat-free liquid egg substitute
2 tablespoons shredded fat-free cheddar cheese
1 tablespoon fat-free sour cream

DIRECTIONS

Spray a large microwave-safe mug with nonstick spray. Add veggies and chicken, sprinkle with fajita seasoning, and stir well. Microwave for 1½ minutes, or until veggies have softened.

Blot away excess moisture. Add egg substitute, stir, and microwave for 1 minute.

Stir in cheese. Microwave for 1 minute, or until set. Stir, top with sour cream, and enjoy!

MAKES 1 SERVING

BUFFALO CHICKEN EGG MUG

180 calories

You'll Need: large microwave-safe mug, nonstick spray | **Prep:** 5 minutes | **Cook:** 5 minutes

Entire recipe:
180 calories, 2.25g fat, 801mg sodium, 6g carbs, 0g fiber, 2g sugars, 33g protein

INGREDIENTS

¾ cup fat-free liquid egg substitute
1 teaspoon dried minced onion
2 ounces cooked and chopped skinless chicken breast
½ tablespoon Frank's RedHot Original Cayenne Pepper Sauce
1 teaspoon light blue cheese dressing
½ teaspoon reduced-fat Parmesan-style grated topping

DIRECTIONS

In a large microwave-safe mug sprayed with nonstick spray, microwave egg substitute and minced onion for 1½ minutes.

Stir in chicken. Microwave for 1 minute, or until set.

Top with hot sauce, blue cheese dressing, and Parm-style topping!

MAKES 1 SERVING

HG ALTERNATIVE!
Don't like blue cheese dressing? Swap it out for light ranch.

CRUNCHY BEEFY TACO EGG MUG

168 calories

You'll Need: large microwave-safe mug, nonstick spray | **Prep:** 5 minutes | **Cook:** 5 minutes

Entire recipe:
168 calories, 0.75g fat, 749mg sodium, 12.5g carbs, 1.75g fiber, 3g sugars, 26.5g protein

INGREDIENTS

¼ cup frozen ground-beef-style soy crumbles
¼ teaspoon taco seasoning mix
¾ cup fat-free liquid egg substitute
1 tablespoon fat-free shredded cheddar cheese
4 baked tortilla chips, roughly crushed
1 tablespoon salsa
1 tablespoon fat-free sour cream

DIRECTIONS

In a large microwave-safe mug sprayed with nonstick spray, microwave soy crumbles for 45 seconds, or until thawed.

Mix in taco seasoning. Add egg substitute, stir, and microwave for 1½ minutes.

Stir in cheese. Microwave for 1 minute, or until set. Top with tortilla chips, salsa, and sour cream!

MAKES 1 SERVING

DENVER OMELETTE IN A MUG

122 calories

You'll Need: large microwave-safe mug, nonstick spray | **Prep:** 5 minutes | **Cook:** 5 minutes

Entire recipe:
122 calories, 0.75g fat, 702mg sodium, 6g carbs, 0.5g fiber, 2.5g sugars, 21.5g protein

INGREDIENTS

¼ cup chopped green bell pepper
2 tablespoons chopped onion
½ cup fat-free liquid egg substitute
1 ounce sliced 97% to 98% fat-free ham (about 2 slices), chopped
2 tablespoons shredded fat-free cheddar cheese

DIRECTIONS

In a large microwave-safe mug sprayed with nonstick spray, microwave pepper and onion for 1½ minutes, or until softened.

Blot away excess moisture. Add egg substitute, stir, and microwave for 1 minute.

Stir in ham and cheese. Microwave for 1 minute, or until set. Eat up!

MAKES 1 SERVING

PIZZA! PIZZA! EGG MUG

134 calories

You'll Need: small bowl, large microwave-safe mug, nonstick spray | **Prep:** 5 minutes | **Cook:** 5 minutes

Entire recipe:
134 calories, 3.25g fat, 746mg sodium, 5g carbs, 0.5g fiber, 3g sugars, 17.5g protein

INGREDIENTS

2 tablespoons canned crushed tomatoes
⅛ teaspoon Italian seasoning
½ cup fat-free liquid egg substitute
1 wedge The Laughing Cow Light Creamy Swiss cheese
6 slices turkey pepperoni, chopped
½ teaspoon reduced-fat Parmesan-style grated topping

DIRECTIONS

In a small bowl, mix crushed tomatoes with Italian seasoning.

In a large microwave-safe mug sprayed with nonstick spray, microwave egg substitute for 1 minute.

Stir in cheese wedge, breaking it into pieces. Microwave for 30 seconds.

Stir in seasoned tomatoes and chopped pepperoni. Microwave for 30 seconds, or until set. Sprinkle with grated topping, stir, and enjoy!

MAKES 1 SERVING

SAY CHEESE! EGG MUG

172 calories

You'll Need: large microwave-safe mug, nonstick spray
Prep: 5 minutes
Cook: 5 minutes

Entire recipe: 172 calories, 5.5g fat, 645mg sodium, 6g carbs, <0.5g fiber, 3g sugars, 22g protein

INGREDIENTS

½ cup fat-free liquid egg substitute

1 piece Mini Babybel Light cheese, chopped

1 wedge The Laughing Cow Light cheese (any flavor)

1 tablespoon light or low-fat ricotta cheese

1 teaspoon dried minced onion

Dash garlic powder

Dash black pepper

½ teaspoon reduced-fat Parmesan-style grated topping

Optional seasonings: additional garlic powder and black pepper

DIRECTIONS

In a large microwave-safe mug sprayed with nonstick spray, microwave egg substitute for 1 minute.

Stir in all remaining ingredients *except* Parm-style topping, breaking the cheese wedge into pieces. Microwave for 1 minute, or until set. Top with Parm-style topping, stir, and enjoy!

MAKES 1 SERVING

MEXI-LICIOUS EGG MUG

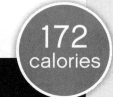

221 calories

You'll Need: large microwave-safe mug, nonstick spray
Prep: 5 minutes
Cook: 5 minutes

Entire recipe: 221 calories, 2.25g fat, 798mg sodium, 28g carbs, 4.5g fiber, 4.5g sugars, 19g protein

INGREDIENTS

2 tablespoons chopped onion

½ cup fat-free liquid egg substitute

One 6-inch corn tortilla

¼ cup fat-free refried beans

2 tablespoons canned diced green chiles (not drained)

1 wedge The Laughing Cow Light Creamy Swiss cheese

Optional topping: fat-free sour cream

DIRECTIONS

In a large microwave-safe mug sprayed with nonstick spray, microwave onion for 1 minute, or until slightly softened.

Blot away excess moisture. Add egg substitute, stir, and microwave for 1 minute.

Stir and microwave for 30 seconds, or until mostly set.

Tear tortilla into bite-sized pieces and add to the mug. Stir in beans, chiles, and cheese wedge, breaking the wedge into pieces.

Microwave for 45 seconds, or until set. Stir and enjoy!

MAKES 1 SERVING

EGG MUG LORRAINE

128 calories

You'll Need: large microwave-safe mug, nonstick spray | **Prep:** 5 minutes | **Cook:** 5 minutes

Entire recipe:
128 calories, 3.5g fat, 680mg sodium, 3.5g carbs, 0g fiber, 2g sugars, 17g protein

INGREDIENTS

½ cup fat-free liquid egg substitute
1 tablespoon precooked real crumbled bacon
1 teaspoon dried minced onion
½ teaspoon Best Foods/Hellmann's Dijonnaise
1 wedge The Laughing Cow Light Creamy
    Swiss cheese

DIRECTIONS

Spray a large microwave-safe mug with nonstick spray. Add all ingredients, breaking cheese wedge into pieces. Stir well. Microwave for 1 minute.

Stir and microwave for 1 more minute, or until set. Stir and eat!

MAKES 1 SERVING

THE HG SPECIAL EGG MUG

125 calories

You'll Need: large microwave-safe mug, nonstick spray | **Prep:** 5 minutes | **Cook:** 5 minutes

Entire recipe:
125 calories, 2.25g fat, 772mg sodium, 3.5g carbs, 0g fiber, 2g sugars, 19.5g protein

INGREDIENTS

½ cup fat-free liquid egg substitute
1 ounce sliced 97% to 98% fat-free turkey breast
    (about 2 slices), roughly chopped
1 wedge The Laughing Cow Light French
    Onion cheese

Optional seasoning: dried minced onion

DIRECTIONS

In a large microwave-safe mug sprayed with nonstick spray, microwave egg substitute for 1 minute.

Stir in turkey and cheese wedge, breaking the wedge into pieces. Microwave for 1 minute, or until set. Stir and dig in!

MAKES 1 SERVING

HG SODIUM TIP:

Save about 250mg of sodium by using cooked and sliced skinless turkey breast as opposed to packaged slices.

IT'S ALL GREEK TO ME EGG MUG

117 calories

You'll Need: large microwave-safe mug, nonstick spray | **Prep:** 5 minutes | **Cook:** 5 minutes

Entire recipe:
117 calories, 2g fat, 459mg sodium, 8g carbs, 1g fiber, 3g sugars, 16g protein

INGREDIENTS

½ cup chopped spinach leaves
¼ cup chopped red onion
½ cup fat-free liquid egg substitute
2 tablespoons diced tomato, patted dry
2 tablespoons crumbled reduced-fat feta cheese
½ tablespoon chopped fresh basil

DIRECTIONS

In a large microwave-safe mug sprayed with nonstick spray, microwave spinach and onion for 1½ minutes, or until softened.

Blot away excess moisture. Add egg substitute, stir, and microwave for 1 minute.

Stir in all remaining ingredients. Microwave for 1 minute, or until set. Dig in!

MAKES 1 SERVING

EGG MUG BURGER-RAMA

205 calories

You'll Need: microwave-safe plate, large microwave-safe mug, nonstick spray
Prep: 5 minutes | **Cook:** 5 minutes

Entire recipe:
205 calories, 2.5g fat, 1,040mg sodium, 15g carbs, 3.5g fiber, 6.5g sugars, 28g protein

INGREDIENTS

1 frozen meatless hamburger-style patty with 100 calories or less
½ cup fat-free liquid egg substitute
1 slice fat-free American cheese, chopped
1 tablespoon ketchup

DIRECTIONS

Microwave burger patty on a microwave-safe plate for 1 minute, or until thawed, and then chop.

Spray a large microwave-safe mug with nonstick spray. Add egg substitute, chopped burger patty, and cheese, and stir well. Microwave for 1 minute.

Stir and microwave for 1 more minute, or until set. Stir, top with ketchup, and enjoy!

MAKES 1 SERVING

ALL-AMERICAN EGG MUG

173 calories

You'll Need: large microwave-safe mug, nonstick spray | **Prep:** 5 minutes | **Cook:** 5 minutes

Entire recipe:
173 calories, 4g fat, 730mg sodium, 7.5g carbs, <0.5g fiber, 2g sugars, 22g protein

INGREDIENTS

1 frozen meatless or turkey sausage patty
    with 80 calories or less
1 tablespoon sugar-free pancake syrup
½ cup fat-free liquid egg substitute
1 slice fat-free American cheese

DIRECTIONS

In a large microwave-safe mug sprayed with nonstick spray, microwave sausage patty until warm. (See package for cook time.)

Crumble sausage into pieces and return to the mug. Add syrup and toss to coat. Add egg substitute, stir, and microwave for 1 minute. Stir and microwave for 1 more minute, or until set.

Tear cheese into pieces and add to the mug. Microwave for 15 seconds, or until cheese has melted. Stir and eat!

MAKES 1 SERVING

BACON-CHEDDAR EGG MUG

184 calories

You'll Need: microwave-safe plate, large microwave-safe mug, nonstick spray
Prep: 5 minutes | **Cook:** 5 minutes

Entire recipe:
184 calories, 7g fat, 643mg sodium, 3.5g carbs, 0g fiber, 1.5g sugars, 26g protein

INGREDIENTS

1 slice center-cut bacon or turkey bacon
¾ cup fat-free liquid egg substitute
3 tablespoons shredded reduced-fat
    cheddar cheese

Optional topping: ketchup

DIRECTIONS

Microwave bacon on a microwave-safe plate for 1½ minutes, or until crisp.

In a large microwave-safe mug sprayed with nonstick spray, microwave egg substitute for 1½ minutes.

Chop or crumble bacon and stir into egg. Microwave for 45 to 50 seconds, until mostly set. Mix in cheese. Microwave for 20 seconds, or until set, and stir. Enjoy!

MAKES 1 SERVING

MEAT LOVER'S EGG MUG

229 calories

You'll Need: microwave-safe plate, large microwave-safe mug, nonstick spray
Prep: 5 minutes
Cook: 10 minutes

Entire recipe: 229 calories, 7g fat, 803mg sodium, 9g carbs, 1g fiber, 4.5g sugars, 29.5g protein

INGREDIENTS

1 slice center-cut bacon or turkey bacon
1 frozen meatless or turkey breakfast sausage link
¼ cup chopped portabella mushrooms
¼ cup chopped onion
½ cup fat-free liquid egg substitute
1 ounce (about 2 slices) no-salt-added turkey breast, chopped
1 wedge The Laughing Cow Light Creamy Swiss cheese

DIRECTIONS

One at a time, microwave bacon and sausage link on a microwave-safe plate. (See packages for cook times.)

In a large microwave-safe mug sprayed with nonstick spray, microwave mushrooms and onion for 1 minute, or until slightly softened.

Blot away excess moisture. Add egg substitute, stir, and microwave for 1½ minutes.

Chop or crumble bacon and sausage and add to the mug. Stir in turkey and cheese wedge, breaking wedge into pieces. Microwave for 1 minute, or until set. Stir and eat!

MAKES 1 SERVING

EGG MUG FLORENTINE

107 calories

You'll Need: small bowl, large microwave-safe mug, nonstick spray
Prep: 5 minutes
Cook: 5 minutes

Entire recipe: 107 calories, 1.5g fat, 525mg sodium, 5g carbs, <0.5g fiber, 2.5g sugars, 14.5g protein

INGREDIENTS

1 teaspoon plain fat-free yogurt
1 teaspoon Best Foods/Hellmann's Dijonnaise
1 drop lemon juice
½ cup chopped spinach leaves
½ cup fat-free liquid egg substitute
1 wedge The Laughing Cow Light Creamy Swiss cheese

DIRECTIONS

In a small bowl, mix yogurt, Dijonnaise, and lemon juice.

In a large microwave-safe mug sprayed with nonstick spray, microwave spinach for 30 seconds, or until slightly wilted.

Blot away excess moisture. Add egg substitute and cheese wedge, breaking the wedge into pieces. Stir and microwave for 1 minute.

Stir and microwave for 1 more minute, or until set. Stir, top with yogurt mixture, and enjoy!

MAKES 1 SERVING

Flip to the photo inserts to see over 100 recipe pics! And for photos of ALL the recipes, go to hungry-girl.com/books.

CHILI CHEESE EGG MUG

195 calories

You'll Need: large microwave-safe mug, nonstick spray
Prep: 5 minutes
Cook: 5 minutes

Entire recipe: 195 calories, 3.5g fat, 692mg sodium, 12.5g carbs, 2g fiber, 4g sugars, 26.5g protein

INGREDIENTS

¾ cup fat-free liquid egg substitute
Dash cumin
Dash cayenne pepper
¼ cup low-fat turkey chili or veggie chili
2 tablespoons shredded reduced-fat cheddar cheese
1 tablespoon fat-free sour cream

DIRECTIONS

In a large microwave-safe mug sprayed with nonstick spray, microwave egg substitute, cumin, and cayenne pepper for 1½ minutes.

Stir in chili. Microwave for 1 minute and 10 seconds, or until mostly set. Mix in cheese. Microwave for 20 seconds, or until set, and stir. Top with sour cream and dig in!

MAKES 1 SERVING

THANKSGIVING IN AN EGG MUG

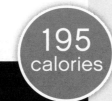

267 calories

You'll Need: 2 large microwave-safe mugs, nonstick spray
Prep: 5 minutes
Cook: 5 minutes

Entire recipe: 267 calories, 1.5g fat, 603mg sodium, 24g carbs, 1.5g fiber, 9.5g sugars, 37g protein

INGREDIENTS

¼ cup dry stuffing mix
¾ cup fat-free liquid egg substitute
1 tablespoon dried minced onion
2 ounces cooked and chopped skinless turkey breast
1 tablespoon sweetened dried cranberries
1 tablespoon fat-free turkey gravy

DIRECTIONS

In a large microwave-safe mug, microwave stuffing mix and 2 tablespoons water for 45 seconds, or until water has absorbed. Fluff with a fork.

In another large microwave-safe mug sprayed with nonstick spray, microwave egg substitute and minced onion for 1½ minutes. Stir in turkey and cranberries. Microwave for 1 minute, or until set.

Stir in stuffing, top with gravy, and gobble up!

MAKES 1 SERVING

HAWAIIAN SCRAMBLE IN A MUG

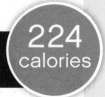
224 calories

You'll Need: large microwave-safe mug, nonstick spray | **Prep:** 5 minutes | **Cook:** 5 minutes

Entire recipe:
224 calories, 2g fat, 830mg sodium, 22g carbs, 1.5g fiber, 14.5g sugars, 25.5g protein

INGREDIENTS

½ cup chopped sweet onion
¾ cup fat-free liquid egg substitute
1 ounce sliced 97% to 98% fat-free ham (about 2 slices), chopped
¼ cup crushed pineapple packed in juice, lightly drained
1 wedge The Laughing Cow Light Creamy Swiss cheese

DIRECTIONS

In a large microwave-safe mug sprayed with nonstick spray, microwave onion for 45 seconds, or until softened.

Blot away excess moisture. Add egg substitute, stir, and microwave for 1½ minutes.

Stir in ham, pineapple, and cheese wedge, breaking wedge into pieces. Microwave for 1½ minutes, or until set. Stir and enjoy!

MAKES 1 SERVING

VEGGIE EGGS-PLOSION MUG

130 calories

You'll Need: large microwave-safe mug, nonstick spray | **Prep:** 5 minutes | **Cook:** 5 minutes

Entire recipe:
130 calories, 1.75g fat, 445mg sodium, 10g carbs, 2g fiber, 5.5g sugars, 16.5g protein

INGREDIENTS

½ cup sliced mushrooms
¼ cup thinly sliced onion
¼ cup chopped asparagus
¼ cup diced tomato, patted dry
½ cup fat-free liquid egg substitute
1 wedge The Laughing Cow Light Creamy Swiss cheese

Optional seasonings: black pepper, garlic powder

DIRECTIONS

In a large microwave-safe mug sprayed with nonstick spray, microwave mushrooms, onion, asparagus, and tomato for 2 minutes, or until softened.

Blot away excess moisture. Add egg substitute, stir, and microwave for 1 minute.

Stir in cheese wedge, breaking it into pieces. Microwave for 1 minute, or until set. Enjoy!

MAKES 1 SERVING

CHEESY CHICKEN & BROCCOLI EGG MUG

224 calories

You'll Need: large microwave-safe mug, nonstick spray | **Prep:** 5 minutes | **Cook:** 5 minutes

Entire recipe:
224 calories, 3g fat, 682mg sodium, 10g carbs, 2.5g fiber, 4g sugars, 37g protein

INGREDIENTS

1 cup small broccoli florets
¾ cup fat-free liquid egg substitute
2 ounces cooked and chopped skinless chicken breast
1 wedge The Laughing Cow Light Creamy Swiss cheese

DIRECTIONS

Place broccoli and 1 tablespoon water in a large microwave-safe mug. Cover and microwave for 1½ minutes, until softened. Remove broccoli and dry mug.

Spray mug with nonstick spray. Add egg substitute, chicken, and broccoli, and microwave for 1½ minutes. Stir and microwave for 45 to 50 seconds, until mostly set.

Mix in cheese wedge, breaking it into pieces. Microwave for 20 seconds, or until set. Stir and enjoy!

MAKES 1 SERVING

CHEESY JALAPEÑO EGG MUG

166 calories

You'll Need: large microwave-safe mug, nonstick spray
Prep: 5 minutes
Cook: 5 minutes

Entire recipe: 166 calories, 1.5g fat, 764mg sodium, 13.5g carbs, 1.5g fiber, 6g sugars, 20.5g protein

INGREDIENTS

½ cup chopped onion
¾ cup fat-free liquid egg substitute
10 jarred jalapeño slices, chopped
1 wedge The Laughing Cow Light Creamy Swiss cheese

DIRECTIONS

In a large microwave-safe mug sprayed with nonstick spray, microwave onion for 45 seconds, or until softened.

Blot away excess moisture. Add egg substitute, stir, and microwave for 1½ minutes.

Mix in jalapeños and cheese wedge, breaking wedge into pieces. Microwave for 1 minute, or until set. Stir and enjoy!

MAKES 1 SERVING

CHICKEN TERIYAKI EGG MUG

188 calories

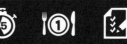

You'll Need: large microwave-safe mug, nonstick spray
Prep: 5 minutes
Cook: 5 minutes

Entire recipe: 188 calories, 1g fat, 725mg sodium, 9g carbs, 1g fiber, 5.5g sugars, 33g protein

INGREDIENTS

1 cup bagged coleslaw mix
¾ cup fat-free liquid egg substitute
2 ounces cooked and chopped skinless chicken breast
2 teaspoons thick teriyaki marinade or sauce

Optional topping: sliced scallions

DIRECTIONS

In a large microwave-safe mug sprayed with nonstick spray, microwave coleslaw mix for 1 minute, or until softened.

Blot away excess moisture. Add egg substitute and stir. Microwave for 1½ minutes.

Stir in chicken. Microwave for 1½ minutes, or until set. Stir and drizzle with teriyaki marinade/sauce. Enjoy!

MAKES 1 SERVING

EGG BAKES

Whip 'em up for a crowd, or keep 'em all for yourself!
These egg-tastic dishes are great—hot out of the oven
or reheated in the microwave!

THE ORIGINAL GINORMOUS EGG BAKE

140 calories PER SERVING

You'll Need: 8-inch by 8-inch baking pan, nonstick spray, large skillet, medium bowl, large bowl, whisk
Prep: 10 minutes | **Cook:** 1 hour 10 minutes

¼th of egg bake:
140 calories, 3g fat, 387mg sodium, 9g carbs, 1g fiber, 5g sugars, 18g protein

INGREDIENTS

1 cup sliced bell pepper
1 cup sliced mushrooms
½ cup sliced onion
2 cups fat-free liquid egg substitute
½ cup fat-free milk
¾ teaspoon garlic powder
⅛ teaspoon black pepper
½ cup sliced tomatoes
½ cup reduced-fat shredded cheese
    (any kind)
1 tablespoon reduced-fat Parmesan-style
    grated topping

Optional toppings: ketchup, salsa, hot sauce

DIRECTIONS

Preheat oven to 375 degrees. Spray an 8-inch by 8-inch baking pan with nonstick spray.

Bring a large skillet sprayed with nonstick spray to medium-high heat. Cook and stir bell pepper, mushrooms, and onion until slightly softened, about 6 minutes. Transfer to a medium bowl and blot away excess moisture.

In a large bowl, combine egg substitute, milk, garlic powder, and black pepper. Whisk thoroughly. Stir in cooked veggies, sliced tomatoes, and shredded cheese.

Transfer mixture to the baking pan. Bake for 30 minutes.

Sprinkle with Parm-style topping. Bake until center is firm, about 30 minutes. Eat up!

MAKES 4 SERVINGS

EGG BAKE OLÉ

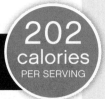

202 calories
PER SERVING

You'll Need: 8-inch by 8-inch baking pan, nonstick spray, large skillet, large bowl, small nonstick pot
Prep: 20 minutes | **Cook:** 1 hour 10 minutes

¼th of egg bake with about ½ cup sauce:
202 calories, <0.5g fat, 812mg sodium, 28g carbs, 3.5g fiber, 8g sugars, 21g protein

INGREDIENTS

Egg Bake
One 10-ounce russet potato, very
    thinly sliced widthwise
⅛ teaspoon each salt and
    black pepper
3 cups fat-free liquid egg substitute
¾ cup diced onion

Sauce
1 cup canned tomato sauce
1 cup diced green bell pepper
½ cup diced onion
½ cup canned fire-roasted
    diced tomatoes
1 teaspoon chopped garlic

DIRECTIONS

Preheat oven to 375 degrees. Spray an 8-inch by 8-inch baking pan with nonstick spray.

Bring a large skillet sprayed with nonstick spray to medium-high heat. Cook potato slices in a single layer for 4 minutes; flip and cook until softened and lightly browned, about 4 minutes. (Work in batches as needed.)

Transfer potato slices to a large bowl, sprinkle with salt and pepper, and toss to mix. Let cool slightly.

Add egg substitute and onion to the bowl. Transfer to the baking pan. Bake until center is firm, about 50 minutes.

Meanwhile, combine sauce ingredients in a small nonstick pot and stir. Bring to a boil and then reduce to a simmer. Cook and stir until veggies are tender, about 12 minutes.

Serve omelette with sauce (reheat as needed) and enjoy!

MAKES 4 SERVINGS

TOTALLY FLY THAI-STYLE EGG BAKE

180 calories
PER SERVING

You'll Need: 8-inch by 8-inch baking pan, nonstick spray, large bowl, whisk | **Prep:** 10 minutes | **Cook:** 1 hour

¼th of egg bake:
180 calories, 1g fat, 718mg sodium, 7g carbs, 1g fiber, 3.5g sugars, 34.5g protein

INGREDIENTS

3 cups fat-free liquid egg substitute
2 tablespoons reduced-sodium/lite soy sauce
8 ounces cooked and chopped skinless
    chicken breast
1½ cups chopped bean sprouts
½ cup chopped scallions

Optional topping: Sriracha chili sauce
    (shelf-stable Asian hot sauce)

DIRECTIONS

Preheat oven to 375 degrees. Spray an 8-inch by 8-inch baking pan with nonstick spray.

In a large bowl, whisk egg substitute with soy sauce. Stir in chicken, sprouts, and ¼ cup scallions. Transfer to the baking pan.

Bake until center is firm, about 1 hour.

Top with remaining ¼ cup scallions and enjoy!

MAKES 4 SERVINGS

EL GINORMO SOUTHWEST EGG BAKE

188 calories PER SERVING

You'll Need: 8-inch by 8-inch baking pan, nonstick spray, large bowl, whisk
Prep: 10 minutes
Cook: 1 hour

¼th of egg bake: 188 calories, 3g fat, 590mg sodium, 17g carbs, 2.5g fiber, 5g sugars, 22g protein

INGREDIENTS

2½ cups fat-free liquid egg substitute
½ cup fat-free milk
1 teaspoon cumin
½ teaspoon taco seasoning mix
½ cup chopped onion
½ cup chopped red bell pepper
1 teaspoon chopped garlic
½ cup canned black beans, drained and rinsed
½ cup canned sweet corn kernels, drained
¼ cup canned diced green chiles
½ cup shredded reduced-fat Mexican-blend cheese

Optional toppings: salsa, fat-free sour cream, chopped scallions

DIRECTIONS

Preheat oven to 375 degrees. Spray an 8-inch by 8-inch baking pan with nonstick spray.

In a large bowl, combine egg substitute, milk, cumin, and taco seasoning. Whisk thoroughly. Stir in onion, bell pepper, and garlic. Transfer to the pan.

Evenly add black beans, corn, and green chiles. Sprinkle with cheese.

Bake until center is firm, about 1 hour. Enjoy!

MAKES 4 SERVINGS

CHEESY-ONION EGG BAKE

205 calories PER SERVING

You'll Need: 8-inch by 8-inch baking pan, nonstick spray, large skillet, large bowl, whisk
Prep: 10 minutes
Cook: 1 hour 10 minutes

¼th of egg bake: 205 calories, 2.5g fat, 829mg sodium, 20g carbs, 1.5g fiber, 7g sugars, 21.5g protein

INGREDIENTS

2 cups chopped onion
4 wedges The Laughing Cow Light Creamy Swiss cheese
3 cups fat-free liquid egg substitute
One 10.75-ounce can Campbell's Healthy Request Cheddar Cheese Condensed Soup

DIRECTIONS

Preheat oven to 375 degrees. Spray an 8-inch by 8-inch baking pan with nonstick spray.

Bring a large skillet sprayed with nonstick spray to medium-high heat. Cook and stir onion until slightly softened, about 6 minutes.

Transfer onion to a large bowl and blot away excess moisture. Add cheese wedges, breaking them into pieces, and stir until melted. Add egg substitute and soup and whisk thoroughly.

Transfer mixture to the baking pan. Bake until center is firm, about 1 hour. Enjoy!

MAKES 4 SERVINGS

HG ALTERNATIVE!

If you can't find the Healthy Request soup, use regular cheddar cheese condensed soup. Then each serving will have 224 calories, 5g fat, 982mg sodium, 19g carbs, 1.5g fiber, 7g sugars, and 22g protein.

For more recipes, tips & tricks, sign up for FREE daily emails at hungry-girl.com!

THE BREAKFAST CLUB EGG BAKE

222 calories PER SERVING

You'll Need: 8-inch by 8-inch baking pan, nonstick spray, large skillet, large bowl, medium bowl, microwave-safe plate (optional)
Prep: 10 minutes
Cook: 1 hour 10 minutes

¼th of egg bake: 222 calories, 7g fat, 597mg sodium, 7.5g carbs, 1.5g fiber, 3.5g sugars, 31g protein

INGREDIENTS

4 cups spinach leaves
8 ounces raw lean ground turkey
¼ teaspoon onion powder
¼ teaspoon garlic powder
⅛ teaspoon each salt and black pepper
5 slices center-cut bacon or turkey bacon
2½ cups fat-free liquid egg substitute
¼ cup bagged sun-dried tomatoes
    (not packed in oil), finely chopped

Optional topping: ketchup

DIRECTIONS

Preheat oven to 375 degrees. Spray an 8-inch by 8-inch baking pan with nonstick spray.

Bring a large skillet sprayed with nonstick spray to medium-high heat. Cook and stir spinach until just wilted, about 2 minutes. Transfer to a large bowl and blot away excess moisture.

In a medium bowl, mix turkey, onion powder, garlic powder, salt, and pepper.

Remove skillet from heat, re-spray, and return to medium-high heat. Cook and crumble turkey for 5 minutes, or until fully cooked. Transfer to the large bowl.

Cook bacon until crispy, either in a large skillet over medium heat or on a microwave-safe plate in the microwave. (See package for cook time.) Chop or crumble and add to the large bowl.

Once contents of the bowl are cool, add egg substitute and tomatoes. Mix well, and transfer to the baking pan.

Bake until center is firm, about 50 minutes. Serve and enjoy!

MAKES 4 SERVINGS

CHEESY BACON-APPLE-BELLA EGG BAKE

207 calories PER SERVING

You'll Need: 8-inch by 8-inch baking pan, nonstick spray, large skillet, microwave-safe plate (optional), large bowl
Prep: 5 minutes
Cook: 1 hour 5 minutes

¼th of egg bake: 207 calories, 4.5g fat, 792mg sodium, 14g carbs, 1.5g fiber, 7.5g sugars, 25g protein

INGREDIENTS

4 slices center-cut bacon or turkey bacon
2 cups chopped portabella mushrooms
1½ cups chopped Fuji apples
2 tablespoons reduced-fat Parmesan-style grated topping
3 wedges The Laughing Cow Light Creamy Swiss cheese
2½ cups fat-free liquid egg substitute
½ cup shredded fat-free cheddar cheese

DIRECTIONS

Preheat oven to 375 degrees. Spray an 8-inch by 8-inch baking pan with nonstick spray.

Cook bacon until crispy, either in a large skillet over medium heat or on a microwave-safe plate in the microwave. (See package for cook time.)

Bring a large skillet sprayed with nonstick spray to medium-high heat. Add mushrooms and apples. Cook and stir until mostly softened, about 7 minutes. Transfer to a large bowl.

Add Parm-style topping and cheese wedges to the bowl, breaking wedges into pieces, and stir until cheese has melted.

Chop or crumble bacon and add to the bowl. Mix in egg substitute. Transfer to the baking pan.

Bake for 40 minutes. Evenly top with cheddar cheese. Bake until center is firm and cheddar cheese has melted, about 10 minutes. Serve and enjoy!

MAKES 4 SERVINGS

BACON BASICS

HG recipes call for center-cut bacon and turkey bacon interchangeably because the stats are very similar and they're equally delicious. Center-cut bacon crisps up best in a skillet, while turkey bacon tastes best when made in the microwave.

GOOD MORNING MEGA QUICHE

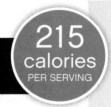

215 calories
PER SERVING

You'll Need: 9-inch by 13-inch baking pan, nonstick spray, large skillet with a lid, microwave-safe plate (optional), large bowl, whisk | **Prep:** 20 minutes | **Cook:** 1 hour 10 minutes

⅛th of quiche:
215 calories, 8g fat, 779mg sodium, 19.5g carbs, 1.5g fiber, 6g sugars, 15g protein

INGREDIENTS

1 package refrigerated Pillsbury Crescent Recipe Creations Seamless Dough Sheet
6 slices center-cut bacon or turkey bacon
2 cups chopped broccoli
2 cups sliced mushrooms
1 cup chopped onion
1 cup chopped red bell pepper
2½ cups fat-free liquid egg substitute
½ cup light plain soymilk
3 wedges The Laughing Cow Light Creamy Swiss cheese, room temperature
½ teaspoon garlic powder
½ teaspoon salt
¼ teaspoon black pepper
½ cup shredded reduced-fat cheddar cheese

DIRECTIONS

Preheat oven to 350 degrees. Spray a 9-inch by 13-inch baking pan with nonstick spray.

Place dough sheet along the bottom of the pan. Firmly press dough into the bottom and corners of the pan. Pierce dough several times with a fork.

Bake until dough just begins to puff up, about 5 minutes. Remove pan, but leave oven on.

Cook bacon until crispy, either in a large skillet over medium heat or on a microwave-safe plate in the microwave. (See package for cook time.)

Bring a large skillet sprayed with nonstick spray to medium-high heat. Add broccoli and ¼ cup water. Cover and cook for about 2 minutes, until broccoli becomes bright green. Uncover and cook until water evaporates, 1 to 2 minutes. Add mushrooms, onion, and bell pepper. Cook and stir until softened, about 8 minutes.

Remove skillet from heat, and blot away excess moisture from veggies.

In a large bowl, combine egg substitute, soymilk, and cheese wedges, breaking cheese wedges into pieces. Add garlic powder, salt, and black pepper. Whisk until mostly smooth. Chop bacon and add to the bowl. Add cooked veggies and stir well.

Evenly pour contents of the bowl over the dough in the pan. Sprinkle with shredded cheese. Bake until egg mixture is cooked through, about 40 minutes. Slice, serve, and enjoy!

MAKES 8 SERVINGS

CHEESY SAUSAGE 'N HASH EGG BAKE

236 calories PER SERVING

You'll Need: 8-inch by 8-inch baking pan, nonstick spray, large skillet, microwave-safe plate (optional), large bowl
Prep: 10 minutes
Cook: 1 hour 5 minutes

¼th of egg bake: 236 calories, 3.5g fat, 789mg sodium, 18g carbs, 2g fiber, 4.5g sugars, 28g protein

INGREDIENTS

3 frozen meatless or turkey sausage patties with 80 calories or less each
1½ cups sliced onion
1½ cups chopped portabella mushrooms
1½ cups frozen shredded hash browns
1½ teaspoons chopped garlic
3 wedges The Laughing Cow Light Creamy Swiss cheese
2½ cups fat-free liquid egg substitute
½ cup shredded fat-free cheddar cheese

DIRECTIONS

Preheat oven to 375 degrees. Spray an 8-inch by 8-inch baking pan with nonstick spray.

Cook sausage patties in a large skillet sprayed with nonstick spray or on a microwave-safe plate in the microwave. (See package for cook time and temperature.)

Bring a large skillet sprayed with nonstick spray to medium-high heat. Add onion, mushrooms, and hash browns. Cook and stir until veggies have slightly softened and hash browns have thawed, about 6 minutes. Transfer to a large bowl.

Add garlic and cheese wedges to the bowl, breaking wedges into pieces, and stir until cheese has melted.

Once sausage patties and contents of the bowl have cooled, chop or crumble sausage patties and add to the bowl. Mix in egg substitute, and transfer to the baking pan.

Bake for 40 minutes. Evenly top with cheddar cheese. Bake until center is firm and cheddar cheese has melted, about 10 minutes. Serve and enjoy!

MAKES 4 SERVINGS

CARAMELIZED ONION 'N SPINACH EGG BAKE

181 calories PER SERVING

You'll Need: 8-inch by 8-inch baking pan, nonstick spray, large skillet, large bowl
Prep: 10 minutes
Cook: 1 hour 30 minutes

¼th of egg bake: 181 calories, 3g fat, 746mg sodium, 14g carbs, 1.5g fiber, 6.5g sugars, 21.5g protein

INGREDIENTS

1 tablespoon light whipped butter or light buttery spread
3 cups thinly sliced sweet onions
¼ teaspoon salt
4 cups spinach leaves
1 teaspoon chopped garlic
4 wedges The Laughing Cow Light Creamy Swiss cheese
3 cups fat-free liquid egg substitute

Optional topping: fat-free sour cream

DIRECTIONS

Preheat oven to 375 degrees. Spray an 8-inch by 8-inch baking pan with nonstick spray.

Place butter in a large skillet and bring to medium-high heat. Add onions and salt. Cook and stir until slightly softened, about 5 minutes.

Reduce heat to medium low. Stirring frequently, cook until caramelized, 25 to 30 minutes. Transfer to a large bowl.

Add spinach to the skillet, still over medium-low heat. Cook and stir until just wilted, about 2 minutes. Transfer to the large bowl.

Add garlic and cheese wedges to the bowl, breaking wedges into pieces, and stir until cheese has melted.

Once contents of the bowl have cooled, mix in egg substitute. Transfer to the baking pan.

Bake until center is firm, about 50 minutes. Enjoy!

MAKES 4 SERVINGS

HAM-IT-UP EGG BAKE

143 calories PER SERVING

You'll Need: 9-inch by 13-inch baking pan, nonstick spray, large bowl, whisk
Prep: 15 minutes
Cook: 45 minutes

¹⁄₁₂th of egg bake: 143 calories, 4.5g fat, 650mg sodium, 12g carbs, 0.5g fiber, 4.5g sugars, 12g protein

INGREDIENTS

1 package refrigerated Pillsbury Crescent Recipe Creations Seamless Dough Sheet
1 cup light or low-fat ricotta cheese, room temperature
4 wedges The Laughing Cow Light Creamy Swiss cheese, room temperature
1 cup fat-free liquid egg substitute
1 pound sliced 97% to 98% fat-free ham, roughly chopped
1 cup scallions sliced into ½-inch pieces
2 tablespoons chopped fresh parsley
¼ teaspoon black pepper

DIRECTIONS

Preheat oven to 350 degrees. Spray a 9-inch by 13-inch baking pan with nonstick spray.

Place dough sheet along the bottom of the pan. Firmly press dough into the bottom and corners of the pan. Pierce dough several times with a fork.

Bake until dough just begins to puff up, about 5 minutes. Remove pan, but leave oven on.

In a large bowl, thoroughly mix ricotta cheese with cheese wedges until smooth and uniform. Add egg substitute and thoroughly whisk until smooth.

Stir in chopped ham, scallions, parsley, and pepper. Evenly pour mixture over the dough in the pan.

Bake until egg mixture is cooked through, about 40 minutes. Eat up!

MAKES 12 SERVINGS

SWEET TREAT A LA SOUFFLÉ

185 calories PER SERVING

You'll Need: 9-inch by 13-inch baking pan, nonstick spray, medium-large bowl, electric mixer
Prep: 10 minutes
Cook: 45 minutes

⅛th of soufflé: 185 calories, 4.5g fat, 436mg sodium, 22.5g carbs, 0g fiber, 11g sugars, 12.5g protein

INGREDIENTS

1 package refrigerated Pillsbury Crescent Creations Seamless Dough Sheet
2½ cups fat-free liquid egg substitute
1 cup fat-free ricotta cheese, room temperature
½ cup fat-free half & half
¼ cup granulated white sugar
1 teaspoon vanilla extract

Optional toppings: sliced strawberries, sugar-free pancake syrup

DIRECTIONS

Preheat oven to 350 degrees. Spray a 9-inch by 13-inch baking pan with nonstick spray.

Place dough sheet along the bottom of the pan. Firmly press dough into the bottom and corners of the pan. Pierce dough several times with a fork.

Bake until dough just begins to puff up, about 5 minutes. Remove pan, but leave oven on.

In a medium-large bowl, combine all remaining ingredients. With an electric mixer set to medium speed, beat until thoroughly mixed, about 2 minutes.

Evenly pour egg mixture over the dough in the pan. Bake until egg mixture is cooked through, about 40 minutes. The mixture may bubble and the dough bottom may rise while baking—this is okay.
Slice 'n serve!

MAKES 8 SERVINGS

HG SWEET ALTERNATIVE!

If made with an equal amount of Splenda No Calorie Sweetener (granulated) in place of the sugar, each serving will have 164 calories, 17g carbs, and 4.5g sugars.

CHAPTER 2

GROWING OATMEAL BOWLS

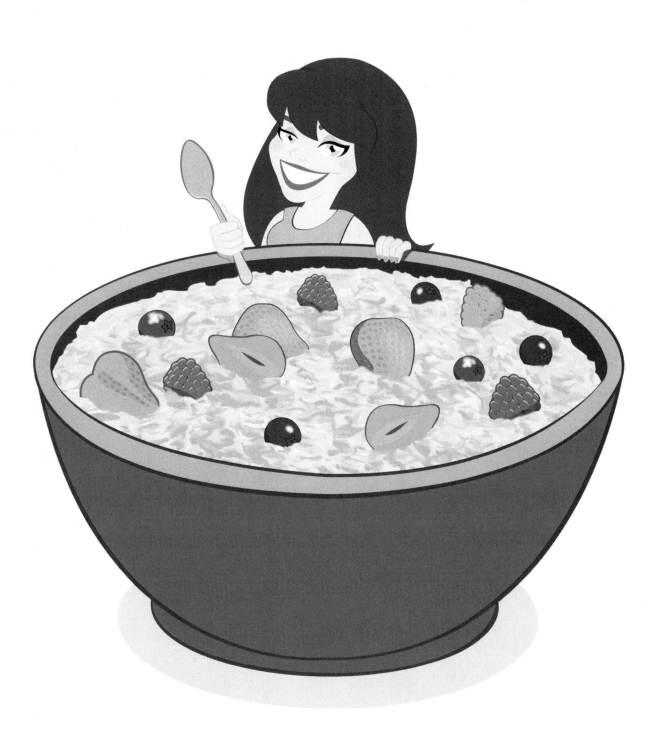

GROWING OATMEAL BOWLS

Banana Split Oatmeal

Happy Trail Mix Oatmeal

PB&J Oatmeal Heaven

S'mores Oatmeal

Large & In Charge Neapolitan Oatmeal

Strawberry Shortcake Oatmeal

Caramel Apple Oatmeal

Choco-Monkey Oatmeal

Maple Bacon Oatmeal

Cinna-Raisin Oatmeal

Skinny Elvis Oatmeal

Piña Colada Oatmeal

Pumpkin Chocolate Chip Oatmeal

Complete & Utter Oatmeal Insanity

Major Mocha Cappuccino Oatmeal

Chocolate Caramel Coconut Oatmeal

Apple Pie Oatmeal Bonanza

PB & Chocolate Oatmeal Blitz

Cranberry-Walnut Maple Oatmeal

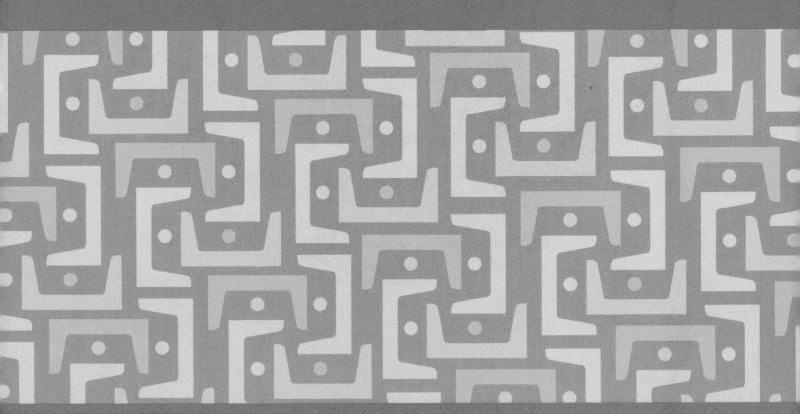

GROWING OATMEAL TIPS & TRICKS . . .

* Use a pot that's wider than it is tall. Don't have a pot like that? Just cook your oatmeal a little longer to allow it to thicken . . .

* This oatmeal cooks for twice as long as standard oatmeal, and it WILL thicken up. So don't worry if it seems like a lot of liquid at the beginning!

* Old-fashioned oats are a must for these recipes. Instant oats won't work here!

YOUR ALMOND BREEZE QUESTIONS ANSWERED!

These recipes call for Unsweetened Vanilla Almond Breeze, made by Blue Diamond, because it's low in calories and deliciously creamy. It's generally found with the shelf-stable boxed milk substitutes at supermarkets. (It can also be ordered online, and it's available in refrigerated form at select markets.) You can use light vanilla soymilk in its place—that has about 25 more calories per cup. And if you do use a sweetened milk swap, nix the sweetener in the recipe and instead sweeten your oatmeal to taste.

A QUICK GUIDE TO SYMBOLS:

15 Minutes or Less

This symbol lets you know a recipe should take you no more than fifteen minutes from start to finish! That includes prep and cook time.

30 Minutes or Less

Just like the 15-minute version, this one points out recipes that take 30 minutes or less to whip up.

Meatless

You guessed it—no meat here! That includes beef, poultry, and fish. Some recipes give the option of a meatless ingredient. If you want your meal without meat, go with the meatless choice.

Single Serving

Pretty straightforward. These are recipes for one.

5 Ingredients or Less

Fans of HG know that we like to keep things simple. And these recipes contain just five ingredients or less!

Photos

These recipes can be seen in one of the book's photo inserts. The number in the symbol tells you which insert. Find photos of all the recipes at hungry-girl.com/books!

GROWING OATMEAL BOWLS

Why would anyone wanna eat a regular bowl of oatmeal when you can enjoy a super-sized one without a lot of extra calories and fat grams?! (Don't bother answering—it's rhetorical.) This section is cram-packed with some of the most DELICIOUS and original breakfast ideas around.

BANANA SPLIT OATMEAL

285 calories

You'll Need: nonstick pot, medium bowl
Prep: 5 minutes
Cook: 20 minutes

Entire recipe: 285 calories, 7.5g fat, 338mg sodium, 51.5g carbs, 6.5g fiber, 12g sugars, 7g protein

INGREDIENTS

½ cup old-fashioned oats
Dash salt
1 cup Unsweetened Vanilla Almond Breeze
1 tablespoon sugar-free strawberry jam/preserves
½ medium banana, thinly sliced
2 tablespoons Fat Free Reddi-wip
1 teaspoon mini semi-sweet chocolate chips

DIRECTIONS

Combine oats and salt in a nonstick pot. Add Almond Breeze and 1 cup water.

Bring to a boil and then reduce to a simmer. Cook and stir until thick and creamy, 12 to 15 minutes.

Transfer to a medium bowl and let slightly cool and thicken. Stir in jam/preserves. Top with banana, Reddi-wip, and chocolate chips!

MAKES 1 SERVING

HAPPY TRAIL MIX OATMEAL

304 calories

You'll Need: nonstick pot, medium bowl
Prep: 5 minutes
Cook: 20 minutes

Entire recipe: 304 calories, 11g fat, 486mg sodium, 45g carbs, 6g fiber, 12.5g sugars, 8.5g protein

INGREDIENTS

½ cup old-fashioned oats
2 no-calorie sweetener packets
⅛ teaspoon salt
1 cup Unsweetened Vanilla Almond Breeze
1 tablespoon raisins, chopped
2 teaspoons sliced almonds, chopped
1 teaspoon peanut butter baking chips, chopped
1 teaspoon mini semi-sweet chocolate chips

DIRECTIONS

Combine oats, sweetener, and salt in a nonstick pot. Add Almond Breeze and 1 cup water.

Bring to a boil and then reduce to a simmer. Cook and stir until thick and creamy, 12 to 15 minutes.

Transfer to a medium bowl and let slightly cool and thicken.

Top with raisins, almonds, peanut butter chips, and chocolate chips. Enjoy!

MAKES 1 SERVING

PB&J OATMEAL HEAVEN

285 calories

You'll Need: nonstick pot, medium bowl, small microwave-safe bowl | **Prep:** 5 minutes | **Cook:** 20 minutes

Entire recipe:
285 calories, 10.25g fat, 417mg sodium, 42g carbs, 6.75g fiber, 5g sugars, 9g protein

INGREDIENTS

Oatmeal
½ cup old-fashioned oats
⅓ cup chopped strawberries
2 teaspoons sugar-free strawberry preserves
1 no-calorie sweetener packet
Dash salt
1 cup Unsweetened Vanilla Almond Breeze

Topping
2 teaspoons Unsweetened Vanilla Almond Breeze
2 teaspoons reduced-fat peanut butter, room temperature

Optional garnish: additional chopped strawberries

DIRECTIONS

Combine all ingredients for oatmeal in a nonstick pot. Mix in 1 cup water.

Bring to a boil and then reduce to a simmer. Cook and stir until thick and creamy, 12 to 15 minutes.

Transfer to a medium bowl and let slightly cool and thicken.

In a small microwave-safe bowl, combine ingredients for topping. Microwave for 10 seconds, or until warm. Stir well.

Drizzle topping over oatmeal. Enjoy!

MAKES 1 SERVING

S'MORES OATMEAL

299 calories

You'll Need: nonstick pot, medium bowl | **Prep:** 5 minutes | **Cook:** 20 minutes

Entire recipe:
299 calories, 9g fat, 512mg sodium, 47.5g carbs, 6.5g fiber, 13g sugars, 8.5g protein

INGREDIENTS

½ cup old-fashioned oats
1 packet hot cocoa mix with 20 to 25 calories
Dash salt
1 cup Unsweetened Vanilla Almond Breeze
2 teaspoons mini semi-sweet chocolate chips
2 tablespoons mini marshmallows
1 low-fat honey graham cracker (¼ sheet), crushed

DIRECTIONS

Combine oats, cocoa mix, and salt in a nonstick pot. Add Almond Breeze and 1 cup water.

Bring to a boil and then reduce to a simmer. Cook and stir until thick and creamy, 12 to 15 minutes.

Remove from heat and stir in 1 teaspoon chocolate chips.

Transfer to a medium bowl and let slightly cool and thicken. Top with marshmallows, crushed graham cracker, and remaining teaspoon chocolate chips. Enjoy!

MAKES 1 SERVING

LARGE & IN CHARGE NEAPOLITAN OATMEAL

275 calories

You'll Need: nonstick pot, medium bowl | **Prep:** 5 minutes | **Cook:** 20 minutes | **Chill:** 2 hours

Entire recipe:
275 calories, 9g fat, 339mg sodium, 42.5g carbs, 7g fiber, 10g sugars, 7g protein

INGREDIENTS

½ cup old-fashioned oats

1 teaspoon sugar-free French vanilla powdered creamer

2 no-calorie sweetener packets

Dash salt

1 cup Unsweetened Vanilla Almond Breeze

¼ teaspoon vanilla extract

½ cup sliced strawberries

½ tablespoon mini semi-sweet chocolate chips

DIRECTIONS

Combine all ingredients *except* strawberries and chocolate chips in a nonstick pot. Mix in 1 cup water.

Bring to a boil and then reduce to a simmer. Cook and stir until just thick and creamy, about 12 minutes. (It will thicken more upon chilling.)

Transfer to a medium bowl and let slightly cool. Cover and refrigerate until chilled, about 2 hours.

Stir oatmeal and top with berries and chocolate chips. Eat up!

MAKES 1 SERVING

STRAWBERRY SHORTCAKE OATMEAL

238 calories

You'll Need: nonstick pot, microwave-safe bowl, medium bowl | **Prep:** 5 minutes | **Cook:** 20 minutes

Entire recipe:
238 calories, 7g fat, 437mg sodium, 38.5g carbs, 5.5g fiber, 7.5g sugars, 6g protein

INGREDIENTS

½ cup old-fashioned oats

2 teaspoons sugar-free French vanilla powdered creamer

⅛ teaspoon salt

¾ cup Unsweetened Vanilla Almond Breeze

3 frozen unsweetened strawberries

1 tablespoon low-sugar strawberry preserves

Optional topping: Fat Free Reddi-wip

DIRECTIONS

Combine oats, creamer, and salt in a nonstick pot. Add Almond Breeze and 1 cup water.

Bring to a boil and then reduce to a simmer. Cook and stir until thick and creamy, 12 to 15 minutes.

Meanwhile, microwave strawberries in a microwave-safe bowl for 50 seconds, or until warm. Do not drain. Add preserves and mash thoroughly.

Once contents of the pot are thick and creamy, stir in strawberry mixture. Transfer to a medium bowl and let slightly cool and thicken. Eat up!

MAKES 1 SERVING

CARAMEL APPLE OATMEAL

309 calories

You'll Need: nonstick pot, medium bowl
Prep: 10 minutes
Cook: 25 minutes

Entire recipe: 309 calories, 7g fat, 687mg sodium, 58g carbs, 8g fiber, 19g sugars, 7g protein

INGREDIENTS

¼ teaspoon cornstarch
2 no-calorie sweetener packets
¼ teaspoon plus ⅛ teaspoon cinnamon
⅛ teaspoon plus 1 dash salt
¾ cup chopped apple
½ cup old-fashioned oats
1 cup Unsweetened Vanilla Almond Breeze
¼ teaspoon vanilla extract
1 tablespoon fat-free or light caramel dip

DIRECTIONS

Combine cornstarch, 1 sweetener packet, ¼ teaspoon cinnamon, and 1 dash salt in a nonstick pot. Add 3 tablespoons cold water and stir to dissolve. Stir in apple and bring to medium heat.

Cook and stir until apple has softened and liquid has thickened, about 7 minutes. Transfer to a medium bowl.

To the empty pot, add oats, remaining sweetener packet, remaining ⅛ teaspoon cinnamon, and remaining ⅛ teaspoon salt. Add Almond Breeze, vanilla extract, and 1 cup water.

Bring to a boil and then reduce to a simmer. Cook and stir for 10 minutes. Stir in apple mixture. Cook and stir until thick and creamy, 2 to 5 minutes.

Transfer to the bowl and let slightly cool and thicken. Drizzle with caramel dip and enjoy!

MAKES 1 SERVING

CHOCO-MONKEY OATMEAL

271 calories

You'll Need: nonstick pot, medium bowl
Prep: 5 minutes
Cook: 20 minutes

Entire recipe: 271 calories, 6.5g fat, 481mg sodium, 47.5g carbs, 7.5g fiber, 11g sugars, 8.5g protein

INGREDIENTS

½ cup old-fashioned oats
1 packet hot cocoa mix with 20 to 25 calories
1 no-calorie sweetener packet
⅛ teaspoon cinnamon
Dash salt
1 cup Unsweetened Vanilla Almond Breeze
¼ cup mashed extra-ripe banana

DIRECTIONS

Combine all ingredients *except* banana in a nonstick pot. Mix in 1 cup water.

Bring to a boil and then reduce to a simmer. Cook and stir for 10 minutes.

Add banana and mix well. Cook and stir until thick and creamy, 2 to 5 minutes.

Transfer to a medium bowl and let slightly cool and thicken. Yum!

MAKES 1 SERVING

※ Flip to the photo inserts to see over 100 recipe pics! And for photos of ALL the recipes, go to hungry-girl.com/books.

MAPLE BACON OATMEAL

231 calories

You'll Need: nonstick pot, skillet or microwave-safe plate, medium bowl
Prep: 5 minutes
Cook: 20 minutes

Entire recipe: 231 calories, 7.5g fat, 497mg sodium, 34g carbs, 5g fiber, 1g sugars, 8.5g protein

INGREDIENTS

½ cup old-fashioned oats
1 no-calorie sweetener packet
Dash cinnamon
Dash salt
¾ cup Unsweetened Vanilla Almond Breeze
⅛ teaspoon maple extract
1 slice center-cut bacon or turkey bacon
2 tablespoons sugar-free pancake syrup

DIRECTIONS

Combine all ingredients *except* bacon and syrup in a nonstick pot. Mix in 1 cup water.

Bring to a boil and then reduce to a simmer. Cook and stir until thick and creamy, 12 to 15 minutes.

Meanwhile, cook bacon until crispy, either in a skillet over medium heat or on a microwave-safe plate in the microwave. (See package for cook time.)

Remove pot from heat and stir in 1 tablespoon syrup. Transfer to a medium bowl and let slightly cool and thicken. Chop or crumble bacon and sprinkle over oatmeal. Top with remaining tablespoon syrup and enjoy!

MAKES 1 SERVING

CINNA-RAISIN OATMEAL

301 calories

You'll Need: nonstick pot, medium bowl
Prep: 5 minutes
Cook: 20 minutes

Entire recipe: 301 calories, 6g fat, 479mg sodium, 55.5g carbs, 6g fiber, 24.5g sugars, 7g protein

INGREDIENTS

½ cup old-fashioned oats
1 tablespoon brown sugar (not packed)
2 no-calorie sweetener packets
¼ teaspoon cinnamon
⅛ teaspoon salt
1 cup Unsweetened Vanilla Almond Breeze
⅛ teaspoon vanilla extract
2 tablespoons raisins, chopped

DIRECTIONS

Combine all ingredients *except* raisins in a nonstick pot. Mix in 1 cup water.

Bring to a boil and then reduce to a simmer. Stir in raisins. Cook and stir until thick and creamy, 12 to 15 minutes.

Transfer to a medium bowl and let slightly cool and thicken. Dig in!

MAKES 1 SERVING

SKINNY ELVIS OATMEAL

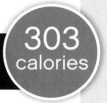
303 calories

You'll Need: nonstick pot, medium bowl | **Prep:** 5 minutes | **Cook:** 20 minutes

Entire recipe:
303 calories, 9.5g fat, 517mg sodium, 49g carbs, 7.5g fiber, 10.5g sugars, 9g protein

INGREDIENTS

½ cup old-fashioned oats
1 no-calorie sweetener packet
⅛ teaspoon cinnamon
⅛ teaspoon salt
1 cup Unsweetened Vanilla Almond Breeze
⅓ cup mashed extra-ripe banana
½ tablespoon reduced-fat peanut butter,
    room temperature

DIRECTIONS

Combine all ingredients *except* banana and peanut butter in a nonstick pot. Mix in 1 cup water.

Bring to a boil and then reduce to a simmer. Cook and stir for 10 minutes. Add banana and mix well. Cook and stir until thick and creamy, 2 to 5 minutes.

Remove from heat and immediately stir in peanut butter. Transfer to a medium bowl and let slightly cool and thicken. Enjoy!

MAKES 1 SERVING

PIÑA COLADA OATMEAL

271 calories

You'll Need: nonstick pot, medium bowl | **Prep:** 5 minutes | **Cook:** 20 minutes

Entire recipe:
271 calories, 8g fat, 347mg sodium, 45g carbs, 6g fiber, 14.5g sugars, 6g protein

INGREDIENTS

½ cup old-fashioned oats
1 no-calorie sweetener packet
Dash salt
1 cup Unsweetened Vanilla Almond Breeze
⅓ cup crushed pineapple packed in juice,
    lightly drained
2 drops coconut extract
2 teaspoons shredded sweetened coconut
1 teaspoon powdered sugar

DIRECTIONS

Combine oats, sweetener, and salt in a nonstick pot. Add Almond Breeze and 1 cup water.

Bring to a boil and then reduce to a simmer. Cook and stir until thick and creamy, 12 to 15 minutes.

Transfer to a medium bowl and let slightly cool and thicken. Stir in pineapple and coconut extract. Sprinkle with shredded coconut and powdered sugar. Enjoy!

MAKES 1 SERVING

PUMPKIN CHOCOLATE CHIP OATMEAL

293 calories

You'll Need: nonstick pot, medium bowl | **Prep:** 5 minutes | **Cook:** 20 minutes

Entire recipe:
293 calories, 9g fat, 477mg sodium, 46.5g carbs, 9.5g fiber, 10g sugars, 8.5g protein

INGREDIENTS

½ cup old-fashioned oats
2 no-calorie sweetener packets
¼ teaspoon pumpkin pie spice
⅛ teaspoon salt
1 cup Unsweetened Vanilla Almond Breeze
½ cup canned pure pumpkin
2 teaspoons mini semi-sweet chocolate chips

Optional topping: Fat Free Reddi-wip

DIRECTIONS

Combine oats, sweetener, pumpkin pie spice, and salt in a nonstick pot. Add Almond Breeze and 1 cup water.

Bring to a boil and then reduce to a simmer. Add pumpkin and cook and stir until thick and creamy, 12 to 15 minutes.

Transfer to a medium bowl and let slightly cool and thicken. Top with chocolate chips and enjoy!

MAKES 1 SERVING

COMPLETE & UTTER OATMEAL INSANITY

248 calories

You'll Need: nonstick pot, medium bowl | **Prep:** 5 minutes | **Cook:** 20 minutes

Entire recipe:
248 calories, 6.5g fat, 420mg sodium, 48g carbs, 13g fiber, 3g sugars, 7.5g protein

INGREDIENTS

½ cup old-fashioned oats
¼ cup Fiber One Original bran cereal
2 tablespoons canned pure pumpkin
1 no-calorie sweetener packet
¼ teaspoon pumpkin pie spice
Dash salt
1 cup Unsweetened Vanilla Almond Breeze
1 tablespoon sugar-free pancake syrup
2 tablespoons Fat Free Reddi-wip

DIRECTIONS

Combine all ingredients *except* syrup and Reddi-wip in a nonstick pot. Mix in ¾ cup water.

Bring to a boil and then reduce to a simmer. Cook and stir until thick and creamy, 12 to 15 minutes.

Remove from heat and stir in syrup. Transfer to a medium bowl and let slightly cool and thicken. Top with Reddi-wip and eat!

MAKES 1 SERVING

MAJOR MOCHA CAPPUCCINO OATMEAL

242 calories

You'll Need: nonstick pot, medium bowl
Prep: 5 minutes
Cook: 20 minutes

Entire recipe: 242 calories, 6.75g fat, 490mg sodium, 37g carbs, 6g fiber, 6g sugars, 7.5g protein

INGREDIENTS

½ cup old-fashioned oats
1 packet hot cocoa mix with 20 to 25 calories
1 teaspoon sugar-free French vanilla powdered creamer
¾ teaspoon instant coffee granules
1 no-calorie sweetener packet
Dash salt
1 cup Unsweetened Vanilla Almond Breeze
¼ cup Fat Free Reddi-wip

DIRECTIONS

Combine all ingredients *except* Reddi-wip in a nonstick pot. Mix in 1 cup water.

Bring to a boil and then reduce to a simmer. Cook and stir until thick and creamy, 12 to 15 minutes.

Transfer to a medium bowl and let slightly cool and thicken. Top with Reddi-wip and enjoy!

MAKES 1 SERVING

CHOCOLATE CARAMEL COCONUT OATMEAL

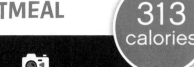

313 calories

You'll Need: nonstick pot, medium bowl
Prep: 5 minutes
Cook: 20 minutes

Entire recipe: 313 calories, 10g fat, 547mg sodium, 50.5g carbs, 6g fiber, 14.5g sugars, 7g protein

INGREDIENTS

½ cup old-fashioned oats
2 no-calorie sweetener packets
⅛ teaspoon salt
1 cup Unsweetened Vanilla Almond Breeze
⅛ teaspoon coconut extract
1 tablespoon shredded sweetened coconut, chopped
1 tablespoon fat-free or light caramel dip
1 teaspoon mini semi-sweet chocolate chips

DIRECTIONS

Combine oats, sweetener, and salt in a nonstick pot. Add Almond Breeze, coconut extract, and 1 cup water.

Bring to a boil and then reduce to a simmer. Stir in 2 teaspoons chopped coconut. Cook and stir until thick and creamy, 12 to 15 minutes.

Transfer to a medium bowl and let slightly cool and thicken. Top with caramel, chocolate chips, and remaining teaspoon chopped coconut. Yum!

MAKES 1 SERVING

For more recipes, tips & tricks, sign up for FREE daily emails at hungry-girl.com!

APPLE PIE
OATMEAL BONANZA

258 calories

You'll Need: nonstick pot, medium bowl
Prep: 5 minutes
Cook: 20 minutes

Entire recipe: 258 calories, 6g fat, 364mg sodium, 44.5g carbs, 7g fiber, 8.5g sugars, 6g protein

INGREDIENTS

½ cup old-fashioned oats
½ cup chopped apple
1 tablespoon sugar-free pancake syrup
1 teaspoon fat-free non-dairy powdered creamer
2 no-calorie sweetener packets
½ teaspoon cinnamon, or more to taste
Dash salt
1 cup Unsweetened Vanilla Almond Breeze
½ teaspoon vanilla extract

DIRECTIONS

Combine all ingredients in a nonstick pot. Mix in 1 cup water.

Bring to a boil and then reduce to a simmer. Cook and stir until thick and creamy, 12 to 15 minutes.

Transfer to a medium bowl and let slightly cool and thicken. Dig in!

MAKES 1 SERVING

PB & CHOCOLATE
OATMEAL BLITZ

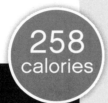

295 calories

You'll Need: nonstick pot, medium bowl
Prep: 5 minutes
Cook: 20 minutes

Entire recipe: 295 calories, 10.5g fat, 515mg sodium, 41g carbs, 6g fiber, 9g sugars, 11g protein

INGREDIENTS

½ cup old-fashioned oats
1 packet hot cocoa mix with 20 to 25 calories
Dash salt
1 cup Unsweetened Vanilla Almond Breeze
1 tablespoon peanut butter baking chips, roughly chopped

DIRECTIONS

Combine all ingredients *except* peanut butter chips in a nonstick pot. Mix in 1 cup water.

Bring to a boil and then reduce to a simmer. Cook and stir until thick and creamy, 12 to 15 minutes.

Remove from heat and stir in peanut butter chips. Transfer to a medium bowl and let slightly cool and thicken. Eat!

MAKES 1 SERVING

CRANBERRY-WALNUT MAPLE OATMEAL

282 calories

You'll Need: nonstick pot, medium bowl | **Prep:** 5 minutes | **Cook:** 20 minutes

Entire recipe:
282 calories, 7.5g fat, 352mg sodium, 48g carbs, 6.5g fiber, 12.5g sugars, 6.5g protein

INGREDIENTS

½ cup old-fashioned oats
2 tablespoons sweetened dried
    cranberries, chopped
1 no-calorie sweetener packet
½ teaspoon cinnamon, or more to taste
Dash salt
¾ cup Unsweetened Vanilla Almond Breeze
½ teaspoon vanilla extract
2 tablespoons sugar-free pancake syrup
½ tablespoon crushed walnuts

DIRECTIONS

Combine all ingredients *except* syrup and walnuts in a nonstick pot. Mix in 1 cup water.

Bring to a boil and then reduce to a simmer. Cook and stir until thick and creamy, 12 to 15 minutes.

Remove from heat and stir in syrup. Transfer to a medium bowl and let slightly cool and thicken. Sprinkle with walnuts, and grab a spoon!

MAKES 1 SERVING

Hungry for More Oatmeal?

Don't stop here—more oat-loaded treats await in the Parfaits chapter!

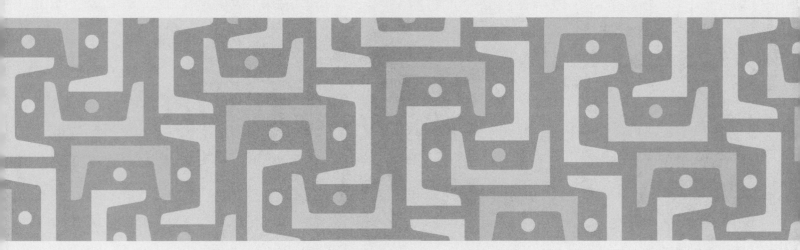

CHAPTER 3

PARFAITS

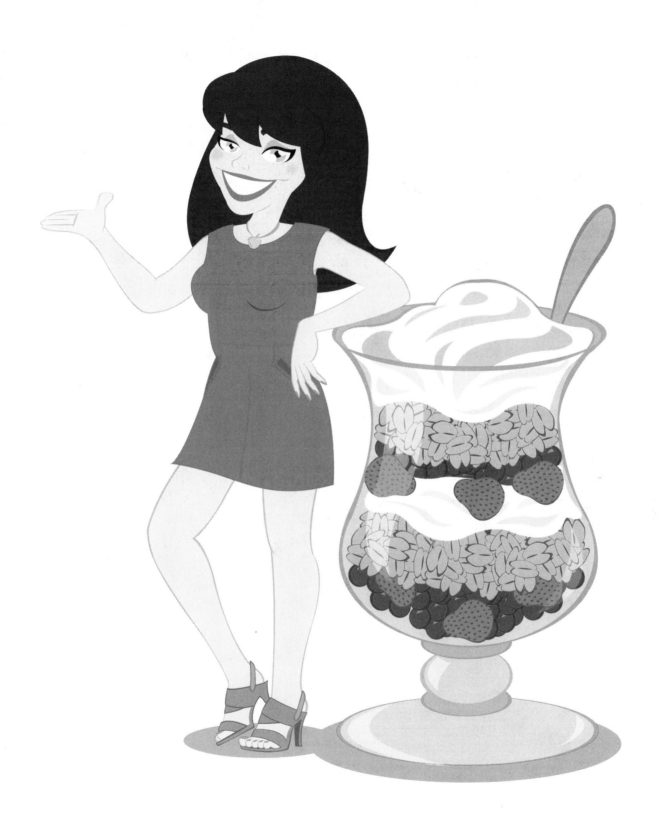

PARFAITS

Magical Maui Oatmeal Parfait

Peaches 'n Cream Oatmeal Parfait

Blueberry Pie Oatmeal Parfait

Bananas Foster Oatmeal Parfait

Pumpkin Pie Oatmeal Parfait

Super-Sized Berry-nana Oatmeal Parfait

PB&J Oatmeal Parfait

Cinn-a-nilla Apple Oatmeal Parfait

Bananas Foster Puddin' Parfait

Peachy Maple–Caramel Crunch Parfait

Creamy Crunchy Freeze-Dried Frenzy

PB&J Yogurt Parfait

Big Black-and-White Berry Parfait

Carnival Parfait

Dessert Island Parfait

Bananas for Brownies Parfait

Pumpkin Pudding Parfait

Very Berry Dreamboat Parfaits

Crunchy Caramel Chocolate Parfaits

Caramel Apple Parfait

Strawberry Shortcake Parfait

Piña Colada Parfait Surprise

Very Berry Vanilla Parfait

Banana Split Yogurt Parfait

Sun-Up Waffle Parfait

Coconut Cream Pie Parfait

Buffalo Chicken Parfait

Thanksgiving Parfaits

Sausage McMuffin Parfait

Cheeseburger Mashed Potato Parfaits

Chicken Nacho Parfait

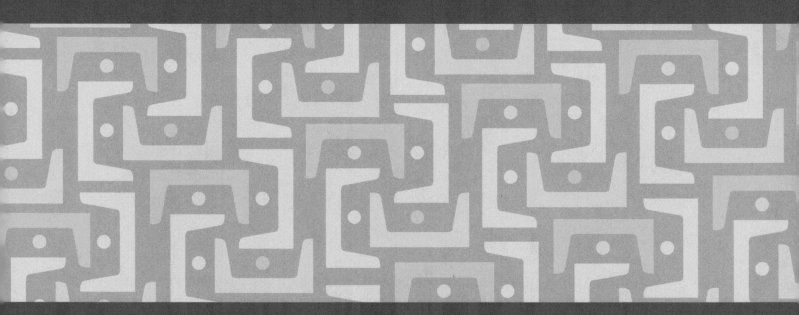

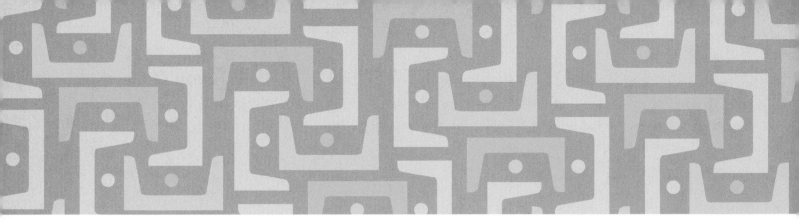

Layered food in a glass rocks.
And that's that.

A QUICK GUIDE TO SYMBOLS:

15 Minutes or Less

This symbol lets you know a recipe should take you no more than fifteen minutes from start to finish! That includes prep and cook time.

30 Minutes or Less

Just like the 15-minute version, this one points out recipes that take 30 minutes or less to whip up.

Meatless

You guessed it—no meat here! That includes beef, poultry, and fish. Some recipes give the option of a meatless ingredient. If you want your meal without meat, go with the meatless choice.

Single Serving

Pretty straightforward. These are recipes for one.

5 Ingredients or Less

Fans of HG know that we like to keep things simple. And these recipes contain just five ingredients or less!

Photos

These recipes can be seen in one of the book's photo inserts. The number in the symbol tells you which insert. Find photos of all the recipes at hungry-girl.com/books!

If you've never enjoyed a Hungry Girl **OATMEAL PARFAIT**, you're missing out. Prepare to be a changed human. These are great as meals AND as snacks. So versatile, so OATY, so AMAZING . . .

MAGICAL MAUI OATMEAL PARFAIT

312 calories

You'll Need: small nonstick pot, medium bowl, small bowl, tall glass
Prep: 5 minutes | **Cook:** 15 minutes | **Chill:** 1 hour 30 minutes

Entire recipe:
312 calories, 10g fat, 556mg sodium, 47g carbs, 6g fiber, 21g sugars, 9.5g protein

INGREDIENTS

Oatmeal
⅓ cup old-fashioned oats
1 no-calorie sweetener packet
⅛ teaspoon cinnamon
⅛ teaspoon salt
¾ cup Unsweetened Vanilla Almond Breeze
¼ cup crushed pineapple packed in juice, lightly drained
⅛ teaspoon vanilla extract

Parfait
½ cup fat-free vanilla yogurt
¼ teaspoon coconut extract
1 tablespoon shredded sweetened coconut
1 tablespoon slivered almonds, chopped

Optional topping: Fat Free Reddi-wip

DIRECTIONS

Combine all oatmeal ingredients in a small nonstick pot. Mix in ¾ cup water.

Bring to a boil and then reduce to a simmer. Cook and stir until somewhat thick and creamy, about 9 minutes. (It will thicken upon chilling.)

Transfer to a medium bowl and let slightly cool. Cover and refrigerate until chilled, at least 1½ hours.

Stir oatmeal. In a small bowl, mix yogurt with coconut extract.

In a tall glass, layer half of each ingredient: oatmeal, yogurt, shredded coconut, and chopped almonds.

Repeat layering with remaining ingredients. Dig in!

MAKES 1 SERVING

OATMEAL PARFAIT TIMESAVING TIP:

Cook your oatmeal the night before, and let it chill overnight.
Then in the morning, just assemble and eat!

PEACHES 'N CREAM OATMEAL PARFAIT

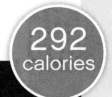

292 calories

You'll Need: small nonstick pot, medium bowl, tall glass
Prep: 5 minutes
Cook: 15 minutes
Chill: 1 hour 30 minutes

Entire recipe: 292 calories, 4.5g fat, 490mg sodium, 54g carbs, 5.5g fiber, 29.5g sugars, 9g protein

INGREDIENTS

Oatmeal
⅓ cup old-fashioned oats
1 no-calorie sweetener packet
¼ teaspoon cinnamon
⅛ teaspoon salt
¾ cup Unsweetened Vanilla Almond Breeze
¼ cup sliced peaches packed in juice, drained and chopped
¼ teaspoon vanilla extract

Parfait
½ cup fat-free vanilla yogurt
½ cup sliced peaches packed in juice, drained and chopped
2 tablespoons Fat Free Reddi-wip

DIRECTIONS

Combine all oatmeal ingredients in a small nonstick pot. Mix in ¾ cup water.

Bring to a boil and then reduce to a simmer. Cook and stir until somewhat thick and creamy, about 9 minutes. (It will thicken upon chilling.)

Transfer to a medium bowl and let slightly cool. Cover and refrigerate until chilled, at least 1½ hours.

Stir oatmeal. In a tall glass, layer half of each ingredient: oatmeal, yogurt, and peaches.

Repeat layering with remaining oatmeal, yogurt, and peaches. Top with Reddi-wip!

MAKES 1 SERVING

BLUEBERRY PIE OATMEAL PARFAIT

253 calories

You'll Need: small nonstick pot, medium bowl, tall glass
Prep: 5 minutes
Cook: 10 minutes
Chill: 1 hour 30 minutes

Entire recipe: 253 calories, 3g fat, 438mg sodium, 46g carbs, 4g fiber, 18.5g sugars, 10g protein

INGREDIENTS

Oatmeal
⅓ cup old-fashioned oats
1 teaspoon sugar-free French vanilla powdered creamer
1 no-calorie sweetener packet
¼ teaspoon cinnamon
⅛ teaspoon almond extract
⅛ teaspoon salt

Parfait
6 ounces (about ¾ cup) fat-free blueberry yogurt
2 low-fat cinnamon graham crackers (½ sheet), crushed

DIRECTIONS

Combine all oatmeal ingredients in a small nonstick pot. Add 1 cup water.

Bring to a boil and then reduce to a simmer. Cook and stir until thick and creamy, 4 to 5 minutes.

Transfer to a medium bowl, cover, and refrigerate until chilled, at least 1½ hours.

Stir oatmeal. In a tall glass, layer half of each ingredient: oatmeal, yogurt, and crushed graham crackers.

Repeat layering with remaining ingredients. Enjoy!

MAKES 1 SERVING

BANANAS FOSTER OATMEAL PARFAIT

  318 calories

You'll Need: small nonstick pot, medium bowl, tall glass
Prep: 5 minutes
Cook: 10 minutes
Chill: 1 hour 30 minutes

Entire recipe: 318 calories, 3g fat, 313mg sodium, 63g carbs, 5g fiber, 32.5g sugars, 11g protein

INGREDIENTS

Oatmeal
⅓ cup old-fashioned oats
1 teaspoon sugar-free French vanilla powdered creamer
1 no-calorie sweetener packet
⅛ teaspoon rum extract
Dash cinnamon
Dash salt

Parfait
Dash cinnamon
6 ounces (about ¾ cup) fat-free banana-cream or vanilla yogurt
½ medium banana, sliced
2 teaspoons fat-free or light caramel dip

Optional topping: Fat Free Reddi-wip

DIRECTIONS

Combine all oatmeal ingredients in a small nonstick pot. Mix in 1 cup water.

Bring to a boil and then reduce to a simmer. Cook and stir until thick and creamy, 4 to 5 minutes.

Transfer to a medium bowl and let slightly cool. Cover and refrigerate until chilled, at least 1½ hours.

Stir oatmeal. Mix cinnamon into yogurt.

In a tall glass, layer half of each ingredient: oatmeal, yogurt, banana slices, and caramel dip.

Repeat layering with remaining ingredients. Enjoy!

MAKES 1 SERVING

PUMPKIN PIE OATMEAL PARFAIT

   292 calories

You'll Need: small nonstick pot, medium bowl, tall glass
Prep: 5 minutes
Cook: 15 minutes
Chill: 1 hour 30 minutes

Entire recipe: 292 calories, 7.25g fat, 542mg sodium, 51g carbs, 7g fiber, 7.5g sugars, 7g protein

INGREDIENTS

Oatmeal
⅓ cup old-fashioned oats
2 no-calorie sweetener packets
¼ teaspoon cinnamon
¼ teaspoon pumpkin pie spice
Dash salt
¾ cup Unsweetened Vanilla Almond Breeze
⅓ cup canned pure pumpkin
¼ teaspoon vanilla extract

Parfait
1 sugar-free vanilla pudding snack with 60 calories or less
1 sheet (4 crackers) low-fat honey graham crackers, roughly crushed

Optional topping: Fat Free Reddi-wip

DIRECTIONS

Combine all oatmeal ingredients in a small nonstick pot. Mix in ¾ cup water.

Bring to a boil and then reduce to a simmer. Cook and stir until somewhat thick and creamy, about 9 minutes. (It will thicken upon chilling.)

Transfer to a medium bowl and let slightly cool. Cover and refrigerate until chilled, at least 1½ hours.

Stir oatmeal. In a tall glass, layer half of each ingredient: oatmeal, pudding, and crushed graham crackers.

Repeat layering with remaining ingredients. Eat up!

MAKES 1 SERVING

SUPER-SIZED BERRY-NANA OATMEAL PARFAIT

285 calories

You'll Need: small nonstick pot, medium bowl, tall glass
Prep: 5 minutes
Cook: 15 minutes
Chill: 1 hour 30 minutes

Entire recipe: 285 calories, 4.5g fat, 359mg sodium, 54g carbs, 6.5g fiber, 21.5g sugars, 9g protein

INGREDIENTS

Oatmeal
⅓ cup old-fashioned oats
1 no-calorie sweetener packet
⅛ teaspoon cinnamon
Dash salt
¾ cup Unsweetened Vanilla Almond Breeze
⅛ teaspoon vanilla extract

Parfait
½ cup fat-free vanilla yogurt
½ cup sliced strawberries
½ medium banana, sliced

DIRECTIONS

Combine all oatmeal ingredients in a small nonstick pot. Mix in ¾ cup water.

Bring to a boil and then reduce to a simmer. Cook and stir until somewhat thick and creamy, about 9 minutes. (It will thicken upon chilling.)

Transfer to a medium bowl and let slightly cool. Cover and refrigerate until chilled, at least 1½ hours.

Stir oatmeal. In a tall glass, layer half of each ingredient: oatmeal, yogurt, strawberries, and banana.

Repeat layering with remaining ingredients. Yum time!

MAKES 1 SERVING

PB&J OATMEAL PARFAIT

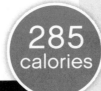
270 calories

You'll Need: small nonstick pot, medium bowl, small microwave-safe bowl, tall glass
Prep: 5 minutes
Cook: 10 minutes
Chill: 1 hour 30 minutes

Entire recipe: 270 calories, 9g fat, 241mg sodium, 41g carbs, 5g fiber, 14g sugars, 7.5g protein

INGREDIENTS

Oatmeal
⅓ cup old-fashioned oats
1 teaspoon sugar-free French vanilla powdered creamer
1 no-calorie sweetener packet
⅛ teaspoon vanilla extract
Dash salt
2 teaspoons reduced-fat peanut butter

Parfait
1 tablespoon low-sugar strawberry preserves
½ cup chopped strawberries
½ tablespoon peanut butter baking chips, chopped

DIRECTIONS

Combine all oatmeal ingredients *except* peanut butter in a small nonstick pot. Add 1 cup water.

Bring to a boil and then reduce to a simmer. Cook and stir until thick and creamy, 4 to 5 minutes.

Stir in peanut butter. Transfer to a medium bowl, cover, and refrigerate until chilled, at least 1½ hours.

Microwave preserves in a small microwave-safe bowl until warm, about 10 seconds. Add strawberries and mix well.

Stir oatmeal. In a tall glass, layer half of each of ingredient: oatmeal, strawberry mixture, and chopped peanut butter chips.

Repeat layering with remaining ingredients. Enjoy!

MAKES 1 SERVING

CINN-A-NILLA APPLE OATMEAL PARFAIT

240 calories

You'll Need: small nonstick pot, medium bowl, small bowl, tall glass
Prep: 5 minutes | **Cook:** 15 minutes | **Chill:** 1 hour 30 minutes

Entire recipe:
240 calories, 4.5g fat, 355mg sodium, 42.5g carbs, 5.75g fiber, 18g sugars, 8g protein

INGREDIENTS

Oatmeal
⅓ cup old-fashioned oats
1 no-calorie sweetener packet
½ teaspoon cinnamon
Dash salt
¾ cup Unsweetened Vanilla
    Almond Breeze
⅛ teaspoon vanilla extract

Parfait
½ cup chopped apple
¼ teaspoon cinnamon
½ cup fat-free vanilla yogurt

DIRECTIONS

Combine all oatmeal ingredients in a small nonstick pot. Mix in ¾ cup water.

Bring to a boil and then reduce to a simmer. Cook and stir until somewhat thick and creamy, about 9 minutes. (It will thicken upon chilling.)

Transfer to a medium bowl and let slightly cool. Cover and refrigerate until chilled, at least 1½ hours.

Stir oatmeal. In a small bowl, sprinkle chopped apple with ⅛ teaspoon cinnamon and toss to coat. Mix remaining ⅛ teaspoon cinnamon into yogurt.

In a tall glass, layer half of each ingredient: oatmeal, yogurt, and cinnamon-coated apple.

Repeat layering with remaining ingredients. Chew!

MAKES 1 SERVING

BANANAS FOSTER PUDDIN' PARFAIT

176 calories

You'll Need: mid-sized glass | **Prep:** 5 minutes

Entire recipe:
176 calories, 2.5g fat, 200mg sodium, 39.5g carbs, 1.75g fiber, 17g sugars, 2g protein

INGREDIENTS

1 sugar-free vanilla pudding snack
    with 60 calories or less
½ large banana, chopped
1 tablespoon fat-free or light caramel dip

Optional topping: cinnamon

DIRECTIONS

In a mid-sized glass, layer half of each ingredient: pudding, chopped banana, and caramel dip.

Repeat layering with remaining ingredients. Add a spoon and eat up!

MAKES 1 SERVING

PEACHY MAPLE–CARAMEL CRUNCH PARFAIT

174 calories

You'll Need: mid-sized glass | **Prep:** 5 minutes

Entire recipe:
174 calories, 0.5g fat, 212mg sodium, 37.5g carbs, 1.5g fiber, 26.5g sugars, 8.5g protein

INGREDIENTS

2 tablespoons sugar-free pancake syrup
6 ounces (about ¾ cup) fat-free vanilla yogurt
½ cup chopped peach
4 caramel-flavored soy crisps or
    mini rice cakes, crushed
Dash cinnamon

DIRECTIONS

Stir pancake syrup into yogurt.

In a mid-sized glass, layer half of each ingredient: yogurt, peach, and crushed soy crisps or mini rice cakes.

Repeat layering with remaining yogurt, peach, and crushed soy crisps or mini rice cakes. Sprinkle with cinnamon!

MAKES 1 SERVING

CREAMY CRUNCHY FREEZE-DRIED FRENZY

165 calories

You'll Need: mid-sized glass
Prep: 5 minutes

Entire recipe: 165 calories, 0.5g fat, 180mg sodium, 40g carbs, 7g fiber, 12g sugars, 11g protein

INGREDIENTS

6 ounces (about ¾ cup) fat-free vanilla yogurt
¼ cup freeze-dried fruit (any variety)
¼ cup Fiber One Original bran cereal

DIRECTIONS

In a mid-sized glass, layer half of each ingredient: yogurt, fruit, and cereal.

Repeat layering with remaining ingredients. Now devour!

MAKES 1 SERVING

PB&J YOGURT PARFAIT

203 calories

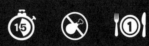

You'll Need: mid-sized glass
Prep: 5 minutes

Entire recipe: 203 calories, 2.25g fat, 190mg sodium, 37.5g carbs, 3g fiber, 26g sugars, 8g protein

INGREDIENTS

6 ounces (about ¾ cup) fat-free strawberry yogurt
½ cup chopped strawberries
¼ cup low-fat peanut butter cereal, lightly crushed
1 teaspoon peanut butter baking chips, crushed

DIRECTIONS

In a mid-sized glass, layer half of each ingredient: yogurt, strawberries, cereal, and crushed peanut butter chips.

Repeat layering with remaining ingredients. Dig in!

MAKES 1 SERVING

BIG BLACK-AND-WHITE BERRY PARFAIT

 196 calories

You'll Need: medium bowl, tall glass
Prep: 5 minutes

Entire recipe: 196 calories, 3g fat, 371mg sodium, 45g carbs, 6g fiber, 11g sugars, 4g protein

INGREDIENTS

1 sugar-free vanilla pudding snack with 60 calories or less
⅓ cup chopped strawberries
⅓ cup blueberries
⅓ cup raspberries
1 sugar-free chocolate pudding snack with 60 calories or less
¼ cup Fat Free Reddi-wip

DIRECTIONS

In a medium bowl, mix vanilla pudding with all the berries.

In a tall glass, layer half of the chocolate pudding followed by half of the vanilla pudding–berry mixture.

Repeat layering with remaining chocolate pudding and vanilla pudding–berry mixture. Top with Reddi-wip and dive in!

MAKES 1 SERVING

CARNIVAL PARFAIT

 284 calories

You'll Need: small microwave-safe bowl, tall glass
Prep: 5 minutes
Cook: 5 minutes

Entire recipe: 284 calories, 2g fat, 112mg sodium, 51g carbs, 3g fiber, 35g sugars, 17g protein

INGREDIENTS

½ tablespoon fat-free or light caramel dip
½ cup chopped Fuji apple
6 ounces (about ⅔ cup) fat-free vanilla Greek yogurt
1 small cake cone, lightly crushed
½ medium banana, thinly sliced
1 teaspoon mini semi-sweet chocolate chips

Optional topping: powdered sugar

DIRECTIONS

In a small microwave-safe bowl, combine caramel dip with ½ teaspoon water and microwave for 15 seconds, or until hot. Mix until smooth. Add apple and toss to coat.

In a tall glass, layer half of each of ingredient: apple mixture, yogurt, crushed cone, sliced banana, and chocolate chips.

Repeat layering with remaining ingredients, and enjoy!

MAKES 1 SERVING

Flip to the photo inserts to see over 100 recipe pics! And for photos of ALL the recipes, go to hungry-girl.com/books.

DESSERT ISLAND PARFAIT

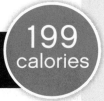
199 calories

You'll Need: mid-sized glass | **Prep:** 5 minutes

Entire recipe:
199 calories, 1g fat, 107mg sodium, 43.5g carbs, 2.75g fiber, 33.5g sugars, 8g protein

INGREDIENTS

3 drops coconut extract
6 ounces (about ¾ cup) fat-free vanilla yogurt
½ medium banana, chopped
¼ cup chopped mango
2 tablespoons Fat Free Reddi-wip
1 teaspoon shredded sweetened coconut

DIRECTIONS

Mix coconut extract into yogurt.

In a mid-sized glass, layer half of each ingredient: yogurt, banana, and mango.

Repeat layering with remaining yogurt and fruit. Top with Reddi-wip and coconut shreds and enjoy!

MAKES 1 SERVING

BANANAS FOR BROWNIES PARFAIT

220 calories

You'll Need: microwave-safe mug, nonstick spray, mid-sized glass | **Prep:** 5 minutes | **Cook:** 5 minutes

Entire recipe:
220 calories, 4g fat, 370mg sodium, 46g carbs, 2.5g fiber, 18.5g sugars, 4.5g protein

INGREDIENTS

2 tablespoons moist-style devil's food cake mix
½ tablespoon fat-free liquid egg substitute
1 sugar-free chocolate pudding snack with 60 calories or less
½ medium banana, sliced
1 teaspoon mini semi-sweet chocolate chips

DIRECTIONS

In a microwave-safe mug sprayed with nonstick spray, mix cake mix, egg substitute, and ½ tablespoon water. Mix in 2 tablespoons pudding (about ⅓rd of the snack).

Microwave for 1 minute. Once cool, crumble with a fork.

In a mid-sized glass, layer half of each ingredient: chocolate crumbles, remaining pudding, sliced banana, and chocolate chips.

Repeat layering with remaining ingredients. Eat!

MAKES 1 SERVING

PUMPKIN PUDDING PARFAIT

172 calories

You'll Need: small bowl, mid-sized glass
Prep: 5 minutes
Chill: 20 minutes

Entire recipe: 172 calories, 2.25g fat, 266mg sodium, 38g carbs, 6g fiber, 7.5g sugars, 3g protein

INGREDIENTS

½ cup canned pure pumpkin
2 tablespoons Cool Whip Free (thawed)
¼ teaspoon pumpkin pie spice
2 no-calorie sweetener packets
Dash cinnamon
1 sugar-free vanilla pudding snack with 60 calories or less
¼ cup Fiber One Caramel Delight cereal, lightly crushed

Optional toppings: Fat Free Reddi-wip, additional cinnamon

DIRECTIONS

In a small bowl, stir pumpkin, Cool Whip, pumpkin pie spice, sweetener, and cinnamon until well mixed. Refrigerate until chilled, at least 20 minutes.

In a mid-sized glass, layer half of each ingredient: pudding, pumpkin mixture, and crushed cereal.

Repeat layering with remaining ingredients. Eat!

MAKES 1 SERVING

VERY BERRY DREAMBOAT PARFAITS

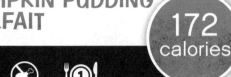

212 calories PER SERVING

You'll Need: medium bowl, 2 mid-sized glasses
Prep: 5 minutes
Chill: 20 minutes

½ of recipe (1 parfait): 212 calories, 2.5g fat, 742mg sodium, 34g carbs, 3g fiber, 12.5g sugars, 11g protein

INGREDIENTS

2 tablespoons Jell-O Sugar Free Fat Free Vanilla Instant pudding mix
2 tablespoons Splenda No Calorie Sweetener (granulated)
¼ teaspoon vanilla extract
1 cup Cool Whip Free (thawed)
½ cup fat-free cream cheese, room temperature
½ cup raspberries
½ cup sliced strawberries
1 sheet (4 crackers) low-fat graham crackers, lightly crushed

Optional topping: Fat Free Reddi-wip

DIRECTIONS

In a medium bowl, combine pudding mix, sweetener, vanilla extract, and ¼ cup cold water. Stir vigorously. Add Cool Whip and cream cheese, and stir until completely smooth. Cover and refrigerate until chilled, at least 20 minutes.

Evenly distribute raspberries between 2 mid-sized glasses. Evenly distribute half of the pudding mixture between the glasses, about ¼ cup each.

Repeat layering with strawberries and the remaining half of the pudding mixture.

Evenly distribute the crushed graham crackers between the glasses. Enjoy!

MAKES 2 SERVINGS

HG SWEET ALTERNATIVE!

Swap out the Splenda for the same amount of granulated white sugar, and each serving will have 254 calories, 45.5g carbs, and 25g sugars.

CRUNCHY CARAMEL CHOCOLATE PARFAITS

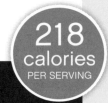

You'll Need: medium bowl, 2 mid-sized glasses
Prep: 5 minutes
Chill: 20 minutes

½ of recipe (1 parfait): 218 calories, 2g fat, 604mg sodium, 44g carbs, 8.5g fiber, 17g sugars, 9.5g protein

INGREDIENTS

1 tablespoon sugar-free fat-free chocolate instant pudding mix
½ tablespoon light chocolate syrup
½ cup Cool Whip Free (thawed)
¼ cup fat-free cream cheese, room temperature
2 Vitalicious VitaTops (any chocolate variety), thawed
8 caramel-flavored mini rice cakes, lightly crushed

Optional toppings: Fat Free Reddi-wip, additional mini rice cakes

DIRECTIONS

In a medium bowl, vigorously stir pudding mix with ¼ cup cold water until mostly smooth and slightly thickened. Mix in chocolate syrup. Add Cool Whip and cream cheese and thoroughly stir until mostly smooth. Cover and refrigerate for at least 20 minutes.

Break one VitaTop into small pieces, and divide between two mid-sized glasses.

Divide half of the pudding mixture between the glasses, about 3 tablespoons each. Divide crushed rice cakes between the glasses.

Break remaining VitaTop into small pieces, and divide between the glasses. Divide remaining pudding mixture between the glasses and enjoy!

MAKES 2 SERVINGS

CARAMEL APPLE PARFAIT

You'll Need: medium microwave-safe bowl, mid-sized glass
Prep: 5 minutes
Cook: 5 minutes

Entire recipe: 250 calories, 4g fat, 176mg sodium, 49g carbs, 3.5g fiber, 34g sugars, 8g protein

INGREDIENTS

1 tablespoon fat-free or light caramel dip
1 cup chopped Fuji apple
6 ounces (about ¾ cup) fat-free vanilla yogurt
2 teaspoons chopped peanuts

DIRECTIONS

In a medium microwave-safe bowl, combine caramel dip with 1 teaspoon water. Microwave for 15 seconds, or until hot. Mix until smooth. Add chopped apple and toss to coat.

To assemble, place half of the apple mixture in a mid-sized glass. Top with all of the yogurt, followed by 1 teaspoon peanuts.

Top with remaining apple mixture, sprinkle with remaining 1 teaspoon peanuts, and dig in!

MAKES 1 SERVING

Cream Cheese Alert!

To avoid lumps, it's crucial for the cream cheese to be room temperature. If you forget to set it out in advance, just microwave it at 50 percent power in 15-second intervals, stirring between intervals, until it reaches room temp.

STRAWBERRY SHORTCAKE PARFAIT

240 calories

You'll Need: medium bowl, small bowl, tall glass | **Prep:** 5 minutes

Entire recipe:
240 calories, 3.5g fat, 239mg sodium, 50g carbs, 1.5g fiber, 22g sugars, 2g protein

INGREDIENTS

½ cup sliced strawberries
¼ cup Cool Whip Free (thawed)
1 tablespoon low-sugar strawberry preserves
6 Reduced Fat Nilla wafers, crushed
1 sugar-free vanilla pudding snack with
    60 calories or less
¼ cup Fat Free Reddi-wip

DIRECTIONS

In a medium bowl, gently mix strawberries with Cool Whip.

In a small bowl, thoroughly mix preserves with 1 tablespoon water.

In a tall glass, layer half of each ingredient: crushed wafers, strawberry/Cool Whip mixture, pudding, and preserves mixture.

Repeat layering with remaining crushed wafers, strawberry/Cool Whip mixture, pudding, and preserves mixture. Top with Fat Free Reddi-wip. Enjoy!

MAKES 1 SERVING

PIÑA COLADA PARFAIT SURPRISE

175 calories

You'll Need: mid-sized glass | **Prep:** 5 minutes

Entire recipe:
175 calories, 0.5g fat, 129mg sodium, 42g carbs, 5g fiber, 28g sugars, 8g protein

INGREDIENTS

¼ teaspoon coconut extract
6 ounces (about ¾ cup) fat-free vanilla yogurt
¼ cup pineapple tidbits packed in juice, drained
¼ cup chopped banana
2 tablespoons Fiber One Original bran cereal

DIRECTIONS

Mix coconut extract into yogurt.

In a mid-sized glass, layer half of each ingredient: yogurt, pineapple tidbits, banana, and cereal.

Repeat layering with remaining ingredients. Eat!

MAKES 1 SERVING

VERY BERRY VANILLA PARFAIT

307 calories

You'll Need: tall glass | **Prep:** 5 minutes

Entire recipe:
307 calories, 1g fat, 145mg sodium, 65.5g carbs, 4g fiber, 50.5g sugars, 8.5g protein

INGREDIENTS

6 ounces (about ¾ cup) fat-free vanilla yogurt
3 full-sized or 10 mini vanilla meringue cookies, lightly crushed
1 cup sliced strawberries
½ cup Cool Whip Free (thawed)

DIRECTIONS

In a tall glass, layer half of each ingredient: yogurt, crushed cookies, strawberries, and Cool Whip.

Repeat layering with remaining ingredients. Eat up!

MAKES 1 SERVING

BANANA SPLIT YOGURT PARFAIT

293 calories

You'll Need: medium bowl, tall glass | **Prep:** 5 minutes

Entire recipe:
293 calories, 4.5g fat, 159mg sodium, 54.5g carbs, 3g fiber, 43g sugars, 9g protein

INGREDIENTS

6 ounces (about ¾ cup) fat-free vanilla yogurt
1 tablespoon low-sugar strawberry preserves
½ medium banana, sliced
1 tablespoon light chocolate syrup
2 teaspoons chopped peanuts
2 teaspoons rainbow sprinkles
2 tablespoons Fat Free Reddi-wip

DIRECTIONS

In a medium bowl, combine yogurt with preserves and mix well.

In a tall glass, layer half of each ingredient: yogurt mixture, banana slices, chocolate syrup, peanuts, and sprinkles.

Repeat layering with remaining yogurt mixture, banana slices, and chocolate syrup.

Top with Reddi-wip and sprinkle with remaining peanuts and sprinkles. Enjoy!

MAKES 1 SERVING

SUN-UP WAFFLE PARFAIT

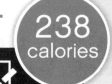

238 calories

You'll Need: tall glass
Prep: 5 minutes
Cook: 5 minutes

Entire recipe: 238 calories, 1.5g fat, 286mg sodium, 49g carbs, 4g fiber, 30g sugars, 9g protein

INGREDIENTS

1 frozen low-fat waffle
Dash cinnamon
6 ounces (about ¾ cup) fat-free peach yogurt
½ cup chopped mango

DIRECTIONS

Toast waffle, and chop into bite-sized pieces. Mix cinnamon into yogurt.

In a tall glass, layer half of each ingredient: waffle pieces, yogurt, and mango.

Repeat layering with remaining ingredients. Yum!

MAKES 1 SERVING

COCONUT CREAM PIE PARFAIT

227 calories

You'll Need: skillet, medium bowl, tall glass
Prep: 5 minutes
Cook: 5 minutes

Entire recipe: 227 calories, 7.5g fat, 301mg sodium, 38g carbs, 3g fiber, 11g sugars, 2.5g protein

INGREDIENTS

2 tablespoons shredded sweetened coconut, chopped
1 sugar-free vanilla pudding snack with 60 calories or less
⅛ teaspoon coconut extract
¼ cup Cool Whip Free (thawed)
1 sheet (4 crackers) low-fat honey graham crackers, roughly crushed

Optional topping: Fat Free Reddi-wip

DIRECTIONS

Bring a skillet to medium heat. Cook and stir 1 tablespoon shredded coconut until lightly browned, 1 to 2 minutes. Allow to cool.

In a medium bowl, mix pudding, remaining 1 tablespoon coconut, and coconut extract. Fold in Cool Whip.

In a tall glass, layer half of each ingredient: crushed graham crackers, pudding mixture, and browned coconut.

Repeat layering with remaining ingredients. Eat up!

MAKES 1 SERVING

Occasionally unconventional and ALWAYS incredibly delicious, **SAVORY HG PARFAITS** are a great way to change things up when it's time to chew. Who says layered food in a glass has to be sweet anyway?

BUFFALO CHICKEN PARFAIT

177 calories

You'll Need: 2 medium bowls, tall glass | **Prep:** 10 minutes

Entire recipe:
177 calories, 3.5g fat, 744mg sodium, 7g carbs, 1.5g fiber, 4g sugars, 29g protein

INGREDIENTS

3 tablespoons fat-free plain Greek yogurt
¼ teaspoon ranch dressing/dip seasoning mix
½ cup shredded lettuce
1 tablespoon crumbled blue cheese
3 ounces cooked and chopped skinless chicken breast
2 teaspoons Frank's RedHot Original Cayenne Pepper Sauce
¼ cup diced carrots
¼ cup diced celery

DIRECTIONS

Mix yogurt with ranch seasoning in a medium bowl. Stir in lettuce and blue cheese.

In another medium bowl, coat chicken with hot sauce.

In a tall glass, layer half of each of ingredient: lettuce mixture, carrots, celery, and saucy chicken.

Repeat layering with remaining ingredients. Enjoy!

MAKES 1 SERVING

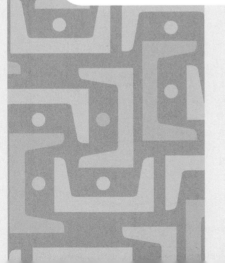

For more recipes, tips & tricks, sign up for FREE daily emails at hungry-girl.com!

THANKSGIVING PARFAITS

216 calories PER SERVING

You'll Need: large microwave-safe bowl, medium microwave-safe bowl, 4 mid-sized glasses
Prep: 10 minutes
Cook: 10 minutes

¼th of recipe (1 parfait): 216 calories, 2g fat, 595mg sodium, 28.5g carbs, 2.5g fiber, 4.5g sugars, 19.5g protein

INGREDIENTS

1½ cups instant mashed potato flakes
¼ teaspoon onion powder
1 tablespoon light whipped butter or light buttery spread
Dash each salt and black pepper, or more to taste
½ cup fat-free turkey gravy
8 ounces cooked and chopped skinless turkey breast
One 14.5-ounce can green beans, drained and chopped
2 tablespoons sweetened dried cranberries

DIRECTIONS

In a large microwave-safe bowl, thoroughly mix potato flakes, onion powder, and 2⅓ cups of water. Cover and microwave for 4 minutes, or until hot.

Once cool enough to handle, stir in butter, salt, and pepper. Re-cover and keep warm.

Place gravy in a medium microwave-safe bowl. Microwave for 2 minutes, or until hot.

Evenly distribute half of the potatoes among 4 mid-sized glasses, about ⅓ cup each.

Evenly distribute the chopped turkey and green beans among the glasses, about ⅓ cup each per glass.

Evenly distribute remaining mashed potatoes, followed by gravy. Top with cranberries and enjoy!

MAKES 4 SERVINGS

HG TIP!
If you like, heat up the turkey and green beans before assembling!

SAUSAGE MCMUFFIN PARFAIT

265 calories

You'll Need: large microwave-safe mug, nonstick spray, tall glass
Prep: 5 minutes
Cook: 5 minutes

Entire recipe: 265 calories, 4.5g fat, 924mg sodium, 27g carbs, 6g fiber, 2.5g sugars, 29g protein

INGREDIENTS

1 frozen meatless or turkey sausage patty with 80 calories or less
½ cup fat-free liquid egg substitute
1 light English muffin
1 slice fat-free American cheese

DIRECTIONS

In a large microwave-safe mug sprayed with nonstick spray, microwave sausage patty for 1 minute, or until hot.

Remove sausage. If needed, rinse and dry mug. Re-spray mug, add egg substitute, and microwave for 1 minute. Lightly stir and microwave for 45 to 60 seconds, until set. Stir to break into pieces.

Toast English muffin and tear into pieces. Chop sausage.

To assemble your parfait, place one-third of the torn muffin in a tall glass and top with half of the egg. Add half of the cheese, tearing it into pieces. Add half of the chopped sausage, followed by another third of the muffin.

Add remaining egg to the glass, followed by the remaining half of the cheese slice, tearing it into pieces. Top with remaining sausage, followed by remaining muffin. Dig in!

MAKES 1 SERVING

CHEESEBURGER MASHED POTATO PARFAITS

168 calories PER SERVING

You'll Need: large microwave-safe bowl, skillet and nonstick spray *or* microwave-safe plate, 4 mid-sized glasses
Prep: 15 minutes | **Cook:** 15 minutes

¼th of recipe (1 parfait):
168 calories, 1.5g fat, 634mg sodium, 29g carbs, 3.25g fiber, 4g sugars, 10g protein

INGREDIENTS

1⅓ cups instant mashed potato flakes
¼ teaspoon onion powder
¼ teaspoon salt
¼ cup fat-free sour cream
2 frozen meatless hamburger-style
   patties with 100 calories or less each
2 slices fat-free American cheese,
   broken into small pieces
½ cup chopped tomatoes
¼ cup chopped onion
4 teaspoons ketchup
4 hamburger dill pickle chips

DIRECTIONS

In a large microwave-safe bowl, thoroughly stir potato flakes, onion powder, salt, and 2⅓ cups water. Cover and microwave for 4 minutes, or until hot.

Stir in sour cream and cover to keep warm.

Cook burger patties in a skillet sprayed with nonstick spray or on a microwave-safe plate in the microwave. (Refer to package for cook time and temperature.) Chop patties into bite-sized pieces.

Scoop ⅓ cup potatoes into each of 4 mid-sized glasses. Evenly distribute chopped burger patties among the glasses, followed by cheese pieces.

Evenly distribute remaining mashed potatoes among the glasses, followed by tomatoes and onion. Top each with 1 teaspoon ketchup and a pickle chip. Enjoy!

MAKES 4 SERVINGS

CHICKEN NACHO PARFAIT

242 calories

You'll Need: 2 microwave-safe bowls, medium bowl, tall glass | **Prep:** 10 minutes | **Cook:** 5 minutes

Entire recipe:
242 calories, 5g fat, 761mg sodium, 25g carbs, 5g fiber, 2.5g sugars, 23.5g protein

INGREDIENTS

2 ounces cooked and chopped
   skinless chicken breast
⅛ teaspoon taco seasoning mix
¼ cup fat-free refried beans
¼ cup diced tomato
2 tablespoons salsa
2 tablespoons shredded reduced-fat
   Mexican-blend cheese
½ ounce (about 8) baked tortilla
   chips, lightly crushed

Optional toppings: fat-free sour
   cream, jarred jalapeño slices

DIRECTIONS

In a microwave-safe bowl, mix chicken with taco seasoning. Microwave for 30 seconds, or until hot.

Place beans in another microwave-safe bowl, cover, and microwave for 45 seconds, or until hot.

In a medium bowl, mix tomato with salsa.

In a tall glass, layer half of each of ingredient: chicken, cheese, beans, tomato-salsa mixture, and chips.

Repeat layering with remaining ingredients. Enjoy!

MAKES 1 SERVING

CHAPTER 4

PANCAKES AND FRENCH TOAST

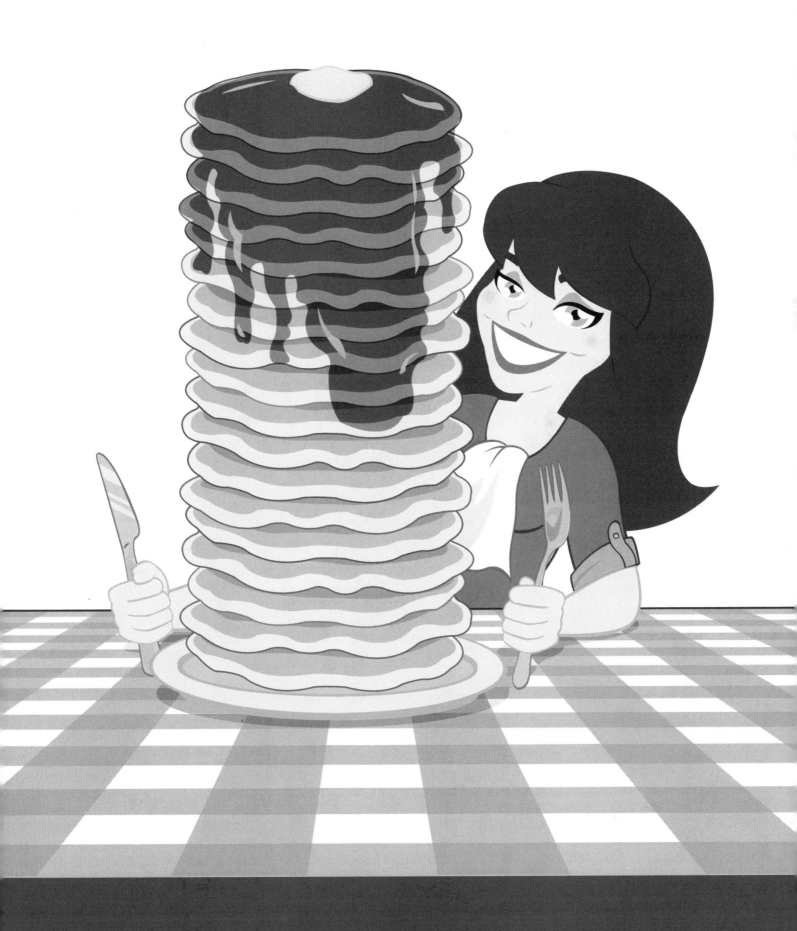

PANCAKES AND FRENCH TOAST

PANCAKES

Crazy-Good Carrot-Cake Pancakes
Banana Pumpkin Pie Pancakes
Gimme S'more Pancakes
Fab-Five Banana Pancake Minis
Oatmeal Raisin Pancakes
Oat-rageous Chocolate Chip Pancake Minis
Hawaiian Pancakes
Rockin' Red Velvet Pancakes
Over the Rainbow Pancakes
Strawberry Short Stack
Banana Chocolate Chip Pancakes
Maple Bacon Pancakes
Apple Cinnamon Sugar Pancakes

FRENCH TOAST

Classic Cinnalicious French Toast
French-Toasted Waffles
Classic Cinnalicious French Toast Nuggets
Pumpkin Cheesecake French Toast Bites
PB&J French Toast Nuggets
Cannoli-Stuffed French Toast Nuggets
Hawaiian French Toast Nuggets
Apple & Cream Cheese Stuffed
   French Toast Nuggets
Overstuffed PB 'n Banana French Toast
Cookies 'n Cream French Toast
Stuffed French-Toasted English Muffin
PB 'n Bacon Stuffed French Toast
Jammed with Cheese Stuffed French Toast
Cinnamon Raisin Stuffed French Toast
The Big Apple French Toast Casserole
Strawberry Banana French Toast Casserole

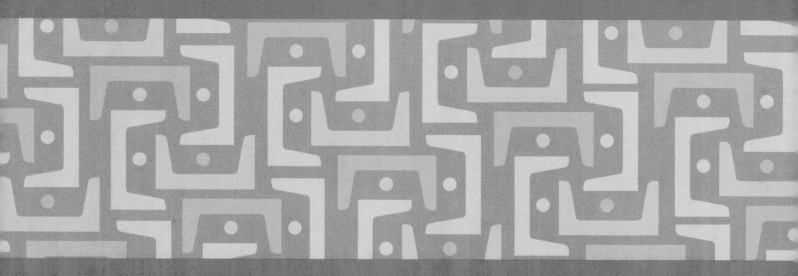

Sweet breakfast foods that are LOW in calories and fat—and HIGH in deliciousness. They're right here!

PANCAKE POINTERS!

* For pancakes packed with goodies like chopped fruit, use a spoon or spatula to even out the batter in the skillet. This way, your pancakes will cook evenly.

* The first pancake generally takes the longest to cook, so keep an eye on that second one; it'll cook faster!

FABULOUS FRENCH TOAST 411:

* Wondering why these recipes call for nonstick spray AND light butter? The spray keeps your food from sticking to the skillet, while the butter's job is to add flavor. It's the perfect way to keep those calories and fat grams in check without sacrificing deliciousness!

* If you prefer egg whites instead of egg sub, swap away! A ¼ cup of egg substitute is equal to about 2 large egg whites.

A QUICK GUIDE TO SYMBOLS:

15 Minutes or Less

This symbol lets you know a recipe should take you no more than fifteen minutes from start to finish! That includes prep and cook time.

30 Minutes or Less

Just like the 15-minute version, this one points out recipes that take 30 minutes or less to whip up.

Meatless

You guessed it—no meat here! That includes beef, poultry, and fish. Some recipes give the option of a meatless ingredient. If you want your meal without meat, go with the meatless choice.

Single Serving

Pretty straightforward. These are recipes for one.

5 Ingredients or Less

Fans of HG know that we like to keep things simple. And these recipes contain just five ingredients or less!

Photos

These recipes can be seen in one of the book's photo inserts. The number in the symbol tells you which insert. Find photos of all the recipes at hungry-girl.com/books!

PANCAKES

Super-fluffy and very yummy—batter up!

CRAZY-GOOD CARROT-CAKE PANCAKES

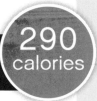
290 calories

You'll Need: small microwave-safe bowl, medium microwave-safe bowl, large bowl, skillet, nonstick spray, plate
Prep: 10 minutes | **Cook:** 15 minutes

Entire recipe (2 glazed pancakes):
290 calories, 1.5g fat, 510mg sodium, 54g carbs, 8g fiber, 15g sugars, 16g protein

INGREDIENTS

Glaze
1 tablespoon light vanilla soymilk
1 no-calorie sweetener packet
½ teaspoon powdered sugar
⅛ teaspoon vanilla extract
1 tablespoon fat-free cream cheese, room temperature

Pancakes
¼ cup shredded carrots, chopped
2 tablespoons canned pure pumpkin
2 tablespoons crushed pineapple packed in juice, drained
2 tablespoons light vanilla soymilk
¼ cup fat-free liquid egg substitute
1 tablespoon raisins
½ teaspoon vanilla extract
⅓ cup whole-wheat flour
1 no-calorie sweetener packet
¾ teaspoon cinnamon
½ teaspoon pumpkin pie spice
¼ teaspoon baking powder
Dash salt

DIRECTIONS

Mix all glaze ingredients *except* cream cheese in a small microwave-safe bowl. Add cream cheese and microwave for 30 seconds, or until softened. Stir until smooth.

Place carrots and 1 tablespoon water in a medium microwave-safe bowl. Cover and microwave for 1 minute, or until softened. Mix in pumpkin, pineapple, soymilk, egg substitute, raisins, vanilla extract, and 2 tablespoons water.

In a large bowl, stir together all other pancake ingredients. Mix in carrot-pumpkin mixture.

Bring a skillet sprayed with nonstick spray to medium-high heat. Add half the batter to form a large pancake. Cook just until it begins to bubble and is solid enough to flip, 2 to 3 minutes. Flip and cook until lightly browned and cooked through, 1 to 2 minutes. Plate pancake and set aside.

Remove skillet from heat, re-spray, and return to medium-high heat. Repeat to make a second pancake. Spread glaze over pancakes and eat up!

MAKES 1 SERVING

BANANA PUMPKIN PIE PANCAKES

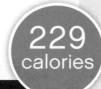

229 calories

You'll Need: medium bowl, skillet, nonstick spray, plate
Prep: 10 minutes
Cook: 10 minutes

Entire recipe (2 pancakes): 229 calories, 2.5g fat, 395mg sodium, 38.5g carbs, 5.5g fiber, 8g sugars, 13g protein

INGREDIENTS

⅓ cup old-fashioned oats
1 tablespoon dry pancake mix
1 no-calorie sweetener packet
¼ teaspoon pumpkin pie spice
¼ teaspoon cinnamon
Dash salt
⅓ cup fat-free liquid egg substitute
3 tablespoons mashed extra-ripe banana
2 tablespoons canned pure pumpkin
¼ teaspoon vanilla extract

DIRECTIONS

In a medium bowl, mix oats, pancake mix, sweetener, pumpkin pie spice, cinnamon, and salt. Mix in all remaining ingredients.

Bring a skillet sprayed with nonstick spray to medium-high heat. Add half the batter to form a large pancake. Cook until it begins to bubble and is solid enough to flip, 2 to 3 minutes. Flip and cook until lightly browned and cooked through, 1 to 2 minutes. Plate pancake and set aside.

Remove skillet from heat, re-spray, and return to medium-high heat. Repeat to make a second pancake. Enjoy!

MAKES 1 SERVING

GIMME S'MORE PANCAKES

281 calories

You'll Need: medium bowl, skillet, nonstick spray, plate
Prep: 10 minutes
Cook: 10 minutes

Entire recipe (2 pancakes): 281 calories, 3.25g fat, 523mg sodium, 52g carbs, 5.5g fiber, 14.5g sugars, 13g protein

INGREDIENTS

⅓ cup whole-wheat flour
½ teaspoon baking powder
1 no-calorie sweetener packet
Dash salt
¼ cup fat-free liquid egg substitute
1 tablespoon light vanilla soymilk
½ tablespoon mini semi-sweet chocolate chips
10 mini marshmallows, halved
½ tablespoon light chocolate syrup
2 tablespoons Fat Free Reddi-wip
2 low-fat honey graham crackers (½ sheet), crushed

DIRECTIONS

In a medium bowl, mix flour, baking powder, sweetener, and salt. Mix in egg substitute, soymilk, and 2 tablespoons water. Fold in chocolate chips and halved marshmallows; make sure marshmallows don't stick together.

Bring a skillet sprayed with nonstick spray to medium-high heat. Add half the batter to form a large pancake. Cook until it begins to bubble and is solid enough to flip, 2 to 3 minutes. Flip and cook until lightly browned and cooked through, 1 to 2 minutes. Plate pancake and set aside.

Remove skillet from heat, re-spray, and return to medium-high heat. Repeat to make a second pancake. Top pancakes with chocolate syrup, Reddi-wip, and crushed graham crackers. Enjoy!

MAKES 1 SERVING

FAB-FIVE BANANA PANCAKE MINIS

185 calories

You'll Need: medium bowl, skillet, nonstick spray
Prep: 10 minutes
Cook: 5 minutes

Entire recipe (5 mini pancakes):
185 calories, 1g fat, 343mg sodium, 37g carbs, 5g fiber, 7.5g sugars, 9.5g protein

INGREDIENTS

¼ cup whole-wheat flour
¼ teaspoon baking powder
1 no-calorie sweetener packet
Dash salt
Dash cinnamon
¼ cup mashed extra-ripe banana
3 tablespoons fat-free liquid egg substitute
1 tablespoon light vanilla soymilk
⅛ teaspoon vanilla extract

DIRECTIONS

In a medium bowl, mix flour, baking powder, sweetener, salt, and cinnamon. Mix in all remaining ingredients.

Bring a skillet sprayed with nonstick spray to medium-high heat. Add batter to form 5 mini pancakes. Cook just until they begin to bubble and are solid enough to flip, about 2 minutes. Flip and cook until lightly browned and cooked through, about 2 more minutes. Enjoy!

MAKES 1 SERVING

OATMEAL RAISIN PANCAKES

299 calories

You'll Need: medium bowl, skillet, nonstick spray, plate
Prep: 10 minutes
Cook: 10 minutes

Entire recipe (2 pancakes): 299 calories, 1.5g fat, 652mg sodium, 59.5g carbs, 7g fiber, 20g sugars, 13g protein

INGREDIENTS

⅓ cup whole-wheat flour
2 tablespoons old-fashioned oats
2 teaspoons brown sugar (not packed)
½ teaspoon baking powder
¼ teaspoon cinnamon
⅛ teaspoon salt
¼ cup fat-free liquid egg substitute
⅛ teaspoon vanilla extract
2 tablespoons raisins (not packed), chopped

Optional toppings: Fat Free Reddi-wip, sugar-free pancake syrup

DIRECTIONS

In a medium bowl, mix flour, oats, brown sugar, baking powder, cinnamon, and salt. Stir in egg substitute, vanilla extract, and ¼ cup water. Fold in raisins; make sure they don't stick together.

Bring a skillet sprayed with nonstick spray to medium-high heat. Add half the batter to form a large pancake. Cook until it begins to bubble and is solid enough to flip, 2 to 3 minutes. Flip and cook until lightly browned and cooked through, 1 to 2 minutes. Plate pancake and set aside.

Remove skillet from heat, re-spray, and return to medium-high heat. Repeat to make a second pancake. Enjoy!

MAKES 1 SERVING

For more recipes, tips & tricks, sign up for FREE daily emails at hungry-girl.com!

OAT-RAGEOUS CHOCOLATE CHIP PANCAKE MINIS

179 calories

You'll Need: medium bowl, skillet, nonstick spray | **Prep:** 5 minutes | **Cook:** 5 minutes

Entire recipe (5 mini pancakes):
179 calories, 3.25g fat, 341mg sodium, 28g carbs, 3.5g fiber, 5g sugars, 9.5g protein

INGREDIENTS

3 tablespoons old-fashioned oats
2 tablespoons whole-wheat flour
¼ teaspoon baking powder
1 no-calorie sweetener packet
Dash salt
3 tablespoons fat-free liquid egg substitute
1 tablespoon light vanilla soymilk
⅛ teaspoon vanilla extract
½ tablespoon mini semi-sweet chocolate chips

DIRECTIONS

In a medium bowl, mix oats, flour, baking powder, sweetener, and salt. Mix in egg substitute, soymilk, vanilla extract, and 1 tablespoon water. Fold in chocolate chips.

Bring a skillet sprayed with nonstick spray to medium-high heat. Add batter to form 5 mini pancakes. Cook just until they begin to bubble and are solid enough to flip, about 2 minutes. Flip and cook until lightly browned and cooked through, about 2 more minutes. Enjoy!

MAKES 1 SERVING

HAWAIIAN PANCAKES

251 calories

You'll Need: medium bowl, skillet, nonstick spray, plate | **Prep:** 5 minutes | **Cook:** 10 minutes

Entire recipe (2 pancakes):
251 calories, 2g fat, 800mg sodium, 41g carbs, 5g fiber, 8.5g sugars, 16.5g protein

INGREDIENTS

⅓ cup whole-wheat flour
½ teaspoon baking powder
1 no-calorie sweetener packet
Dash salt
¼ cup fat-free liquid egg substitute
⅛ teaspoon vanilla extract
1 ounce (about 2 slices) Canadian
   bacon, chopped
¼ cup crushed pineapple packed in juice,
   lightly drained

DIRECTIONS

In a medium bowl, mix flour, baking powder, sweetener, and salt. Mix in egg substitute, vanilla extract, and ¼ cup water. Stir in Canadian bacon and pineapple.

Bring a skillet sprayed with nonstick spray to medium-high heat. Add half the batter to form a large pancake. Cook until it begins to bubble and is solid enough to flip, 2 to 3 minutes. Flip and cook until lightly browned and cooked through, 1 to 2 minutes. Plate pancake and set aside.

Remove skillet from heat, re-spray, and return to medium-high heat. Repeat to make a second pancake. Enjoy!

MAKES 1 SERVING

ROCKIN' RED VELVET PANCAKES

273 calories

You'll Need: small microwave-safe bowl, tall glass, medium bowl, skillet, nonstick spray, plate
Prep: 10 minutes
Cook: 10 minutes

Entire recipe (2 iced pancakes): 273 calories, 3g fat, 717mg sodium, 46g carbs, 7.5g fiber, 9g sugars, 17.5g protein

INGREDIENTS

Icing
2 tablespoons Cool Whip Free (thawed)
1 tablespoon fat-free cream cheese, room temperature
1 no-calorie sweetener packet

Pancakes
1 packet hot cocoa mix with 20 to 25 calories
1 tablespoon unsweetened cocoa powder
1 teaspoon mini semi-sweet chocolate chips
⅓ cup whole-wheat flour
½ teaspoon baking powder
2 no-calorie sweetener packets
Dash salt
¼ cup fat-free liquid egg substitute
1 tablespoon light vanilla soymilk
3 drops red food coloring

DIRECTIONS

In a small microwave-safe bowl, mix all icing ingredients until smooth.

Place cocoa mix, cocoa powder, and ½ teaspoon chocolate chips in a tall glass. Add ¼ cup very hot water and stir until mostly dissolved.

In a medium bowl, mix flour, baking powder, sweetener, and salt. Stir in cocoa mixture, egg substitute, soymilk, and food coloring. Fold in remaining ½ teaspoon chocolate chips.

Bring a skillet sprayed with nonstick spray to medium-high heat. Add half the batter to form a large pancake. Cook until it begins to bubble and is solid enough to flip, 2 to 3 minutes. Flip and cook until lightly browned and cooked through, 1 to 2 minutes. Plate pancake and set aside.

Remove skillet from heat, re-spray, and return to medium-high heat. Repeat to make a second pancake.

Microwave icing for 20 seconds, or until warm. Spread over pancakes and eat up!

MAKES 1 SERVING

OVER THE RAINBOW PANCAKES

267 calories

You'll Need: medium bowl, whisk, skillet, nonstick spray, plate
Prep: 5 minutes
Cook: 10 minutes

Entire recipe (2 pancakes): 267 calories, 3g fat, 501mg sodium, 49g carbs, 3.5g fiber, 16g sugars, 10.5g protein

INGREDIENTS

¼ cup whole-wheat flour
2 tablespoons moist-style yellow cake mix
½ teaspoon baking powder
1 no-calorie sweetener packet
¼ cup fat-free liquid egg substitute
⅛ teaspoon almond extract
2 teaspoons rainbow sprinkles

Optional topping: Fat Free Reddi-wip

DIRECTIONS

In a medium bowl, mix flour, cake mix, baking powder, and sweetener. Add egg substitute, almond extract, and ¼ cup water. Whisk until smooth. Stir in sprinkles.

Bring a skillet sprayed with nonstick spray to medium-high heat. Add half the batter to form a large pancake. Cook until it begins to bubble and is solid enough to flip, 2 to 3 minutes. Flip and cook until lightly browned and cooked through, 1 to 2 minutes. Plate pancake and set aside.

Remove skillet from heat, re-spray, and return to medium-high heat. Repeat to make a second pancake. Enjoy!

MAKES 1 SERVING

STRAWBERRY SHORT STACK

289 calories

You'll Need: 2 medium bowls, small microwave-safe bowl, skillet, nonstick spray, plate
Prep: 10 minutes | **Cook:** 15 minutes

Entire recipe:
289 calories, 1.75g fat, 471mg sodium, 60.5g carbs, 7.5g fiber, 7g sugars, 14g protein

INGREDIENTS

⅓ cup whole-wheat flour
2 tablespoons old-fashioned oats
½ teaspoon baking powder
1 no-calorie sweetener packet
Dash salt
¼ cup fat-free liquid egg substitute
1 tablespoon light vanilla soymilk
2 tablespoons sugar-free
    strawberry jam/preserves
½ cup sliced strawberries
¼ cup Cool Whip Free (thawed)

Optional toppings: Fat Free Reddi-wip,
    sugar-free pancake syrup

DIRECTIONS

In a medium bowl, mix flour, oats, baking powder, sweetener, and salt. Stir in egg substitute, soymilk, and 2 tablespoons water.

In a small microwave-safe bowl, microwave jam/preserves for 20 seconds, or until softened. Stir into the medium bowl.

Bring a skillet sprayed with nonstick spray to medium-high heat. Add half the batter to form a large pancake. Cook until it begins to bubble and is solid enough to flip, 2 to 3 minutes. Flip and cook until lightly browned and cooked through, 1 to 2 minutes. Plate pancake and set aside.

Remove skillet from heat, re-spray, and return to medium-high heat. Repeat to make a second pancake. Plate and let slightly cool.

In another medium bowl, lightly mix strawberries with Cool Whip. Evenly spoon mixture over one pancake and lightly top with the other pancake. Woohoo!

MAKES 1 SERVING

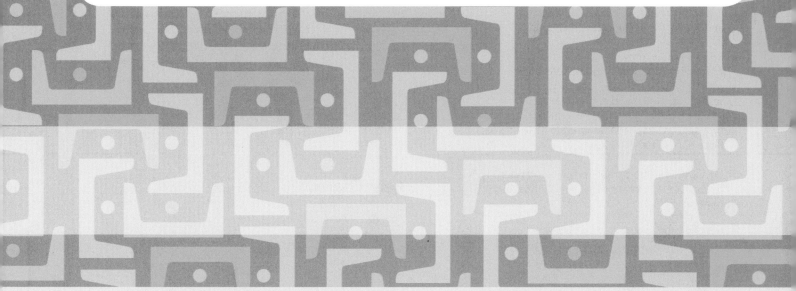

BANANA CHOCOLATE CHIP PANCAKES

328 calories

You'll Need: medium bowl, skillet, nonstick spray, plate
Prep: 10 minutes
Cook: 10 minutes

Entire recipe (2 pancakes): 328 calories, 4.5g fat, 648mg sodium, 61g carbs, 8g fiber, 14.5g sugars, 13.5g protein

INGREDIENTS

⅓ cup whole-wheat flour
2 tablespoons old-fashioned oats
½ teaspoon baking powder
1 no-calorie sweetener packet
⅛ teaspoon salt
Dash cinnamon
¼ cup fat-free liquid egg substitute
⅓ cup mashed extra-ripe banana
⅛ teaspoon vanilla extract
2 teaspoons mini semi-sweet chocolate chips

Optional toppings: Fat Free Reddi-wip, sugar-free pancake syrup

DIRECTIONS

In a medium bowl, mix flour, oats, baking powder, sweetener, salt, and cinnamon. Mix in egg substitute, banana, vanilla extract, and ¼ cup water. Stir in chocolate chips.

Bring a skillet sprayed with nonstick spray to medium-high heat. Add half the batter to form a large pancake. Cook until it begins to bubble and is solid enough to flip, 2 to 3 minutes. Flip and cook until lightly browned and cooked through, 1 to 2 minutes. Plate pancake and set aside.

Remove skillet from heat, re-spray, and return to medium-high heat. Repeat to make a second pancake. Enjoy!

MAKES 1 SERVING

MAPLE BACON PANCAKES

217 calories

You'll Need: skillet, microwave-safe plate (optional), medium bowl, nonstick spray, plate
Prep: 5 minutes
Cook: 15 minutes

Entire recipe (2 pancakes): 217 calories, 3g fat, 685mg sodium, 34.5g carbs, 5g fiber, 1g sugars, 14g protein

INGREDIENTS

1 slice center-cut bacon or turkey bacon
⅓ cup whole-wheat flour
½ teaspoon baking powder
1 no-calorie sweetener packet
Dash salt
¼ cup fat-free liquid egg substitute
1 tablespoon sugar-free pancake syrup
¼ teaspoon maple extract

DIRECTIONS

Cook bacon until crispy, either in a skillet over medium heat or on a microwave-safe plate in the microwave. (See package for cook time.) Finely chop or crumble.

In a medium bowl, mix flour, baking powder, sweetener, and salt. Mix in egg substitute, syrup, maple extract, and 3 tablespoons water.

Bring a skillet sprayed with nonstick spray to medium-high heat. Add half the batter to form a large pancake. Evenly top with half of the bacon. Cook until it begins to bubble and is solid enough to flip, 2 to 3 minutes. Flip and cook until lightly browned and cooked through, 1 to 2 minutes. Plate pancake and set aside.

Remove skillet from heat, re-spray, and return to medium-high heat. Repeat to make a second pancake. Enjoy!

MAKES 1 SERVING

APPLE CINNAMON SUGAR PANCAKES

255 calories

You'll Need: microwave-safe bowl, medium bowl, skillet, nonstick spray, plate
Prep: 10 minutes | **Cook:** 15 minutes

Entire recipe (2 pancakes):
255 calories, 1g fat, 671mg sodium, 51g carbs, 6.5g fiber, 16g sugars, 11.5g protein

INGREDIENTS

½ teaspoon cornstarch
½ cup chopped apple
1 tablespoon brown sugar (not packed)
¼ teaspoon plus 1 dash cinnamon
2 dashes salt
⅓ cup whole-wheat flour
½ teaspoon baking powder
1 no-calorie sweetener packet
¼ cup fat-free liquid egg substitute
⅛ teaspoon vanilla extract

Optional toppings: sugar-free pancake
    syrup, Fat Free Reddi-wip

DIRECTIONS

In a microwave-safe bowl, mix cornstarch with 2 teaspoons water. Add apple, brown sugar, ¼ teaspoon cinnamon, and a dash salt. Toss to coat. Cover and microwave for 1 minute, or until softened. Mix well.

In a medium bowl, mix flour, baking powder, sweetener, remaining dash cinnamon, and remaining dash salt. Stir in egg substitute, vanilla extract, and ¼ cup water. Fold in apple mixture.

Bring a skillet sprayed with nonstick spray to medium-high heat. Add half the batter to form a large pancake. Cook until it begins to bubble and is solid enough to flip, 2 to 3 minutes. Flip and cook until lightly browned and cooked through, 1 to 2 minutes. Plate pancake and set aside.

Remove skillet from heat, re-spray, and return to medium-high heat. Repeat to make a second pancake. Enjoy!

MAKES 1 SERVING

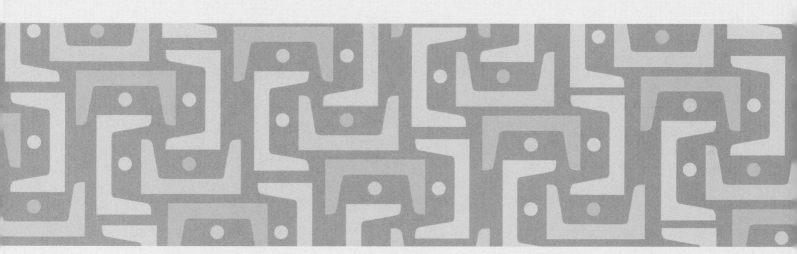

FRENCH TOAST

French toast is typically a calorie-and-fat-fest, but we do things differently in HG Land . . .

CLASSIC CINNALICIOUS FRENCH TOAST

226 calories

You'll Need: wide bowl, large skillet, nonstick spray | **Prep:** 5 minutes | **Cook:** 5 minutes

Entire recipe:
226 calories, 4.5g fat, 549mg sodium, 31g carbs, 8g fiber, 4g sugars, 18g protein

INGREDIENTS

½ cup fat-free liquid egg substitute
½ teaspoon cinnamon
¼ teaspoon vanilla extract
1 no-calorie sweetener packet
2 teaspoons light whipped butter or light buttery spread
3 slices light bread

DIRECTIONS

In a wide bowl, mix egg substitute, ¼ teaspoon cinnamon, vanilla extract, and sweetener.

Bring a large skillet sprayed with nonstick spray to medium-high heat. Add butter and let it coat the bottom. Meanwhile, coat bread on all sides with egg mixture.

Cook bread until golden brown, 1 to 2 minutes per side.

Top with remaining ¼ teaspoon cinnamon and enjoy!

MAKES 1 SERVING

Flip to the photo inserts to see over 100 recipe pics! And for photos of ALL the recipes, go to **hungry-girl.com/books**.

FRENCH-TOASTED WAFFLES

274 calories

You'll Need: wide bowl, skillet, nonstick spray | **Prep:** 5 minutes | **Cook:** 10 minutes

Entire recipe (2 waffles):
274 calories, 6g fat, 807mg sodium, 41.5g carbs, 3.25g fiber, 6.5g sugars, 16g protein

INGREDIENTS

2 frozen low-fat waffles

½ cup fat-free liquid egg substitute

½ teaspoon vanilla extract

¼ teaspoon cinnamon

2 teaspoons light whipped butter or light buttery spread

¼ cup sugar-free pancake syrup

1 teaspoon powdered sugar

DIRECTIONS

Lightly toast waffles. In a wide bowl, mix egg substitute, vanilla extract, and cinnamon.

Bring a skillet sprayed with nonstick spray to medium-high heat. Add butter and let it coat the bottom. Meanwhile, coat waffles on all sides with egg mixture.

Cook waffles until golden brown, 3 to 4 minutes per side.

Top with syrup, sprinkle with powdered sugar, and enjoy!

MAKES 1 SERVING

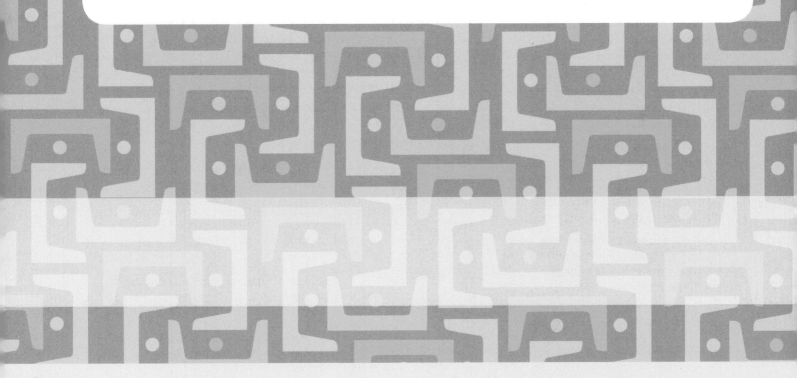

HG **French toast nuggets** are made with HOT DOG buns. Weird? Sorta. But they're AMAZING . . .

CLASSIC CINNALICIOUS FRENCH TOAST NUGGETS

147 calories

You'll Need: wide bowl, skillet, nonstick spray
Prep: 5 minutes
Cook: 5 minutes

Entire recipe (8 nuggets): 147 calories, 4.5g fat, 360mg sodium, 19.5g carbs, 5g fiber, 3g sugars, 10g protein

INGREDIENTS

½ teaspoon sugar-free French vanilla powdered creamer
¼ cup fat-free liquid egg substitute
1 dash cinnamon
1 light hot dog bun
2 teaspoons light whipped butter or light buttery spread

Optional topping: sugar-free pancake syrup

DIRECTIONS

In a wide bowl, mix powdered creamer with ½ tablespoon hot water and stir to dissolve. Add egg substitute and cinnamon. Stir well.

Split bun in half. Cut each half widthwise into 4 pieces, leaving you with 8 "nuggets."

Bring a skillet sprayed with nonstick spray to medium-high heat. Add butter and let it coat the bottom. Meanwhile, coat nuggets on all sides with egg mixture.

Cook nuggets, flipping occasionally, until golden brown on all sides, 3 to 4 minutes. Enjoy!

MAKES 1 SERVING

NUGGET-FLIPPIN' TIP!
Tongs are a good tool . . . Try 'em!

PUMPKIN CHEESECAKE FRENCH TOAST BITES

182 calories

You'll Need: wide bowl, small bowl, skillet, nonstick spray
Prep: 10 minutes
Cook: 5 minutes

Entire recipe (4 nuggets): 182 calories, 4.5g fat, 520mg sodium, 24.5g carbs, 3.5g fiber, 5g sugars, 12.5g protein

INGREDIENTS

¼ cup fat-free liquid egg substitute
¾ teaspoon vanilla extract
½ teaspoon cinnamon
1 no-calorie sweetener packet
2 tablespoons fat-free cream cheese, room temperature
1 tablespoon canned pure pumpkin
¼ teaspoon pumpkin pie spice
1 light hot dog bun
2 teaspoons light whipped butter or light buttery spread
2 tablespoons Fat Free Reddi-wip

Optional dip: sugar-free pancake syrup

DIRECTIONS

In a wide bowl, mix egg substitute, ½ teaspoon vanilla extract, ¼ teaspoon cinnamon, and half of sweetener.

In a small bowl, thoroughly mix cream cheese, pumpkin, pumpkin pie spice, remaining ¼ teaspoon vanilla extract, remaining ¼ teaspoon cinnamon, and remaining half of sweetener.

Open bun without separating the halves. Spread cream cheese mixture onto one half and lightly press to seal. Slice into four "nuggets."

Bring a skillet sprayed with nonstick spray to medium-high heat. Add butter and let it coat the bottom. Meanwhile, coat nuggets on all sides with egg mixture.

Cook nuggets, flipping occasionally, until golden brown on all sides, 3 to 4 minutes.

Serve topped with Reddi-wip!

MAKES 1 SERVING

PB&J FRENCH TOAST NUGGETS

267 calories

You'll Need: wide bowl, skillet, nonstick spray
Prep: 5 minutes
Cook: 5 minutes

Entire recipe (4 nuggets): 267 calories, 10g fat, 448mg sodium, 32.5g carbs, 6.5g fiber, 10.5g sugars, 13.5g protein

INGREDIENTS

¼ cup fat-free liquid egg substitute
½ teaspoon vanilla extract
¼ teaspoon cinnamon
1 light hot dog bun
1 tablespoon reduced-fat peanut butter, room temperature
1 tablespoon low-sugar grape jelly or strawberry preserves
2 teaspoons light whipped butter or light buttery spread

Optional toppings: powdered sugar, sugar-free pancake syrup

DIRECTIONS

In a wide bowl, mix egg substitute, vanilla extract, and cinnamon.

Open bun without separating the halves. Spread peanut butter onto one half, top with jelly or preserves, and lightly press to seal. Slice into four "nuggets."

Bring a skillet sprayed with nonstick spray to medium-high heat. Add butter and let it coat the bottom. Meanwhile, coat nuggets on all sides with egg mixture.

Cook nuggets, flipping occasionally, until golden brown on all sides, 3 to 4 minutes. Enjoy!

MAKES 1 SERVING

CANNOLI-STUFFED FRENCH TOAST NUGGETS

228 calories

You'll Need: wide bowl, small bowl, skillet, nonstick spray
Prep: 10 minutes
Cook: 5 minutes

Entire recipe (4 nuggets): 228 calories, 6.5g fat, 395mg sodium, 31g carbs, 3g fiber, 10.5g sugars, 12.5g protein

INGREDIENTS

¼ cup fat-free liquid egg substitute
¼ teaspoon cinnamon
1 teaspoon vanilla extract
3 tablespoons fat-free ricotta cheese
1 no-calorie sweetener packet
2 teaspoons mini semi-sweet chocolate chips
1 light hot dog bun
2 teaspoons light whipped butter or light buttery spread
½ teaspoon powdered sugar

Optional topping: sugar-free pancake syrup

DIRECTIONS

In a wide bowl, mix egg substitute, cinnamon, and ½ teaspoon vanilla extract.

In a small bowl, mix ricotta cheese, sweetener, and remaining ½ teaspoon vanilla extract. Fold in chocolate chips.

Open bun without separating the halves. Spoon ricotta mixture onto one half and lightly press to seal. Slice into four "nuggets."

Bring a skillet sprayed with nonstick spray to medium-high heat. Add butter and let it coat the bottom. Meanwhile, coat nuggets on all sides with egg mixture.

Cook nuggets, flipping occasionally, until golden brown on all sides, 3 to 4 minutes.

Serve sprinkled with powdered sugar and enjoy!

MAKES 1 SERVING

Can't find 80-calorie light buns?

Just get the lowest-calorie hot dog buns you see and adjust the calorie count accordingly. Bonus points if they have fiber!

HAWAIIAN FRENCH TOAST NUGGETS

259 calories

You'll Need: wide bowl, small bowl, skillet, nonstick spray | **Prep:** 5 minutes | **Cook:** 5 minutes

Entire recipe (4 nuggets):
259 calories, 6.5g fat, 570mg sodium, 37.5g carbs, 7g fiber, 17.5g sugars, 14.5g protein

INGREDIENTS

¼ cup fat-free liquid egg substitute
½ teaspoon coconut extract
¼ teaspoon cinnamon
¼ cup crushed pineapple packed in juice, drained, blotted dry
2 tablespoons fat-free cream cheese, room temperature
1 tablespoon shredded sweetened coconut
1 teaspoon brown sugar (not packed)
1 light hot dog bun
2 teaspoons light whipped butter or light buttery spread

Optional toppings: powdered sugar, sugar-free pancake syrup

DIRECTIONS

In a wide bowl, mix egg substitute, coconut extract, and cinnamon.

In a small bowl, mix pineapple, cream cheese, shredded coconut, and brown sugar.

Open bun without separating the halves. Spoon pineapple mixture onto one half and lightly press to seal. Slice into four "nuggets."

Bring a skillet sprayed with nonstick spray to medium-high heat. Add butter and let it coat the bottom. Meanwhile, coat nuggets on all sides with egg mixture.

Cook nuggets, flipping occasionally, until golden brown on all sides, 3 to 4 minutes. Enjoy!

MAKES 1 SERVING

APPLE & CREAM CHEESE STUFFED FRENCH TOAST NUGGETS

206 calories

You'll Need: wide bowl, small microwave-safe bowl, skillet, nonstick spray | **Prep:** 5 minutes | **Cook:** 10 minutes

Entire recipe (4 nuggets):
206 calories, 4.5g fat, 533mg sodium, 28.5g carbs, 6.5g fiber, 8.5g sugars, 13.5g protein

INGREDIENTS

¼ cup fat-free liquid egg substitute
1 teaspoon vanilla extract
½ teaspoon cinnamon
¼ cup diced apple
1 no-calorie sweetener packet
2 tablespoons fat-free cream cheese, room temperature
1 light hot dog bun
2 teaspoons light whipped butter or light buttery spread

Optional topping: sugar-free pancake syrup

DIRECTIONS

In a wide bowl, mix egg substitute, vanilla extract, and ¼ teaspoon cinnamon.

In a small microwave-safe bowl, top apple with sweetener and remaining ¼ teaspoon cinnamon; toss to coat. Microwave for 1 minute, or until softened. Mix in cream cheese.

Open bun without separating the halves. Spoon apple mixture onto one half and lightly press to seal. Slice into four "nuggets."

Bring a skillet sprayed with nonstick spray to medium-high heat. Add butter and let it coat the bottom of the skillet. Meanwhile, coat nuggets on all sides with egg mixture.

Cook nuggets, flipping occasionally, until golden brown on all sides, 3 to 4 minutes

MAKES 1 SERVING

OVERSTUFFED PB 'N BANANA FRENCH TOAST

327 calories

You'll Need: wide bowl, small bowl, skillet, nonstick spray
Prep: 10 minutes
Cook: 10 minutes

Entire recipe: 327 calories, 8.5g fat, 700mg sodium, 48.5g carbs, 7.25g fiber, 11g sugars, 18g protein

INGREDIENTS

⅓ cup fat-free liquid egg substitute
1¼ teaspoons vanilla extract
½ teaspoon plus 1 dash cinnamon
1 no-calorie sweetener packet
1 tablespoon fat-free cream cheese, room temperature
2 teaspoons reduced-fat peanut butter, room temperature
2 slices light white bread
½ small banana, sliced
2 teaspoons light whipped butter or light buttery spread
¼ cup sugar-free pancake syrup

DIRECTIONS

In a wide bowl, mix egg substitute, 1 teaspoon vanilla extract, ¼ teaspoon cinnamon, and half of the sweetener.

In a small bowl, thoroughly mix cream cheese, peanut butter, remaining ¼ teaspoon vanilla extract, ¼ teaspoon cinnamon, and remaining half of sweetener. Gently spread mixture onto one slice of bread. Top with banana, remaining dash cinnamon, and the other bread slice. Lightly press to seal.

Bring a skillet sprayed with nonstick spray to medium-high heat. Add butter and let it coat the bottom. Meanwhile, coat sandwich on all sides with egg mixture.

Cook sandwich until golden brown, 2 to 3 minutes per side.

Serve with syrup for dipping. Enjoy!

MAKES 1 SERVING

COOKIES 'N CREAM FRENCH TOAST

237 calories

You'll Need: wide bowl, small bowl, skillet, nonstick spray, plate
Prep: 5 minutes
Cook: 10 minutes

Entire recipe: 237 calories, 5.5g fat, 611mg sodium, 31.5g carbs, 5g fiber, 9.5g sugars, 16g protein

INGREDIENTS

¼ cup fat-free liquid egg substitute
2 tablespoons fat-free cream cheese, room temperature
2 chocolate graham crackers (½ sheet), crushed
¼ teaspoon vanilla extract
1 no-calorie sweetener packet
2 slices light bread
2 teaspoons light whipped butter or light buttery spread
1 teaspoon light chocolate syrup
½ teaspoon powdered sugar

DIRECTIONS

Place egg substitute in a wide bowl.

In a small bowl, mix cream cheese, crushed graham crackers, vanilla extract, and sweetener. Spread onto one slice of bread. Top with the other bread slice and lightly press to seal.

Bring a skillet sprayed with nonstick spray to medium-high heat. Add butter and let it coat the bottom. Meanwhile, coat sandwich on all sides with egg substitute.

Cook sandwich until golden brown, 2 to 3 minutes per side. Plate and top with chocolate syrup and powdered sugar!

MAKES 1 SERVING

STUFFED FRENCH-TOASTED ENGLISH MUFFIN

208 calories

You'll Need: wide bowl, small bowl, skillet, nonstick spray
Prep: 5 minutes
Cook: 10 minutes

Entire recipe: 208 calories, 4.5g fat, 409mg sodium, 35g carbs, 6.5g fiber, 9g sugars, 11g protein

INGREDIENTS

1 light English muffin
3 tablespoons fat-free liquid egg substitute
½ teaspoon vanilla extract
¼ teaspoon cinnamon
1 tablespoon fat-free cream cheese, room temperature
½ teaspoon powdered sugar
1 tablespoon low-sugar preserves/jelly/jam (any flavor)
2 teaspoons light whipped butter or light buttery spread

Optional topping: sugar-free pancake syrup

DIRECTIONS

Split English muffin and lightly toast.

In a wide bowl, mix egg substitute, vanilla extract, and cinnamon.

In a small bowl, mix cream cheese with powdered sugar. Evenly spread on split sides of English muffin halves.

Spread preserves/jelly/jam over cream cheese on one muffin half. Top with the other muffin half, split-side down.

Bring a skillet sprayed with nonstick spray to medium-high heat. Add butter and let it coat the bottom. Meanwhile, coat sandwich on all sides with egg mixture.

Cook sandwich until golden brown, 2 to 3 minutes per side. Eat up!

MAKES 1 SERVING

PB 'N BACON STUFFED FRENCH TOAST

281 calories

You'll Need: skillet, microwave-safe plate (optional), wide bowl, small bowl, nonstick spray
Prep: 5 minutes
Cook: 10 minutes

Entire recipe: 281 calories, 11g fat, 668mg sodium, 27g carbs, 6g fiber, 5g sugars, 19g protein

INGREDIENTS

1 slice center-cut bacon or turkey bacon
¼ cup fat-free liquid egg substitute
1 teaspoon vanilla extract
¼ teaspoon plus 1 dash cinnamon
1 tablespoon fat-free cream cheese, room temperature
2 teaspoons reduced-fat peanut butter, room temperature
1 no-calorie sweetener packet
2 slices light bread
2 teaspoons light whipped butter or light buttery spread

Optional topping: sugar-free pancake syrup

DIRECTIONS

Cook bacon until crispy, either in a skillet over medium heat or on a microwave-safe plate in the microwave. (See package for cook time.) Chop or crumble.

In a wide bowl, mix egg substitute, vanilla extract, and ¼ teaspoon cinnamon.

In a small bowl, mix cream cheese, peanut butter, sweetener, and remaining dash cinnamon. Gently spread mixture onto one slice of bread. Top with bacon and the other bread slice. Lightly press to seal.

Bring a skillet sprayed with nonstick spray to medium-high heat. Add butter and let it coat the bottom. Meanwhile, coat sandwich on all sides with egg mixture.

Cook sandwich until golden brown, 2 to 3 minutes per side. Enjoy!

MAKES 1 SERVING

JAMMED WITH CHEESE STUFFED FRENCH TOAST

263 calories

You'll Need: wide bowl, skillet, nonstick spray
Prep: 10 minutes
Cook: 10 minutes

Entire recipe: 263 calories, 5.5g fat, 810mg sodium, 42g carbs, 5.25g fiber, 4g sugars, 18.5g protein

INGREDIENTS

½ cup fat-free liquid egg substitute
½ teaspoon vanilla extract
¼ teaspoon cinnamon
2 slices light white bread
1 wedge The Laughing Cow Light Creamy Swiss cheese
2 tablespoons sugar-free strawberry jam/preserves
2 teaspoons light whipped butter or light buttery spread
¼ cup sugar-free pancake syrup

DIRECTIONS

In a wide bowl, mix egg substitute, vanilla extract, and cinnamon.

Lay bread slices flat and spread both with the cheese wedge. Spread jam/preserves over one slice and top with the other slice, cheese-side down. Lightly press to seal.

Bring a skillet sprayed with nonstick spray to medium-high heat. Add butter and let it coat the bottom. Meanwhile, coat sandwich on all sides with egg mixture.

Cook sandwich until golden brown, 2 to 3 minutes per side.

Serve with syrup for dipping and enjoy!

MAKES 1 SERVING

CINNAMON RAISIN STUFFED FRENCH TOAST

237 calories

You'll Need: wide bowl, small bowl, skillet, nonstick spray
Prep: 5 minutes
Cook: 10 minutes

Entire recipe: 237 calories, 4.5g fat, 557mg sodium, 31.5g carbs, 6g fiber, 12g sugars, 16g protein

INGREDIENTS

¼ cup fat-free liquid egg substitute
1¼ teaspoons vanilla extract
¼ teaspoon plus ⅛ teaspoon cinnamon
2 tablespoons fat-free cream cheese, room temperature
1 tablespoon raisins, chopped
1 no-calorie sweetener packet
2 slices light bread
2 teaspoons light whipped butter or light buttery spread

Optional topping: sugar-free pancake syrup

DIRECTIONS

In a wide bowl, mix egg substitute, 1 teaspoon vanilla extract, and ¼ teaspoon cinnamon.

In a small bowl, mix cream cheese, raisins, sweetener, remaining ¼ teaspoon vanilla extract, and remaining ⅛ teaspoon cinnamon. Gently spread onto one slice of bread. Top with the other bread slice and lightly press to seal.

Bring a skillet sprayed with nonstick spray to medium-high heat. Add butter and let it coat the bottom. Meanwhile, coat sandwich on all sides with egg mixture.

Cook sandwich until golden brown, 2 to 3 minutes per side. Enjoy!

MAKES 1 SERVING

These **French toast casseroles** are big, baked, and BEAUTEOUS…

THE BIG APPLE FRENCH TOAST CASSEROLE

220 calories
PER SERVING

You'll Need: 8-inch by 8-inch baking pan, nonstick spray, small microwave-safe bowl, large bowl, medium bowl
Prep: 30 minutes | **Cook:** 55 minutes

¼th of casserole:
220 calories, 4.5g fat, 674mg sodium, 31g carbs, 6g fiber, 8.5g sugars, 17g protein

INGREDIENTS

2 tablespoons light whipped butter or light buttery spread
1 cup light vanilla soymilk
1 cup fat-free liquid egg substitute
¼ cup plus 2 tablespoons sugar-free pancake syrup
2 tablespoons Splenda No Calorie Sweetener (granulated)
1¼ teaspoons cinnamon
⅛ teaspoon salt
8 slices light bread
1 cup peeled and diced apple
Half an 8-ounce tub fat-free cream cheese, room temperature
¼ teaspoon vanilla extract

HG SWEET ALTERNATIVE!

Swap out the Splenda for the same amount of granulated white sugar, and each serving will have 241 calories, 36.5g carbs, and 14.5g sugars.

DIRECTIONS

Preheat oven to 350 degrees. Spray an 8-inch by 8-inch baking pan with nonstick spray.

In a small microwave-safe bowl, microwave butter for 20 seconds, or until melted. In a large bowl, mix melted butter, soymilk, egg substitute, 2 tablespoons syrup, ½ tablespoon sweetener, 1 teaspoon cinnamon, and salt.

Cut bread into cubes. Stir bread cubes and diced apple into the mixture in the large bowl.

In a medium bowl, thoroughly mix cream cheese, vanilla extract, remaining 1½ tablespoons sweetener, and remaining ¼ teaspoon cinnamon.

Spoon half of the bread mixture into the baking pan. Dollop with cream cheese mixture. Top with remaining bread mixture.

Bake until firm and set, about 55 minutes.

Top or serve with syrup and enjoy!

MAKES 4 SERVINGS

STRAWBERRY BANANA FRENCH TOAST CASSEROLE

245 calories
PER SERVING

You'll Need: 8-inch by 8-inch baking pan, nonstick spray, small microwave-safe bowl, large bowl, medium bowl
Prep: 30 minutes | **Cook:** 55 minutes

¼th of casserole:
245 calories, 4.5g fat, 628mg sodium, 36.5g carbs, 7g fiber, 11g sugars, 17.5g protein

INGREDIENTS

2 tablespoons light whipped butter or
    light buttery spread
1 cup light vanilla soymilk
1 cup fat-free liquid egg substitute
3 tablespoons Splenda No Calorie
    Sweetener (granulated)
1¼ teaspoons cinnamon
⅛ teaspoon salt
8 slices light bread
1 medium banana, sliced into coins
1 cup sliced strawberries
Half an 8-ounce tub fat-free cream cheese,
    room temperature
¼ teaspoon vanilla extract
¼ cup sugar-free pancake syrup

HG SWEET ALTERNATIVE!

Swap out the Splenda for the same amount of granulated white sugar, and each serving will have 277 calories, 45g carbs, and 20.5g sugars.

DIRECTIONS

Preheat oven to 350 degrees. Spray an 8-inch by 8-inch baking pan with nonstick spray.

In a small microwave-safe bowl, microwave butter for 20 seconds, or until melted. In a large bowl, mix melted butter, soymilk, egg substitute, 1½ tablespoons sweetener, 1 teaspoon cinnamon, and salt.

Cut bread into cubes. Stir bread, banana, and strawberries into the mixture in the large bowl.

In a medium bowl, thoroughly mix cream cheese, vanilla extract, remaining 1½ tablespoons sweetener, and remaining ¼ teaspoon cinnamon.

Spoon half of the bread mixture into the baking pan. Dollop with cream cheese mixture. Top with remaining bread mixture.

Bake until firm and set, about 55 minutes.

Top or serve with syrup and enjoy!

MAKES 4 SERVINGS

Hungry for More Decadent Breakfast Goodies?
Skip ahead to Chapter 16 for sticky buns, muffins, Danishes, and more!

CHAPTER 5

FAUX-FRYS: POPPERS, ONION RINGS, CHICKEN NUGGETS & MORE

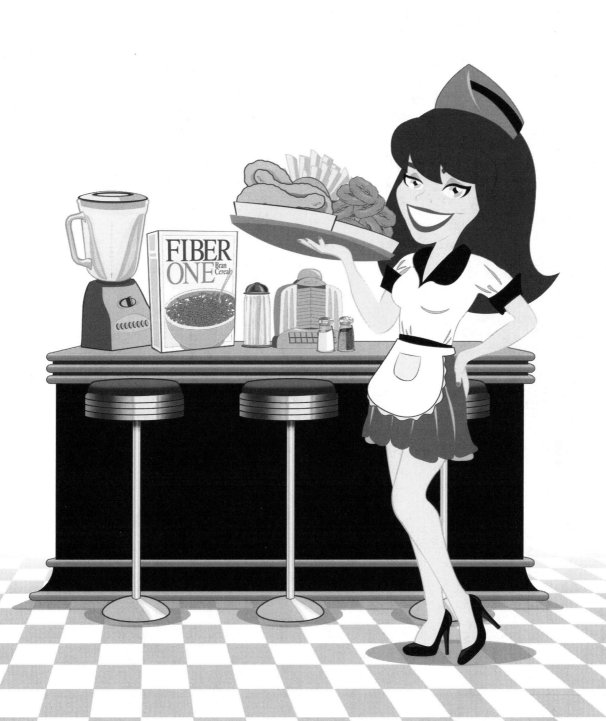

FAUX-FRYS: POPPERS, ONION RINGS, CHICKEN NUGGETS & MORE

Jalapeño Swappers

Jalapeño 'n Onion Poppers

Big Blue Buffalo Jala' Poppers

Mexi-Crab Stuffed Poppers

Stuffed Mushroom Jalapeño Poppers

Lord of the Onion Rings

Mexi-licious Onion Loops with Queso

Honey Yum Mustard Onion Rings

Hot 'n Spicy Onion Rings

Onion Rings Parm

Hungry Cowgirl Onion Rings

Sour Cream & Onion Rings with Dip

Chili-ed Up Onion Rings

Bloomin' Blossom

Sweet 'n Sassy Boneless Hot Wings

H-O-T Hot Boneless Buffalo Wings

Ranch-ified Chicken Nuggets

Taco-Flavored Chicken Nuggets

Fiber-ific Fried Chicken Strips

Onion Chicken Fingers

Kickin' Buttermilk Faux-Fried Chicken

BBQ Chicken Fingers

Planet Hungrywood Cap'n Crunchy Chicken

Crispity Crunchity Drumsticks

Pan-Fried Chicken Parm

Chicken Parm Rollup

Flounder Parm

Chicken Parm Dunkers

Pork Parmesan

Shrimp Parmesan

No-Harm Eggplant Parm

Jalapeño Popper Chicken

De-lish Faux-Fried Fish

Buffalicious Shrimp

Faux-Fried & Fabulous Calamari

Sweet Coconut Crunch Shrimp

Swapcorn Shrimp

Dy-no-mite Dream Shrimp

Here at Hungry Girl, we don't believe in grease or deep fryers. Instead, we use unconventional coatings and BAKE our creations. CLEVER!!! We call it "faux-frying"...

FIBER ONE, WE'RE CRUSHING ON YOU! TIPS & TRICKS . . .

It's difficult to grind small amounts of Fiber One Original bran cereal in a full-sized blender. This is why recipes with ¼ cup or less call for it already crushed in the ingredients. If you have a small blender or food processor, use it. If you don't, you have two equally easy options . . .

Crush it in a sealable bag.
Place the cereal in the bag, squeeze out the air, and seal. Using the flat end of a meat mallet, pound the cereal through the bag on a flat surface. No mallet? A rolling pin or any heavy kitchen utensil with a flat surface will do.

Grind up a bunch at once.
Blend up a large amount of cereal at once, and store it in an airtight container or sealable bag. Then use this handy-dandy conversion chart for recipes.

* ¼ cup Fiber One Original bran cereal, finely crushed = **2 tablespoons pre-ground crumbs**

* ⅓ cup Fiber One Original bran cereal (crushed in directions) = **2 tablespoons plus 2 teaspoons pre-ground crumbs**

* ½ cup Fiber One Original bran cereal (crushed in directions) = **¼ cup pre-ground crumbs**

A QUICK GUIDE TO SYMBOLS:

15 Minutes or Less	**30 Minutes or Less**	**Meatless**	**Single Serving**	**5 Ingredients or Less**	**Photos**
This symbol lets you know a recipe should take you no more than fifteen minutes from start to finish! That includes prep and cook time.	Just like the 15-minute version, this one points out recipes that take 30 minutes or less to whip up.	You guessed it—no meat here! That includes beef, poultry, and fish. Some recipes give the option of a meatless ingredient. If you want your meal without meat, go with the meatless choice.	Pretty straightforward. These are recipes for one.	Fans of HG know that we like to keep things simple. And these recipes contain just five ingredients or less!	These recipes can be seen in one of the book's photo inserts. The number in the symbol tells you which insert. Find photos of all the recipes at hungry-girl.com/books!

Our original Jalapeño Swappers were so in demand that we had to create a whole SLEW of recipes for **JALAPEÑO POPPERS**. Guess you could say they're "popper-ular!" (But don't, unless you wanna lose respect from friends and family members.)

JALAPEÑO QUICK TIP!

Use a spoon to seed your jalapeños. When handling jalapeños, don't touch your eyes— that pepper juice can STING. And wash your hands well immediately afterward.

JALAPEÑO SWAPPERS

50 calories
PER SERVING

You'll Need: baking sheet, nonstick spray, blender or food processor, 2 wide bowls, small bowl
Prep: 30 minutes
Cook: 30 minutes

⅕th of recipe (2 poppers): 50 calories, 0.5g fat, 170mg sodium, 8.5g carbs, 3g fiber, 1.5g sugars, 5.5g protein

INGREDIENTS

½ cup Fiber One Original bran cereal
Dash each salt and black pepper, or more to taste
Dash garlic powder, or more to taste
¼ cup fat-free cream cheese, room temperature
¼ cup shredded fat-free cheddar cheese
5 jalapeño peppers, halved lengthwise, seeds and stems removed
¼ cup fat-free liquid egg substitute

DIRECTIONS

Preheat oven to 350 degrees. Spray a baking sheet with nonstick spray.

In a blender or food processor, grind cereal into crumbs. Transfer to a wide bowl and mix in seasonings.

In a small bowl, thoroughly mix cream cheese with shredded cheddar cheese. Evenly spoon and spread mixture into pepper halves.

Place egg substitute in another wide bowl. One at a time, coat pepper halves with egg substitute, shake to remove excess, and coat with crumbs. Evenly place on the baking sheet, stuffed sides up.

Bake until outside is crispy and pepper halves have softened, 25 to 30 minutes.

MAKES 5 SERVINGS

JALAPEÑO 'N ONION POPPERS

87 calories PER SERVING

You'll Need: baking sheet, nonstick spray, blender or food processor, 2 wide bowls, skillet, medium bowl
Prep: 30 minutes
Cook: 40 minutes

¼th of recipe (3 poppers): 87 calories, 2g fat, 388mg sodium, 15g carbs, 5g fiber, 4.5g sugars, 4.5g protein

INGREDIENTS

½ cup Fiber One Original bran cereal
1 tablespoon (about ¼th of a 1-ounce packet) onion soup/dip seasoning mix
1 cup chopped onion
4 wedges The Laughing Cow Light Creamy Swiss cheese
6 jalapeño peppers, halved lengthwise, seeds and stems removed
⅓ cup fat-free liquid egg substitute

DIRECTIONS

Preheat oven to 350 degrees. Spray a baking sheet with nonstick spray.

In a blender or food processor, grind cereal into crumbs. Transfer to a wide bowl and mix in seasoning mix.

Bring a skillet sprayed with nonstick spray to medium-high heat. Cook and stir onion until softened and browned, about 6 minutes.

Transfer onion to a medium bowl. Add cheese wedges, breaking them into pieces, and stir until smooth. Evenly spoon and spread mixture into pepper halves.

Place egg substitute in another wide bowl. One at a time, coat pepper halves with egg substitute, shake to remove excess, and coat with crumbs. Evenly place on the baking sheet, stuffed sides up.

Bake until outside is crispy and pepper halves have softened, 25 to 30 minutes.

MAKES 4 SERVINGS

BIG BLUE BUFFALO JALA' POPPERS

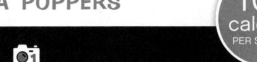**106 calories** PER SERVING

You'll Need: baking sheet, nonstick spray, blender or food processor, 2 wide bowls, small bowl
Prep: 30 minutes
Cook: 30 minutes

¼th of recipe (3 poppers): 106 calories, 3.5g fat, 639mg sodium, 14g carbs, 4.5g fiber, 4.5g sugars, 6.5g protein

INGREDIENTS

½ cup Fiber One Original bran cereal
¼ teaspoon onion powder
¼ teaspoon garlic powder
Dash cayenne pepper
4 wedges The Laughing Cow Light Creamy Swiss cheese
2 tablespoons Frank's RedHot Original Cayenne Pepper Sauce
3 tablespoons crumbled blue cheese
6 jalapeño peppers, halved lengthwise, seeds and stems removed
¼ cup fat-free liquid egg substitute

DIRECTIONS

Preheat oven to 350 degrees. Spray a baking sheet with nonstick spray.

In a blender or food processor, grind cereal into crumbs. Transfer to a wide bowl and mix in seasonings.

In a small bowl, thoroughly mix cheese wedges with 1 tablespoon hot sauce. Stir in blue cheese. Evenly spoon and spread mixture into the pepper halves.

In another wide bowl, mix egg substitute with remaining 1 tablespoon hot sauce. One at a time, coat pepper halves with egg mixture, shake to remove excess, and coat with crumbs. Evenly place on the baking sheet, stuffed sides up.

Bake until outside is crispy and pepper halves have softened, 25 to 30 minutes. Mmmm!

MAKES 4 SERVINGS

MEXI-CRAB STUFFED POPPERS

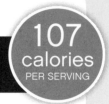

107 calories
PER SERVING

You'll Need: baking sheet, nonstick spray, 2 wide bowls, medium bowl
Prep: 30 minutes | **Cook:** 30 minutes

¼th of recipe (3 poppers):
107 calories, 1.5g fat, 315mg sodium, 19g carbs, 3.5g fiber, 4.5g sugars, 6.5g protein

INGREDIENTS

¼ cup Fiber One Original bran cereal, finely crushed

3 tablespoons yellow cornmeal

1 teaspoon taco seasoning mix

2 ounces (about ⅓ cup) roughly chopped imitation crabmeat

2 tablespoons canned black beans, drained and rinsed

2 tablespoons frozen sweet corn kernels, thawed

Dash cayenne pepper

2 wedges The Laughing Cow Light Creamy Swiss cheese

6 jalapeño peppers, halved lengthwise, seeds and stems removed

¼ cup fat-free liquid egg substitute

DIRECTIONS

Preheat oven to 350 degrees. Spray a baking sheet with nonstick spray.

In a wide bowl, mix crushed cereal, cornmeal, and taco seasoning.

In a medium bowl, thoroughly mix crabmeat, black beans, corn kernels, cayenne pepper, and cheese wedges, breaking cheese wedges into pieces as you add them. Evenly spoon and spread filling into pepper halves.

Place egg substitute in another wide bowl. One at a time, coat pepper halves with egg substitute, shake to remove excess, and coat with crumbs. Evenly place on the baking sheet, stuffed sides up.

Bake until outside is crispy and pepper halves have softened, 25 to 30 minutes.

MAKES 4 SERVINGS

CRUMB-COATING TIPS & TRICKS

Wipe your hands often. This'll help keep your egg mixture crumb-free and your crumbs clump-free.

Try the two-handed method. Use one hand to coat your food items in egg substitute, shake off the excess, and then use the other hand to coat the items with crumbs. This way you won't transport the excess egg on your fingers into the crumb mixture.

Crumb-coating alternative: the seal-and-shake method. Place your crumbs in a sealable container. After coating the food items with egg and shaking off the excess, add the items to the container and seal. Then shake it until all the items are coated! You can also do this in a sealable plastic bag.

STUFFED MUSHROOM JALAPEÑO POPPERS

67 calories
PER SERVING

You'll Need: baking sheet, nonstick spray, small bowl, skillet, medium bowl
Prep: 30 minutes | **Cook:** 35 minutes

¼th of recipe (3 poppers):
67 calories, 2g fat, 329mg sodium, 8.5g carbs, 2.5g fiber, 3g sugars, 4g protein

INGREDIENTS

¼ cup Fiber One Original bran cereal, finely crushed

1 tablespoon reduced-fat Parmesan-style grated topping

⅛ teaspoon each salt and black pepper

1½ cups chopped mushrooms

½ teaspoon chopped garlic

¼ teaspoon onion powder

4 wedges The Laughing Cow Light Creamy Swiss cheese

6 jalapeño peppers, halved lengthwise, seeds and stems removed

DIRECTIONS

Preheat oven to 350 degrees. Spray a baking sheet with nonstick spray.

In a small bowl, mix crushed cereal, Parm-style topping, salt, and black pepper.

Bring a skillet sprayed with nonstick spray to medium-high heat. Cook and stir mushrooms and garlic until softened and browned, about 4 minutes.

Transfer mushroom-garlic mixture to a medium bowl. Add onion powder and cheese wedges, breaking wedges into pieces. Mix well. Evenly spoon and spread mixture into pepper halves.

Sprinkle cereal-Parm mixture over the filling in each pepper half. Evenly place on the baking sheet, stuffed sides up.

Bake until topping is crispy and pepper halves have softened, 25 to 30 minutes.

MAKES 4 SERVINGS

✳ Flip to the photo inserts to see over 100 recipe pics! And for photos of ALL the recipes, go to **hungry-girl.com/books**.

HG's Lord of the Onion Rings started it all . . .
and our **ONION RING RECIPES** keep
getting better and better!

HG FYI:

Most large onions
yield about 30 whole
rings. If you have
more (or fewer) rings,
just continue coating
until you run out of
rings, egg mixture,
or crumbs.

LORD OF THE ONION RINGS

155 calories

You'll Need: 2 baking sheets, nonstick spray, blender or food processor, 2 wide bowls
Prep: 20 minutes
Cook: 25 minutes

Entire recipe (about 30 rings):
155 calories, 1g fat, 515mg sodium,
41g carbs, 16g fiber, 7g sugars, 9g protein

INGREDIENTS

1 large onion
½ cup Fiber One Original bran cereal
¼ teaspoon garlic powder, or more to taste
⅛ teaspoon onion powder, or more to taste
⅛ teaspoon salt, or more to taste
Dash black pepper, or more to taste
½ cup fat-free liquid egg substitute

DIRECTIONS

Preheat oven to 375 degrees. Spray 2 baking sheets with nonstick spray.

Slice off onion's ends and remove outer layer. Cut into ½-inch-wide slices, and separate into rings.

In a blender or food processor, grind cereal into crumbs. Transfer to a wide bowl and mix in seasonings.

Place egg substitute in another wide bowl. One at a time, dunk rings in the egg substitute, shake to remove excess, and coat with crumbs. Evenly lay rings on the baking sheets.

Bake for 10 minutes. Flip rings. Continue to bake until outside is crispy and inside is soft, 10 to 15 minutes. Yum!

MAKES 1 SERVING

MEXI-LICIOUS ONION LOOPS WITH QUESO

183 calories
PER SERVING

You'll Need: 2 baking sheets, nonstick spray, blender or food processor, 2 wide bowls, microwave-safe bowl
Prep: 25 minutes | **Cook:** 25 minutes

½ of recipe (about 15 rings with ⅓ cup dip):
183 calories, 3g fat, 857mg sodium, 37.5g carbs, 10g fiber, 6.5g sugars, 7.5g protein

INGREDIENTS

1 large onion
½ cup Fiber One Original bran cereal
1 ounce (about 15) baked tortilla chips
1 teaspoon taco seasoning mix
½ cup fat-free liquid egg substitute
½ cup salsa
2 wedges The Laughing Cow Light Creamy Swiss cheese

DIRECTIONS

Preheat oven to 375 degrees. Spray 2 baking sheets with nonstick spray.

Slice off onion's ends and remove outer layer. Cut into ½-inch-wide slices, and separate into rings.

In a blender or food processor, grind cereal and chips into crumbs. Transfer to a wide bowl and mix in taco seasoning.

Place egg substitute in another wide bowl. One at a time, dunk rings in the egg substitute, shake to remove excess, and coat with crumbs. Evenly lay rings on the baking sheets.

Bake for 10 minutes. Flip rings. Continue to bake until outside is crispy and inside is soft, 10 to 15 minutes.

Meanwhile, in a microwave-safe bowl, mix salsa with cheese wedges, breaking cheese wedges into pieces as you add them. Microwave for 1 minute, or until hot. Thoroughly stir until uniform.

Serve rings with sauce for dunking—YUM!

MAKES 2 SERVINGS

RINGMASTER TRICKS!

Use tongs or a fork to handle the rings.
Then there's less chance of eggy hands leading to eggy crumbs, which can cause clumps. If you use a fork, don't pierce the rings with it; just balance them on it.

Set aside half of the crumb mixture in advance.
This way, you'll have a fresh batch of crumbs to use after coating the first half of your rings.

HONEY YUM MUSTARD ONION RINGS

135 calories PER SERVING

You'll Need: 2 baking sheets, nonstick spray, blender or food processor, 2 wide bowls
Prep: 25 minutes | **Cook:** 25 minutes

½ of recipe (about 15 rings):
135 calories, 3g fat, 353mg sodium, 31.5g carbs, 8.5g fiber, 6g sugars, 3g protein

INGREDIENTS

1 large onion
½ cup Fiber One Original bran cereal
2½ tablespoons yellow cornmeal
¼ teaspoon onion powder, or more to taste
⅛ teaspoon garlic powder, or more to taste
⅛ teaspoon salt, or more to taste
Dash black pepper, or more to taste
¼ cup Newman's Own Lite Honey Mustard dressing (or another light honey mustard dressing)
2 tablespoons fat-free liquid egg substitute

Optional dip: additional honey mustard dressing

DIRECTIONS

Preheat oven to 375 degrees. Spray 2 baking sheets with nonstick spray.

Slice off onion's ends and remove outer layer. Cut into ½-inch-wide slices, and separate into rings.

In a blender or food processor, grind cereal into crumbs. Transfer to a wide bowl and mix in cornmeal and seasonings.

In another wide bowl, thoroughly mix dressing with egg substitute. One at a time, dunk rings in the dressing-egg mixture, shake to remove excess, and coat with crumbs. Evenly lay rings on the baking sheets.

Bake for 10 minutes. Flip rings. Bake until outside is crispy and inside is soft, 10 to 15 minutes.

MAKES 2 SERVINGS

HOT 'N SPICY ONION RINGS

141 calories PER SERVING

You'll Need: 2 baking sheets, nonstick spray, blender or food processor, 2 wide bowls
Prep: 25 minutes | **Cook:** 25 minutes

½ of recipe (about 15 rings):
141 calories, 3g fat, 761mg sodium, 31.5g carbs, 9g fiber, 5g sugars, 5g protein

INGREDIENTS

1 large onion
½ cup Fiber One Original bran cereal
1 ounce (about 15) reduced-fat BBQ-flavored potato chips
1 teaspoon garlic powder
⅛ teaspoon each salt and black pepper
¼ cup fat-free liquid egg substitute
2 tablespoons Frank's RedHot Original Cayenne Pepper Sauce

DIRECTIONS

Preheat oven to 375 degrees. Spray 2 baking sheets with nonstick spray.

Slice off onion's ends and remove outer layer. Cut into ½-inch-wide slices, and separate into rings.

In a blender or food processor, grind cereal and chips into crumbs. Transfer to a wide bowl and mix in garlic powder, salt, and pepper.

In another wide bowl, mix egg substitute with hot sauce. One at a time, dunk rings in egg mixture, shake to remove excess, and lightly coat with crumbs. Evenly lay rings on the baking sheets.

Bake for 10 minutes. Flip rings. Bake until outside is crispy and inside is soft, 10 to 15 minutes. Enjoy!

MAKES 2 SERVINGS

ONION RINGS PARM

176 calories PER SERVING

You'll Need: 2 baking sheets, nonstick spray, blender or food processor, 2 wide bowls
Prep: 25 minutes
Cook: 25 minutes

½ of recipe (about 15 rings and ¼ cup sauce): 176 calories, 3g fat, 723mg sodium, 37g carbs, 11g fiber, 7.5g sugars, 8.5g protein

INGREDIENTS

1 large onion
½ cup Fiber One Original bran cereal
2 tablespoons whole-wheat flour
2 tablespoons reduced-fat Parmesan-style grated topping
1 tablespoon dried basil
1 teaspoon garlic powder
1 teaspoon dried oregano
¼ teaspoon each salt and black pepper
½ cup fat-free liquid egg substitute
½ cup low-fat marinara sauce

DIRECTIONS

Preheat oven to 375 degrees. Spray 2 baking sheets with nonstick spray.

Slice off onion's ends and remove outer layer. Cut into ½-inch-wide slices, and separate into rings.

In a blender or food processor, grind cereal into crumbs. Transfer to a wide bowl and mix in flour, Parm-style topping, and seasonings.

Place egg substitute in another wide bowl. One at a time, dunk rings in the egg substitute, shake to remove excess, and coat with crumbs. Evenly lay rings on the baking sheets.

Bake for 10 minutes. Flip rings. Bake until outside is crispy and inside is soft, 10 to 15 minutes. Serve with marinara for dipping!

MAKES 2 SERVINGS

HUNGRY COWGIRL ONION RINGS

148 calories PER SERVING

You'll Need: 2 baking sheets, nonstick spray, blender or food processor, 2 wide bowls, whisk
Prep: 25 minutes
Cook: 25 minutes

½ of recipe (about 15 rings): 148 calories, 3g fat, 441mg sodium, 34g carbs, 8.5g fiber, 6.5g sugars, 5g protein

INGREDIENTS

1 large onion
½ cup Fiber One Original bran cereal
1 ounce (about 15) reduced-fat BBQ-flavored potato chips
1 teaspoon dried minced onion
1 teaspoon ranch dressing/dip seasoning mix
½ cup fat-free liquid egg substitute
1 tablespoon BBQ sauce with 45 calories or less per 2-tablespoon serving

DIRECTIONS

Preheat oven to 375 degrees. Spray 2 baking sheets with nonstick spray.

Slice off onion's ends and remove outer layer. Cut into ½-inch-wide slices, and separate into rings.

In a blender or food processor, grind cereal and chips into crumbs. Transfer to a wide bowl and mix in minced onion and ranch mix.

In another wide bowl, whisk egg substitute with BBQ sauce. One at a time, dunk rings in the egg mixture, shake to remove excess, and coat with crumbs. Evenly lay rings on the baking sheets.

Bake for 10 minutes. Flip rings. Continue to bake until outside is crispy and inside is soft, 10 to 15 minutes. Chew, you!

MAKES 2 SERVINGS

SOUR CREAM & ONION RINGS WITH DIP

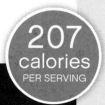
207 calories PER SERVING

You'll Need: 2 baking sheets, nonstick spray, blender or food processor, 2 wide bowls, small bowl
Prep: 30 minutes
Cook: 25 minutes

½ of recipe (about 15 rings with ¼ cup dip): 207 calories, 4g fat, 746mg sodium, 41g carbs, 9g fiber, 9.5g sugars, 8.5g protein

INGREDIENTS

1 large onion
½ cup Fiber One Original bran cereal
1 ounce (about 15) reduced-fat sour cream & onion potato chips
1 tablespoon dried minced onion
½ teaspoon garlic powder
¼ teaspoon each salt and black pepper
½ cup fat-free liquid egg substitute
½ cup fat-free sour cream
2 teaspoons onion soup/dip seasoning mix

DIRECTIONS

Preheat oven to 375 degrees. Spray 2 baking sheets with nonstick spray.

Slice off onion's ends and remove outer layer. Cut into ½-inch-wide slices, and separate into rings.

In a blender or food processor, grind cereal and chips into crumbs. Transfer to a wide bowl and mix in minced onion, garlic powder, salt, and black pepper.

Place egg substitute in another wide bowl. One at a time, dunk rings in the egg substitute, shake to remove excess, and coat with crumbs. Evenly lay rings on the baking sheets.

Bake for 10 minutes. Flip rings. Bake until outside is crispy and inside is soft, 10 to 15 minutes.

In a small bowl, mix onion soup/dip mix into sour cream. Serve with onion rings for dipping!

MAKES 2 SERVINGS

CHILI-ED UP ONION RINGS

119 calories PER SERVING

You'll Need: 2 baking sheets, nonstick spray, blender or food processor, 2 wide bowls
Prep: 25 minutes
Cook: 25 minutes

½ of recipe (about 15 rings): 119 calories, 1g fat, 414mg sodium, 29.5g carbs, 9.5g fiber, 4g sugars, 6g protein

INGREDIENTS

1 large onion
½ cup Fiber One Original bran cereal
2½ tablespoons yellow cornmeal
¾ teaspoon ground cumin
¾ teaspoon chili powder
½ teaspoon garlic powder
¼ teaspoon salt
⅛ teaspoon black pepper
½ cup fat-free liquid egg substitute

Optional dips: salsa, fat-free sour cream

DIRECTIONS

Preheat oven to 375 degrees. Spray 2 baking sheets with nonstick spray.

Slice off onion's ends and remove outer layer. Cut into ½-inch-wide slices, and separate into rings.

In a blender or food processor, grind cereal into crumbs. Transfer to a wide bowl and mix in cornmeal and seasonings.

Place egg substitute in another wide bowl. One at a time, dunk rings in the egg substitute, shake to remove excess, and coat with crumbs. Evenly lay rings on the baking sheets.

Bake for 10 minutes. Flip rings. Bake until outside is crispy and inside is soft, 10 to 15 minutes. Yum!

MAKES 2 SERVINGS

BLOOMIN' BLOSSOM

192 calories PER SERVING

You'll Need: baking pan, nonstick spray, blender or food processor, medium bowl, 2 large bowls, small bowl
Prep: 35 minutes | **Cook:** 40 minutes

½ of recipe:
192 calories, 1.75g fat, 700mg sodium, 54g carbs, 17g fiber, 13g sugars, 7g protein

INGREDIENTS

Onion
1 jumbo sweet onion (not peeled)
1 cup Fiber One Original bran cereal
¼ teaspoon seasoned salt
¼ teaspoon garlic powder
⅛ teaspoon black pepper
½ cup fat-free liquid egg substitute

Sauce
3 tablespoons fat-free mayonnaise
2 teaspoons ketchup
⅛ teaspoon seasoned salt
Dash chili powder

DIRECTIONS

Preheat oven to 400 degrees. Spray a baking pan with nonstick spray.

Slice off the top half-inch of the onion. Leaving the bottom root intact, carefully peel off the outside layer.

Cut down and across the middle, stopping a half-inch from the root. Repeat to make a criss-cross, cutting down the middle and stopping a half-inch from the bottom, yielding 4 sections attached at the bottom. Cut each section down the middle, stopping a half-inch before the root.

Place the onion in a large bowl, cut side down, and cover with ice water. Let stand for 10 minutes, until "petals" open up.

Meanwhile, in a blender or food processor, grind cereal into crumbs. Transfer to a medium bowl and mix in seasoned salt, garlic powder, and pepper.

Remove onion from the bowl, and use your hands to gently pry the petals open. Discard water. Dry onion and bowl, and return onion to the bowl. Cover and thoroughly coat onion with egg substitute, making sure to get in between the petals. Gently shake to remove excess egg substitute and transfer onion to another large bowl.

Sprinkle onion with crumb mixture and thoroughly coat entire surface and in between petals, repositioning onion as needed.

Place onion in the baking pan, cut side up. Bake until outside is crispy and inside is soft, about 40 minutes. Meanwhile, in a small bowl, thoroughly mix sauce ingredients.

If you like, carefully cut out the center of the onion so petals are easier to remove. Serve with sauce and enjoy!

MAKES 2 SERVINGS

For more recipes, tips & tricks, sign up for FREE daily emails at **hungry-girl.com**!

These **BONELESS WINGS, CHICKEN NUGGETS, AND CHICKEN FINGERS** are great as snacks, meals, and party foods!

SWEET 'N SASSY BONELESS HOT WINGS

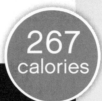

267 calories

You'll Need: baking sheet, nonstick spray, 2 wide bowls, medium bowl
Prep: 10 minutes
Cook: 20 minutes

Entire recipe (8 wings): 267 calories, 1.5g fat, 775mg sodium, 30g carbs, 2g fiber, 15g sugars, 31g protein

INGREDIENTS

2 tablespoons whole-wheat flour
Dash each salt and black pepper
4 ounces raw boneless skinless chicken breast, cut into 8 nuggets
2 tablespoons fat-free liquid egg substitute
2 tablespoons sweet Asian chili sauce
1 teaspoon seasoned rice vinegar
¼ teaspoon red pepper flakes

DIRECTIONS

Preheat oven to 375 degrees. Spray a baking sheet with nonstick spray.

In a wide bowl, mix flour, salt, and black pepper.

Place chicken nuggets in another wide bowl, top with egg substitute, and toss to coat.

One at a time, shake nuggets to remove excess egg and coat with seasoned flour. Evenly lay on the baking sheet.

Bake for 10 minutes. Flip chicken. Bake until outside is lightly browned and chicken is cooked through, about 6 minutes.

In a medium bowl, mix chili sauce, vinegar, and red pepper flakes. Add cooked nuggets and toss to coat. Yum!

MAKES 1 SERVING

H-O-T HOT BONELESS BUFFALO WINGS

175 calories
PER SERVING

You'll Need: baking sheet, nonstick spray, blender or food processor, wide bowl, large bowl
Prep: 15 minutes
Cook: 20 minutes

½ of recipe (5 wings): 175 calories, 1.5g fat, 1,153mg sodium, 14g carbs, 4g fiber, <1g sugars, 27g protein

INGREDIENTS

¼ cup Fiber One Original bran cereal
1 ounce (about 15 crisps) Pringles Light Fat Free BBQ Potato Crisps (or another fat-free BBQ-flavored potato chip)
Dash onion powder
Dash garlic powder
Dash cayenne pepper
Dash each salt and black pepper
8 ounces raw boneless skinless chicken breast, cut into 10 nuggets
3 tablespoons Frank's RedHot Original Cayenne Pepper Sauce

DIRECTIONS

Preheat oven to 375 degrees. Spray a baking sheet with nonstick spray.

In a blender or food processor, grind cereal and chips into crumbs. Transfer to a wide bowl and mix in seasonings.

Place chicken nuggets in a large bowl. Top with sauce and toss to coat.

One at a time, shake nuggets to remove excess sauce and coat with crumbs. Evenly lay on the baking sheet.

Bake for 10 minutes. Flip chicken. Bake until cooked through and crispy, about 6 minutes. Eat!

MAKES 2 SERVINGS

HG FYI:
You probably won't use all the hot sauce to coat the chicken, but we included it in the nutritional info. Actual sodium count likely will be lower.

RANCH-IFIED CHICKEN NUGGETS

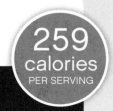

259 calories
PER SERVING

You'll Need: baking sheet, nonstick spray, blender or food processor, wide bowl, large bowl, whisk
Prep: 20 minutes
Cook: 20 minutes

½ of recipe (8 nuggets): 259 calories, 4g fat, 790mg sodium, 19.5g carbs, 4g fiber, 1.5g sugars, 36.5g protein

INGREDIENTS

¼ cup Fiber One Original bran cereal
1 ounce (about 19) ranch-flavored mini rice cakes or soy crisps
2 teaspoons ranch dressing/dip seasoning mix
2 tablespoons fat-free liquid egg substitute
2 tablespoons fat-free ranch dressing
10 ounces raw boneless skinless chicken breast, cut into 16 nuggets
⅛ teaspoon each salt and black pepper

DIRECTIONS

Preheat oven to 375 degrees. Spray a baking sheet with nonstick spray.

In a blender or food processor, grind cereal and mini rice cakes or soy crisps into crumbs. Transfer to a wide bowl and mix in ranch seasoning mix.

In a large bowl, whisk egg substitute with ranch dressing. Season chicken nuggets with salt and pepper, add to the large bowl, and toss to coat.

One at a time, shake nuggets to remove excess egg mixture and coat with crumbs. Evenly lay on the baking sheet.

Bake for 10 minutes. Flip chicken. Bake until chicken is crispy and cooked through, about 6 minutes.

Enjoy!

MAKES 2 SERVINGS

TACO-FLAVORED CHICKEN NUGGETS

230 calories
PER SERVING

You'll Need: baking sheet, nonstick spray, wide bowl, small bowl, large bowl
Prep: 15 minutes
Cook: 20 minutes

½ of recipe (8 nuggets): 230 calories, 2g fat, 696mg sodium, 14g carbs, 2g fiber, 1g sugars, 36g protein

INGREDIENTS

¼ cup whole-wheat flour
2 teaspoons taco seasoning mix
¼ teaspoon each salt and black pepper
2 tablespoons fat-free liquid egg substitute
2 tablespoons taco sauce
10 ounces raw boneless skinless chicken breast, cut into 16 nuggets

Optional seasoning: cayenne pepper

DIRECTIONS

Preheat oven to 375 degrees. Spray a baking sheet with nonstick spray.

In a wide bowl, mix flour, taco seasoning, and ⅛ teaspoon each salt and black pepper. If you like, add a dash of cayenne pepper.

In a small bowl, mix egg substitute with taco sauce.

Place chicken nuggets in a large bowl and season with remaining ⅛ teaspoon each salt and black pepper. Top with egg mixture and toss to coat.

One at a time, shake nuggets to remove excess egg and coat with seasoned flour. Evenly lay on the baking sheet.

Bake for 10 minutes. Flip chicken. Bake until outside is lightly browned and chicken is cooked through, about 6 minutes. Olé!

MAKES 2 SERVINGS

FIBER-IFIC FRIED CHICKEN STRIPS

277 calories

You'll Need: baking sheet, nonstick spray, blender or food processor, 2 wide bowls
Prep: 10 minutes | **Cook:** 20 minutes

Entire recipe (8 strips):
277 calories, 3g fat, 696mg sodium, 26g carbs, 14g fiber, 0g sugars, 47g protein

INGREDIENTS

½ cup Fiber One Original bran cereal
¼ teaspoon garlic salt
¼ cup fat-free liquid egg substitute
6 ounces raw boneless skinless
   chicken breast, cut into 8 strips

Optional seasoning: black pepper

DIRECTIONS

Preheat oven to 375 degrees. Spray a baking sheet with nonstick spray.

In a blender or food processor, grind cereal into crumbs. Transfer to a wide bowl and mix in garlic salt.

Place egg substitute in another wide bowl. One at a time, dunk chicken strips in the egg substitute, shake to remove excess, and coat with crumbs. Evenly lay on the baking sheet.

Bake for 10 minutes. Flip chicken. Bake until cooked through and crispy, about 8 minutes. Eat!

MAKES 1 SERVING

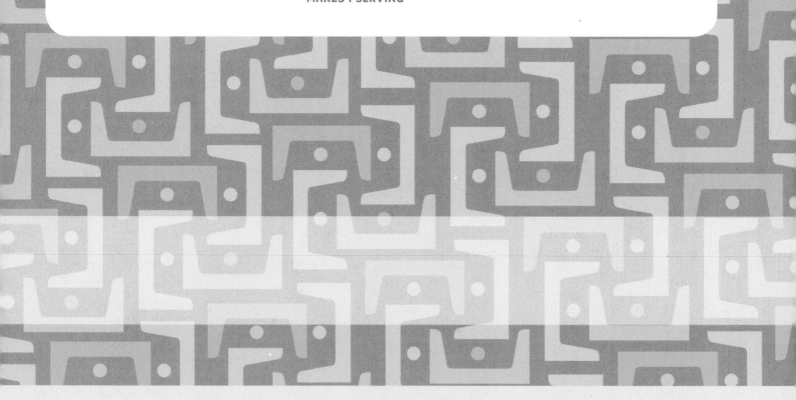

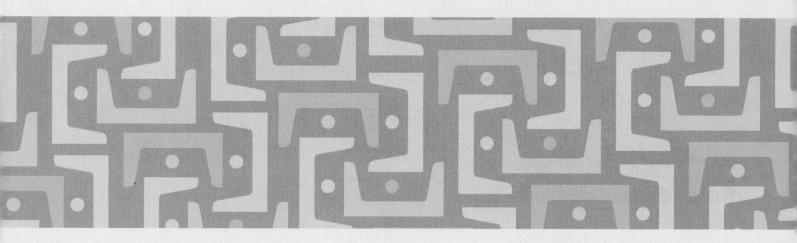

ONION CHICKEN FINGERS

211 calories PER SERVING

You'll Need: baking sheet, nonstick spray, blender or food processor, 2 wide bowls
Prep: 15 minutes | **Cook:** 20 minutes

½ of recipe (4 chicken fingers):
211 calories, 2.5g fat, 590mg sodium, 16g carbs, 7.5g fiber, 1g sugars, 36g protein

INGREDIENTS

½ cup Fiber One Original bran cereal
1 tablespoon onion soup/dip seasoning mix
    (about ¼th of a 1-ounce packet)
½ teaspoon dried minced onion
½ teaspoon onion powder
⅓ cup fat-free liquid egg substitute
10 ounces raw boneless skinless
    chicken breast, cut into 8 long strips
⅛ teaspoon each salt and black pepper

Optional dip: ketchup

DIRECTIONS

Preheat oven to 375 degrees. Spray a baking sheet with nonstick spray.

In a blender or food processor, grind cereal into crumbs. Transfer to a wide bowl and mix in onion soup/dip mix, minced onion, and onion powder.

Place egg substitute in another wide bowl. Season chicken with salt and pepper. One at a time, dunk chicken strips in the egg substitute, shake to remove excess, and coat with crumbs. Evenly lay on the baking sheet.

Bake for 10 minutes. Flip chicken. Bake until cooked through and crispy, about 8 minutes. Eat!

MAKES 2 SERVINGS

KICKIN' BUTTERMILK FAUX-FRIED CHICKEN

315 calories PER SERVING

You'll Need: large sealable plastic bag, baking sheet, nonstick spray, blender or food processor, wide bowl
Prep: 10 minutes
Marinate: 1 hour
Cook: 20 minutes

½ of recipe (5 strips): 315 calories, 5g fat, 586mg sodium, 25.5g carbs, 5g fiber, 3g sugars, 43g protein

INGREDIENTS

⅓ cup reduced-fat buttermilk
⅛ teaspoon paprika
12 ounces raw boneless skinless chicken breast, cut into 10 long strips
⅓ cup Fiber One Original bran cereal
⅓ cup panko breadcrumbs
1 tablespoon onion soup/dip seasoning mix

Optional seasoning: salt

DIRECTIONS

In a large sealable plastic bag, mix buttermilk with paprika. Add chicken and coat completely. Seal and marinate in the fridge for 1 hour.

Preheat oven to 375 degrees. Spray a baking sheet with nonstick spray.

In a blender or food processor, grind cereal into crumbs. Transfer to a wide bowl and mix in panko breadcrumbs, onion soup/dip mix and, if you like, a dash of salt.

One at a time, shake chicken strips to remove excess marinade and coat with crumbs. Evenly lay on the baking sheet.

Bake for 10 minutes. Flip chicken. Bake until cooked through and crispy, about 8 minutes. CRUNCH time!

MAKES 2 SERVINGS

BBQ CHICKEN FINGERS

264 calories PER SERVING

You'll Need: baking sheet, nonstick spray, blender or food processor, 2 wide bowls, whisk
Prep: 20 minutes
Cook: 20 minutes

½ of recipe (4 chicken fingers): 264 calories, 4.5g fat, 825mg sodium, 23g carbs, 5.5g fiber, 4g sugars, 35.5g protein

INGREDIENTS

⅓ cup Fiber One Original bran cereal
1 ounce (about 15) reduced-fat BBQ potato chips
1 teaspoon BBQ seasoning mix/rub
¼ teaspoon each salt and black pepper
3 tablespoons fat-free liquid egg substitute
3 tablespoons BBQ sauce with 45 calories or less per 2-tablespoon serving
10 ounces raw boneless skinless chicken breast, cut into 8 long strips

Optional dip: BBQ sauce with 45 calories or less per 2-tablespoon serving

DIRECTIONS

Preheat oven to 375 degrees. Spray a baking sheet with nonstick spray.

In a blender or food processor, grind cereal and chips into crumbs. Transfer to a wide bowl and mix in BBQ seasoning mix/rub and ⅛ teaspoon each salt and pepper.

In another wide bowl, whisk egg substitute with BBQ sauce.

Season chicken with remaining ⅛ teaspoon each salt and pepper. One at a time, dunk chicken strips in the egg mixture, shake to remove excess, and coat with crumbs. Evenly lay on the baking sheet.

Bake for 10 minutes. Flip chicken. Bake until cooked through and crispy, about 8 minutes. Eat!

MAKES 2 SERVINGS

PLANET HUNGRYWOOD CAP'N CRUNCHY CHICKEN

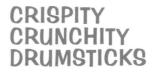

You'll Need: 2 wide bowls, large skillet, nonstick spray, small bowl
Prep: 15 minutes
Cook: 10 minutes

½ **of recipe (2 strips with 2 tablespoons sauce):**
234 calories, 2g fat, 617mg sodium, 23.5g carbs, 4g fiber, 10g sugars, 29g protein

INGREDIENTS

¼ cup Fiber One Original bran cereal, finely crushed
½ cup Cap'n Crunch cereal (original), coarsely crushed
⅛ teaspoon onion powder
⅛ teaspoon garlic powder
Dash each salt and black pepper
3 tablespoons fat-free liquid egg substitute
8 ounces raw boneless skinless chicken breast, cut into 4 long strips
2 tablespoons Best Foods/Hellmann's Dijonnaise
2 tablespoons honey mustard

DIRECTIONS

In a wide bowl, mix both crushed cereals with seasonings.

Place egg substitute in another wide bowl. One at a time, dunk chicken strips in the egg substitute, shake to remove excess, and coat with crumbs.

Bring a large skillet sprayed with nonstick spray to medium heat. Evenly lay coated strips in the skillet and cook for 5 minutes. Flip strips and cook until outside is crispy and chicken is cooked through, about 4 minutes.

In a small bowl, mix Dijonnaise with honey mustard. Serve with chicken for dipping!

MAKES 2 SERVINGS

CRISPITY CRUNCHITY DRUMSTICKS

You'll Need: baking sheet, nonstick spray, blender or food processor, wide bowl, large bowl
Prep: 15 minutes
Cook: 35 minutes

⅓**rd of recipe (2 drumsticks):**
184 calories, 5g fat, 567mg sodium, 10.5g carbs, 5g fiber, <0.5g sugars, 28g protein

INGREDIENTS

½ cup Fiber One Original bran cereal
1¼ teaspoons black pepper
¾ teaspoon garlic powder
¾ teaspoon onion powder
¾ teaspoon dried oregano
¼ teaspoon chili powder
½ teaspoon salt
6 raw chicken drumsticks, skin removed
¼ cup fat-free liquid egg substitute

DIRECTIONS

Preheat oven to 400 degrees. Spray a baking sheet with nonstick spray.

In a blender or food processor, grind cereal into crumbs. Transfer to a wide bowl and mix in pepper, garlic powder, onion powder, oregano, chili powder, and ¼ teaspoon salt.

Place drumsticks in a large bowl and season with remaining ¼ teaspoon salt. Top and coat with egg substitute.

One at a time, shake drumsticks to remove excess egg and coat with crumbs. Evenly lay on the baking sheet.

Bake for 20 minutes. Flip drumsticks. Bake until cooked through and crispy, about 15 minutes. Enjoy!

MAKES 3 SERVINGS

Yup, HG PARMESAN DISHES are AWESOME . . . Cheesy, hot, and happenin'!

POUND FOR POUND: A TWO-STEP CHICKEN CUTLET TUTORIAL

1. Either lay the cutlet between two pieces of plastic wrap or place it in a sealable bag and squeeze out the air before sealing.

2. Starting with the thickest point, pound the cutlet with a meat mallet until it's the desired thickness. Don't have a mallet? Any heavy kitchen utensil with a flat surface will do.

PAN-FRIED CHICKEN PARM

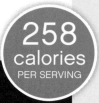
258 calories PER SERVING

You'll Need: blender or food processor, 2 wide bowls, small bowl, large skillet with a lid, nonstick spray
Prep: 20 minutes
Cook: 15 minutes

½ of recipe (1 cutlet): 258 calories, 6g fat, 684mg sodium, 16.5g carbs, 7g fiber, 1g sugars, 38.5g protein

INGREDIENTS

½ cup Fiber One Original bran cereal
1½ teaspoons Italian seasoning, or more to taste
½ teaspoon garlic powder, or more to taste
½ teaspoon onion powder, or more to taste
⅛ teaspoon salt, or more to taste
¼ cup canned tomato sauce with Italian seasonings
¼ cup fat-free liquid egg substitute
Two 4-ounce raw boneless skinless chicken breast
  cutlets, pounded to ½-inch thickness
½ cup shredded part-skim mozzarella cheese

Optional seasoning: black pepper

DIRECTIONS

In a blender or food processor, grind cereal into crumbs. Transfer to a wide bowl and mix in Italian seasoning, ¼ teaspoon garlic powder, ¼ teaspoon onion powder, and salt.

In a small bowl, mix tomato sauce with remaining ¼ teaspoon garlic powder and remaining ¼ teaspoon onion powder.

Place egg substitute in another wide bowl. One at a time, coat cutlets with egg, shake to remove excess, and coat with crumbs.

Bring a large skillet sprayed with nonstick spray to medium-high heat. Lay coated cutlets in the skillet and cook for 4 minutes per side, or until chicken is cooked through.

Evenly spread sauce over chicken cutlets, still in the skillet. Sprinkle with mozzarella cheese.

Reduce heat to low and cover skillet. Cook until cheese has melted, 2 to 3 minutes. Enjoy!

MAKES 2 SERVINGS

CHICKEN PARM ROLLUP

293 calories

You'll Need: baking pan, nonstick spray, blender or food processor (optional), small bowl, toothpicks (optional), aluminum foil
Prep: 15 minutes
Cook: 35 minutes

Entire recipe: 293 calories, 6g fat, 750mg sodium, 19.5g carbs, 7.5g fiber, 2g sugars, 43g protein

INGREDIENTS

1 stick light string cheese
¼ cup Fiber One Original bran cereal, finely crushed
1 tablespoon reduced-fat Parmesan-style grated topping
¼ teaspoon Italian seasoning
⅛ teaspoon garlic powder
⅛ teaspoon onion powder
One 5-ounce raw boneless skinless chicken breast cutlet, pounded to ½-inch thickness
Dash each salt and black pepper
¼ cup canned stewed tomatoes with Italian seasonings (about 3 pieces), patted dry
1 tablespoon fat-free liquid egg substitute

Optional dip: low-fat marinara sauce

DIRECTIONS

Preheat oven to 350 degrees. Spray a baking pan with nonstick spray.

Break string cheese into thirds and place in a blender or food processor—blend at high speed until shredded. (Or pull into shreds and roughly chop.)

In a small bowl, mix crushed cereal, ½ tablespoon Parm-style topping, Italian seasoning, garlic powder, and onion powder.

Season chicken with salt and pepper and lay on a dry surface. Place stewed tomatoes in the center of the cutlet. Sprinkle with shredded string cheese and remaining ½ tablespoon Parm-style topping. Roll up cutlet over the filling. (It will be STUFFED!) If needed, secure with toothpicks.

Lightly cover with egg substitute and evenly coat with crumbs. Place in the baking pan. Cover pan with foil and bake for 20 minutes.

Remove foil and bake until chicken is cooked through, about 15 minutes. Eat up!

MAKES 1 SERVING

FLOUNDER PARM

231 calories
PER SERVING

You'll Need: blender or food processor, medium bowl, plate, wide bowl, large skillet with a lid, nonstick spray
Prep: 15 minutes
Cook: 10 minutes

½ of recipe (1 fillet): 231 calories, 9g fat, 907mg sodium, 18.5g carbs, 7.5g fiber, 2g sugars, 25g protein

INGREDIENTS

½ cup Fiber One Original bran cereal
¼ teaspoon Italian seasoning
¼ teaspoon garlic powder
¼ teaspoon onion powder
⅛ teaspoon each salt and black pepper
¼ cup fat-free liquid egg substitute
Two 4-ounce raw flounder fillets
¼ cup low-fat marinara sauce
½ cup shredded part-skim mozzarella cheese
1 tablespoon reduced-fat Parmesan-style grated topping

DIRECTIONS

In a blender or food processor, grind cereal into crumbs. Transfer to a medium bowl and mix in seasonings. Spread onto a plate.

Place egg substitute in a wide bowl. One at a time, coat fillets with egg, gently shake to remove excess, and coat with crumbs.

Bring a large skillet sprayed with nonstick spray to medium-high heat. Cook fillets for 2 minutes per side, or until just cooked through.

Still in the skillet, spread sauce on fillets. Sprinkle with shredded cheese and Parm-style topping.

Reduce heat to low and cover skillet. Cook until cheese has melted, 2 to 3 minutes. Eat up!

MAKES 2 SERVINGS

CHICKEN PARM DUNKERS

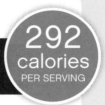

292 calories PER SERVING

You'll Need: baking sheet, nonstick spray, blender or food processor, wide bowl, large bowl, microwave-safe bowl
Prep: 20 minutes | **Cook:** 20 minutes

½ of recipe (8 nuggets with ¼ cup sauce):
292 calories, 7g fat, 827mg sodium, 20.5g carbs, 8g fiber, 4g sugars, 42g protein

INGREDIENTS

½ cup Fiber One Original bran cereal

2 teaspoons reduced-fat Parmesan-style grated topping

1 teaspoon Italian seasoning

½ teaspoon garlic powder

¼ teaspoon salt

10 ounces raw boneless skinless chicken breast, cut into 16 nuggets

⅛ teaspoon black pepper

¼ cup fat-free liquid egg substitute

⅓ cup shredded part-skim mozzarella cheese

½ cup low-fat marinara sauce

DIRECTIONS

Preheat oven to 375 degrees. Spray a baking sheet with nonstick spray.

In a blender or food processor, grind cereal into crumbs. Transfer to a wide bowl. Mix in Parm-style topping, Italian seasoning, garlic powder, and ⅛ teaspoon salt.

Place chicken nuggets in a large bowl and season with pepper and remaining ⅛ teaspoon salt. Top with egg substitute and toss to coat.

One at a time, shake nuggets to remove excess egg and coat with crumbs. Evenly lay on the baking sheet.

Bake for 10 minutes. Flip chicken. Bake until cooked through and slightly crispy, about 6 minutes.

Remove from oven and set oven to broil.

Closely arrange nuggets in two groups on the sheet. Top each group with mozzarella cheese. Broil until cheese has melted, 1 to 2 minutes.

In a microwave-safe bowl, microwave marinara sauce for 45 seconds, or until warm. Serve with chicken for dippin'!

MAKES 2 SERVINGS

Flip to the photo inserts to see over 100 recipe pics! And for photos of ALL the recipes, go to **hungry-girl.com/books.**

PORK PARMESAN

 311 calories PER SERVING

You'll Need: blender or food processor, medium bowl, plate, wide bowl, extra-large skillet with a lid, nonstick spray
Prep: 15 minutes
Cook: 15 minutes

½ of recipe (1 cutlet): 311 calories, 10g fat, 760mg sodium, 24g carbs, 11g fiber, 3g sugars, 39g protein

INGREDIENTS

⅔ cup Fiber One Original bran cereal
2 teaspoons dried basil
1 teaspoon dried oregano
1 teaspoon garlic powder
¼ teaspoon each salt and black pepper
¼ cup fat-free liquid egg substitute
Two 5-ounce raw boneless pork tenderloin cutlets, very thinly pounded (about ¼-inch thick)
⅓ cup low-fat marinara sauce
⅓ cup shredded part-skim mozzarella cheese
2 teaspoons reduced-fat Parmesan-style grated topping

DIRECTIONS

In a blender or food processor, grind cereal into crumbs. Transfer to a medium bowl and mix in basil, oregano, garlic powder, and ⅛ teaspoon each salt and pepper. Spread onto a plate.

Place egg substitute in a wide bowl. Season pork with remaining ⅛ teaspoon each salt and pepper. One at a time, coat cutlets with egg, shake to remove excess, and coat with crumbs.

Bring an extra-large skillet sprayed with nonstick spray to medium-high heat. Cook cutlets for 5 minutes per side, or until just cooked through.

Reduce heat to low. Spread sauce on cutlets, and sprinkle with shredded cheese and Parm-style topping. Cover and cook until cheese has melted, 2 to 3 minutes. Eat up!

MAKES 2 SERVINGS

SHRIMP PARMESAN

314 calories PER SERVING

You'll Need: baking sheet, nonstick spray, blender or food processor, wide bowl, large bowl
Prep: 15 minutes
Cook: 15 minutes

½ of recipe (about 9 shrimp): 314 calories, 9g fat, 967mg sodium, 26g carbs, 10g fiber, 4g sugars, 39g protein

INGREDIENTS

⅔ cup Fiber One Original bran cereal
¼ teaspoon Italian seasoning
¼ teaspoon garlic powder
¼ teaspoon onion powder
⅛ teaspoon black pepper
10 ounces (about 18) raw large shrimp, peeled, tails removed, deveined
⅓ cup fat-free liquid egg substitute
½ cup low-fat marinara sauce
½ cup shredded part-skim mozzarella cheese
1 tablespoon reduced-fat Parmesan-style grated topping

DIRECTIONS

Preheat oven to 375 degrees. Spray a baking sheet with nonstick spray.

In a blender or food processor, grind cereal into crumbs. Transfer to a wide bowl and mix in seasonings.

Place shrimp in a large bowl and pat dry. Top with egg substitute and toss to coat.

One at a time, shake shrimp to remove excess egg and coat with crumbs. Evenly lay on the baking sheet.

Bake for 5 minutes. Flip shrimp. Bake until cooked through and slightly crispy, about 5 more minutes.

Remove pan and set oven to broil.

Closely arrange shrimp in two groups on the sheet. Evenly top each group with sauce, shredded cheese, and Parm-style topping. Broil until cheese melts, about 2 minutes. Dig in!

MAKES 2 SERVINGS

NO-HARM EGGPLANT PARM

213 calories
PER SERVING

You'll Need: baking sheet, nonstick spray, blender or food processor, 2 very wide bowls, 8-inch by 8-inch baking pan, aluminum foil
Prep: 10 minutes
Cook: 1 hour and 5 minutes

¼th of recipe: 213 calories, 7.5g fat, 811mg sodium, 30g carbs, 13g fiber, 6.5g sugars, 15g protein

INGREDIENTS

1 cup Fiber One Original bran cereal
½ teaspoon garlic powder
⅛ teaspoon each salt and black pepper
½ cup fat-free liquid egg substitute
1 large eggplant, ends removed
1 cup canned tomato sauce with Italian seasonings
1 cup shredded part-skim mozzarella cheese
¼ cup reduced-fat Parmesan-style grated topping

Optional seasonings: dried basil, oregano

DIRECTIONS

Preheat oven to 375 degrees. Spray a baking sheet with nonstick spray.

In a blender or food processor, grind cereal into crumbs. Transfer to a very wide bowl and mix in seasonings.

Place egg substitute in another very wide bowl.

Cut eggplant lengthwise into ½-inch slices. Pat dry. One at a time, dunk eggplant slices in the egg substitute, shake to remove excess, and coat with crumbs. Evenly lay slices on the baking sheet.

Bake for 30 minutes. Flip slices. Bake until crispy, about 10 minutes. Remove sheet, but leave oven on.

Spray an 8-inch by 8-inch baking pan with nonstick spray. Spread ¼ cup sauce along the bottom, and evenly top with half of the eggplant slices.

Continue to layer ingredients in this order: ¼ cup sauce, ½ cup mozzarella cheese, 2 tablespoons Parm-style topping, ¼ cup sauce, remaining eggplant slices, remaining ¼ cup sauce, remaining ½ cup mozzarella cheese, and remaining 2 tablespoons Parm-style topping.

Cover pan with aluminum foil and bake for 25 minutes, or until hot. Devour!

MAKES 4 SERVINGS

JALAPEÑO POPPER CHICKEN

233 calories

You'll Need: baking pan, nonstick spray, small bowl, toothpicks (optional), aluminum foil
Prep: 15 minutes
Cook: 35 minutes

Entire recipe: 233 calories, 4g fat, 764mg sodium, 15g carbs, 7g fiber, 1.5g sugars, 36.5g protein

INGREDIENTS

¼ cup Fiber One Original bran cereal, finely crushed
⅛ teaspoon garlic powder
⅛ teaspoon onion powder
Dash cayenne pepper
One 5-ounce raw boneless skinless chicken breast cutlet, pounded to ½-inch thickness
Dash each salt and black pepper
1 wedge The Laughing Cow Light Creamy Swiss cheese
1½ tablespoons chopped jarred jalapeño slices (about 5 slices)
1 tablespoon fat-free liquid egg substitute

DIRECTIONS

Preheat oven to 350 degrees. Spray a baking pan with nonstick spray.

In a small bowl, mix crushed cereal, garlic powder, onion powder, and cayenne pepper.

Season chicken with salt and black pepper and lay cutlet flat on a dry surface. Spread with cheese and top with chopped jalapeño. Roll up cutlet over the filling and, if needed, secure with toothpicks.

Lightly cover with egg substitute and evenly coat with crumbs. Place in the baking pan. Cover pan with foil and bake for 20 minutes.

Remove foil and bake until chicken is cooked through, about 15 minutes. Dig in!

MAKES 1 SERVING

DE-LISH FAUX-FRIED FISH

201 calories

You'll Need: broiler pan (or toaster oven), nonstick spray, 2 wide bowls
Prep: 10 minutes | **Cook:** 15 minutes

Entire recipe (2 strips):
201 calories, 1.5g fat, 653mg sodium, 13g carbs, 3.5g fiber, 1g sugars, 34.5g protein

INGREDIENTS

2 tablespoons Fiber One Original bran cereal, finely crushed
2 tablespoons panko breadcrumbs
¼ teaspoon garlic powder, or more to taste
¼ teaspoon Old Bay Seasoning, or more to taste
⅛ teaspoon onion powder, or more to taste
⅛ teaspoon salt, or more to taste
2 tablespoons fat-free liquid egg substitute
6 ounces raw cod, cut into two strips

Optional seasoning: black pepper
Optional dip: fat-free tartar sauce

DIRECTIONS

Preheat oven to 450 degrees, and spray a broiler pan with nonstick spray. (Or spray a toaster-oven rack with nonstick spray, and preheat toaster oven to 450 degrees.)

In a wide bowl, mix crushed cereal, panko breadcrumbs, and seasonings.

Place egg substitute in another wide bowl. One at a time, coat cod strips with egg, gently shake to remove excess, and coat with crumbs.

Place coated strips on the broiler pan (or toaster-oven rack) and bake until crispy on the outside and flaky and cooked through on the inside, about 15 minutes. Eat up!

MAKES 1 SERVING

BUFFALICIOUS SHRIMP

165 calories PER SERVING

You'll Need: baking sheet, nonstick spray, small microwave-safe bowl, 2 wide bowls, medium bowl
Prep: 10 minutes
Cook: 10 minutes

½ of recipe (about 7 shrimp): 165 calories, 3.5g fat, 725mg sodium, 7g carbs, 0.5g fiber, <0.5g sugars, 25.5g protein

INGREDIENTS

Sauce
1½ tablespoons Frank's RedHot Original Cayenne Pepper Sauce
½ tablespoon light whipped butter or light buttery spread
Dash garlic powder

Shrimp
2 tablespoons whole-wheat flour
Dash salt
Dash garlic powder
Dash onion powder
8 ounces (about 14) raw large shrimp, peeled, tails removed, deveined
2 tablespoons fat-free liquid egg substitute

DIRECTIONS

Preheat oven to 375 degrees. Spray a baking sheet with nonstick spray.

In a small microwave-safe bowl, mix sauce ingredients with 1 tablespoon water.

In a wide bowl, mix flour with seasonings.

Place shrimp in another wide bowl and pat dry. Top with egg substitute and toss to coat. One at a time, shake shrimp to remove excess egg and coat with seasoned flour. Evenly lay on the baking sheet.

Lightly mist shrimp with nonstick spray. Bake for 5 minutes. Flip shrimp. Bake until cooked through and slightly crispy, about 5 more minutes.

Microwave sauce mixture for 30 seconds, or until hot. Stir until smooth.

Place cooked shrimp in a medium bowl, top with sauce, and toss to coat. Enjoy!

MAKES 2 SERVINGS

FAUX-FRIED & FABULOUS CALAMARI

236 calories

You'll Need: baking sheet, nonstick spray, 2 wide bowls
Prep: 15 minutes
Cook: 15 minutes

Entire recipe: 236 calories, 4g fat, 779mg sodium, 31.5g carbs, 7g fiber, 1g sugars, 23g protein

INGREDIENTS

¼ cup Fiber One Original bran cereal, finely crushed
3 tablespoons panko breadcrumbs
¼ teaspoon garlic powder
¼ teaspoon onion powder
¼ teaspoon Italian seasoning
¼ teaspoon salt
Dash black pepper, or more to taste
4 ounces raw calamari rings (not breaded)
2 tablespoons fat-free liquid egg substitute

Optional: reduced-fat Parmesan-style grated topping, lemon wedges, low-fat marinara sauce

DIRECTIONS

Preheat oven to 350 degrees. Spray a baking sheet with nonstick spray.

In a wide bowl, mix crushed cereal, panko breadcrumbs, and seasonings.

Place calamari rings in another wide bowl and pat dry. Top with egg substitute and toss to coat. One at a time, shake rings to remove excess egg and coat with crumbs. Evenly lay on the baking sheet.

Bake for 10 minutes. Flip rings. Bake until firm and cooked through, about 5 minutes. If you like, sprinkle with Parm-style topping and serve with lemon wedges and marinara sauce. YUM!

MAKES 1 SERVING

SWEET COCONUT CRUNCH SHRIMP

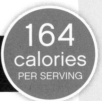

164 calories PER SERVING

You'll Need: baking sheet, nonstick spray, wide bowl, large bowl | **Prep:** 20 minutes | **Cook:** 15 minutes

¼th of recipe (about 5 shrimp):
164 calories, 4.5g fat, 266mg sodium, 12g carbs, 2g fiber, 3.5g sugars, 19.5g protein

INGREDIENTS

¼ cup Fiber One Original bran cereal, finely crushed
⅓ cup shredded sweetened coconut
3 tablespoons panko breadcrumbs
¼ teaspoon chili powder
⅛ teaspoon garlic powder
⅛ teaspoon black pepper
Dash salt
12 ounces (about 20) raw large shrimp, peeled, tails removed, deveined
3 tablespoons fat-free liquid egg substitute

DIRECTIONS

Preheat oven to 400 degrees. Spray a baking sheet with nonstick spray.

In a wide bowl, mix crushed cereal, coconut, panko breadcrumbs, and seasonings.

Place shrimp in a large bowl and pat dry. Top with egg substitute and toss to coat.

One at a time, shake shrimp to remove excess egg and coat with crumbs. Evenly lay on the baking sheet.

Bake until cooked through and crispy, 10 to 12 minutes. Serve and enjoy!

MAKES 4 SERVINGS

SWAPCORN SHRIMP

180 calories

You'll Need: baking sheet, nonstick spray, blender or food processor, 2 wide bowls
Prep: 10 minutes | **Cook:** 10 minutes

Entire recipe (about 12 shrimp):
180 calories, 2.5g fat, 636mg sodium, 27g carbs, 14g fiber, 0g sugars, 25g protein

INGREDIENTS

½ cup Fiber One Original bran cereal
⅛ teaspoon each salt and black pepper
3 ounces (about 12) small raw shrimp, peeled, tails removed, deveined
¼ cup fat-free liquid egg substitute

DIRECTIONS

Preheat oven to 350 degrees. Spray a baking sheet with nonstick spray.

In a blender or food processor, grind cereal into crumbs. Transfer to a wide bowl and mix in salt and pepper.

Place shrimp in another wide bowl and pat dry. Top with egg substitute and toss to coat. One at a time, shake shrimp to remove excess egg and coat with crumbs. Evenly lay on the baking sheet.

Bake for 5 minutes. Flip shrimp. Bake until cooked through and crispy, about 5 more minutes. Enjoy!

MAKES 1 SERVING

DY-NO-MITE DREAM SHRIMP

230 calories PER SERVING

You'll Need: baking sheet, nonstick spray, 2 wide bowls, microwave-safe bowl
Prep: 15 minutes | **Cook:** 15 minutes

½ of recipe (about 7 shrimp with 2 tablespoons sauce):
230 calories, 3g fat, 691mg sodium, 24.5g carbs, 1g fiber, 4.5g sugars, 26.5g protein

INGREDIENTS

Shrimp

⅓ cup panko breadcrumbs

2 tablespoons whole-wheat flour

⅛ **teaspoon** salt

⅛ teaspoon garlic powder

⅛ teaspoon onion powder

8 ounces (about 14) raw large tail-on shrimp, peeled, deveined

2 tablespoons fat-free liquid egg substitute

Sauce

3 tablespoons fat-free mayonnaise

½ tablespoon sweet Asian chili sauce

½ tablespoon Sriracha chili sauce (shelf-stable Asian hot sauce)

DIRECTIONS

Preheat oven to 350 degrees. Spray a baking sheet with nonstick spray.

In a wide bowl, mix panko breadcrumbs, flour, and seasonings.

Place shrimp in another wide bowl and pat dry. Top with egg substitute and toss to coat.

One at a time, shake shrimp to remove excess egg and coat with crumbs. Evenly lay on the baking sheet.

Bake for 8 minutes. Flip shrimp. Bake until cooked through and crispy, about 6 minutes.

Meanwhile, mix sauce ingredients in a microwave-safe bowl. Microwave for 30 seconds, or until hot. Stir until smooth.

Serve shrimp with sauce for dipping, or evenly spoon sauce over the shrimp. Enjoy!

MAKES 2 SERVINGS

For more recipes, tips & tricks, sign up for FREE daily emails at **hungry-girl.com!**

CHAPTER 6

SWAPPUCCINOS & SHAKES

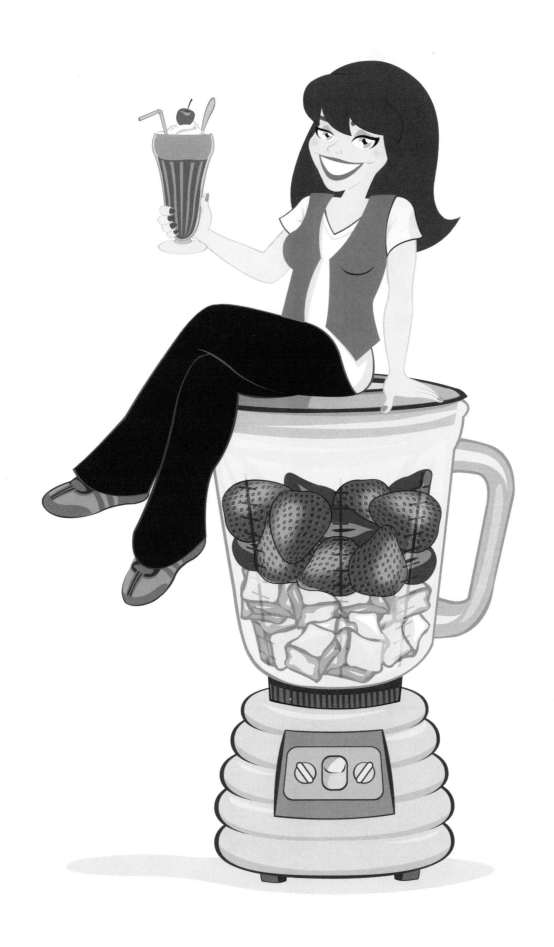

SWAPPUCCINOS & SHAKES

SWAPPUCCINOS

Double-O-Cinnamon Swappuccino
Salted Caramel Cocoa-ccino
Joe Cool Java Freeze
Mint Chocolate Chip Freeze
Espress' Yourself Swappuccino
Vanilla-Chilla Coffee Float
Mocha-Coco Swappuccino
Cara-mellow Coffee Freeze
Frozen Fudge Chip Freeze
Banana-Berry Cloud
Strawberry Cloud
Green Tea Crème Swappuccino
Raspberry Mocha Madness Swappuccino
Vanillalicious Cafe Freeze

SHAKES

Cravin' Cap'n Crunch Shake
Key Lime Pie Shake
Slurpable Split Shake
Frozen S'mores Hot Cocoa
PB&J Super-Shake
Chocolate-Banana Smoothie
Dreamsicle Shiver
Happy Monkey Banana Shake
Chilla in Vanilla Milkshake
Ginormous Chocolate Shake
Cookie-rific Ice Cream Freeze
Cookie Crisp Puddin' Shake
Chocolate-Covered-Cherries Freeze
Caramel Apple Frappe
Minty Cookie-rific Ice Cream Freeze
Froot Loops Freeze
Eggnog Freeze
Freakishly Good Frozen Hot Chocolate
Cinnamon-Toast-Crunch Shake
Shamrock 'n Roll Shake
Peach Cobbler Shake

Dust off your blender. It's about to get busy . . .

SHAKE THINGS UP . . .

* If your freezy beverage stops blending, turn off the machine and remove the blender from the base. Stir it up and blend again.

* Ice is important, and pre-crushed ice is best. Make sure your ice isn't old or freezer-burned.

SUGAR-FREE CALORIE-FREE SYRUP 411

* Torani Sugar Free Syrups are the best, hands down. Find popular flavors like vanilla in the coffee aisle . . . Just make sure they're the zero-calorie, sugar-free ones (they make sugary versions too!). They can also be found at specialty stores like Cost Plus World Market and BevMo!

A QUICK GUIDE TO SYMBOLS:

15 Minutes or Less	30 Minutes or Less	Meatless	Single Serving	5 Ingredients or Less	Photos
This symbol lets you know a recipe should take you no more than fifteen minutes from start to finish! That includes prep and cook time.	Just like the 15-minute version, this one points out recipes that take 30 minutes or less to whip up.	You guessed it—no meat here! That includes beef, poultry, and fish. Some recipes give the option of a meatless ingredient. If you want your meal without meat, go with the meatless choice.	Pretty straightforward. These are recipes for one.	Fans of HG know that we like to keep things simple. And these recipes contain just five ingredients or less!	These recipes can be seen in one of the book's photo inserts. The number in the symbol tells you which insert. Find photos of all the recipes at hungry-girl.com/books!

SWAPPUCCINOS

These are BETTER than the blended beverages made at coffee stores—with an itty-bitty fraction of the calories and fat. They're less expensive, too!

DOUBLE-O-CINNAMON SWAPPUCCINO

76 calories

You'll Need: tall glass, blender | **Prep:** 5 minutes

Entire recipe:
76 calories, 3.5g fat, 68mg sodium, 8g carbs, 1g fiber, 2.5g sugars, 3g protein

INGREDIENTS

1 tablespoon sugar-free French vanilla powdered creamer
1 teaspoon instant coffee granules
2 no-calorie sweetener packets
½ cup light vanilla soymilk
½ teaspoon cinnamon
1½ cups crushed ice *or* 8 to 12 ice cubes

Optional toppings: Fat Free Reddi-wip, additional cinnamon

DIRECTIONS

In a tall glass, combine creamer, coffee granules, and sweetener. Add 2 tablespoons hot water and stir to dissolve.

Transfer mixture to a blender. Add soymilk, cinnamon, and 2 tablespoons cold water. Add ice and blend at high speed until smooth. Pour and enjoy!

MAKES 1 SERVING

SALTED CARAMEL COCOA-CCINO

111 calories

You'll Need: tall glass, blender | **Prep:** 5 minutes

Entire recipe:
111 calories, 0.5g fat, 575mg sodium, 24g carbs, 1.5g fiber, 17g sugars, 3.5g protein

INGREDIENTS

2 packets hot cocoa mix with 20 to 25 calories each
3 teaspoons fat-free or light caramel dip
1½ cups crushed ice *or* 8 to 12 ice cubes
¼ cup Fat Free Reddi-wip
2 dashes ground sea salt
1 dash granulated white sugar or Splenda No Calorie Sweetener (granulated)

DIRECTIONS

In a tall glass, combine cocoa mix with ⅓ cup hot water and stir to dissolve. Add 2 teaspoons caramel dip and stir until melted.

Transfer mixture to a blender. Add ⅓ cup cold water and ice, and blend at high speed until smooth.

Pour and top with Reddi-wip and remaining 1 teaspoon caramel dip. Sprinkle with salt and sugar or Splenda and enjoy!

MAKES 1 SERVING

JOE COOL JAVA FREEZE

68 calories

You'll Need: tall glass, blender | **Prep:** 5 minutes

Entire recipe:
68 calories, 3.75g fat, 55mg sodium, 6.5g carbs, <0.5g fiber, 1g sugars, 1.5g protein

INGREDIENTS

4 teaspoons sugar-free French vanilla
 powdered creamer
1 teaspoon instant coffee granules
2 no-calorie sweetener packets
¼ cup light vanilla soymilk
1½ cups crushed ice *or* 8 to 12 ice cubes

DIRECTIONS

In a tall glass, combine creamer, coffee granules, and sweetener. Add ¼ cup hot water and stir to dissolve.

Transfer mixture to a blender. Add soymilk and ½ cup cold water. Add ice and blend at high speed until just blended. Pour and enjoy!

MAKES 1 SERVING

MINT CHOCOLATE CHIP FREEZE

87 calories

You'll Need: tall glass, blender
Prep: 5 minutes

Entire recipe: 87 calories, 4.75g fat, 36mg sodium, 12g carbs, 0g fiber, 3g sugars, <0.5g protein

INGREDIENTS

1 tablespoon sugar-free French vanilla
 powdered creamer
2 no-calorie sweetener packets
1 teaspoon instant coffee granules
1 tablespoon sugar-free chocolate syrup
1 teaspoon mini semi-sweet chocolate chips
1 drop peppermint extract
1 cup crushed ice *or* 5 to 8 ice cubes
2 tablespoons Chocolate Reddi-wip

DIRECTIONS

In a tall glass, combine creamer, sweetener, and coffee granules. Add 2 tablespoons hot water and stir to dissolve.

Transfer mixture to a blender, and add ¾ cup cold water. Add all remaining ingredients *except* Reddi-wip and blend at high speed until smooth.

Pour and top with Reddi-wip!

MAKES 1 SERVING

ESPRESS' YOURSELF SWAPPUCCINO

   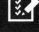

76 calories

You'll Need: tall glass, blender
Prep: 5 minutes

Entire recipe: 76 calories, 3.5g fat, 68mg sodium, 7.5g carbs, <0.5g fiber, 2.5g sugars, 3.5g protein

INGREDIENTS

1 tablespoon sugar-free French vanilla
 powdered creamer
1 tablespoon instant coffee granules
2 no-calorie sweetener packets
½ cup light vanilla soymilk
1½ cups crushed ice *or* 8 to 12 ice cubes

Optional topping: Fat Free Reddi-wip

DIRECTIONS

In a tall glass, combine creamer, coffee granules, and sweetener. Add 2 tablespoons hot water and stir to dissolve.

Transfer mixture to a blender. Add soymilk and 2 tablespoons cold water. Add ice and blend at high speed until smooth. Pour, sip, and smile!

MAKES 1 SERVING

VANILLA-CHILLA COFFEE FLOAT

111 calories

You'll Need: tall glass, blender | **Prep:** 5 minutes

Entire recipe:
111 calories, 3g fat, 111mg sodium, 17.5g carbs, 0g fiber, 6.5g sugars, 3g protein

INGREDIENTS

1 teaspoon instant coffee granules
1 teaspoon sugar-free French vanilla powdered creamer
1 no-calorie sweetener packet
½ cup light vanilla soymilk
2 tablespoons sugar-free calorie-free vanilla-flavored syrup
1½ cups crushed ice *or* 8 to 12 ice cubes
One ½-cup scoop Cool Whip Free (not thawed)

DIRECTIONS

In a tall glass, combine coffee granules, powdered creamer, and sweetener. Add 2 tablespoons hot water and stir to dissolve.

Transfer mixture to a blender. Add soymilk, syrup, and ice, and blend at high speed until smooth.

Pour, top with Cool Whip, and enjoy!

MAKES 1 SERVING

MOCHA-COCO SWAPPUCCINO

120 calories

You'll Need: skillet, tall glass, blender | **Prep:** 10 minutes | **Cook:** 5 minutes

Entire recipe:
120 calories, 4.5g fat, 24mg sodium, 21g carbs, 4g fiber, 8g sugars, 2.5g protein

INGREDIENTS

2 teaspoons shredded sweetened coconut, roughly chopped
2 tablespoons unsweetened cocoa powder
1 tablespoon fat-free non-dairy powdered creamer
1 teaspoon instant coffee granules
1 teaspoon mini semi-sweet chocolate chips
2 no-calorie sweetener packets, or more to taste
⅛ teaspoon coconut extract
2 cups crushed ice *or* 10 to 16 ice cubes
2 tablespoons Fat Free Reddi-wip
1 teaspoon light chocolate syrup

DIRECTIONS

In a skillet over medium heat, cook and stir chopped coconut until lightly browned, about 2 minutes.

In a tall glass, combine cocoa powder, creamer, coffee granules, chocolate chips, and sweetener. Add ½ cup very hot water, and stir until mostly dissolved.

Stir in coconut extract and transfer mixture to a blender. Add ice and blend at high speed until smooth.

Pour, top with Reddi-wip, and drizzle with chocolate syrup. Sprinkle with lightly browned coconut and enjoy!

MAKES 1 SERVING

CARA-MELLOW COFFEE FREEZE

158 calories

You'll Need: tall glass, blender
Prep: 5 minutes

Entire recipe: 158 calories, 2g fat, 289mg sodium, 34g carbs, <0.5g fiber, 13.5g sugars, 2.5g protein

INGREDIENTS

1 teaspoon instant coffee granules
2 no-calorie sweetener packets
1 tablespoon plus 1 teaspoon fat-free or light caramel dip
¼ cup light vanilla soymilk
1 sugar-free caramel pudding snack with 60 calories or less
1½ cups crushed ice *or* 8 to 12 ice cubes
2 tablespoons Fat Free Reddi-wip

DIRECTIONS

In a tall glass, combine coffee granules, sweetener, and 1 tablespoon caramel dip. Add ¼ cup hot water and stir to dissolve.

Transfer mixture to a blender. Add soymilk, pudding, and ice, and blend at high speed until smooth.

Pour and top with Reddi-wip and remaining teaspoon caramel dip. Mmmm . . .

MAKES 1 SERVING

FROZEN FUDGE CHIP FREEZE

134 calories

You'll Need: tall glass, blender
Prep: 5 minutes

Entire recipe: 134 calories, 4.5g fat, 184mg sodium, 21g carbs, 1.5g fiber, 13g sugars, 4g protein

INGREDIENTS

1 packet hot cocoa mix with 20 to 25 calories
1 no-calorie sweetener packet
¼ cup light vanilla soymilk
1 tablespoon sugar-free chocolate syrup
1 tablespoon mini semi-sweet chocolate chips
1 cup crushed ice *or* 5 to 8 ice cubes
2 tablespoons Fat Free Reddi-wip

DIRECTIONS

In a tall glass, combine cocoa mix with sweetener. Add ¼ cup hot water and stir to dissolve.

Transfer mixture to a blender. Add all remaining ingredients *except* Reddi-wip, and blend at high speed until smooth.

Pour, top with Reddi-wip, and slurp!

MAKES 1 SERVING

BANANA-BERRY CLOUD

146 calories

You'll Need: tall glass, blender | **Prep:** 5 minutes

Entire recipe:
146 calories, 1.5g fat, 348mg sodium, 29g carbs, 3g fiber, 14g sugars, 4.5g protein

INGREDIENTS

⅔ cup light vanilla soymilk
1 tablespoon sugar-free fat-free banana instant pudding mix
Half a 2-serving packet (about ½ teaspoon) sugar-free strawberry powdered drink mix
4 frozen unsweetened strawberries, partially thawed
½ medium banana, sliced into coins and frozen
1½ cups crushed ice *or* 8 to 12 ice cubes
2 tablespoons Fat Free Reddi-wip

DIRECTIONS

In a tall glass, combine soymilk, pudding mix, and drink mix, and stir until mostly dissolved.

Transfer mixture to a blender. Add all remaining ingredients *except* Reddi-wip and blend at high speed until smooth.

Pour and top with Reddi-wip!

MAKES 1 SERVING

STRAWBERRY CLOUD

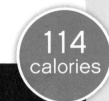

114 calories

You'll Need: tall glass, blender
Prep: 5 minutes

Entire recipe: 114 calories, 2.5g fat, 105mg sodium, 17g carbs, 2g fiber, 11g sugars, 4g protein

INGREDIENTS

2 teaspoons sugar-free French vanilla powdered creamer
3 no-calorie sweetener packets
⅔ cup frozen unsweetened strawberries
5 ounces light vanilla soymilk
1 ounce sugar-free calorie-free strawberry-flavored syrup
½ cup crushed ice *or* 3 to 4 ice cubes
2 tablespoons Fat Free Reddi-wip

DIRECTIONS

In a tall glass, combine creamer with sweetener. Add 2 tablespoons hot water and stir to dissolve.

Transfer mixture to a blender. Add all remaining ingredients *except* Reddi-wip and blend at high speed until smooth.

Pour, top with Reddi-wip, and enjoy!

MAKES 1 SERVING

GREEN TEA CRÈME SWAPPUCCINO

75 calories

You'll Need: tall glass, blender
Prep: 5 minutes

Entire recipe: 75 calories, 2.5g fat, 96mg sodium, 8g carbs, 1g fiber, 4g sugars, 3g protein

INGREDIENTS

2 teaspoons sugar-free French vanilla powdered creamer
1 heaping teaspoon matcha green tea powder
2 no-calorie sweetener packets
½ cup light vanilla soymilk
2 tablespoons sugar-free calorie-free vanilla-flavored syrup
1½ cups crushed ice *or* 8 to 12 ice cubes
2 tablespoons Fat Free Reddi-wip

DIRECTIONS

In a tall glass, combine creamer, green tea powder, and sweetener. Add 2 tablespoons hot water and stir to dissolve.

Transfer mixture to a blender, and add 2 tablespoons cold water. Add all remaining ingredients *except* Reddi-wip and blend at high speed until smooth.

Pour and top with Reddi-wip. Yum!

MAKES 1 SERVING

HG FYI:
Find matcha green tea powder in tea shops, at select markets, and online.

Flip to the photo inserts to see over 100 recipe pics! And for photos of ALL the recipes, go to **hungry-girl.com/books.**

RASPBERRY MOCHA MADNESS SWAPPUCCINO

82 calories

You'll Need: tall glass, blender | **Prep:** 5 minutes

Entire recipe:
82 calories, 1.75g fat, 80mg sodium, 15.5g carbs, 1g fiber, 8g sugars, 3g protein

INGREDIENTS

1½ teaspoons instant coffee granules

1 teaspoon sugar-free French vanilla powdered creamer

1 teaspoon unsweetened cocoa powder

2 no-calorie sweetener packets

½ cup light chocolate soymilk

¼ cup sugar-free calorie-free raspberry-flavored syrup

1½ cups crushed ice *or* 8 to 12 ice cubes

2 tablespoons Fat Free Reddi-wip

DIRECTIONS

In a tall glass, combine coffee granules, creamer, cocoa powder, and sweetener. Add 2 tablespoons hot water and stir to dissolve.

Transfer mixture to a blender. Add soymilk, syrup, and ice, and blend at high speed until smooth.

Pour and top with Reddi-wip!

MAKES 1 SERVING

VANILLALICIOUS CAFE FREEZE

96 calories

You'll Need: tall glass, blender | **Prep:** 5 minutes

Entire recipe:
96 calories, 3.5g fat, 121mg sodium, 11g carbs, 0g fiber, 4.5g sugars, 4g protein

INGREDIENTS

1 tablespoon sugar-free French vanilla powdered creamer

3 no-calorie sweetener packets

5 ounces light vanilla soymilk

1 ounce sugar-free calorie-free vanilla-flavored syrup

1 teaspoon instant coffee granules

1 cup crushed ice *or* 5 to 8 ice cubes

2 tablespoons Fat Free Reddi-wip

DIRECTIONS

In a tall glass, combine creamer with sweetener. Add 2 tablespoons hot water and stir to dissolve.

Transfer mixture to a blender. Add all remaining ingredients *except* Reddi-wip and blend at high speed until smooth.

Pour and top with Reddi-wip. Yum!

MAKES 1 SERVING

SHAKES

Thick, creamy, and guilt-free. The way a shake should be . . .

CRAVIN' CAP'N CRUNCH SHAKE

192 calories

You'll Need: tall glass, blender | **Prep:** 5 minutes

Entire recipe:
192 calories, 2.75g fat, 219mg sodium, 35g carbs, 2.5g fiber, 17g sugars, 7g protein

INGREDIENTS

1 teaspoon sugar-free French vanilla powdered creamer

2 no-calorie sweetener packets

⅔ cup light vanilla soymilk

½ cup fat-free vanilla ice cream

¼ cup Cap'n Crunch cereal (original)

2 tablespoons sugar-free calorie-free vanilla-flavored syrup

¼ teaspoon vanilla extract

¾ cup crushed ice *or* 4 to 6 ice cubes

Optional topping: Fat Free Reddi-wip

DIRECTIONS

In a tall glass, combine powdered creamer with sweetener. Add 1 tablespoon warm water and stir to dissolve. Transfer to a blender.

Add all remaining ingredients and blend at high speed until smooth. Yummm!

MAKES 1 SERVING

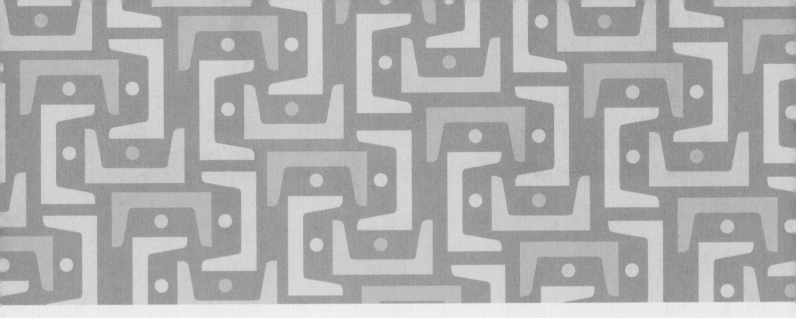

KEY LIME PIE SHAKE

124 calories

You'll Need: blender, tall glass | **Prep:** 5 minutes

Entire recipe:
124 calories, 1.25g fat, 122mg sodium, 24g carbs, 1.5g fiber, 13g sugars, 4.5g protein

INGREDIENTS

½ cup light vanilla soymilk

¼ cup fat-free vanilla ice cream

2 tablespoons crushed pineapple packed in juice

2 tablespoons sugar-free calorie-free vanilla-flavored syrup

1 tablespoon lime juice

1 no-calorie sweetener packet

¾ cup crushed ice *or* 4 to 6 ice cubes

2 tablespoons Fat Free Reddi-wip

1 low-fat honey graham cracker (¼ sheet), crushed

DIRECTIONS

Place all ingredients *except* Reddi-wip and graham cracker in a blender. Blend at high speed until smooth.

Pour into a tall glass, and top with Reddi-wip and crushed graham cracker!

MAKES 1 SERVING

SLURPABLE SPLIT SHAKE

220 calories

You'll Need: small microwave-safe bowl, tall glass, blender
Prep: 5 minutes

Entire recipe: 220 calories, 2g fat, 100mg sodium, 47g carbs, 4g fiber, 22g sugars, 5.5g protein

INGREDIENTS

3 frozen unsweetened strawberries
1 teaspoon sugar-free strawberry jam/preserves
1 teaspoon sugar-free French vanilla powdered creamer
1 no-calorie sweetener packet
½ cup light vanilla soymilk
1 small banana
¼ cup fat-free vanilla ice cream
1 cup crushed ice *or* 5 to 8 ice cubes
2 tablespoons Fat Free Reddi-wip
½ tablespoon light chocolate syrup

Optional topping: maraschino cherry

DIRECTIONS

In a small microwave-safe bowl, microwave strawberries for 30 seconds, or until mostly thawed. Thoroughly mash and mix in jam/preserves.

In a tall glass, combine creamer with sweetener. Add 1 tablespoon hot water and stir to dissolve. Transfer to a blender.

To the blender, add soymilk, banana, ice cream, and ice. Blend at high speed until smooth.

Pour and top with strawberry mixture, Reddi-wip, and chocolate syrup. Enjoy!

MAKES 1 SERVING

FROZEN S'MORES HOT COCOA

169 calories

You'll Need: tall glass, blender
Prep: 5 minutes

Entire recipe: 169 calories, 4.5g fat, 202mg sodium, 30g carbs, 1.5g fiber, 18.5g sugars, 2.5g protein

INGREDIENTS

1 packet hot cocoa mix with 20 to 25 calories
1 tablespoon mini semi-sweet chocolate chips
1 teaspoon fat-free non-dairy powdered creamer
1 no-calorie sweetener packet
1½ cups crushed iced *or* 8 to 12 ice cubes
15 mini marshmallows
2 low-fat honey graham crackers (½ sheet), coarsely crushed
2 tablespoons Fat Free Reddi-wip

DIRECTIONS

In a tall glass, combine cocoa mix, chocolate chips, powdered creamer, and sweetener. Add ¼ cup very hot water and stir until mostly dissolved.

Transfer mixture to a blender, and add ¼ cup cold water. Add ice and blend at high speed until smooth.

Pour, stir in marshmallows and crushed graham crackers, and top with Reddi-wip!

MAKES 1 SERVING

PB&J SUPER-SHAKE

199 calories

You'll Need: blender, tall glass | **Prep:** 5 minutes

Entire recipe:
199 calories, 7.25g fat, 291mg sodium, 29.5g carbs, 3g fiber, 12g sugars, 6g protein

INGREDIENTS

⅔ cup Unsweetened Original Almond Breeze
⅓ cup fat-free vanilla ice cream
¼ cup Reese's Puffs cereal
2 frozen unsweetened strawberries, partially thawed
2 teaspoons reduced-fat peanut butter
1 no-calorie sweetener packet
⅔ cup crushed ice *or* 3 to 5 ice cubes

Optional topping: Fat Free Reddi-wip

DIRECTIONS

Place all ingredients in a blender and blend at high speed until thoroughly mixed. Pour into a tall glass. PB-rific!

MAKES 1 SERVING

CHOCOLATE-BANANA SMOOTHIE

164 calories

You'll Need: tall glass, blender
Prep: 5 minutes

Entire recipe: 164 calories, 1.5g fat, 137mg sodium, 35.5g carbs, 3.75g fiber, 18g sugars, 3g protein

INGREDIENTS

1 packet hot cocoa mix with 20 to 25 calories
2 teaspoons fat-free non-dairy powdered creamer
1 teaspoon mini semi-sweet chocolate chips
1 no-calorie sweetener packet
1 small banana, sliced into coins and frozen
1 cup crushed ice *or* 5 to 8 ice cubes

DIRECTIONS

In a tall glass, combine cocoa mix, creamer, chocolate chips, and sweetener. Add ¼ cup very hot water and stir to dissolve.

Transfer mixture to a blender, and add ½ cup cold water. Add frozen banana slices and ice, and blend at medium speed until smooth. Enjoy!

MAKES 1 SERVING

DREAMSICLE SHIVER

164 calories

You'll Need: tall glass, blender
Prep: 5 minutes

Entire recipe: 164 calories, <0.5g fat, 65mg sodium, 38g carbs, 1g fiber, 20g sugars, 3g protein

INGREDIENTS

2 teaspoons fat-free non-dairy powdered creamer
1 no-calorie sweetener packet
1 cup Trop50 No Pulp orange juice beverage
½ cup fat-free vanilla ice cream
1½ cups crushed ice *or* 8 to 12 ice cubes

DIRECTIONS

In a tall glass, combine creamer with sweetener. Add 2 tablespoons hot water and stir to dissolve.

Transfer mixture to a blender. Add all remaining ingredients and blend at high speed until smooth. Slurp away!

MAKES 1 SERVING

HAPPY MONKEY BANANA SHAKE

211 calories

You'll Need: tall glass, blender
Prep: 5 minutes

Entire recipe: 211 calories, 2g fat, 371mg sodium, 45g carbs, 3g fiber, 20g sugars, 5.5g protein

INGREDIENTS

1 teaspoon fat-free non-dairy powdered creamer
1 no-calorie sweetener packet
½ cup light vanilla soymilk
1 tablespoon Jell-O Sugar Free Fat Free Vanilla Instant pudding mix
¼ cup fat-free vanilla ice cream
½ medium banana, sliced into coins and frozen
1 cup crushed ice *or* 5 to 8 ice cubes
2 Reduced Fat Nilla Wafers
2 tablespoons Fat Free Reddi-wip
1 maraschino cherry

DIRECTIONS

In a tall glass, combine creamer with sweetener. Add 1 tablespoon hot water and stir to dissolve. Add soymilk and pudding mix, and stir until mostly dissolved.

Transfer mixture to a blender. Add ice cream, frozen banana coins, and ice, and blend at high speed until smooth.

Pour, break wafers into pieces, and stir them into the shake. Top with Reddi-wip and cherry!

MAKES 1 SERVING

HG ALTERNATIVE!

If you like, leave out the wafer cookies. Still awesome (and under 200 calories)!

CHILLA IN VANILLA MILKSHAKE

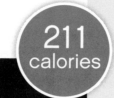

162 calories

You'll Need: tall glass, blender
Prep: 5 minutes

Entire recipe: 162 calories, 2.25g fat, 127mg sodium, 28.5g carbs, 1g fiber, 8g sugars, 6g protein

INGREDIENTS

½ tablespoon sugar-free French vanilla powdered creamer
2 no-calorie sweetener packets
½ cup light vanilla soymilk
½ cup fat-free vanilla ice cream
⅛ teaspoon vanilla extract
1 cup crushed ice *or* 5 to 8 ice cubes
2 tablespoons Fat Free Reddi-wip

Optional topping: maraschino cherry

DIRECTIONS

In a tall glass, combine creamer with sweetener. Add 1 tablespoon hot water and stir to dissolve.

Transfer mixture to a blender. Add all remaining ingredients *except* Reddi-wip and blend at high speed until smooth.

Pour, top with Reddi-wip, and dive in!

MAKES 1 SERVING

GINORMOUS CHOCOLATE SHAKE

206 calories

You'll Need: very tall glass, blender | **Prep:** 5 minutes

Entire recipe:
206 calories, <1g fat, 244mg sodium, 48g carbs, 7g fiber, 30g sugars, 6g protein

INGREDIENTS

1 packet hot cocoa mix with 20 to 25 calories
2 no-calorie sweetener packets
1½ tablespoons light chocolate syrup
¾ cup fat-free chocolate ice cream
2 cups crushed ice *or* 10 to 16 ice cubes

Optional toppings: Fat Free Reddi-wip, maraschino cherry

DIRECTIONS

In a very tall glass, combine cocoa mix with sweetener. Add ¼ cup hot water and stir to dissolve.

Transfer mixture to a blender. Add syrup and ¾ cup cold water. Add ice cream and ice, and blend at medium speed until smooth. Enjoy!

MAKES 1 SERVING

COOKIE-RIFIC ICE CREAM FREEZE

159 calories

You'll Need: tall glass, blender | **Prep:** 5 minutes

Entire recipe:
159 calories, 3.25g fat, 164mg sodium, 26.5g carbs, 1.5g fiber, 12g sugars, 6g protein

INGREDIENTS

1 teaspoon sugar-free French vanilla powdered creamer
2 no-calorie sweetener packets
5 ounces light vanilla soymilk
½ pack Nabisco 100 Cal Oreo Thin Crisps *or* 3 chocolate graham crackers (¾ sheet), broken into pieces
¼ cup fat-free vanilla ice cream
1½ cups crushed ice *or* 8 to 12 ice cubes

Optional topping: Fat Free Reddi-wip

DIRECTIONS

In a tall glass, combine creamer with sweetener. Add 2 tablespoons hot water and stir to dissolve.

Transfer to a blender. Add all remaining ingredients and blend at high speed until smooth. Mmmmmm!

MAKES 1 SERVING

COOKIE CRISP PUDDIN' SHAKE

198 calories

You'll Need: blender, tall glass | **Prep:** 5 minutes

Entire recipe:
198 calories, 3.75g fat, 321mg sodium, 37g carbs, 1g fiber, 16.5g sugars, 5g protein

INGREDIENTS

1 sugar-free vanilla pudding snack with 60 calories or less
⅔ cup light chocolate soymilk
⅓ cup Cookie Crisp cereal (original)
1 teaspoon mini semi-sweet chocolate chips
1 no-calorie sweetener packet
¾ cup crushed ice *or* 4 to 6 ice cubes

Optional toppings: Fat Free Reddi-wip, additional mini semi-sweet chocolate chips

DIRECTIONS

Place all ingredients in a blender. Blend at high speed until smooth. Pour into a tall glass. Cookie-licious!

MAKES 1 SERVING

CHOCOLATE-COVERED-CHERRIES FREEZE

160 calories

You'll Need: tall glass, blender | **Prep:** 5 minutes

Entire recipe:
160 calories, 4g fat, 163mg sodium, 28g carbs, 3g fiber, 21.5g sugars, 3.5g protein

INGREDIENTS

1 packet hot cocoa mix with 20 to 25 calories
1 tablespoon mini semi-sweet chocolate chips
1 no-calorie sweetener packet
12 frozen unsweetened pitted dark sweet cherries
1½ cups crushed ice *or* 8 to 12 ice cubes
2 tablespoons Fat Free Reddi-wip

DIRECTIONS

In a tall glass, combine cocoa mix, chocolate chips, and sweetener. Add ¼ cup very hot water and stir to dissolve.

Transfer mixture to a blender and add ¼ cup cold water. Add cherries and ice and blend at high speed until smooth.

Pour, top with Reddi-wip, and sip!

MAKES 1 SERVING

CARAMEL APPLE FRAPPE

199 calories

You'll Need: blender, tall glass
Prep: 5 minutes

Entire recipe: 199 calories, 1g fat, 250mg sodium, 45g carbs, 2g fiber, 23.5g sugars, 2.5g protein

INGREDIENTS

1 sugar-free caramel pudding snack with 60 calories or less
½ cup apple cider
¼ cup freeze-dried apple pieces
¼ cup fat-free vanilla ice cream
¼ teaspoon cinnamon
⅛ teaspoon vanilla extract
1 cup crushed ice *or* 5 to 8 ice cubes
2 tablespoons Fat Free Reddi-wip

DIRECTIONS

Place all ingredients *except* Reddi-wip in a blender. Blend at high speed until smooth.

Pour into a tall glass, top with Reddi-wip, and enjoy!

MAKES 1 SERVING

MINTY COOKIE-RIFIC ICE CREAM FREEZE

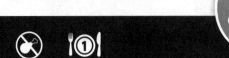

159 calories

You'll Need: tall glass, blender
Prep: 5 minutes

Entire recipe: 159 calories, 3.25g fat, 164mg sodium, 26.5g carbs, 1.5g fiber, 12g sugars, 6g protein

INGREDIENTS

1 teaspoon sugar-free French vanilla powdered creamer
2 no-calorie sweetener packets
5 ounces light vanilla soymilk
½ pack Nabisco 100 Cal Oreo Thin Crisps *or* 3 chocolate graham crackers (¾ sheet), broken into pieces
¼ cup fat-free vanilla ice cream
¼ teaspoon peppermint extract
2 drops green food coloring
1½ cups crushed ice *or* 8 to 12 ice cubes

Optional topping: Fat Free Reddi-wip

DIRECTIONS

In a tall glass, combine creamer with sweetener. Add 2 tablespoons hot water and stir to dissolve.

Transfer mixture to a blender. Add all remaining ingredients and blend at high speed until smooth. Mmmmmm!

MAKES 1 SERVING

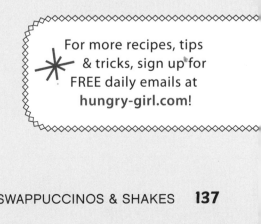
For more recipes, tips & tricks, sign up for FREE daily emails at hungry-girl.com!

FROOT LOOPS FREEZE

154 calories

You'll Need: tall glass, blender | **Prep:** 5 minutes

Entire recipe:
154 calories, 3.5g fat, 140mg sodium, 25g carbs, 1.5g fiber, 14.5g sugars, 5g protein

INGREDIENTS

1 tablespoon sugar-free French vanilla powdered creamer
1 no-calorie sweetener packet
½ cup light vanilla soymilk
¼ cup fat-free vanilla ice cream
⅓ cup Froot Loops cereal
1 cup crushed ice *or* 5 to 8 ice cubes
2 tablespoons Fat Free Reddi-wip

DIRECTIONS

In a tall glass, combine creamer with sweetener. Add 2 tablespoons hot water and stir to dissolve.

Transfer mixture to a blender. Add soymilk, ice cream, cereal, and ice, and blend at high speed until smooth.

Pour and top with Reddi-wip!

MAKES 1 SERVING

EGGNOG FREEZE

110 calories

You'll Need: tall glass, blender | **Prep:** 5 minutes

Entire recipe:
110 calories, 1g fat, 310mg sodium, 19.5g carbs, 0.5g fiber, 10.5g sugars, 4.5g protein

INGREDIENTS

1 tablespoon Jell-O Sugar Free Fat Free Vanilla Instant pudding mix
1 no-calorie sweetener packet
½ cup light vanilla soymilk
¼ cup fat-free vanilla ice cream
⅛ teaspoon rum extract
1 dash ground nutmeg
1 cup crushed ice *or* 5 to 8 ice cubes
2 tablespoons Fat Free Reddi-wip

Optional topping: cinnamon

DIRECTIONS

In a tall glass, combine pudding mix, sweetener, and soymilk, and stir until mostly dissolved.

Transfer mixture to a blender. Add all remaining ingredients *except* Reddi-wip and blend at high speed until smooth.

Pour and top with Reddi-wip!

MAKES 1 SERVING

FREAKISHLY GOOD FROZEN HOT CHOCOLATE

58 calories

You'll Need: tall glass, blender
Prep: 5 minutes

Entire recipe: 58 calories, 0.5g fat, 184mg sodium, 10g carbs, 1g fiber, 5g sugars, 3g protein

INGREDIENTS

1 packet hot cocoa mix with 20 to 25 calories
2 no-calorie sweetener packets
¼ cup light vanilla soymilk
1 tablespoon sugar-free calorie-free vanilla-flavored syrup
1 teaspoon sugar-free chocolate syrup
1 cup crushed ice *or* 5 to 8 ice cubes
2 tablespoons Fat Free Reddi-wip

DIRECTIONS

In a tall glass, combine cocoa mix with sweetener. Add 2 tablespoons hot water and stir to dissolve.

Transfer mixture to a blender and add 2 tablespoons cold water. Add all remaining ingredients *except* Reddi-wip and blend at high speed until smooth.

Pour, top with Reddi-wip, and indulge!

MAKES 1 SERVING

CINNAMON-TOAST-CRUNCH SHAKE

160 calories

You'll Need: tall glass, blender
Prep: 5 minutes

Entire recipe: 160 calories, 4.5g fat, 168mg sodium, 25g carbs, 1g fiber, 14g sugars, 5g protein

INGREDIENTS

1 tablespoon sugar-free French vanilla powdered creamer
1 no-calorie sweetener packet
½ cup light vanilla soymilk
¼ cup fat-free vanilla ice cream
¼ cup Cinnamon Toast Crunch cereal
1 cup crushed ice *or* 5 to 8 ice cubes
2 tablespoons Fat Free Reddi-wip

Optional topping: cinnamon

DIRECTIONS

In a tall glass, combine creamer with sweetener. Add 2 tablespoons hot water and stir to dissolve.

Transfer mixture to a blender. Add soymilk, ice cream, cereal, and ice, and blend at high speed until smooth.

Pour and top with Reddi-wip!

MAKES 1 SERVING

HG ALTERNATIVE!
Reserve a few squares of cereal for topping off your shake!

SHAMROCK 'N ROLL SHAKE

175 calories

You'll Need: tall glass, blender
Prep: 5 minutes

Entire recipe: 175 calories, 4g fat, 150mg sodium, 29g carbs, 2g fiber, 13.5g sugars, 7.5g protein

INGREDIENTS

1 tablespoon sugar-free French vanilla powdered creamer
1 no-calorie sweetener packet
¾ cup light vanilla soymilk
½ cup fat-free vanilla ice cream
¼ teaspoon peppermint extract
2 drops green food coloring
1½ cups crushed ice *or* 8 to 12 ice cubes

DIRECTIONS

In a tall glass, combine creamer with sweetener. Add 1 tablespoon hot water and stir to dissolve.

Transfer mixture to a blender. Add all remaining ingredients and blend at high speed until smooth. Cheers!

MAKES 1 SERVING

PEACH COBBLER SHAKE

191 calories

You'll Need: tall glass, blender
Prep: 5 minutes

Entire recipe: 191 calories, 2.5g fat, 132mg sodium, 39g carbs, 3.5g fiber, 24.5g sugars, 6g protein

INGREDIENTS

1 teaspoon sugar-free French vanilla powdered creamer
1 no-calorie sweetener packet
½ cup light vanilla soymilk
¼ cup fat-free vanilla ice cream
1 cup frozen sliced unsweetened peaches, partially thawed
1 cup crushed ice *or* 5 to 8 ice cubes
½ teaspoon plus 1 dash cinnamon
2 low-fat cinnamon graham crackers (½ sheet), crushed
2 tablespoons Fat Free Reddi-wip

Optional topping: additional cinnamon

DIRECTIONS

In a tall glass, combine creamer with sweetener. Add 2 tablespoons hot water and stir to dissolve.

Transfer mixture to a blender. Add soymilk and 2 tablespoons cold water. Add ice cream, peaches, ice, and ½ teaspoon cinnamon, and blend at high speed until smooth.

Pour, stir in crushed graham crackers, and top with Reddi-wip and remaining dash cinnamon!

MAKES 1 SERVING

Thirsty for More?

If you want a drink with a kick, many cocktails await you in the Party Foods, Cocktails & Holiday chapter.

SWAPS FOR SOYMILK

We call for light vanilla soymilk because it's sweet and creamy, with fewer calories than regular milk (even the fat-free kind). A cup of light vanilla soymilk has about 70 calories and 2g fat. But if you avoid soy, check out these swaps . . .

✳ **Blue Diamond Unsweetened Vanilla Almond Breeze**

Super-low in calories (40 per cup!) and extremely delicious. Depending on your taste buds, you might want to add a no-calorie sweetener packet since this is unsweetened, unlike most vanilla soymilk.

✳ **So Delicious Unsweetened Coconut Milk Beverage**

A little higher in fat, but it's creamy and amazing and has just 50 calories per cup. Feel free to zazzle it up with some calorie-free sweetener.

✳ **Fat-Free Dairy Milk**

It has about 20 extra calories per cup, but it'll work. It will save you some fat and add a little protein, but it isn't as creamy as the others. Add a small amount of calorie-free sweetener.

CHAPTER 7

FOIL PACKS

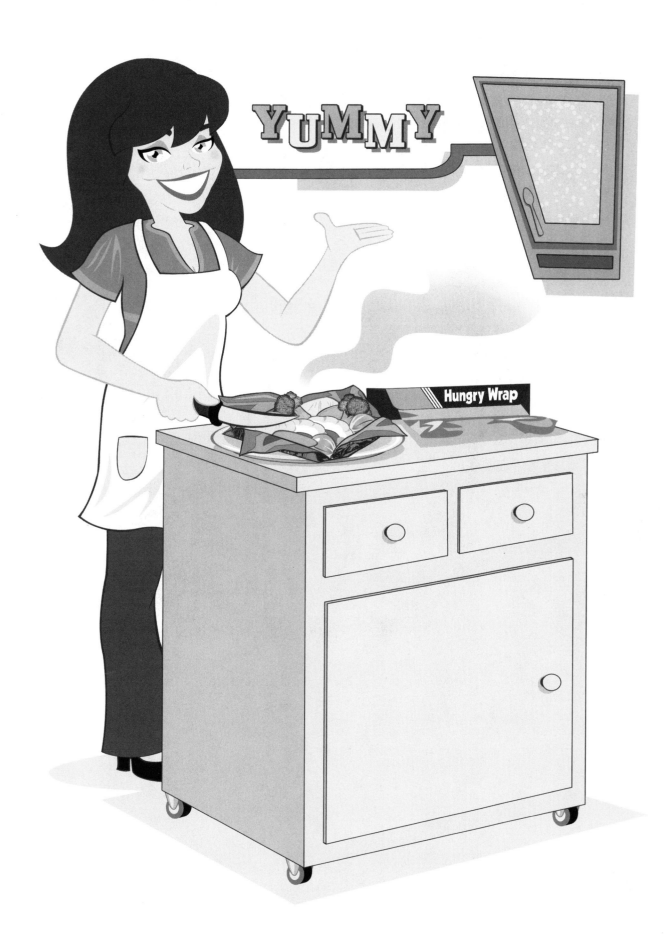

FOIL PACKS

Winner Winner Chicken Dinner

Chicken Cacciatore

Glaze-of-Sunshine Apricot Chicken

Stuffed 'n Squashed Mushroom Pack

Portabella Parmesan

Buffalo Chicken Portabella Pack

Mexi-licious Stuffed Portabella

Dreamy Butternut Chicken

Fajitas in a Foil Pack

Colossal Asian Veggie 'n Chicken Pack

Fruity Fish Foil Pack

Hustle 'n Brussels Pack Attack

Chicken-with-a-Kick Pack

So-Fancy Fish Pack

Rockin' Chicken Ratatouille

Mom-Style Creamy Chicken 'n Veggies

Sesame Salmon & Snap Peas

Cha-Cha-Cherry BBQ Chicken

Crazy Pineapple Salmon Teriyaki

The Rat(atouille) Pack

Do the Cabbage Pack!

Woohoo! Bayou Fish Pack

Sweet Potato Apple Pack

Steamy Creamy Squash

Jump for Choy! Fish Pack

Mega-mazing Veggie Pack

Spinach Artichoke Chicken

Spicy Shrimp 'n Veggies

Ragin' Cajun Shrimp

Apple Raisin Chicken

Flounder L'Orange

Mango Chicken

Sweet & Sour Cabbage

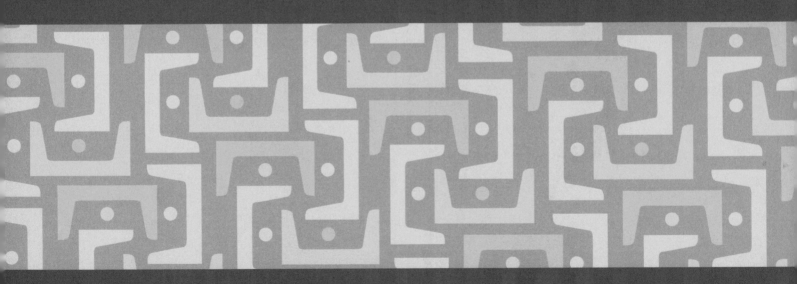

Some of the simplest and tastiest HG dishes of all time—entrées AND sides. Just foil, fold, bake, and chew . . . YES!!!

AVERT FOIL-PACK DISASTERS!

* When you fold up your foil, form a tightly sealed package—you don't want any heat escaping—with a little extra room at the top for the steaming action to take place.

* Hot steam will be released when you open your foil pack. So let it cool for a few minutes, and then slice the foil to let some steam escape.

WANNA GRILL YOUR FOIL PACK?

Cook it for about half the given time, and keep the grill cover down.

Temperature conversions:

375 degrees in oven—medium heat on grill
400 degrees in oven—medium-high heat on grill
425 degrees in oven—high heat on grill

And have a baking sheet or large plate ready to place the pack on once it's cooked!

A QUICK GUIDE TO SYMBOLS:

15 Minutes or Less

This symbol lets you know a recipe should take you no more than fifteen minutes from start to finish! That includes prep and cook time.

30 Minutes or Less

Just like the 15-minute version, this one points out recipes that take 30 minutes or less to whip up.

Meatless

You guessed it—no meat here! That includes beef, poultry, and fish. Some recipes give the option of a meatless ingredient. If you want your meal without meat, go with the meatless choice.

Single Serving

Pretty straightforward. These are recipes for one.

5 Ingredients or Less

Fans of HG know that we like to keep things simple. And these recipes contain just five ingredients or less!

Photos

These recipes can be seen in one of the book's photo inserts. The number in the symbol tells you which insert. Find photos of all the recipes at hungry-girl.com/books!

WINNER WINNER CHICKEN DINNER

251 calories

You'll Need: heavy-duty aluminum foil, baking sheet, nonstick spray, medium microwave-safe bowl
Prep: 15 minutes | **Cook:** 25 minutes

Entire recipe:
251 calories, 4.5g fat, 340mg sodium, 16g carbs, 3.75g fiber, 7g sugars, 35.5g protein

INGREDIENTS

½ tablespoon light whipped butter or light buttery spread

¾ cup sliced onion

½ cup sliced mushrooms

1 small yellow summer squash, ends removed, sliced

1 teaspoon onion soup/dip seasoning mix

One 5-ounce raw boneless skinless chicken breast cutlet, pounded to ½-inch thickness

Optional seasonings: salt and black pepper

DIRECTIONS

Preheat oven to 375 degrees. Lay a large piece of heavy-duty foil on a baking sheet and spray with nonstick spray.

In a medium microwave-safe bowl, microwave butter for 15 seconds, or until melted. Add onion, mushrooms, and squash, and ½ teaspoon onion soup/dip mix. Stir well and distribute onto the center of the foil.

Season chicken with remaining ½ teaspoon onion soup/dip mix and place over the veggie mixture. Cover with another large piece of foil.

Fold together and seal all four edges of the foil pieces, forming a well-sealed packet. Bake for 25 minutes, or until chicken is cooked through and veggies are tender.

Cut packet to release steam before opening entirely. Yum!

MAKES 1 SERVING

For more recipes, tips & tricks, sign up for FREE daily emails at **hungry-girl.com!**

CHICKEN CACCIATORE

240 calories

You'll Need: heavy-duty aluminum foil, baking sheet, nonstick spray, medium bowl
Prep: 20 minutes
Cook: 25 minutes

Entire recipe: 240 calories, 2g fat, 779mg sodium, 18.5g carbs, 4g fiber, 10g sugars, 36g protein

INGREDIENTS

¾ cup canned diced tomatoes (not drained)
⅓ cup chopped red bell pepper
⅓ cup sliced mushrooms
⅓ cup chopped onion
1 teaspoon chopped garlic
¼ teaspoon dried oregano
¼ teaspoon dried basil
One 5-ounce raw boneless skinless chicken breast cutlet, pounded to ½-inch thickness
⅛ teaspoon each salt and black pepper

DIRECTIONS

Preheat oven to 375 degrees. Lay a large piece of heavy-duty foil on a baking sheet and spray with nonstick spray.

In a medium bowl, mix all ingredients *except* chicken, salt, and black pepper.

Season chicken with salt and black pepper and place on the center of the foil. Top with veggie mixture and cover with another large piece of foil.

Fold together and seal all four edges of the foil pieces, forming a well-sealed packet. Bake for 25 minutes, or until chicken is cooked through and veggies are tender.

Cut packet to release steam before opening entirely. Enjoy!

MAKES 1 SERVING

GLAZE-OF-SUNSHINE APRICOT CHICKEN

233 calories
PER SERVING

You'll Need: heavy-duty aluminum foil, baking sheet, nonstick spray, small microwave-safe bowl, large bowl
Prep: 15 minutes
Cook: 25 minutes

½ of pack: 233 calories, 3.5g fat, 274mg sodium, 13g carbs, 0g fiber, <0.5g sugars, 39g protein

INGREDIENTS

½ tablespoon light whipped butter or light buttery spread
1 tablespoon cider vinegar
½ tablespoon cornstarch
¼ cup sugar-free apricot preserves, room temperature
½ tablespoon onion soup/dip seasoning mix
Two 6-ounce raw boneless skinless chicken breast cutlets, pounded to ½-inch thickness

Optional seasonings: salt and black pepper

DIRECTIONS

Preheat oven to 375 degrees. Lay a large piece of heavy-duty foil on a baking sheet and spray with nonstick spray.

In a small microwave-safe bowl, microwave butter for 15 seconds, or until just melted.

In a large bowl, combine vinegar with cornstarch and stir to dissolve. Mix in preserves, melted butter, and soup/dip mix. Add chicken and flip to coat. Place chicken on the center of the foil and top with any remaining preserves mixture. Cover with another large piece of foil.

Fold together and seal all four edges of the foil pieces, forming a well-sealed packet. Bake for 25 minutes, or until chicken is cooked through.

Cut packet to release steam before opening entirely. Enjoy!

MAKES 2 SERVINGS

STUFFED 'N SQUASHED MUSHROOM PACK

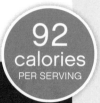

92 calories PER SERVING

You'll Need: heavy-duty aluminum foil, baking sheet, nonstick spray, medium bowl
Prep: 15 minutes
Cook: 25 minutes

½ of pack (1 stuffed mushroom): 92 calories, 2.25g fat, 397mg sodium, 11.5g carbs, 3.25g fiber, 4g sugars, 6g protein

INGREDIENTS

2 large portabella mushrooms, stems chopped and reserved
2 wedges The Laughing Cow Light Creamy Swiss cheese
½ teaspoon chopped garlic
½ teaspoon dried minced onion
⅛ teaspoon salt, or more to taste
Dash ground thyme, or more to taste
1 summer squash (yellow or green), ends removed, finely diced
½ tablespoon reduced-fat Parmesan-style grated topping

DIRECTIONS

Preheat oven to 375 degrees. Lay a large piece of heavy-duty foil on a baking sheet and spray with nonstick spray.

Place mushroom caps on the sheet with rounded sides down.

In a medium bowl, thoroughly mix cheese wedges, garlic, minced onion, salt, and thyme. Stir in chopped mushroom stems and diced squash. Divide mixture between the mushroom caps and sprinkle with Parm-style topping. Cover with another large piece of foil.

Fold together and seal all four edges of the foil pieces, forming a well-sealed packet. Bake for 25 minutes, or until mushrooms are tender.

Cut packet to release steam before opening entirely. Enjoy!

MAKES 2 SERVINGS

PORTABELLA PARMESAN

113 calories PER SERVING

You'll Need: heavy-duty aluminum foil, baking sheet, nonstick spray, medium bowl
Prep: 15 minutes
Cook: 25 minutes

½ of pack (1 stuffed mushroom): 113 calories, 4.5g fat, 435mg sodium, 12.5g carbs, 2.5g fiber, 5.5g sugars, 7.5g protein

INGREDIENTS

2 large portabella mushrooms, stems chopped and reserved
½ cup low-fat marinara sauce
1 teaspoon dried minced onion
½ teaspoon chopped garlic
Dash each salt and black pepper
1 tablespoon reduced-fat Parmesan-style grated topping
¼ cup shredded part-skim mozzarella cheese

DIRECTIONS

Preheat oven to 375 degrees. Lay a large piece of heavy-duty foil on a baking sheet and spray with nonstick spray.

Place mushroom caps on the sheet with rounded sides down.

In a medium bowl, mix chopped mushroom stems, sauce, minced onion, garlic, salt, black pepper, and 2 teaspoons Parm-style topping.

Spoon mixture into caps. Evenly top with remaining 1 teaspoon Parm-style topping, followed by mozzarella cheese. Cover with another large piece of foil.

Fold together and seal all four edges of the foil pieces, forming a well-sealed packet. Bake for 25 minutes, or until mushrooms are tender.

Cut packet to release steam before opening entirely. Enjoy!

MAKES 2 SERVINGS

BUFFALO CHICKEN PORTABELLA PACK

131 calories PER SERVING

You'll Need: heavy-duty aluminum foil, baking sheet, nonstick spray, medium bowl
Prep: 15 minutes
Cook: 25 minutes

½ of pack (1 stuffed mushroom): 131 calories, 3g fat, 778mg sodium, 9g carbs, 1.5 fiber, 3.5g sugars, 16g protein

INGREDIENTS

2 large portabella mushrooms, stems chopped and reserved
2 wedges The Laughing Cow Light Creamy Swiss cheese
1½ tablespoons Frank's RedHot Original Cayenne Pepper Sauce
3 ounces cooked and finely chopped skinless chicken breast
¼ cup finely chopped onion
1 tablespoon reduced-fat Parmesan-style grated topping

DIRECTIONS

Preheat oven to 375 degrees. Lay a large piece of heavy-duty foil on a baking sheet and spray with nonstick spray.

Place mushroom caps on the sheet with the rounded sides down.

In a medium bowl, stir cheese wedges with hot sauce until smooth and uniform. Stir in chopped mushroom stems, chicken, and onion. Spoon mixture into the mushroom caps. Sprinkle with Parm-style topping. Cover with another large piece of foil.

Fold together and seal all four edges of the foil pieces, forming a well-sealed packet. Bake for 25 minutes, or until mushrooms are soft and tender.

Cut packet to release steam before opening entirely. Chew!

MAKES 2 SERVINGS

MEXI-LICIOUS STUFFED PORTABELLA

100 calories PER SERVING

You'll Need: heavy-duty aluminum foil, baking sheet, nonstick spray, medium bowl
Prep: 15 minutes
Cook: 25 minutes

½ of pack (1 stuffed mushroom): 100 calories, 3.5g fat, 483mg sodium, 10g carbs, 2.5g fiber, 2.5g sugars, 9.5g protein

INGREDIENTS

2 large portabella mushrooms, stems chopped and reserved
⅓ cup frozen ground-beef-style soy crumbles, thawed, patted dry
½ teaspoon taco seasoning mix
¼ cup red enchilada sauce
2 tablespoons salsa
¼ cup shredded reduced-fat Mexican-blend cheese

Optional topping: fat-free sour cream

DIRECTIONS

Preheat oven to 375 degrees. Lay a large piece of heavy-duty foil on a baking sheet and spray with nonstick spray.

Place mushroom caps on the sheet with rounded sides down.

In a medium bowl, mix chopped mushroom stems, soy crumbles, and taco seasoning. Stir in sauce and salsa.

Spoon mixture into caps. Evenly top with cheese. Cover with another large piece of foil.

Fold together and seal all four edges of the foil pieces, forming a well-sealed packet. Bake for 25 minutes, or until mushrooms are tender.

Cut packet to release steam before opening entirely. Enjoy!

MAKES 2 SERVINGS

DREAMY BUTTERNUT CHICKEN

292 calories PER SERVING

You'll Need: heavy-duty aluminum foil, baking sheet, nonstick spray, large bowl
Prep: 15 minutes
Cook: 35 minutes

½ of pack (about 2 cups): 292 calories, 3.25g fat, 575mg sodium, 35.5g carbs, 6g fiber, 10g sugars, 32g protein

INGREDIENTS

½ cup canned 98% fat-free cream of chicken condensed soup
¼ cup fat-free sour cream
1 teaspoon chopped garlic
2 cups peeled and sliced butternut squash
1½ cups chopped cauliflower
¾ cup chopped onion
8 ounces raw boneless skinless chicken breast, cut into bite-sized pieces
⅛ teaspoon each salt and black pepper

DIRECTIONS

Preheat oven to 375 degrees. Lay a large piece of heavy-duty foil on a baking sheet and spray with nonstick spray.

In a large bowl, mix condensed soup, sour cream, and garlic. Stir in squash, cauliflower, and onion. Distribute onto the center of the foil.

Season chicken with salt and pepper and place over the veggie mixture. Cover with another large piece of foil.

Fold together and seal all four edges of the foil pieces, forming a well-sealed packet. Bake for 35 minutes, or until chicken is cooked through and veggies are tender.

Cut packet to release steam before opening entirely. Mix well and enjoy!

MAKES 2 SERVINGS

FAJITAS IN A FOIL PACK

244 calories PER SERVING

You'll Need: heavy-duty aluminum foil, baking sheet, nonstick spray, large bowl
Prep: 15 minutes
Cook: 25 minutes

½ of pack: 244 calories, 2.5g fat, 716mg sodium, 13g carbs, 3g fiber, 5.5g sugars, 41.5g protein

INGREDIENTS

1½ tablespoons lime juice
1 teaspoon cornstarch
1 teaspoon garlic powder
1 teaspoon onion powder
1 teaspoon chili powder
½ teaspoon salt
⅛ teaspoon ground cumin
12 ounces raw boneless skinless chicken breast, sliced into thin strips
1 cup sliced bell pepper
1 small zucchini, ends removed, sliced into thin strips
1 cup sliced onion

DIRECTIONS

Preheat oven to 375 degrees. Lay a large piece of heavy-duty foil on a baking sheet and spray with nonstick spray.

In a large bowl, combine lime juice with cornstarch and stir to dissolve. Stir in all the seasonings to form a thick paste. Add chicken and veggies and stir to coat.

Distribute chicken-veggie mixture onto the center of the foil, and cover with another large piece of foil.

Fold together and seal all four edges of the foil pieces, forming a well-sealed packet. Bake for 25 minutes, or until chicken is cooked through and veggies are tender.

Cut packet to release steam before opening entirely. Mix and enjoy!

MAKES 2 SERVINGS

COLOSSAL ASIAN VEGGIE 'N CHICKEN PACK

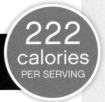

222 calories PER SERVING

You'll Need: heavy-duty aluminum foil, baking sheet, nonstick spray, small bowl
Prep: 15 minutes | **Cook:** 35 minutes

¼th of pack (about 1½ cups):
222 calories, 1.5g fat, 811mg sodium, 19g carbs, 3.25g fiber, 9.5g sugars, 30.5g protein

INGREDIENTS

1 tablespoon seasoned rice vinegar
½ tablespoon cornstarch
3 tablespoons oyster sauce
1 teaspoon chopped garlic
⅛ teaspoon ground ginger
3 cups thinly sliced cabbage
2 cups bean sprouts
1½ cups sugar snap peas
1 cup sliced mushrooms
½ cup matchstick-cut carrots
One 8-ounce can sliced water chestnuts, drained
12 ounces raw boneless skinless chicken
    breast, cut into bite-sized pieces

DIRECTIONS

Preheat oven to 375 degrees. Lay a large piece of heavy-duty foil on a baking sheet and spray with nonstick spray.

In a small bowl, combine vinegar with cornstarch and stir to dissolve. Mix in oyster sauce, garlic, and ginger.

Distribute all veggies onto the center of the foil and top with chicken. Drizzle with sauce mixture and cover with another large piece of foil.

Fold together and seal all four edges of the foil pieces, forming a well-sealed packet. Bake for 35 minutes, or until chicken is cooked through and veggies are tender.

Cut packet to release steam before opening entirely. Stir and enjoy!

MAKES 4 SERVINGS

FRUITY FISH FOIL PACK

204 calories PER SERVING

You'll Need: heavy-duty aluminum foil, baking sheet, nonstick spray | **Prep:** 5 minutes | **Cook:** 15 minutes

½ of pack (1 fillet):
204 calories, 3g fat, 358mg sodium, 10.5g carbs, 0.5g fiber, 6g sugars, 34g protein

INGREDIENTS

Two 6-ounce raw tilapia fillets
½ cup pineapple or mango salsa
¼ cup sliced red onion

DIRECTIONS

Preheat oven to 375 degrees. Lay a large piece of heavy-duty foil on a baking sheet and spray with nonstick spray.

Lay fish on the center of the foil, and top with salsa and onion. Cover with another large piece of foil.

Fold together and seal all four edges of the foil pieces, forming a well-sealed packet. Bake for 15 minutes, or until fish is cooked through.

Cut packet to release steam before opening entirely. Mmmmm!

MAKES 2 SERVINGS

HUSTLE 'N BRUSSELS PACK ATTACK

182 calories PER SERVING

You'll Need: heavy-duty aluminum foil, baking sheet, nonstick spray, medium bowl
Prep: 10 minutes | **Cook:** 35 minutes

½ of pack:
182 calories, 2.75g fat, 513mg sodium, 35.5g carbs, 6.5g fiber, 5g sugars, 6g protein

INGREDIENTS

10 Brussels sprouts (or 14, if small), halved
10 ounces baby red potatoes, cut to same size as halved sprouts
½ cup chopped onion
1 teaspoon olive oil
1 teaspoon dried rosemary
½ teaspoon chopped garlic
½ teaspoon coarse salt

DIRECTIONS

Preheat oven to 400 degrees. Lay a large piece of heavy-duty foil on a baking sheet and spray with nonstick spray.

Mix all ingredients in a medium bowl. Distribute onto the center of the foil, and cover with another large piece of foil.

Fold together and seal all four edges of the foil pieces, forming a well-sealed packet. Bake for 30 to 35 minutes, or until veggies are tender.

Cut packet to release steam before opening entirely. Serve and eat!

MAKES 2 SERVINGS

CHICKEN-WITH-A-KICK PACK

245 calories

You'll Need: heavy-duty aluminum foil, baking sheet, nonstick spray, medium bowl
Prep: 10 minutes | **Cook:** 20 minutes

Entire recipe:
245 calories, 2g fat, 923mg sodium, 24.5g carbs, 5g fiber, 4.5g sugars, 31.5g protein

INGREDIENTS

4 ounces raw boneless skinless chicken breast, chopped
⅓ cup canned tomato sauce
¼ cup canned seasoned black beans, lightly drained
¼ cup canned sweet corn kernels, drained
¼ cup chopped green bell pepper
1 teaspoon hot sauce

Optional seasoning: salt

DIRECTIONS

Preheat oven to 375 degrees. Lay a large piece of heavy-duty foil on a baking sheet and spray with nonstick spray.

In a medium bowl, mix all ingredients. Distribute onto the center of the foil, and cover with another large piece of foil.

Fold together and seal all four edges of the foil pieces, forming a well-sealed packet. Bake for 20 minutes, or until chicken is cooked through.

Cut packet to release steam before opening entirely. Enjoy!

MAKES 1 SERVING

HG TIP:
Shave about 480mg sodium off this recipe by using no-salt-added tomato sauce and fresh or frozen corn.

SO-FANCY FISH PACK

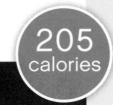

You'll Need: heavy-duty aluminum foil, baking sheet, nonstick spray, small bowl
Prep: 10 minutes
Cook: 15 minutes

Entire recipe: 205 calories, 4g fat, 412mg sodium, 6g carbs, 2.75g fiber, 3g sugars, 35g protein

INGREDIENTS

1 teaspoon light whipped butter or light buttery spread
½ teaspoon chopped fresh parsley
½ teaspoon crushed garlic
⅛ teaspoon salt
8 thin (or 6 thick) asparagus stalks, tough ends removed
One 6-ounce raw tilapia fillet
2 slices lemon

DIRECTIONS

Preheat oven to 375 degrees. Lay a large piece of heavy-duty foil on a baking sheet and spray with nonstick spray.

In a small bowl, mix butter, parsley, garlic, and salt.

Line up asparagus stalks on the center of the foil and top with fish. Spread with butter mixture and top with lemon slices. Cover with another large piece of foil.

Fold together and seal all four edges of the foil pieces, forming a well-sealed packet. Bake for 15 minutes, or until fish is cooked through and asparagus is tender.

Cut packet to release steam before opening entirely. Eat!

MAKES 1 SERVING

ROCKIN' CHICKEN RATATOUILLE

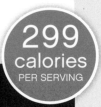

You'll Need: heavy-duty aluminum foil, baking sheet, nonstick spray, medium bowl, large bowl
Prep: 20 minutes
Cook: 30 minutes

½ of pack (about 2¼ cups): 299 calories, 2g fat, 660mg sodium, 32.5g carbs, 9.75g fiber, 18g sugars, 37.5g protein

INGREDIENTS

1 cup canned fire-roasted diced tomatoes, drained
½ cup tomato paste
¼ cup finely chopped fresh basil
1 teaspoon chopped garlic
⅛ teaspoon red pepper flakes
10 ounces raw boneless skinless chicken breast, cubed
⅛ teaspoon each salt and black pepper
1½ cups cubed eggplant
¾ cup chopped red bell pepper
¾ cup sliced and halved zucchini
¾ cup coarsely chopped onion

DIRECTIONS

Preheat oven to 375 degrees. Lay a large piece of heavy-duty foil on a baking sheet and spray with nonstick spray.

In a medium bowl, mix tomatoes, tomato paste, basil, garlic, and red pepper flakes.

Place chicken in a large bowl and season with salt and black pepper. Add all veggies, top with tomato mixture, and stir to coat.

Distribute mixture onto the center of the foil, and cover with another large piece of foil.

Fold together and seal all four edges of the foil pieces, forming a well-sealed packet. Bake for 30 minutes, or until chicken is cooked through and veggies are tender.

Cut packet to release steam before opening entirely. Eat up!

MAKES 2 SERVINGS

MOM-STYLE CREAMY CHICKEN 'N VEGGIES

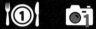

307 calories

You'll Need: heavy-duty aluminum foil, baking sheet, nonstick spray, large bowl
Prep: 10 minutes
Cook: 40 minutes

Entire recipe: 307 calories, 4g fat, 881mg sodium, 26g carbs, 5.25g fiber, 10.5g sugars, 40g protein

INGREDIENTS

¼ cup canned 98% fat-free cream of mushroom condensed soup
¼ cup fat-free sour cream
½ teaspoon chopped garlic
1 cup frozen cauliflower florets
½ cup frozen petite mixed vegetables
¼ cup canned sliced mushrooms, drained
One 5-ounce raw boneless skinless chicken breast cutlet

Optional seasonings: salt and black pepper

DIRECTIONS

Preheat oven to 375 degrees. Lay a large piece of heavy-duty foil on a baking sheet and spray with nonstick spray.

In a large bowl, mix condensed soup, sour cream, and garlic. Add cauliflower, mixed veggies, and mushrooms, and stir to coat.

Season chicken with salt and pepper, if you like, and place on the center of the foil. Top with veggie mixture, and cover with another large piece of foil.

Fold together and seal all four edges of the foil pieces, forming a well-sealed packet. Bake for 35 to 40 minutes, or until chicken is cooked through.

Cut packet to release steam before opening entirely. Now dig in!

MAKES 1 SERVING

HG ALTERNATIVE!
Thaw your frozen veggies first, and reduce your cook time to 25 minutes or so!

SESAME SALMON & SNAP PEAS

275 calories

You'll Need: heavy-duty aluminum foil, baking sheet, nonstick spray, wide bowl
Marinate: 15 minutes
Prep: 10 minutes
Cook: 15 minutes

Entire recipe: 275 calories, 15g fat, 460mg sodium, 10g carbs, 2g fiber, 6.5g sugars, 24.5g protein

INGREDIENTS

2 tablespoons low-fat sesame ginger dressing
⅛ teaspoon chopped garlic
Dash ground ginger
One 4-ounce raw skinless salmon fillet
1 cup sugar snap peas
½ teaspoon sesame seeds

DIRECTIONS

Preheat oven to 375 degrees. Lay a large piece of heavy-duty foil on a baking sheet and spray with nonstick spray.

In a wide bowl, mix dressing, garlic, and ginger. Add salmon and flip to coat. Cover and marinate in the fridge for 15 minutes.

Place snap peas onto the center of the foil and top with salmon. Drizzle with remaining marinade, and cover with another large piece of foil.

Fold together and seal all four edges of the foil pieces, forming a well-sealed packet. Bake for 15 minutes, or until salmon is cooked through and snap peas are tender.

Cut packet to release steam before opening entirely. Sprinkle with sesame seeds and enjoy!

MAKES 1 SERVING

CHA-CHA-CHERRY BBQ CHICKEN

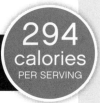

294 calories
PER SERVING

You'll Need: heavy-duty aluminum foil, baking sheet, nonstick spray, medium bowl
Prep: 10 minutes | **Cook:** 25 minutes

½ of pack (about 1 cup):
294 calories, 2g fat, 874mg sodium, 33.5g carbs, 1.5g fiber, 24.5g sugars, 34g protein

INGREDIENTS

10 ounces raw boneless skinless
chicken breast, cut into strips
⅛ teaspoon each salt and black pepper
1 cup sliced onion
½ cup frozen unsweetened pitted dark sweet
cherries, thawed, roughly chopped
½ cup BBQ sauce with 45 calories or
less per 2-tablespoon serving

DIRECTIONS

Preheat oven to 375 degrees. Lay a large piece of heavy-duty foil on a baking sheet and spray with nonstick spray.

Season chicken strips with salt and pepper. Distribute onto the center of the foil and top with onion.

In a medium bowl, mix chopped cherries with BBQ sauce. Pour mixture over the onion and chicken. Cover with another large piece of foil.

Fold together and seal all four edges of the foil pieces, forming a well-sealed packet. Bake for 25 minutes, or until chicken is cooked through.

Cut packet to release steam before opening entirely. Time to chew!

MAKES 2 SERVINGS

CRAZY PINEAPPLE SALMON TERIYAKI

347 calories

You'll Need: heavy-duty aluminum foil, baking sheet, nonstick spray, small bowl
Prep: 5 minutes | **Cook:** 20 minutes

Entire recipe:
347 calories, 15.5g fat, 349mg sodium, 22g carbs, 0.75g fiber, 19g sugars, 28.5g protein

INGREDIENTS

½ tablespoon teriyaki marinade or sauce
½ tablespoon sweet Asian chili sauce
One 5-ounce raw skinless salmon fillet
2 pineapple rings packed in juice, drained
Dash cayenne pepper

DIRECTIONS

Preheat oven to 375 degrees. Lay a large piece of heavy-duty foil on a baking sheet and spray with nonstick spray.

In a small bowl, mix teriyaki marinade/sauce with chili sauce.

Place salmon on the center of the foil, top with the sauce mixture, and flip to coat. Top with pineapple slices and sprinkle with cayenne pepper. Cover with another large piece of foil.

Fold together and seal all four edges of the foil pieces, forming a well-sealed packet. Bake for 20 minutes, or until fish is cooked through.

Cut packet to release steam before opening entirely. YUM!

MAKES 1 SERVING

THE RAT(ATOUILLE) PACK

168 calories

You'll Need: heavy-duty aluminum foil, baking sheet, nonstick spray, medium bowl
Prep: 20 minutes
Cook: 30 minutes

Entire recipe: 168 calories, 0.5g fat, 682mg sodium, 37.5g carbs, 10.5g fiber, 20g sugars, 7g protein

INGREDIENTS

¼ cup tomato paste
2 tablespoons finely chopped fresh basil
½ teaspoon chopped garlic
⅛ teaspoon salt, or more to taste
Dash red pepper flakes, or more to taste
Dash black pepper, or more to taste
1 cup cubed eggplant
½ cup chopped red bell pepper
½ cup sliced and halved zucchini
½ cup canned fire-roasted diced tomatoes, drained
½ cup coarsely chopped onion

DIRECTIONS

Preheat oven to 375 degrees. Lay a large piece of heavy-duty foil on a baking sheet and spray with nonstick spray.

In a medium bowl, mix tomato paste, basil, garlic, salt, red pepper flakes, and black pepper. Add all remaining ingredients and stir to coat. Distribute mixture onto the center of the foil. Cover with another large piece of foil.

Fold together and seal all four edges of the foil pieces, forming a well-sealed packet. Bake for 30 minutes, or until veggies are tender.

Cut packet to release steam before opening entirely. Mmmm!

MAKES 1 SERVING

DO THE CABBAGE PACK!

88 calories
PER SERVING

You'll Need: heavy-duty aluminum foil, baking sheet, nonstick spray
Prep: 10 minutes
Cook: 35 minutes

¼th of pack: 88 calories, 4.5g fat, 292mg sodium, 8g carbs, 2.5g fiber, 4.5g sugars, 5g protein

INGREDIENTS

½ head cabbage, cored
1 small onion, sliced
2 tablespoons light whipped butter or light buttery spread
¼ cup precooked real crumbled bacon
1 teaspoon chopped garlic
Dash each salt and black pepper, or more to taste
Dash paprika, or more to taste

DIRECTIONS

Preheat oven to 400 degrees. Lay a large piece of heavy-duty foil on a baking sheet and spray with nonstick spray.

Slice cabbage half into 4 thin wedges. Halve each wedge, leaving you with 8 "chunks." Distribute cabbage onto the center of the foil and top with onion. Dollop with butter and sprinkle with bacon, garlic, and seasonings. Cover with another large piece of foil.

Fold together and seal all four edges of the foil pieces, forming a well-sealed packet. Bake for 35 minutes, or until veggies are soft.

Cut packet to release steam before opening entirely. Mix well and eat up!

MAKES 4 SERVINGS

WOOHOO! BAYOU FISH PACK

270 calories PER SERVING

You'll Need: heavy-duty aluminum foil, baking sheet, nonstick spray, large bowl, small bowl
Prep: 10 minutes | **Cook:** 20 minutes

½ of pack:
270 calories, 2g fat, 592mg sodium, 32.5g carbs, 9.5g fiber, 8g sugars, 31g protein

INGREDIENTS

1 cup canned red kidney beans, drained and rinsed

½ cup finely chopped green bell pepper

½ cup finely chopped onion

½ cup finely chopped celery

¼ cup tomato paste

½ teaspoon Cajun seasoning

½ teaspoon chopped garlic

⅛ teaspoon ground thyme

⅛ teaspoon each salt and black pepper

Two 4-ounce raw flounder fillets

Optional topping: hot sauce

DIRECTIONS

Preheat oven to 350 degrees. Lay a large piece of heavy-duty foil on a baking sheet and spray with nonstick spray.

In a large bowl, mix beans, bell pepper, onion, and celery.

In a small bowl, mix tomato paste, ¼ teaspoon Cajun seasoning, garlic, thyme, salt, and black pepper. Add to the large bowl and stir to coat. Distribute mixture onto the center of the foil.

Season flounder with remaining ¼ teaspoon Cajun seasoning and place over the mixture on the foil. Cover with another large piece of foil.

Fold together and seal all four edges of the foil pieces, forming a well-sealed packet. Bake for 20 minutes, or until flounder is cooked through and veggies are tender.

Cut packet to release steam before opening it entirely. Enjoy!

MAKES 2 SERVINGS

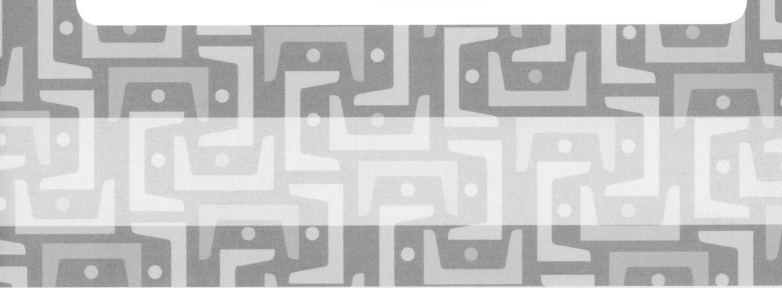

SWEET POTATO APPLE PACK

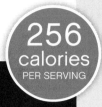

256 calories PER SERVING

You'll Need: heavy-duty aluminum foil, baking sheet, nonstick spray
Prep: 10 minutes
Cook: 25 minutes

½ of pack (1 heaping cup): 256 calories, 4g fat, 288mg sodium, 55g carbs, 7.25g fiber, 29g sugars, 2.5g protein

INGREDIENTS

9 ounces sweet potato, peeled and cut into bite-sized chunks
1 large Fuji apple, cored and cut into bite-sized chunks
2 tablespoons dried sweetened cranberries
1½ tablespoons light whipped butter or light buttery spread
1½ tablespoons brown sugar (not packed)
¼ teaspoon cinnamon, or more to taste
⅛ teaspoon salt, or more to taste
Dash ground nutmeg, or more to taste

DIRECTIONS

Preheat oven to 350 degrees. Lay a large piece of heavy-duty foil on a baking sheet and spray with nonstick spray.

Distribute potato, apple, and cranberries onto the center of the foil. Dollop with butter and sprinkle with brown sugar, cinnamon, salt, and nutmeg. Cover with another large piece of foil.

Fold together and seal all four edges of the foil pieces, forming a well-sealed packet. Bake for 25 minutes, or until potato and apple are tender.

Cut packet to release steam before opening entirely. Mix well and enjoy!

MAKES 2 SERVINGS

STEAMY CREAMY SQUASH

80 calories PER SERVING

You'll Need: heavy-duty aluminum foil, baking sheet, nonstick spray, medium bowl, small microwave-safe bowl
Prep: 10 minutes
Cook: 20 minutes

½ of pack (about 1 cup): 80 calories, 2.75g fat, 232mg sodium, 11g carbs, 3g fiber, 5g sugars, 3.5g protein

INGREDIENTS

2 zucchini (or yellow summer squash), stem ends removed
½ cup thinly sliced onion
2 teaspoons light whipped butter or light buttery spread
⅛ teaspoon dried oregano
Dash each salt and black pepper, or more to taste
½ teaspoon chopped garlic
1 wedge The Laughing Cow Light Creamy Swiss cheese

DIRECTIONS

Preheat oven to 375 degrees. Lay a large piece of heavy-duty foil on a baking sheet and spray with nonstick spray.

Thinly slice zucchini lengthwise into wide, flat strips. Cut strips in half widthwise and distribute onto the center of the foil. Top with onion, dollop with butter, and sprinkle with oregano, salt, pepper, and garlic. Cover with another large piece of foil.

Fold together and seal all four edges of the foil pieces, forming a well-sealed packet. Bake for 20 minutes, or until veggies are tender.

Cut packet to release steam before opening entirely. Transfer veggies to a medium bowl.

In a small microwave-safe bowl, microwave cheese wedge for 20 seconds, or until warm. Stir until smooth, add to veggies, and stir to coat. EAT!

MAKES 2 SERVINGS

JUMP FOR CHOY! FISH PACK

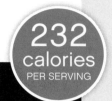
232 calories PER SERVING

You'll Need: heavy-duty aluminum foil, baking sheet, nonstick spray, small bowl
Prep: 10 minutes
Cook: 20 minutes

½ of pack: 232 calories, 2g fat, 656mg sodium, 19.5g carbs, 3g fiber, 13g sugars, 35g protein

INGREDIENTS

1 pound baby bok choy, ends removed, separated into leaves

1 cup zucchini cut into 1/2-inch chunks

12 ounces raw cod (two 6-ounce fillets or four 3-ounce fillets)

2 tablespoons thick teriyaki marinade or sauce

2 tablespoons low-sugar or sugar-free orange marmalade

Optional seasonings: salt and black pepper

DIRECTIONS

Preheat oven to 375 degrees. Lay a large piece of heavy-duty foil on a baking sheet and spray with nonstick spray.

Distribute bok choy onto the center of the foil and top with zucchini. Lay cod over the veggies.

In a small bowl, thoroughly mix teriyaki marinade or sauce with orange marmalade. Evenly spoon mixture over the cod and veggies. Cover with another large piece of foil.

Fold together and seal all four edges of the foil pieces, forming a well-sealed packet. Bake for 20 minutes, or until cod is cooked through and veggies are tender.

Cut packet to release steam before opening entirely. Eat up!

MAKES 2 SERVINGS

MEGA-MAZING VEGGIE PACK

97 calories PER SERVING

You'll Need: heavy-duty aluminum foil, baking sheet, nonstick spray, small bowl
Prep: 10 minutes
Cook: 20 minutes

¼th of pack (about ¾ cup): 97 calories, 0.5g fat, 359mg sodium, 22g carbs, 3g fiber, 11g sugars, 2.5g protein

INGREDIENTS

6 ounces kale leaves, torn or cut into large pieces

2 cups chopped red bell peppers

One 8-ounce can sliced water chestnuts, drained

¼ cup sweet Asian chili sauce

1 tablespoon seasoned rice vinegar

1 teaspoon chopped garlic

⅛ teaspoon each salt and black pepper

DIRECTIONS

Preheat oven to 375 degrees. Lay a large piece of heavy-duty foil on a baking sheet and spray with nonstick spray.

Distribute kale onto the center of the foil. Top with bell peppers and water chestnuts.

In a small bowl, mix chili sauce, rice vinegar, and garlic. Drizzle over veggies. Cover with another large piece of foil.

Fold together and seal all four edges of the foil pieces, forming a well-sealed packet. Bake for 20 minutes, or until veggies are tender.

Cut packet to release steam before opening entirely. Season with salt and black pepper, mix well, and enjoy!

MAKES 4 SERVINGS

SPINACH ARTICHOKE CHICKEN

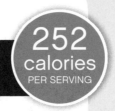

252 calories
PER SERVING

You'll Need: heavy-duty aluminum foil, baking sheet, nonstick spray, skillet, medium microwave-safe bowl
Prep: 10 minutes | **Cook:** 30 minutes

½ of pack (1 cutlet):
252 calories, 4.5g fat, 836mg sodium, 12g carbs, 3g fiber, 3.5g sugars, 38g protein

INGREDIENTS

2 cups chopped spinach leaves
2 wedges The Laughing Cow Light
    Creamy Swiss cheese
1 tablespoon fat-free mayonnaise
2 artichoke hearts packed in water,
    drained and chopped
1 tablespoon reduced-fat Parmesan-style
    grated topping
1 teaspoon garlic powder
Two 5-ounce raw boneless skinless chicken
    breast cutlets
⅛ teaspoon each salt and black pepper
½ cup sliced onion

Optional seasoning: cayenne pepper

DIRECTIONS

Preheat oven to 375 degrees. Lay a large piece of heavy-duty foil on a baking sheet and spray with nonstick spray.

Bring a skillet sprayed with nonstick spray to medium heat. Cook and stir spinach until wilted, about 3 minutes. Remove from heat and thoroughly blot to remove excess moisture.

In a medium microwave-safe bowl, microwave cheese wedges for 20 seconds, or until warm. Add mayo and thoroughly mix. Stir in spinach, artichoke hearts, Parm-style topping, garlic powder and, if you like, a dash or two of cayenne pepper.

Season chicken cutlets with salt and pepper, and place side by side on the center of the foil. Evenly top with onion and spinach-artichoke mixture. Cover with another large piece of foil.

Fold together and seal all four edges of the foil pieces, forming a well-sealed packet. Bake for 25 minutes, or until chicken is cooked through.

Cut packet to release steam before opening entirely. Enjoy!

MAKES 2 SERVINGS

Flip to the photo inserts to see over 100 recipe pics! And for photos of ALL the recipes, go to **hungry-girl.com/books.**

SPICY SHRIMP 'N VEGGIES

   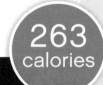

263 calories

You'll Need: heavy-duty aluminum foil, baking sheet, nonstick spray, large bowl
Prep: 15 minutes
Cook: 15 minutes

Entire recipe: 263 calories, 2g fat, 804mg sodium, 28g carbs, 8g fiber, 12g sugars, 32.5g protein

INGREDIENTS

¾ cup canned crushed tomatoes
1 teaspoon chopped garlic
¼ teaspoon red pepper flakes
⅛ teaspoon black pepper
5 ounces raw shrimp, peeled, tails removed, deveined
1 cup small broccoli florets
½ cup chopped bell pepper
¼ cup chopped onion

Optional seasonings: salt and black pepper

DIRECTIONS

Preheat oven to 375 degrees. Lay a large piece of heavy-duty foil on a baking sheet and spray with nonstick spray.

In a large bowl, mix crushed tomatoes, garlic, red pepper flakes, and black pepper. Stir in remaining ingredients. Distribute onto the center of the foil, and cover with another large piece of foil.

Fold together and seal all four edges of the foil pieces, forming a well-sealed packet. Bake for 15 minutes, or until shrimp are cooked through and veggies are tender.

Cut packet to release steam before opening entirely. Yum!

MAKES 1 SERVING

HG ALTERNATIVE!
Use just a dash of red pepper flakes for less heat.

RAGIN' CAJUN SHRIMP

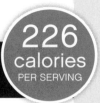

226 calories PER SERVING

You'll Need: heavy-duty aluminum foil, baking sheet, nonstick spray, small microwave-safe bowl, large bowl
Prep: 15 minutes
Cook: 20 minutes

½ of pack: 226 calories, 6.5g fat, 587mg sodium, 12g carbs, 2g fiber, 5g sugars, 27g protein

INGREDIENTS

2 tablespoons lime juice
2 tablespoons light whipped butter or light buttery spread
1 teaspoon cornstarch
1½ teaspoons Cajun seasoning
10 ounces raw shrimp, peeled, tails removed, deveined
⅛ teaspoon garlic powder
1 cup sliced bell pepper cut into 2-inch strips
1 cup sliced onion cut into 2-inch strips

Optional seasonings: salt and black pepper

DIRECTIONS

Preheat oven to 375 degrees. Lay a large piece of heavy-duty foil on a baking sheet and spray with nonstick spray.

In a small microwave-safe bowl, microwave lime juice with butter for 30 seconds, or until butter is mostly melted. Mix in cornstarch and 1 teaspoon Cajun seasoning.

Place shrimp in a large bowl and sprinkle with garlic powder and remaining ½ teaspoon Cajun seasoning. Add veggies and lime-butter mixture, and toss to coat. Distribute onto the center of the foil, and cover with another large piece of foil.

Fold together and seal all four edges of the foil pieces, forming a well-sealed packet. Bake for 20 minutes, or until shrimp are cooked through and veggies are tender.

Cut packet to release steam before opening entirely. Eat up!

MAKES 2 SERVINGS

APPLE RAISIN CHICKEN

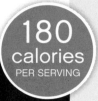

301 calories
PER SERVING

You'll Need: heavy-duty aluminum foil, baking sheet, nonstick spray, large bowl, medium bowl, whisk
Prep: 15 minutes
Cook: 25 minutes

½ of pack: 301 calories, 2g fat, 297mg sodium, 35g carbs, 3g fiber, 25g sugars, 34g protein

INGREDIENTS

10 ounces raw boneless skinless chicken breast, cut into strips
⅛ teaspoon each salt and black pepper
1 cup chopped onion
1 cup chopped apple
2 tablespoons raisins, chopped
¼ cup balsamic vinegar
1 tablespoon brown sugar (not packed)
1½ teaspoons cornstarch
1 teaspoon Dijon mustard

DIRECTIONS

Preheat oven to 375 degrees. Lay a large piece of heavy-duty foil on a baking sheet and spray with nonstick spray.

Season chicken strips with salt and pepper and distribute onto the center of the foil.

In a large bowl, mix onion, apple, and raisins. In a medium bowl, whisk all remaining ingredients until cornstarch has dissolved. Pour contents of the small bowl into the large bowl and toss to coat.

Evenly spoon mixture over chicken. Cover with another large piece of foil.

Fold together and seal all four edges of the foil pieces, forming a well-sealed packet. Bake for 25 minutes, or until chicken is fully cooked and onion and apple are tender.

Cut packet to release steam before opening entirely. Chew!

MAKES 2 SERVINGS

FLOUNDER L'ORANGE

180 calories
PER SERVING

You'll Need: heavy-duty aluminum foil, baking sheet, nonstick spray, small bowl
Prep: 10 minutes
Cook: 15 minutes

½ of pack (1 fillet with veggies):
180 calories, 5g fat, 602mg sodium, 17g carbs, 3.5g fiber, 9.5g sugars, 16.5g protein

INGREDIENTS

2 tablespoons low-sugar orange marmalade
1 tablespoon light whipped butter or light buttery spread
1 teaspoon Dijon mustard
2 cups bagged broccoli cole slaw
1 cup thinly sliced onion
Two 4-ounce raw flounder fillets
⅛ teaspoon each salt and black pepper

DIRECTIONS

Preheat oven to 375 degrees. Lay a large piece of heavy-duty foil on a baking sheet and spray with nonstick spray.

In a small bowl, mix marmalade, butter, and mustard.

Distribute broccoli slaw onto the center of the foil and top with onion. Season fillets with salt and pepper and place over the veggies. Evenly top with marmalade mixture. Cover with another large piece of foil.

Fold together and seal all four edges of the foil pieces, forming a well-sealed packet. Bake for 15 minutes, or until fish is cooked through and veggies are tender.

Cut packet to release steam before opening entirely. Eat!

MAKES 2 SERVINGS

MANGO CHICKEN

318 calories

You'll Need: heavy-duty aluminum foil, baking sheet, nonstick spray, medium bowl
Prep: 15 minutes
Cook: 25 minutes

Entire recipe: 318 calories, 2g fat, 863mg sodium, 36.5g carbs, 5g fiber, 19g sugars, 37.5g protein

INGREDIENTS

One 5-ounce raw boneless skinless
    chicken breast cutlet, pounded to
    ½-inch thickness
1 teaspoon onion soup/dip seasoning mix
¼ teaspoon onion powder
¼ teaspoon garlic powder
¾ cup sliced onion
½ cup cubed mango
¼ cup canned black beans, drained
    and rinsed
1½ teaspoons chopped cilantro
1 teaspoon seasoned rice vinegar
⅛ teaspoon each salt and black pepper

DIRECTIONS

Preheat oven to 375 degrees. Lay a large piece of heavy-duty foil on a baking sheet and spray with nonstick spray.

Season chicken with onion seasoning mix, onion powder, and garlic powder and lay cutlets on the center of the foil. Top with onion and mango.

In a medium bowl, mix all remaining ingredients. Evenly spoon over contents of the foil. Cover with another large piece of foil.

Fold together and seal all four edges of the foil pieces, forming a well-sealed packet. Bake for 25 minutes, or until chicken is cooked through and onion is tender.

Cut packet to release steam before opening entirely. Yum!

MAKES 1 SERVING

SWEET & SOUR CABBAGE

154 calories PER SERVING

You'll Need: heavy-duty aluminum foil, baking sheet, nonstick spray, medium microwave-safe bowl
Prep: 25 minutes
Cook: 30 minutes

¼th of pack (about 1¾ cups): 154 calories, <0.5g fat, 492mg sodium, 37g carbs, 4.5g fiber, 25.5g sugars, 3g protein

INGREDIENTS

Two 8-ounce cans pineapple chunks packed
    in juice (not drained)
1 tablespoon cornstarch
3 tablespoons seasoned rice vinegar
1 tablespoon ketchup
1 tablespoon reduced-sodium/lite soy sauce
½ teaspoon chopped garlic
¼ teaspoon red pepper flakes
⅛ teaspoon ground ginger
½ head cabbage, cored and chopped
2 cups chopped onion

Optional seasonings: salt and black pepper

DIRECTIONS

Preheat oven to 375 degrees. Lay a large piece of heavy-duty foil on a baking sheet and spray with nonstick spray.

Drain and discard juice from one can of pineapple. Drain juice from the other can into a medium microwave-safe bowl. Set pineapple chunks aside.

To make the sauce, add cornstarch to the microwave-safe bowl of juice and stir to dissolve. Mix in vinegar, ketchup, soy sauce, garlic, red pepper flakes, and ginger. Microwave for 1½ minutes, or until slightly thickened. Mix well.

Distribute cabbage, onion, and pineapple chunks onto the center of the foil. Evenly top with sauce, and cover with another large piece of foil.

Fold together and seal all four edges of the foil pieces, forming a well-sealed packet. Bake for 25 minutes, or until veggies have softened.

Cut packet to release steam before opening entirely. Mix well and dive in!

MAKES 4 SERVINGS

CHAPTER 8

CROCK POTS

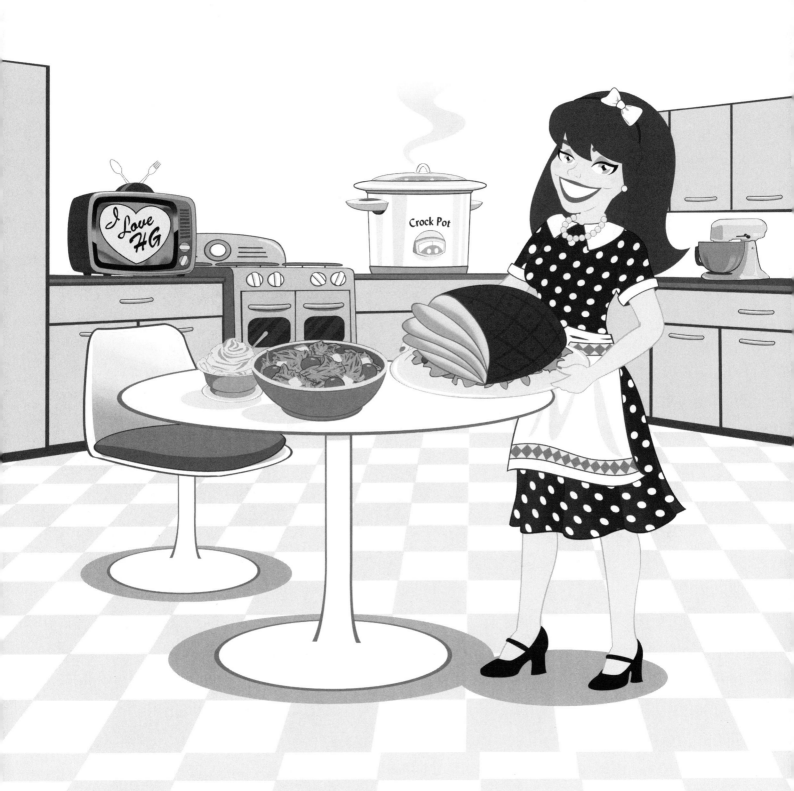

CROCK POTS

Very VERY Veggie Stew

Dan-Good Cioppino

Chicken and Sausage Gumbo

Hungry Chick Chunky Soup

Thick 'n Hearty Big Bean Soup

Asian Beef Noodle Soup

Split Pea Soup

Zesty Garden Zuppa

Beefy Chili

Chunky Veggie Pumpkin Chili

Chicken Chili Surprise

EZ as 1-2-3-Alarm Turkey Chili

Crazy-Delicious Seafood Corn Chowder

Spicy Southwest Chicken Chowder

Ten-Alarm Southwestern Corn Chowder

Slow-Cookin' BBQ Chicken

Slow-Cookin' Mexican Chicken

'Cue the Pulled Pork

Pulled BBQ Beef

Pump-Up-the-Jam Cocktail Weenies

Flaming Cocktail Weenies

Peach-BBQ Cocktail Weenies

Sweet-Hot Steak Bites

Crock-Pot Fake-Baked Beans

Fruity & Tangy Cocktail Meatballs

Turkey-rific Taco Bean Dip

Glaze-of-Glory Candied Carrots

Pump-Up-the-Jam Chicken

Turkey Mushroom Surprise

Crock-Pot Roast

Crock-Pot Coq Au Vin

Cheeseburger Mac Attack

Outside-In Turkey Tamale Pie

Cranberry & Apple Chicken

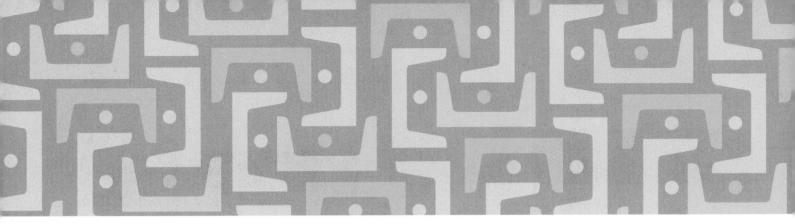

Crock-pot cooking is hugely popular because of how simple it is . . . and how AWESOME the results are. Here are over thirty recipes for you slow-cooker fans out there . . .

READY TO CROCK?

For these recipes, make sure your crock pot has at least a 4-quart capacity.

A QUICK GUIDE TO SYMBOLS:

15 Minutes or Less

This symbol lets you know a recipe should take you no more than fifteen minutes from start to finish! That includes prep and cook time.

30 Minutes or Less

Just like the 15-minute version, this one points out recipes that take 30 minutes or less to whip up.

Meatless

You guessed it—no meat here! That includes beef, poultry, and fish. Some recipes give the option of a meatless ingredient. If you want your meal without meat, go with the meatless choice.

Single Serving

Pretty straightforward. These are recipes for one.

5 Ingredients or Less

Fans of HG know that we like to keep things simple. And these recipes contain just five ingredients or less!

Photos

These recipes can be seen in one of the book's photo inserts. The number in the symbol tells you which insert. Find photos of all the recipes at hungry-girl.com/books!

VERY VERY VEGGIE STEW

100 calories PER SERVING

You'll Need: crock pot, large bowl
Prep: 15 minutes
Cook: 3 to 4 hours *or* 7 to 8 hours

⅛th **of recipe (about 1 cup):** 100 calories, 1g fat, 296mg sodium, 20g carbs, 6g fiber, 7g sugars, 4g protein

INGREDIENTS

1 cup canned chickpeas, drained and rinsed
1 eggplant, peeled and cut into ½-inch cubes
2 cups coarsely chopped zucchini
1 cup coarsely chopped carrots
1 cup cubed butternut squash
1 cup chopped onion
1 tomato, coarsely chopped
1½ cups fat-free vegetable broth
One 6-ounce can tomato paste
1 tablespoon chopped garlic
1 teaspoon olive oil
1 teaspoon dried basil
⅓ teaspoon cinnamon
¼ teaspoon salt, or more to taste
⅛ teaspoon paprika
⅛ teaspoon ground ginger
1 no-calorie sweetener packet

DIRECTIONS

Place the chickpeas and all the veggies in a crock pot.

In a large bowl, combine all other ingredients. Mix well and pour evenly over the contents of the crock pot. Gently stir to allow the sauce to coat the veggies.

Cover and cook on high for 3 to 4 hours *or* on low for 7 to 8 hours. Enjoy!

MAKES 8 SERVINGS

DAN-GOOD CIOPPINO

169 calories PER SERVING

You'll Need: crock pot
Prep: 10 minutes
Cook: 3 to 4 hours

⅛th **of recipe (about 1 cup):** 169 calories, 3g fat, 794mg sodium, 18.5g carbs, 1.25g fiber, 10.5g sugars, 16.5g protein

INGREDIENTS

Four 14.5-ounce cans (about 7 cups) creamy tomato soup with 4g fat or less per serving
One 10-ounce can whole baby clams, drained
One 6-ounce can lump crabmeat, drained
8 ounces raw large scallops, quartered
8 ounces raw shrimp, peeled, tails removed, deveined
4 cloves fresh garlic, crushed
2 dried bay leaves

DIRECTIONS

Place all ingredients in a crock pot and stir.

Cover and cook on low for 3 to 4 hours, until scallops and shrimp are cooked through.

Remove and discard bay leaves. EAT!

MAKES 9 SERVINGS

WHO'S DAN?

Dan is my super-talented husband. He came up with this recipe!

CHICKEN AND SAUSAGE GUMBO

117 calories PER SERVING

You'll Need: crock pot, large bowl
Prep: 10 minutes
Cook: 3 to 4 hours *or* 7 to 8 hours

¹⁄₁₀th of recipe (about 1 cup): 117 calories, 3.5g fat, 523mg sodium, 8g carbs, 2g fiber, 3.5g sugars, 13g protein

INGREDIENTS

8 ounces raw boneless skinless chicken breast cutlets

⅛ teaspoon each salt and black pepper

12 ounces (about 4 links) fully cooked chicken sausage, sliced into ¼-inch coins

One 14.5-ounce can diced tomatoes with green chiles (not drained)

3 cups (24 ounces) reduced-sodium fat-free chicken broth

2 cups frozen cut okra

1½ cups chopped celery

1 green bell pepper, stem removed, seeded, chopped

1 large onion, chopped

1½ teaspoons Cajun seasoning

1 teaspoon chopped garlic

1 teaspoon Worcestershire sauce

1 teaspoon ground thyme

DIRECTIONS

Season chicken with salt and pepper, and place it in a crock pot. Add all remaining ingredients and lightly stir.

Cover and cook on high for 3 to 4 hours *or* on low for 7 to 8 hours, until chicken is fully cooked.

Remove chicken and place in a large bowl. Shred with two forks—one to hold the chicken in place and the other to scrape across and shred it.

Return shredded chicken to the crock pot, and give your gumbo a stir. Serve it up!

MAKES 10 SERVINGS

HUNGRY CHICK CHUNKY SOUP

150 calories PER SERVING

You'll Need: crock pot, large bowl
Prep: 20 minutes
Cook: 3 to 4 hours *or* 7 to 8 hours

¹⁄₁₀th of recipe (about 1 cup): 150 calories, 1g fat, 570mg sodium, 15g carbs, 4.25g fiber, 5g sugars, 20.5g protein

INGREDIENTS

1½ pounds raw boneless skinless chicken breasts, halved

½ teaspoon salt

⅛ teaspoon black pepper

Two 14.5-ounce cans (about 3½ cups) fat-free chicken broth

One 15-ounce can cannellini (white kidney) beans, drained and rinsed

One 14.5-ounce can stewed tomatoes (not drained)

2 cups bagged coleslaw mix

2 carrots, chopped

1 small onion, finely diced

1 cup frozen peas

¼ teaspoon ground thyme

1 dried bay leaf

DIRECTIONS

Season chicken with ¼ teaspoon salt and the pepper. Place all ingredients *except* remaining salt in a crock pot and stir. Cover and cook on high for 3 to 4 hours *or* on low for 7 to 8 hours, until chicken is fully cooked.

Remove and discard the bay leaf. Transfer chicken to a large bowl. Shred with two forks—one to hold the chicken in place and the other to scrape across and shred it.

Stir shredded chicken and remaining ¼ teaspoon salt into the soup in the crock pot. Serve up and enjoy!

MAKES 10 SERVINGS

THICK 'N HEARTY BIG BEAN SOUP

176 calories PER SERVING

You'll Need: crock pot, blender | **Prep:** 20 minutes | **Cook:** 3 to 4 hours *or* 7 to 8 hours

⅛th of recipe (1 heaping cup):
176 calories, 1g fat, 774mg sodium, 33g carbs, 9g fiber, 5.5g sugars, 9.5g protein

INGREDIENTS

One 15.5-ounce can cannellini (white kidney) beans, drained and rinsed

One 15-ounce can chickpeas/garbanzo beans, drained and rinsed

One 15-ounce can black beans, drained and rinsed

4 cups (32 ounces) fat-free vegetable broth

3 cups chopped portabella mushrooms

2 cups chopped onion

1¼ cups chopped carrots

½ tablespoon chopped garlic

¼ teaspoon ground cumin

¼ teaspoon each salt and black pepper

DIRECTIONS

Add all ingredients to a crock pot and stir well.

Cover and cook on high for 3 to 4 hours *or* on low for 7 to 8 hours, until veggies are soft.

Stir well. Transfer 2 cups to a blender and let slightly cool. Blend at high speed until smooth. Stir mixture into the contents of crock pot. Enjoy!

MAKES 8 SERVINGS

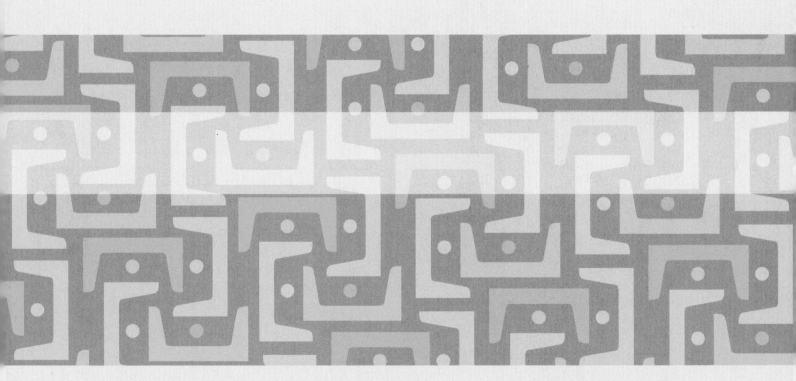

ASIAN BEEF NOODLE SOUP

89 calories
PER SERVING

You'll Need: strainer, large microwave-safe bowl, crock pot
Prep: 20 minutes
Cook: 3 to 4 hours *or* 7 to 8 hours

⅒th of recipe (about 1 cup): 89 calories, 2g fat, 632mg sodium, 6.5g carbs, 2.5g fiber, 1.5g sugars, 11g protein

INGREDIENTS

2 bags House Foods Tofu Shirataki Fettuccine Shaped Noodle Substitute
12 ounces raw lean beefsteak, cut into small pieces
⅛ teaspoon each salt and black pepper
5 cups (40 ounces) fat-free beef broth
One 15-ounce can straw mushrooms, drained
One 8-ounce can bamboo shoots, drained
1 cup chopped onion
1 cup shredded carrots
2½ teaspoons reduced-sodium/lite soy sauce
2 teaspoons chopped garlic
1 teaspoon chopped fresh ginger
1 teaspoon red pepper flakes

DIRECTIONS

Use a strainer to rinse and drain noodles. Pat dry. In a large microwave-safe bowl, microwave noodles for 2 minutes. Drain excess liquid and thoroughly pat dry. Roughly cut noodles and place in a crock pot.

Season beef with salt and pepper, and add to the crock pot. Add all remaining ingredients and stir.

Cover and cook on high for 3 to 4 hours *or* on low for 7 to 8 hours, until beef is fully cooked. Serve and enjoy!

MAKES 10 SERVINGS

HG FYI:
Flip to page 192 for the Tofu Shirataki 411!

SPLIT PEA SOUP

157 calories
PER SERVING

You'll Need: crock pot, blender
Prep: 25 minutes
Cook: 5 to 6 hours

⅐th of recipe (about 1 cup): 157 calories, 0.5g fat, 699mg sodium, 29g carbs, 9.5g fiber, 6.5g sugars, 9.5g protein

INGREDIENTS

1¼ cups dried split peas, rinsed
2 cups finely chopped onion
2 cups finely chopped celery
1½ tablespoons chopped garlic
5 cups (40 ounces) fat-free vegetable broth
½ teaspoon salt, or more to taste
¼ teaspoon black pepper, or more to taste

Optional seasonings: cayenne pepper, garlic powder

DIRECTIONS

Evenly layer peas, onion, celery, and garlic in a crock pot. Pour in broth. Do *not* stir. Cover and cook on high for 5 to 6 hours, until peas are soft.

Add salt and black pepper and thoroughly stir. Carefully transfer half of the mixture (about 3½ cups) to a blender and let slightly cool. Pulse until smooth.

Return mixture to the crock pot and stir well. Eat!

MAKES 7 SERVINGS

For more recipes, tips & tricks, sign up for FREE daily emails at **hungry-girl.com!**

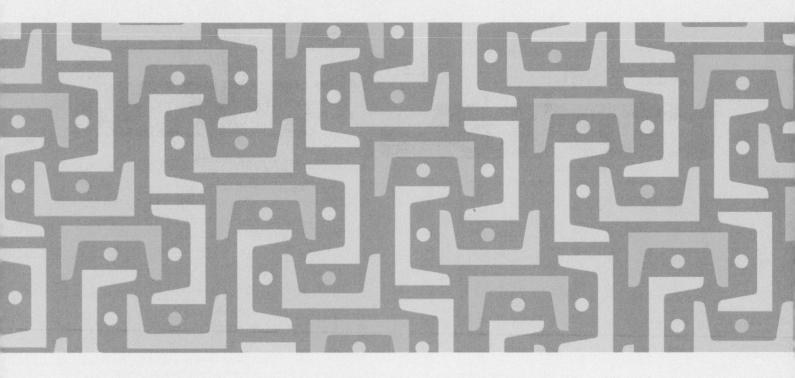

ZESTY GARDEN ZUPPA

135 calories PER SERVING

You'll Need: crock pot | **Prep:** 25 minutes | **Cook:** 3 to 4 hours *or* 7 to 8 hours

⅛th of recipe (about 1 cup):
135 calories, 3.5g fat, 645mg sodium, 16.5g carbs, 2g fiber, 4g sugars, 9g protein

INGREDIENTS

12 ounces red potatoes, halved and sliced

4 cups (32 ounces) fat-free chicken broth

3 cups chopped kale leaves

2 cups chopped onion

1 cup chopped red bell pepper

½ tablespoon chopped garlic

¼ teaspoon each salt and black pepper

¼ teaspoon red pepper flakes

3 links uncooked sweet Italian turkey sausage with 10g fat or less each

½ cup fat-free half & half

Optional topping: fresh chopped parsley

DIRECTIONS

Place all ingredients *except* sausage and half & half in a crock pot and stir well.

Remove and discard sausage casings, and cut sausage into bite-sized pieces. Evenly top contents of the crock pot with sausage pieces.

Cover and cook on high for 3 to 4 hours *or* on low for 7 to 8 hours, until veggies are soft and sausage is fully cooked.

Stir in half & half. Serve it up!

MAKES 8 SERVINGS

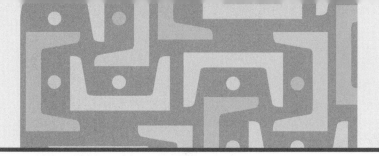

SODIUM-SLASHING SWAPS

* **Broth:**
  Using no-salt-added broth instead of regular will save 400mg of sodium per cup.

* **Salsa:**
  Swap premade versions for chopped tomatoes, onions, and herbs to save 700mg of sodium per ½ cup.

* **Deli Meat:**
  Look for reduced-sodium or no-salt-added slices. Or bake your own poultry and slice it thin to save 250mg of sodium per ounce.

* **Canned Beans:**
  Rinsing them (as called for in these recipes) saves you about 20 percent of the sodium amount listed on the can. Seek out no-salt-added beans and save another 500mg of sodium per cup.

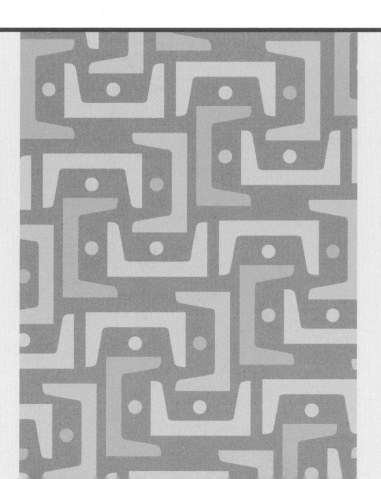

BEEFY CHILI

209 calories PER SERVING

You'll Need: crock pot
Prep: 30 minutes
Cook: 3 to 4 hours *or* 7 to 8 hours

⅒th **of recipe (about 1 cup):** 209 calories, 3.5g fat, 808mg sodium, 28g carbs, 7g fiber, 8g sugars, 16.5g protein

INGREDIENTS

One 1-pound raw lean beef tenderloin roast, trimmed of excess fat, quartered

¼ teaspoon each salt and black pepper

One 29-ounce can tomato sauce

One 15-ounce can chili beans (pinto beans in chili sauce), not drained

One 15-ounce can red kidney beans, drained and rinsed

One 14.5-ounce can diced tomatoes, drained

2 cups chopped onion

1 cup chopped green bell pepper

1 cup frozen sweet corn kernels

2 tablespoons chopped canned chipotle peppers in adobo sauce

2 teaspoons chopped garlic

1 teaspoon chili powder

1 teaspoon ground cumin

Optional topping: fat-free sour cream

DIRECTIONS

Season beef with salt and black pepper and place in a crock pot. Add remaining ingredients and gently mix; make sure beef stays at the bottom of the crock pot.

Cover and cook on high for 3 to 4 hours *or* on low for 7 to 8 hours, until beef is fully cooked.

Remove beef and cut into bite-sized pieces. Stir into the chili and enjoy!

MAKES 10 SERVINGS

CHUNKY VEGGIE PUMPKIN CHILI

131 calories PER SERVING

You'll Need: crock pot
Prep: 15 minutes
Cook: 3 to 4 hours *or* 7 to 8 hours

1/11th **of recipe (about 1 cup):** 131 calories, 1g fat, 515mg sodium, 25g carbs, 6.5g fiber, 7g sugars, 6.5g protein

INGREDIENTS

One 28-ounce can crushed tomatoes

One 15-ounce can pure pumpkin

2 teaspoons chopped garlic

½ tablespoon cayenne pepper, or more to taste

1 teaspoon chili powder

1 teaspoon pumpkin pie spice

½ teaspoon ground cumin

¼ teaspoon salt, or more to taste

One 15-ounce can chili beans (pinto beans in chili sauce), not drained

One 15-ounce can black beans, drained and rinsed

One 14.5-ounce can diced tomatoes

2 cups chopped portabella mushrooms

1½ cups chopped zucchini

1½ cups chopped onion

½ cup canned diced green chiles

DIRECTIONS

Add crushed tomatoes, pumpkin, garlic, and all the seasonings to a crock pot. Mix well.

Add all remaining ingredients and stir thoroughly.

Cover and cook on high for 3 to 4 hours *or* on low for 7 to 8 hours. Enjoy!

MAKES 11 SERVINGS

CHICKEN CHILI SURPRISE

175 calories PER SERVING

You'll Need: blender or food processor, crock pot, large bowl
Prep: 20 minutes
Cook: 3 to 4 hours *or* 7 to 8 hours

¹⁄₁₀th of recipe (about 1 cup): 175 calories, 1.25g fat, 531mg sodium, 19g carbs, 4.75g fiber, 2g sugars, 22g protein

INGREDIENTS

Two 15-ounce cans cannellini (white kidney) beans, drained and rinsed
4 cups (32 ounces) fat-free chicken broth
1½ pounds raw boneless skinless chicken breasts, halved
¼ teaspoon each salt and black pepper
One 7-ounce can diced green chiles, lightly drained
1 small onion, chopped
1 cup finely chopped celery
1 cup frozen white corn kernels
1 tablespoon chopped garlic
1 teaspoon chili powder
½ teaspoon ground cumin
½ teaspoon hot sauce
½ teaspoon dried oregano

Optional toppings: salsa, fat-free sour cream

DIRECTIONS

Place 1 can's worth of beans in a blender or food processor. Add 1 cup broth and puree until smooth. Transfer to a crock pot.

Season chicken with salt and pepper and add to the crock pot. Add remaining can's worth of beans, remaining 3 cups broth, and all other ingredients.

Cover and cook on high for 3 to 4 hours *or* on low for 7 to 8 hours, until chicken is fully cooked.

Transfer chicken to a large bowl. Shred with two forks—one to hold the chicken in place and the other to scrape across and shred it. Return the shredded chicken to the crock pot, and stir into the chili. Eat up!

MAKES 10 SERVINGS

EZ AS 1-2-3-ALARM TURKEY CHILI

176 calories PER SERVING

You'll Need: large bowl, crock pot
Prep: 20 minutes
Cook: 3 to 4 hours *or* 7 to 8 hours

¹⁄₁₂th of recipe (about 1 cup): 176 calories, 3g fat, 765mg sodium, 23g carbs, 5.5g fiber, 6g sugars, 13g protein

INGREDIENTS

One 29-ounce can tomato sauce
One 15-ounce can chili beans (pinto beans in chili sauce), not drained
One 15-ounce can red kidney beans, drained and rinsed
One 14.5-ounce can diced tomatoes, drained
2 bell peppers (different colors), stems removed, seeded, chopped
1 large onion, chopped
1 cup frozen sliced or chopped carrots
1 cup frozen sweet corn kernels
1 to 3 canned chipotle peppers in adobo sauce, chopped, sauce reserved
2 teaspoons chopped garlic
1 teaspoon chili powder
1 teaspoon ground cumin
1 pound raw lean ground turkey

Optional seasoning: salt
Optional topping: fat-free sour cream

DIRECTIONS

Combine all ingredients *except* turkey in a large bowl. Add 2 teaspoons adobo sauce from the canned chipotle peppers. Mix to combine and coat all beans and veggies with sauce.

Place turkey in the bottom of a crock pot and break up into small chunks. Pour chili mixture on top and mix.

Cover and cook on high for 3 to 4 hours *or* on low for 7 to 8 hours, until turkey is fully cooked and veggies have softened. Stir well and enjoy!

MAKES 12 SERVINGS

CRAZY-DELICIOUS SEAFOOD CORN CHOWDER

138 calories PER SERVING

You'll Need: crock pot, large bowl
Prep: 10 minutes
Cook: 3 to 4 hours *or* 7 to 8 hours

⅑th of recipe (1 heaping cup):
138 calories, 1.5g fat, 553mg sodium,
16.5g carbs, 1.5g fiber, 5g sugars,
14.5g protein

INGREDIENTS

Two 14.5-ounce cans (about 3½ cups)
    fat-free chicken broth
One 14.75-ounce can cream-style corn
Two 6-ounce cans lump crabmeat,
    thoroughly drained
One 6-ounce frozen fillet tilapia,
    cod, or other mild white fish
2 cups (about 7 ounces) frozen cooked
    ready-to-eat shrimp
1 cup frozen sweet corn kernels
1 red bell pepper, stem removed,
    seeded, chopped
½ cup finely chopped onion
½ cup light plain soymilk
½ teaspoon chopped garlic
½ cup instant mashed potato flakes
¼ cup fat-free sour cream

Optional seasonings: salt and black pepper

DIRECTIONS

Place all ingredients *except* potato flakes and
sour cream in a crock pot, and mix well. (Yup,
that fish fillet goes in whole!)

Cover and cook on high for 3 to 4 hours
or on low for 7 to 8 hours, until fish is
cooked through.

Stir to break up the fish fillet. Add potato flakes
and sour cream, and stir thoroughly. Enjoy!

MAKES 9 SERVINGS

SPICY SOUTHWEST CHICKEN CHOWDER

163 calories PER SERVING

You'll Need: crock pot, large bowl
Prep: 25 minutes
Cook: 3 to 4 hours *or* 7 to 8 hours

⅒th of recipe (about 1 cup): 163 calories,
1.5g fat, 654mg sodium, 18.5g carbs, 3g fiber,
4.5g sugars, 18.5g protein

INGREDIENTS

Two 14.5-ounce cans (about 3½ cups) fat-free
    chicken broth
One 15-ounce can black beans, drained and rinsed
One 14.75-ounce can cream-style corn
1 cup chopped red bell pepper
1 cup chopped onion
2 tablespoons chopped canned chipotle peppers in
    adobo sauce (about 2 peppers)
½ cup light plain soymilk
1 teaspoon chopped garlic
¼ teaspoon ground cumin
1½ pounds raw boneless skinless chicken breast, halved
½ teaspoon each salt and black pepper
½ cup instant mashed potato flakes
¼ cup fat-free sour cream
¼ cup chopped cilantro

DIRECTIONS

In a crock pot, combine broth, beans, corn, bell pepper,
onion, chipotle peppers, soymilk, garlic, and cumin.
Stir well.

Season chicken with salt and black pepper and place in
the crock pot. Cover and cook on high for 3 to 4 hours *or*
on low for 7 to 8 hours, until chicken is cooked through.

Transfer chicken to a large bowl. Shred with two forks—
one to hold chicken in place and the other to scrape across
and shred.

Stir shredded chicken into the soup in the crock pot. Stir in
potato flakes, sour cream,
and cilantro. Enjoy!

MAKES 10 SERVINGS

HG ALTERNATIVE!
Skip the chipotle peppers
for a deliciously mild
chicken chowder.

TEN-ALARM SOUTHWESTERN CORN CHOWDER

119 calories PER SERVING

You'll Need: crock pot | **Prep:** 15 minutes | **Cook:** 3 to 4 hours *or* 7 to 8 hours

⅛th **of recipe (1 heaping cup):**
119 calories, 1g fat, 367mg sodium, 24.5g carbs, 2.75g fiber, 7g sugars, 4g protein

INGREDIENTS

Two 14.5-ounce cans (about 3½ cups) fat-free chicken or vegetable broth

One 14.75-ounce can cream-style corn

2 cups frozen sweet corn kernels

2 plum tomatoes, chopped

1 red bell pepper, stem removed, seeded, chopped

1 green bell pepper, stem removed, seeded, chopped

1 onion, finely chopped

½ cup light plain soymilk

1 tablespoon chopped canned chipotle peppers in adobo sauce

1 teaspoon chopped garlic

¼ teaspoon ground cumin

¾ cup instant mashed potato flakes

¼ cup fat-free sour cream

Optional seasonings: salt and black pepper
Optional topping: chopped fresh cilantro

DIRECTIONS

Place all ingredients *except* the potato flakes and sour cream in a crock pot. Mix well.

Cover and cook on high for 3 to 4 hours *or* on low for 7 to 8 hours.

Add potato flakes and sour cream. Stir thoroughly. Slurpin' time!

MAKES 8 SERVINGS

HG TIP!
For no-alarm chowder, leave out the chipotle peppers in sauce . . .

* Flip to the photo inserts to see over 100 recipe pics! And for photos of ALL the recipes, go to **hungry-girl.com/books**.

SLOW-COOKIN' BBQ CHICKEN

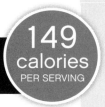

149 calories
PER SERVING

You'll Need: crock pot, large bowl | **Prep:** 10 minutes | **Cook:** 3 to 4 hours *or* 7 to 8 hours

⅐th of recipe (about ½ cup):
149 calories, 1g fat, 462mg sodium, 10g carbs, <0.5g fiber, 9g sugars, 22.5g protein

INGREDIENTS

1 cup canned tomato sauce
½ cup ketchup
2 tablespoons plus 2 teaspoons brown sugar (not packed)
2 tablespoons plus 2 teaspoons cider vinegar
2 teaspoons garlic powder
1½ pounds raw boneless skinless chicken breasts, halved

Optional seasoning: red pepper flakes

DIRECTIONS

In a crock pot, mix all ingredients *except* chicken. Add chicken and stir to coat.

Cover and cook on high for 3 to 4 hours *or* on low for 7 to 8 hours, until chicken is fully cooked.

Transfer chicken to a large bowl. Shred with two forks—one to hold the chicken in place and the other to scrape across and shred it. Return shredded chicken to the crock pot and mix well. Eat up!

MAKES 7 SERVINGS

SLOW-COOKIN' MEXICAN CHICKEN

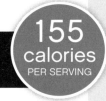

155 calories
PER SERVING

You'll Need: crock pot, large bowl | **Prep:** 10 minutes | **Cook:** 3 to 4 hours *or* 7 to 8 hours

⅙th of recipe (about ⅔ cup):
155 calories, 1.25g fat, 339mg sodium, 5.5g carbs, <0.5g fiber, 2.5g sugars, 27g protein

INGREDIENTS

1 cup canned crushed tomatoes
½ cup roasted red peppers packed in water, drained and chopped
¼ cup canned diced green chiles
1 tablespoon taco seasoning mix
½ tablespoon garlic powder
¼ teaspoon red pepper flakes, or more to taste
⅛ teaspoon black pepper, or more to taste
1½ pounds raw boneless skinless chicken breasts, halved

Optional seasoning: salt

DIRECTIONS

In a crock pot, mix all ingredients *except* chicken. Add chicken and stir to coat.

Cover and cook on high for 3 to 4 hours *or* on low for 7 to 8 hours, until chicken is fully cooked.

Transfer chicken to a large bowl. Shred with two forks—one to hold the chicken in place and the other to scrape across and shred it. Return the shredded chicken to the crock pot and mix well. Enjoy!

MAKES 6 SERVINGS

'CUE THE PULLED PORK

220 calories PER SERVING

You'll Need: crock pot, large bowl
Prep: 15 minutes
Cook: 3 to 4 hours *or* 7 to 8 hours

⅙th of recipe (about ⅔ cup): 220 calories, 6g fat, 637mg sodium, 16g carbs, 1g fiber, 12g sugars, 24g protein

INGREDIENTS

1 cup canned tomato sauce
½ cup ketchup
2 tablespoons plus 2 teaspoons cider vinegar
2 tablespoons plus 2 teaspoons brown sugar (not packed)
2 teaspoons garlic powder
12 ounces raw lean boneless pork tenderloin, trimmed of excess fat
12 ounces raw boneless pork shoulder (the leanest piece you can find), trimmed of excess fat
¼ teaspoon salt
⅛ teaspoon black pepper
2 cups roughly chopped onion

Optional seasoning: red pepper flakes

DIRECTIONS

In a crock pot, mix tomato sauce, ketchup, vinegar, sugar, and garlic powder. Season both types of pork with salt and pepper and add to the pot. Top with onion and lightly stir.

Cover and cook on high for 3 to 4 hours *or* on low for 7 to 8 hours, until pork is cooked through.

Transfer pork to a large bowl. Shred with two forks—one to hold the meat in place and one to scrape across and shred it. Return shredded pork to the crock pot and mix well. Mmmm . . .

MAKES 6 SERVINGS

PULLED BBQ BEEF

224 calories PER SERVING

You'll Need: crock pot, large bowl
Prep: 15 minutes
Cook: 3 to 4 hours *or* 7 to 8 hours

⅙th of recipe (about ¾ cup): 224 calories, 4.5g fat, 607mg sodium, 19g carbs, 1.5g fiber, 13.5g sugars, 27g protein

INGREDIENTS

1 cup canned tomato sauce
½ cup ketchup
2 tablespoons plus 2 teaspoons cider vinegar
2 tablespoons plus 2 teaspoons brown sugar (not packed)
2 teaspoons garlic powder
1½ pounds raw boneless top sirloin beef, trimmed of excess fat
¼ teaspoon salt
⅛ teaspoon black pepper
2 cups roughly chopped onion

DIRECTIONS

In a crock pot, mix tomato sauce, ketchup, vinegar, sugar, and garlic powder. Season beef with salt and pepper and add to the pot. Top with onion and lightly stir.

Cover and cook on high for 3 to 4 hours *or* on low for 7 to 8 hours, until beef is cooked through.

Transfer beef to a large bowl. Shred with two forks—one to hold the meat in place and one to scrape across and shred it. Return shredded beef to the crock pot and mix well. Yum time!

MAKES 6 SERVINGS

PUMP-UP-THE-JAM COCKTAIL WEENIES

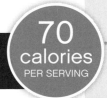

88 calories
PER SERVING

You'll Need: crock pot, medium bowl | **Prep:** 10 minutes | **Cook:** 3 to 4 hours

¹⁄₁₄th of recipe (3 weenies with sauce):
88 calories, 1g fat, 692mg sodium, 14.5g carbs, 0g fiber, 8.5g sugars, 5.5g protein

INGREDIENTS

14 hot dogs with about 40 calories and 1g fat or less each

¾ cup very finely chopped yellow onion

1 cup chili sauce (the kind stocked near the ketchup)

¾ cup low-sugar grape jelly

1 ½ teaspoons Dijon mustard

DIRECTIONS

Cut each hot dog into thirds, for cocktail-sized franks. Place franks and onion in a crock pot.

In a medium bowl, combine chili sauce, jelly, and mustard; mix well. Add to the crock pot and gently stir to coat.

Cover and cook on low for 3 to 4 hours.

Stir well and then serve up the hot dogs with extra sauce on top!

MAKES 14 SERVINGS

FLAMING COCKTAIL WEENIES

70 calories
PER SERVING

You'll Need: medium bowl, whisk, crock pot | **Prep:** 10 minutes | **Cook:** 3 to 4 hours

¹⁄₁₄th of recipe (3 weenies with sauce):
70 calories, 1.5g fat, 524mg sodium, 8.5g carbs, 0g fiber, 4.5g sugars, 5.5g protein

INGREDIENTS

¼ cup red wine vinegar

¼ cup reduced-fat Parmesan-style grated topping

3 tablespoons honey

2 tablespoons Dijon mustard

1 tablespoon Mexican hot sauce

2 teaspoons light whipped butter or light buttery spread, room temperature

14 hot dogs with about 40 calories and 1g fat or less each

DIRECTIONS

Place all ingredients *except* hot dogs in a medium bowl. Add 2 tablespoons water and thoroughly whisk. Transfer to a crock pot.

Cut each hot dog into thirds, for cocktail-sized franks, and add to the crock pot. Stir to coat.

Cover and cook on low for 3 to 4 hours. Stir well and serve!

MAKES 14 SERVINGS

PEACH-BBQ COCKTAIL WEENIES

75 calories PER SERVING

You'll Need: small food processor or blender, crock pot
Prep: 10 minutes
Cook: 3 to 4 hours

¹⁄₁₄th of recipe (3 weenies with sauce):
75 calories, 1g fat, 595mg sodium, 11g carbs, <0.5g fiber, 7g sugars, 5.5g protein

INGREDIENTS

Half a 15-ounce can (about 1 cup) sliced peaches packed in juice, drained
¾ cup canned tomato sauce
½ cup ketchup
1 tablespoon brown sugar (not packed)
1 tablespoon cider vinegar
1 tablespoon molasses
2 teaspoons garlic powder
14 hot dogs with about 40 calories and 1g fat or less each

DIRECTIONS

Puree peaches in a small food processor or blender. Transfer to a crock pot. Add all ingredients *except* hot dogs and thoroughly mix.

Cut each hot dog into thirds, for cocktail-sized franks, and add to the crock pot. Stir to coat.

Cover and cook on low for 3 to 4 hours. Stir well and serve!

MAKES 14 SERVINGS

SWEET-HOT STEAK BITES

196 calories PER SERVING

You'll Need: crock pot
Prep: 10 minutes
Cook: 3 to 4 hours *or* 7 to 8 hours

⅕th of recipe (about 6 "bites" with sauce):
196 calories, 4.5g fat, 313mg sodium, 18g carbs, 0.5g fiber, 15g sugars, 19.5g protein

INGREDIENTS

One 8-ounce can crushed pineapple packed in juice, lightly drained
⅓ cup sweet Asian chili sauce
½ teaspoon reduced-sodium/lite soy sauce
¼ teaspoon red pepper flakes, or more to taste
1 pound raw lean beefsteak, cut into about 30 bite-sized pieces
⅛ teaspoon each salt and black pepper
1 onion, finely chopped

DIRECTIONS

Place pineapple, chili sauce, soy sauce, and red pepper flakes in a crock pot. Mix well.

Season beef with salt and black pepper and add to the crock pot. Add onion and stir to coat.

Cover and cook on high for 3 to 4 hours *or* on low for 7 to 8 hours, until beef is cooked through and onion has softened.

Yum!

MAKES 5 SERVINGS

For more recipes, tips & tricks, sign up for FREE daily emails at hungry-girl.com!

CROCK-POT FAKE-BAKED BEANS

174 calories PER SERVING

You'll Need: medium bowl, crock pot
Prep: 20 minutes
Cook: 3 to 4 hours *or* 7 to 8 hours

¹⁄₁₀th of recipe (about ¾ cup): 174 calories, 0.75g fat, 473mg sodium, 36.5g carbs, 9g fiber, 12g sugars, 7.5g protein

INGREDIENTS

One 6-ounce can tomato paste
¼ cup molasses
2 tablespoons cider vinegar
1 tablespoon yellow mustard
1 teaspoon chopped garlic
½ teaspoon salt
One 15-ounce can black beans, drained and rinsed
One 15-ounce can pinto beans, drained and rinsed
One 15-ounce can red kidney beans, drained and rinsed
3 cups finely chopped onion
2 cups finely chopped red bell pepper
1 cup finely chopped Fuji apple

DIRECTIONS

In a medium bowl, combine tomato paste, molasses, vinegar, mustard, garlic, and salt. Mix thoroughly.

Place all remaining ingredients in a crock pot. Add the tomato paste mixture and toss to coat.

Cover and cook on high for 3 to 4 hours *or* on low for 7 to 8 hours.

Stir well and then serve it up!

MAKES 10 SERVINGS

FRUITY & TANGY COCKTAIL MEATBALLS

135 calories PER SERVING

You'll Need: large baking sheet, nonstick spray, large bowl, blender or food processer, crock pot, toothpicks
Prep: 15 minutes
Cook: 10 minutes plus 3 to 4 hours

⅛th of recipe (3 meatballs with about 2 tablespoons sauce): 135 calories, 2.5g fat, 191mg sodium, 15g carbs, 0.5g fiber, 14g sugars, 12g protein

INGREDIENTS

Meatballs
1 pound raw extra-lean ground beef
½ cup finely diced mango
2 tablespoons ketchup
1 teaspoon dried minced onion
¼ teaspoon salt

Sauce
One 15-ounce can peach slices packed in juice, drained
½ cup low-sugar or sugar-free apricot preserves
¼ cup cider vinegar
1 tablespoon Sriracha chili sauce (shelf-stable Asian hot sauce)

DIRECTIONS

Preheat oven to 450 degrees. Spray a large baking sheet with nonstick spray.

In a large bowl, combine all meatball ingredients. Mix thoroughly with your hands. Form 24 evenly sized meatballs and place on the baking sheet, evenly spaced.

Bake until meatballs are just cooked, 8 to 10 minutes.

Meanwhile, in a blender or food processor, pulse peaches until mostly smooth. Transfer to a crock pot. Add all remaining sauce ingredients to the crock pot and mix well.

Carefully transfer meatballs to the crock pot. Stir to coat. Cover and cook on low for 3 to 4 hours.

Stir well and serve up meatballs with toothpicks and the extra sauce from the crock pot!

MAKES 8 SERVINGS

TURKEY-RIFIC TACO BEAN DIP

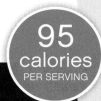

95 calories PER SERVING

You'll Need: large skillet, nonstick spray, crock pot
Prep: 10 minutes
Cook: 10 minutes plus 3 to 4 hours *or* 7 to 8 hours

¹⁄₁₆th **of recipe (about ⅓ cup):** 95 calories, 2g fat, 332mg sodium, 11.5g carbs, 3g fiber, 2g sugars, 7.5g protein

INGREDIENTS

10 ounces raw lean ground turkey
1½ teaspoons taco seasoning mix
2 cups diced plum tomatoes
1 cup diced onion
Two 16-ounce cans fat-free refried beans
Two 4-ounce cans diced green chiles
½ cup shredded reduced-fat
    Mexican-blend cheese

Serving suggestions: baked tortilla chips,
    sliced bell peppers

DIRECTIONS

Bring a large skillet sprayed with nonstick spray to medium-high heat. Add turkey and sprinkle with taco seasoning. Cook and finely crumble for about 6 minutes, until turkey is fully cooked. Drain any excess liquid and transfer turkey to a crock pot.

Evenly top turkey with tomatoes, onion, beans, and chiles.

Cover and cook on high for 3 to 4 hours *or* on low for 7 to 8 hours.

Turn off crock pot and remove lid. Add cheese and stir well.

Serve with your guilt-free dippers of choice and enjoy!

MAKES 16 SERVINGS

GLAZE-OF-GLORY CANDIED CARROTS

102 calories PER SERVING

You'll Need: 2 small bowls, crock pot
Prep: 15 minutes
Cook: 3 to 4 hours *or* 7 to 8 hours plus 15 minutes

⅐th **of recipe (about 1 cup):** 102 calories, 1.5g fat, 286mg sodium, 22g carbs, 3g fiber, 13g sugars, 1.5g protein

INGREDIENTS

¼ cup low-sugar apricot preserves
2 tablespoons brown sugar (not packed)
1½ tablespoons light whipped butter or
    light buttery spread
1 teaspoon cinnamon
½ teaspoon salt, or more to taste
¼ teaspoon ground nutmeg
One 32-ounce bag (about 6 cups) baby carrots
1 onion, sliced
1 yellow bell pepper, stem removed, seeded, and sliced
1 red bell pepper, stem removed, seeded, and sliced
1 tablespoon cornstarch

Optional seasonings: black pepper, cayenne pepper,
    ground ginger

DIRECTIONS

To make the glaze, in a small bowl, combine preserves, brown sugar, butter, cinnamon, salt, and nutmeg. Stir well.

Put all of the veggies in a crock pot and top with the glaze.

Use a large spoon to stir the contents of the crock pot up a bit. (Don't worry if the preserves mixture isn't evenly distributed.)

Cover and cook on high for 3 to 4 hours *or* on low for 7 to 8 hours.

Once the veggies are cooked, in another small bowl, combine cornstarch with 2 tablespoons cold water, and stir until the cornstarch has dissolved. Add to the crock pot and mix well.

Turn off the pot and leave uncovered until sauce has thickened, about 15 minutes. Stir and enjoy!

MAKES 7 SERVINGS

PUMP-UP-THE-JAM CHICKEN

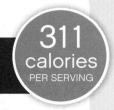

311 calories PER SERVING

You'll Need: crock pot, medium bowl, small bowl
Prep: 15 minutes | **Cook:** 3 to 4 hours *or* 7 to 8 hours plus 10 minutes

¼th of recipe (about 1 cup):
311 calories, 2g fat, 882mg sodium, 30g carbs, 0.5g fiber, 20g sugars, 40g protein

INGREDIENTS

1½ pounds raw boneless skinless chicken breast, cut into 2-inch chunks
⅛ teaspoon each salt and black pepper
½ cup chili sauce (the kind stocked near the ketchup)
½ cup low-sugar grape jelly
½ teaspoon onion powder
2 cups sliced onion
1 tablespoon cornstarch

DIRECTIONS

Season chicken with salt and pepper and place in a crock pot.

In a medium bowl, thoroughly mix remaining ingredients *except* sliced onion and cornstarch.

Top chicken with onion. Pour jam mixture over onion and chicken and lightly stir.

Cover and cook on high for 3 to 4 hours *or* on low for 7 to 8 hours, until chicken is fully cooked.

Turn off crock pot. In a small bowl, dissolve cornstarch in 1 tablespoon cold water. Stir into the liquid in the crock pot. Let sit, uncovered, until slightly thickened, about 10 minutes.

Stir and enjoy!

MAKES 4 SERVINGS

TURKEY MUSHROOM SURPRISE

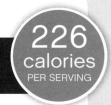

226 calories PER SERVING

You'll Need: crock pot | **Prep:** 10 minutes | **Cook:** 3 to 4 hours *or* 7 to 8 hours plus 5 minutes

⅕th of recipe (1 heaping cup):
226 calories, 8.5g fat, 670mg sodium, 10.5g carbs, 1g fiber, 2.5g sugars, 27.5g protein

INGREDIENTS

1¼ pounds raw lean ground turkey
One 12-ounce jar fat-free turkey gravy
5 cups sliced mushrooms
1 onion, thinly sliced
1 tablespoon onion soup/dip seasoning mix
1 tablespoon cornstarch

DIRECTIONS

In a crock pot, thoroughly mix all ingredients *except* onion soup/dip mix and cornstarch.

Cover and cook on high for 3 to 4 hours *or* on low for 7 to 8 hours, until turkey is fully cooked and mushrooms have softened.

If needed, reduce heat to low. Thoroughly stir onion soup/dip mix and cornstarch into the crock pot. Let sit, uncovered, until slightly thickened, about 5 minutes. Enjoy!

MAKES 5 SERVINGS

CROCK-POT ROAST

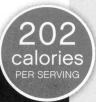

206 calories PER SERVING

You'll Need: large skillet, nonstick spray, crock pot, small bowl
Prep: 15 minutes
Cook: 10 minutes plus 3 to 4 hours *or* 7 to 8 hours

1/12th of recipe (about 2 ½ ounces cooked meat with ⅔ cup broth and veggies): 206 calories, 7g fat, 447mg sodium, 11g carbs, 2g fiber, 4.5g sugars, 25.5g protein

INGREDIENTS

One 3-pound raw boneless chuck beef roast (trimmed of excess fat)
1 teaspoon each salt and black pepper
One 14-ounce can fat-free beef broth
4 cups carrots cut into ½-inch coins
3 cups roughly chopped onion
2 cups sliced mushrooms
1 cup celery cut into ½-inch pieces
2 tablespoons tomato paste
1 tablespoon Worcestershire sauce
2 sprigs fresh thyme
1 teaspoon chopped garlic
2 tablespoons cornstarch

DIRECTIONS

Bring a large skillet sprayed with nonstick spray to high heat. Season roast with ¼ teaspoon each salt and pepper. Cook and rotate until all sides are browned, about 5 minutes. Place in a crock pot.

Add all remaining ingredients *except* cornstarch to the crock pot, including the remaining ¾ teaspoon each salt and black pepper. Gently stir.

Cook on high for 3 to 4 hours *or* on low for 7 to 8 hours, until roast is cooked through.

Turn off crock pot. In a small bowl, dissolve cornstarch in 2 tablespoons cold water. Stir into the liquid in the crock pot. Let sit, uncovered, until slightly thickened, about 5 minutes.

Remove and discard thyme sprigs. Slice meat and serve topped with veggies and sauce!

MAKES 12 SERVINGS

HG TIP!
If the roast breaks into pieces when you trim away the fat, just cook each piece in the skillet until browned—the smaller pieces will take less time. Tongs are great for rotating the meat when browning.

CROCK-POT COQ AU VIN

202 calories PER SERVING

You'll Need: skillet or microwave-safe plate, crock pot
Prep: 10 minutes
Cook: 10 minutes plus 3 to 4 hours *or* 7 to 8 hours

⅙th of recipe (about 1 cup): 202 calories, 3g fat, 330mg sodium, 9g carbs, 1.25g fiber, 3.5g sugars, 29g protein

INGREDIENTS

4 slices center-cut bacon or turkey bacon
1 cup fat-free low-sodium chicken broth
½ cup red wine
1 tablespoon cornstarch
½ tablespoon chopped garlic
2 sprigs fresh thyme, chopped
1½ pounds raw boneless skinless chicken breast tenders
¼ teaspoon each salt and black pepper
2 cups sliced mushrooms
1½ cups baby carrots
1½ cups sliced onion

DIRECTIONS

Cook bacon until crispy, either in a skillet over medium heat or on a microwave-safe plate in the microwave. (See package for cook time.) Crumble or chop.

In a crock pot, thoroughly mix broth, wine, cornstarch, garlic, and thyme. Season chicken with salt and pepper and add to the pot. Add bacon and veggies and thoroughly stir.

Cover and cook on high for 3 to 4 hours *or* on low for 7 to 8 hours, until chicken is cooked through. Stir well and enjoy!

MAKES 6 SERVINGS

CHEESEBURGER MAC ATTACK

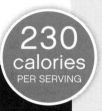

179 calories PER SERVING

You'll Need: large pot, strainer, large bowl, crock pot
Prep: 5 minutes
Cook: 10 minutes plus 3 to 4 hours *or* 7 to 8 hours

⅛th **of recipe (about 1 cup):** 179 calories, 5.75g fat, 512mg sodium, 19g carbs, 2g fiber, 3.5g sugars, 12.5g protein

INGREDIENTS

5 ounces (about 1⅓ cups) uncooked high-fiber elbow macaroni
10 ounces raw lean ground turkey
2 tablespoons ketchup
1 teaspoon onion powder
24 ounces (about 6 cups) frozen cauliflower and low-fat cheese sauce
2 scallions, thinly sliced
3 wedges The Laughing Cow Light Creamy Swiss cheese

Optional seasonings: salt and black pepper

DIRECTIONS

In a large pot, cook pasta until very al dente, about half of the time indicated on the package. Drain well.

In a large bowl, mix turkey, ketchup, onion powder, and frozen cauliflower and cheese sauce. Transfer mixture to a crock pot.

Stir in cooked pasta. Cover and cook on high for 3 to 4 hours *or* on low for 7 to 8 hours, until turkey is fully cooked.

Add scallions and cheese wedges, breaking the wedges into pieces, and thoroughly stir. Dig in!

MAKES 8 SERVINGS

OUTSIDE-IN TURKEY TAMALE PIE

230 calories PER SERVING

You'll Need: large skillet, nonstick spray, crock pot, medium bowl, whisk
Prep: 20 minutes
Cook: 10 minutes plus 3 to 4 hours *or* 7 to 8 hours

⅐th **of recipe (about 1 cup):** 230 calories, 7.5g fat, 481mg sodium, 21g carbs, 3g fiber, 3g sugars, 19g protein

INGREDIENTS

1¼ pounds raw lean ground turkey
¾ cup yellow cornmeal
1 cup fat-free chicken or vegetable broth
One 14.5-ounce can diced tomatoes with chiles (not drained)
1 small onion, chopped
¾ cup canned sweet corn kernels, drained
½ cup canned red kidney beans, drained and rinsed
½ cup sliced black olives
2 teaspoons chili powder
1 teaspoon ground cumin

Optional toppings: fat-free shredded cheddar cheese, fat-free sour cream

DIRECTIONS

Bring a large skillet sprayed with nonstick spray to medium-high heat. Cook and crumble turkey for about 6 minutes, until browned and fully cooked. Drain excess liquid and transfer turkey to a crock pot.

In a medium bowl, whisk cornmeal with broth. Let stand for 5 minutes.

Add cornmeal mixture to the crock pot along with all other ingredients. Mix thoroughly.

Cover and cook on high for 3 to 4 hours *or* on low for 7 to 8 hours. Mmmmmm!!!

MAKES 7 SERVINGS

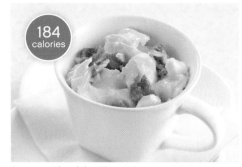

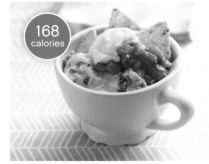

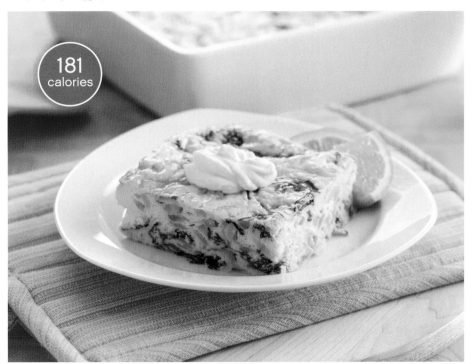

Bacon-Cheddar Egg Mug, p. 21

Caramelized Onion 'n Spinach Egg Bake, p. 31

Crunchy Beefy Taco Egg Mug, p. 16

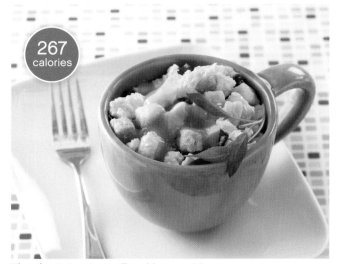

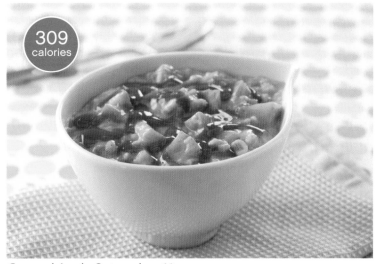

Thanksgiving in an Egg Mug, p. 23

Caramel Apple Oatmeal, p. 41

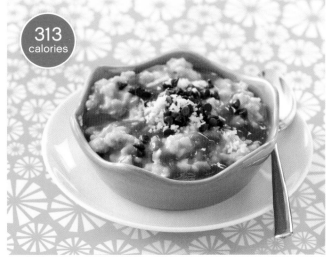

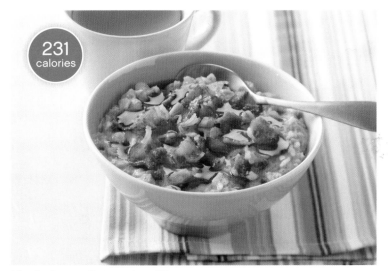

Chocolate Caramel Coconut Oatmeal, p. 45

Maple Bacon Oatmeal, p. 42

PARFAITS * PANCAKES AND FRENCH TOAST * FAUX-FRYS

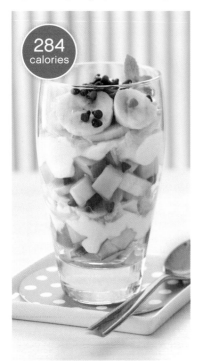

284 calories

Carnival Parfait, p. 58

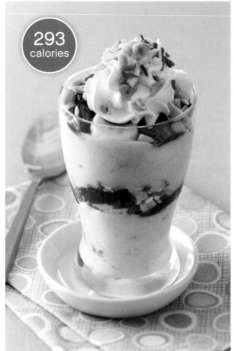

293 calories

Banana Split Yogurt Parfait, p. 63

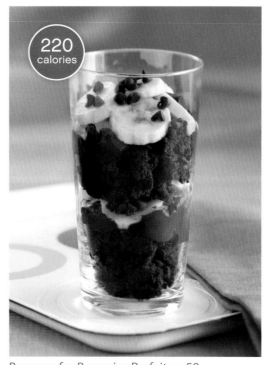

220 calories

Bananas for Brownies Parfait, p. 59

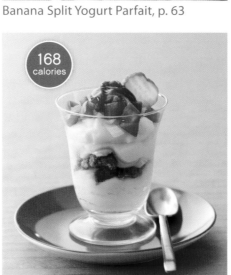

168 calories

Cheeseburger Mashed Potato Parfait, p. 67

177 calories

Buffalo Chicken Parfait, p. 65

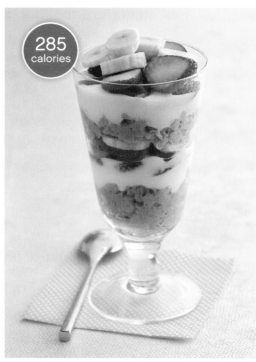

285 calories

Super-Sized Berry-nana Oatmeal Parfait, p. 55

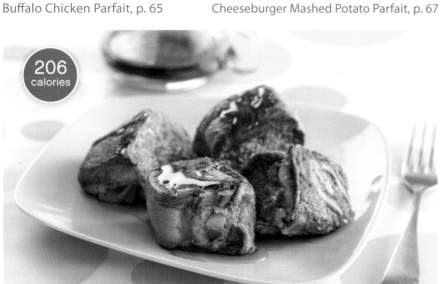

206 calories

Apple & Cream Cheese Stuffed French Toast Nuggets, p. 84

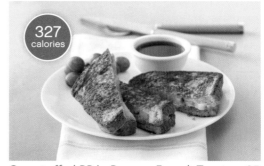

327 calories

Overstuffed PB 'n Banana French Toast, p. 85

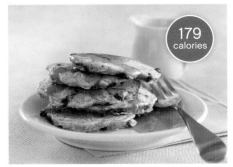

179 calories

Oat-rageous Chocolate Chip Pancake Minis, p. 75

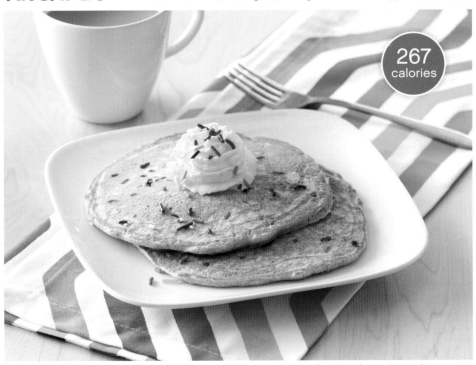

267 calories

Over the Rainbow Pancakes, p. 76

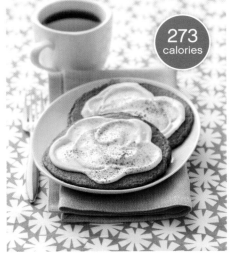

273 calories

Rockin' Red Velvet Pancakes, p. 76

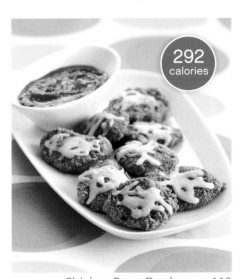

292 calories

Chicken Parm Dunkers, p. 112

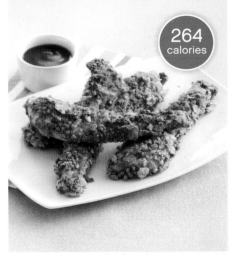

264 calories

BBQ Chicken Fingers, p. 108

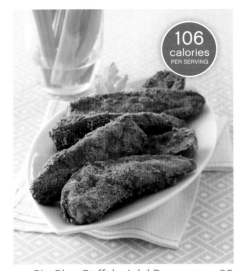

106 calories PER SERVING

Big Blue Buffalo Jala' Poppers, p. 95

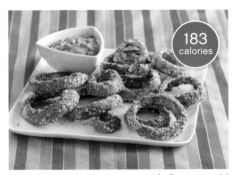

183 calories

Mexi-licious Onion Loops with Queso, p. 99

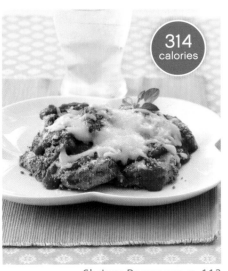

314 calories

Shrimp Parmesan, p. 113

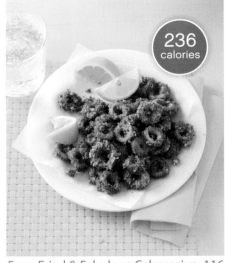

236 calories

Faux-Fried & Fabulous Calamari, p. 116

SWAPPUCCINOS & SHAKES

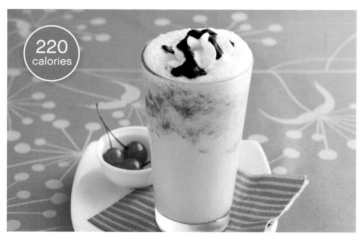

220 calories

Slurpable Split Shake, p. 132

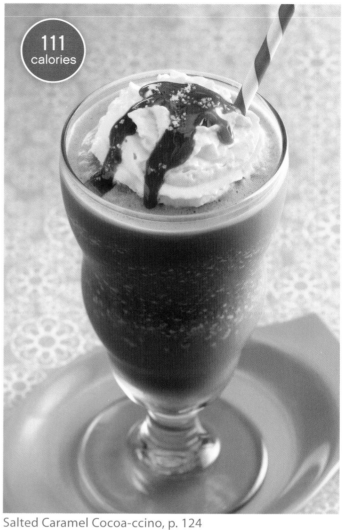

111 calories

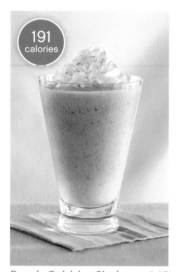

191 calories

Peach Cobbler Shake, p. 140

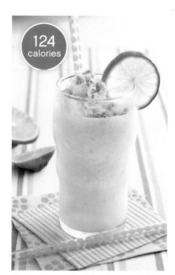

124 calories

Key Lime Pie Shake, p. 131

Salted Caramel Cocoa-ccino, p. 124

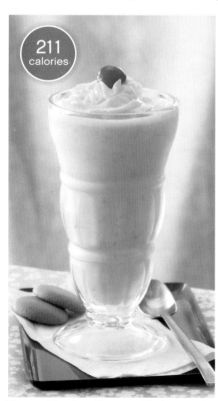

211 calories

Happy Monkey Banana Shake, p. 134

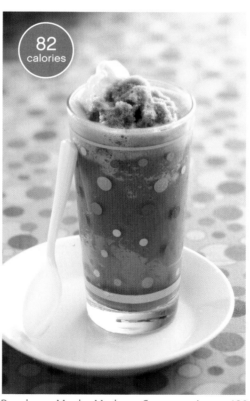

82 calories

Raspberry Mocha Madness Swappuccino, p. 129

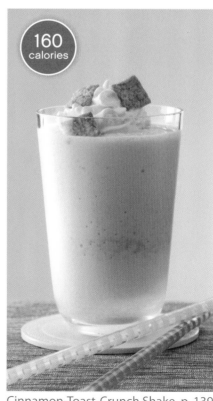

160 calories

Cinnamon-Toast-Crunch Shake, p. 139

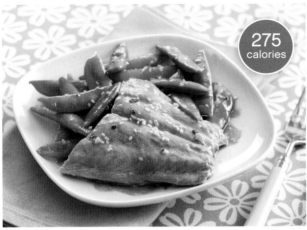

275 calories

Sesame Salmon & Snap Peas, p. 154

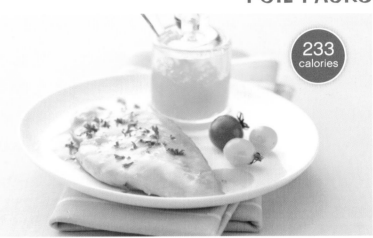

233 calories

Glaze-of-Sunshine Apricot Chicken, p. 147

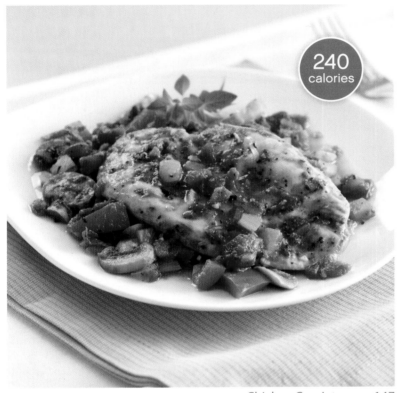

240 calories

Chicken Cacciatore, p. 147

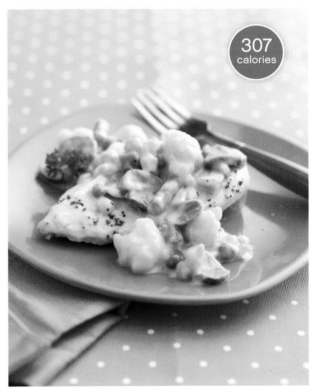

307 calories

Mom-Style Creamy Chicken 'n Veggies, p. 154

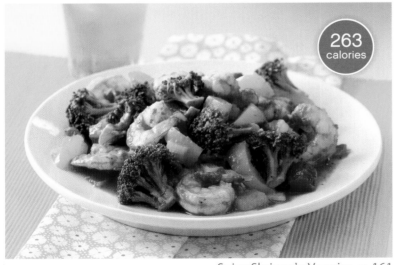

263 calories

Spicy Shrimp 'n Veggies, p. 161

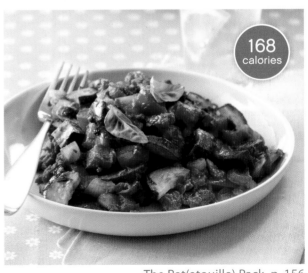

168 calories

The Rat(atouille) Pack, p. 156

CROCK POTS

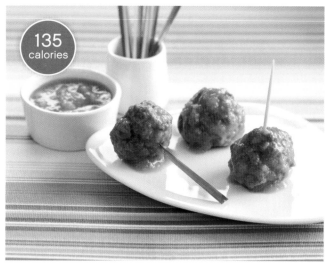

135 calories

Fruity & Tangy Cocktail Meatballs, p. 182

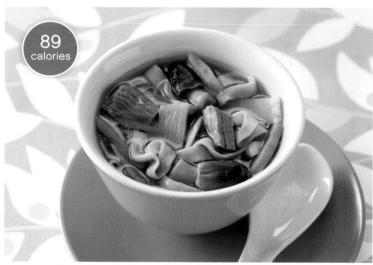

89 calories

Asian Beef Noodle Soup, p. 171

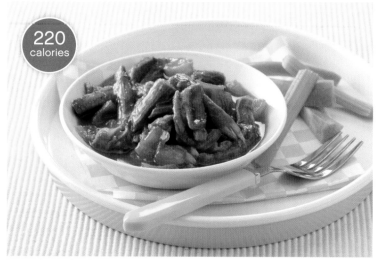

220 calories

'Cue the Pulled Pork, p. 179

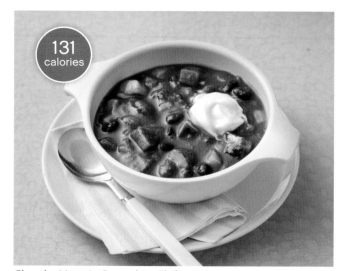

131 calories

Chunky Veggie Pumpkin Chili, p. 174

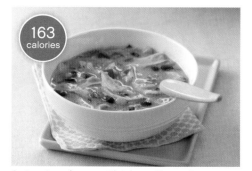

163 calories

Spicy Southwest Chicken Chowder, p. 176

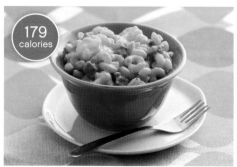

179 calories

Cheeseburger Mac Attack, p. 186

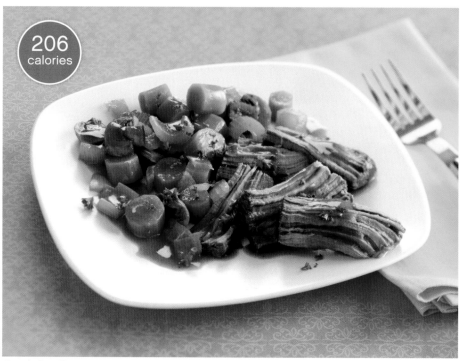

206 calories

Crock-Pot Roast, p. 185

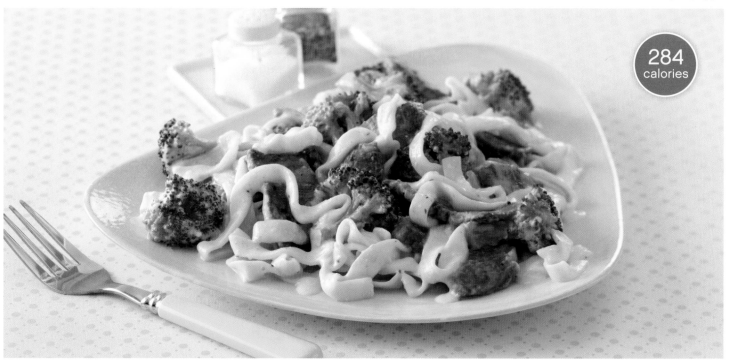

284 calories

Steak Lover's Girlfredo, p. 194

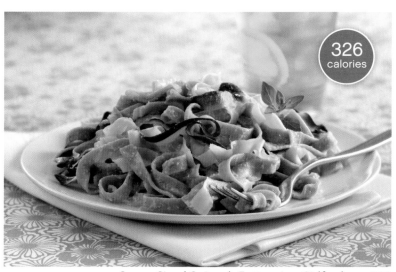

326 calories

Super-Sized Spinach Fettuccine Girlfredo, p. 218

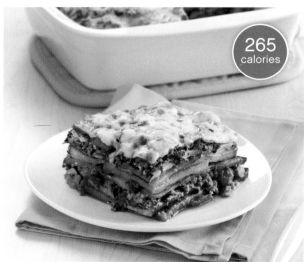

265 calories

Veggie-rific Noodle-Free Lasagna, p. 210

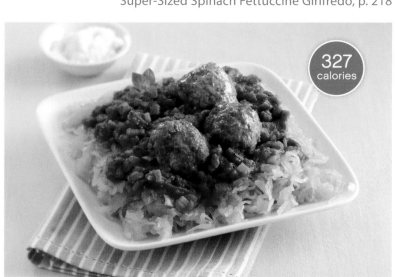

327 calories

Spaghetti Swap & Meatballs, p. 204

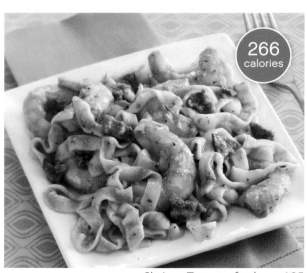

266 calories

Shrimp Tomato-fredo, p. 195

PIZZA

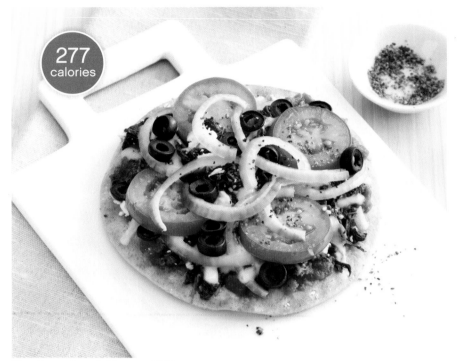

277 calories

The Great Greek Pizza, p. 227

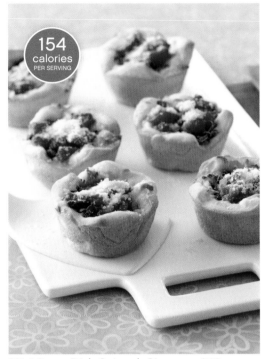

154 calories PER SERVING

Mini Deep Dish Spinach Pizzas, p. 242

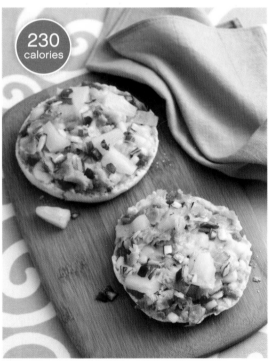

230 calories

Pizza Luau, p. 235

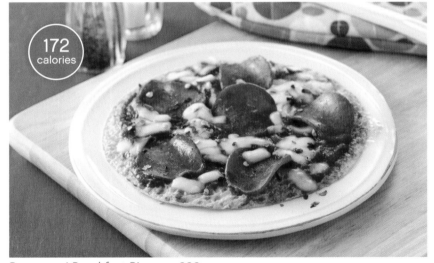

172 calories

Pepperoni Breakfast Pizza, p. 232

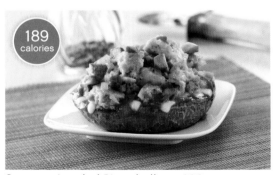

189 calories

Sausage-Loaded Pizza-bella, p. 239

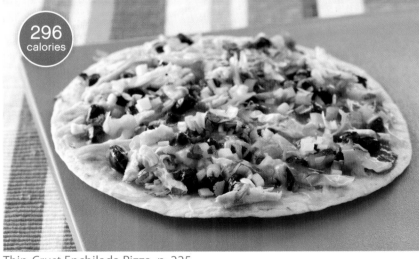

296 calories

Thin-Crust Enchilada Pizza, p. 225

CRANBERRY & APPLE CHICKEN

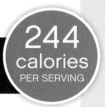
244 calories
PER SERVING

You'll Need: crock pot, small microwave-safe bowl | **Prep:** 20 minutes | **Cook:** 3 to 4 hours *or* 7 to 8 hours

¼th of recipe (about ¾ cup):
244 calories, 2.5g fat, 254mg sodium, 27g carbs, 2.5g fiber, 21.5g sugars, 26.5g protein

INGREDIENTS

1½ cups chopped Fuji apple
1 cup sliced onion
½ cup chopped celery
½ cup dried sweetened cranberries
1 teaspoon garlic
1 pound raw boneless skinless chicken breast, cut into strips
¼ teaspoon each salt and black pepper
1 tablespoon light whipped butter or light buttery spread
1 teaspoon lemon juice
2 tablespoons brown sugar (not packed)

DIRECTIONS

Place apple, onion, celery, cranberries, and garlic in a crock pot. Season chicken with salt and pepper and add to the pot.

In a small microwave-safe bowl, combine butter, lemon juice, and 2 tablespoons water. Microwave for 15 seconds, or until butter has melted and liquid is hot. Add sugar and stir to dissolve. Add mixture to the crock pot and gently stir to coat.

Cover and cook on high for 3 to 4 hours or on low for 7 to 8 hours, until chicken is fully cooked. Stir and enjoy!

MAKES 4 SERVINGS

QUICK Q&A WITH HG:

Why do you specify Fujis in most of your recipes that call for apples?

Because Fujis are the BEST. They're the perfect blend of crisp, sweet, and tart. They work in just about any apple recipe, and they're great for snacking. If you can't find Fujis, go for any sweet apple, like Honeycrisp, Pink Lady, or Gala.

CHAPTER 9

PASTA

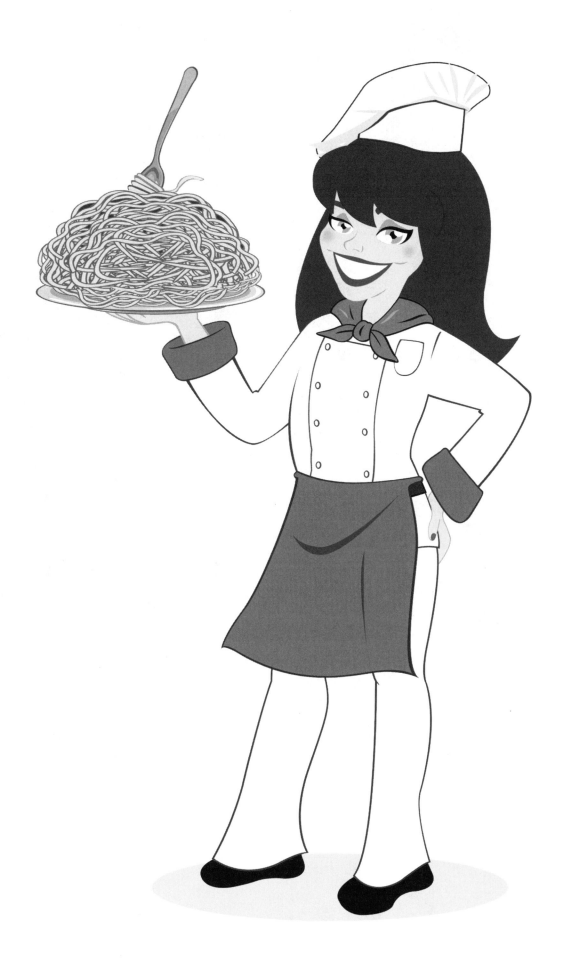

PASTA

Fettuccine Hungry Girlfredo

Hungry Girlfredo Veggie Explosion

Seafood Girlfredo

Steak Lover's Girlfredo

Shrimp Tomato-fredo

Fettuccine Hungry Chick-fredo

Super-Schmancy Hungry Girlfredo

Italian-Style Bacon Girlfredo

Buffalo Veggie Hungry Girlfredo

Creamy Salmon Girlfredo

Cin-sational Cincinnati Chili

Beef Strogataki

Simply the Pesto Spaghetti

Clam-tastic Shirataki Pasta

Chicken Carbonara a la Hungry Girl

Spicy Southern Shrimp Fettuccine

Vodka Impasta

Super-Delicious Shrimp Scampi

Chicken Florentine

Vampire-Proof Chicken 'n Veggie Pasta

Spaghetti Swap & Meatballs

Cheesy-Peasy Spaghetti Squash

Spaghetti Squash 'n Shrimp Arrabbiata

Buttery Garlic Spaghetti Squash

Pepperoni Spaghetti Squash

Mediterranean Spaghetti Squash

EZ Cheesy Lasagna for Two

Hungry Girlfredo White Lasagna

Veggie-rific Noodle-Free Lasagna

Pumpkin Lasagna

Slaw and Order

Chicken Amore Pasta Swap

Broccoli Slaw Turkey Bolognese

Takes-the-Cake Ziti Bake

Funkadelic Chili Mac

Super-Sized Pesto Pasta

Roasted Veggie Fettuccine

Chunky Eggplant Penne for Two

Super-Sized Spinach Fettuccine Girlfredo

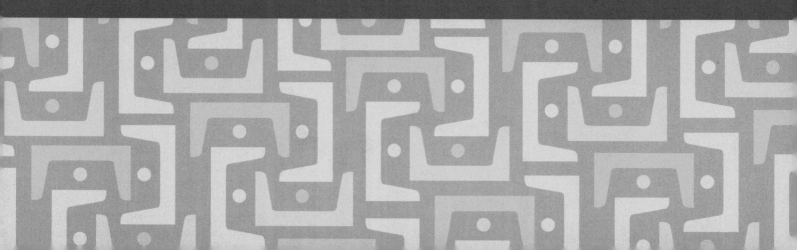

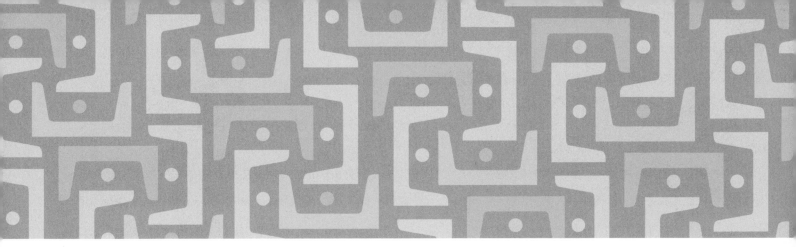

In the Hungry Girl world, "pasta" can be achieved
with ingredients other than traditional flour-based noodles . . .
Prepare to be WOWED!

A QUICK GUIDE TO SYMBOLS:

15 Minutes or Less

This symbol lets you know a recipe should take you no more than fifteen minutes from start to finish! That includes prep and cook time.

30 Minutes or Less

Just like the 15-minute version, this one points out recipes that take 30 minutes or less to whip up.

Meatless

You guessed it—no meat here! That includes beef, poultry, and fish. Some recipes give the option of a meatless ingredient. If you want your meal without meat, go with the meatless choice.

Single Serving

Pretty straightforward. These are recipes for one.

5 Ingredients or Less

Fans of HG know that we like to keep things simple. And these recipes contain just five ingredients or less!

Photos

These recipes can be seen in one of the book's photo inserts. The number in the symbol tells you which insert. Find photos of all the recipes at hungry-girl.com/books!

FETTUCCINE HUNGRY GIRLFREDO has become an HG classic. These variations all feature the now-famous "it couple" when it comes to creamy pasta swaps: Tofu Shirataki and The Laughing Cow Light cheese wedges!

THE TOFU SHIRATAKI 411 . . .

Find 'em with the tofu.
House Foods Tofu Shirataki noodles can be found in the refrigerated section of the market, near the tofu. And they come floating in a bag of liquid. Yup, it's all true.

Doppelganger alert!
Don't confuse these with plain shirataki noodles. The texture's not quite as similar to pasta.

Top tofu shirataki tip: Dry them WELL!
Drain and rinse the noodles VERY well in a strainer. Shake the strainer to get rid of ALL the excess liquid. THOROUGHLY pat the noodles dry with paper towels. This is VERY important. Soggy noodles = watery dishes.

Cut 'em up.
Why? Because the noodles are usually very long. So give them a rough chop, with a knife or with kitchen shears.

FETTUCCINE HUNGRY GIRLFREDO

99 calories

You'll Need: strainer, skillet, nonstick spray | **Prep:** 10 minutes | **Cook:** 5 minutes

Entire recipe:
99 calories, 3.5g fat, 323mg sodium, 9.5g carbs, 4g fiber, 1.5g sugars, 5g protein

INGREDIENTS

1 bag House Foods Tofu Shirataki Fettuccine Shaped Noodle Substitute
1 wedge The Laughing Cow Light Creamy Swiss cheese
2 teaspoons reduced-fat Parmesan-style grated topping
1 teaspoon fat-free sour cream

Optional seasonings: salt and black pepper

DIRECTIONS

Use a strainer to rinse and drain noodles. Thoroughly pat dry. Roughly cut noodles.

Bring a skillet sprayed with nonstick spray to medium heat. Add all ingredients, breaking the cheese wedge into pieces. Cook and stir until cheese has melted, mixed with sour cream, and coated noodles, 2 to 3 minutes. Enjoy!

MAKES 1 SERVING

HUNGRY GIRLFREDO VEGGIE EXPLOSION

151 calories

You'll Need: strainer, microwave-safe bowl, skillet, nonstick spray
Prep: 10 minutes
Cook: 10 minutes

Entire recipe: 151 calories, 4g fat, 357mg sodium, 20g carbs, 7g fiber, 7g sugars, 8.5g protein

INGREDIENTS

1 bag House Foods Tofu Shirataki Fettuccine Shaped Noodle Substitute
½ cup small broccoli florets
½ cup red bell pepper chunks
½ cup zucchini chunks
1 tablespoon fat-free sour cream
1 wedge The Laughing Cow Light Creamy Swiss cheese
2 teaspoons reduced-fat Parmesan-style grated topping

Optional seasonings: salt, black pepper, garlic powder, chili powder

DIRECTIONS

Use a strainer to rinse and drain noodles. Thoroughly pat dry. Roughly cut noodles.

Place all veggies in a microwave-safe bowl with 2 tablespoons water. Cover and microwave for 2 to 3 minutes, until veggies are tender. Drain or blot away excess water.

Bring a skillet sprayed with nonstick spray to medium heat. Add noodles, sour cream, and cheese wedge, breaking the wedge into pieces. Cook and stir until cheese has melted, mixed with sour cream, and coated noodles, 2 to 3 minutes.

Stir in veggies and Parm-style topping. Cook and stir until hot, 1 to 2 minutes. Eat!

MAKES 1 SERVING

SEAFOOD GIRLFREDO

266 calories

You'll Need: strainer, skillet, nonstick spray
Prep: 15 minutes
Cook: 10 minutes

Entire recipe: 266 calories, 5.5g fat, 1,049mg sodium, 19g carbs, 4.5g fiber, 3g sugars, 31.5g protein

INGREDIENTS

1 bag House Foods Tofu Shirataki Fettuccine Shaped Noodle Substitute
4 ounces raw shrimp, peeled, tails removed, deveined
½ cup sliced mushrooms
1 teaspoon fat-free sour cream
¼ teaspoon lemon juice
¼ teaspoon chopped garlic
1 wedge The Laughing Cow Light Creamy Swiss cheese
2 teaspoons reduced-fat Parmesan-style grated topping
2 ounces (about ⅓ cup) roughly chopped imitation crabmeat

Optional seasonings: salt and black pepper

DIRECTIONS

Use a strainer to rinse and drain noodles. Thoroughly pat dry. Roughly cut noodles.

Bring a skillet sprayed with nonstick spray to medium heat. Cook and stir shrimp and mushrooms until shrimp are just cooked through, about 4 minutes.

Remove shrimp and mushrooms and set aside. If needed, clean skillet. Remove from heat, re-spray, and return to medium heat. To the skillet, add noodles, sour cream, lemon juice, chopped garlic, and cheese wedge, breaking the wedge into pieces. Cook and stir until cheese has melted, mixed with sour cream, and coated noodles, 2 to 3 minutes.

Stir in Parm-style topping, shrimp, mushrooms, and crab. Cook and stir until hot, 1 to 2 minutes. Yum!

MAKES 1 SERVING

STEAK LOVER'S GIRLFREDO

284 calories

You'll Need: strainer, skillet with a lid, nonstick spray | **Prep:** 10 minutes | **Cook:** 15 minutes

Entire recipe:
284 calories, 8g fat, 594mg sodium, 17.5g carbs, 6.5g fiber, 4g sugars, 34g protein

INGREDIENTS

1 bag House Foods Tofu Shirataki Fettuccine Shaped Noodle Substitute

4 ounces thinly sliced raw lean beefsteak filet (freeze slightly before slicing)

⅛ teaspoon black pepper

⅛ teaspoon garlic powder

Dash salt

1 cup small broccoli florets

1 tablespoon fat-free sour cream

1 wedge The Laughing Cow Light Creamy Swiss cheese

2 teaspoons reduced-fat Parmesan-style grated topping

Optional seasonings: additional salt and black pepper

DIRECTIONS

Use a strainer to rinse and drain noodles. Thoroughly pat dry. Roughly cut noodles.

Bring a skillet sprayed with nonstick spray to medium-high heat. Add beef and sprinkle with seasonings. Cook and stir for about 2 minutes, until just cooked through.

Remove beef and set aside. If needed, clean skillet. Remove from heat, re-spray, and return to medium-high heat. Add broccoli and ¼ cup water. Cover and cook for 4 to 5 minutes, until softened. Uncover and cook and stir until water has evaporated, about 1 minute.

Add noodles, sour cream, and cheese wedge, breaking the wedge into pieces. Cook and stir until cheese has melted, mixed with sour cream, and coated noodles, 2 to 3 minutes.

Stir in beef and Parm-style topping. Cook and stir until hot, 1 to 2 minutes. Eat!

MAKES 1 SERVING

SHIRATAKI NOODLE SWAPPIN'!

We know not *everyone* loves the taste and texture of Tofu Shirataki. If you want to enjoy these recipes with regular noodles, just prepare 2 ounces uncooked high-fiber fettuccine or spaghetti per package instructions, and use that instead of a bag of Tofu Shirataki. This'll add about 150 calories and 35 grams of carbs to the recipe. Still WAY better than restaurant versions!

SHRIMP TOMATO-FREDO

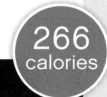
266 calories

You'll Need: strainer, skillet, nonstick spray
Prep: 10 minutes
Cook: 10 minutes

Entire recipe: 266 calories, 5.5g fat, 817mg sodium, 22g carbs, 7g fiber, 8.5g sugars, 28g protein

INGREDIENTS

1 bag House Foods Tofu Shirataki Fettuccine Shaped Noodle Substitute

4 ounces raw shrimp, peeled, tails removed, deveined

3 tablespoons low-fat marinara sauce

1 wedge The Laughing Cow Light Creamy Swiss cheese

2 tablespoons bagged sun-dried tomatoes (not packed in oil), chopped

2 teaspoons reduced-fat Parmesan-style grated topping

½ teaspoon dried basil

¼ teaspoon dried minced onion

⅛ teaspoon black pepper

DIRECTIONS

Use a strainer to rinse and drain noodles. Thoroughly pat dry. Roughly cut noodles.

Bring a skillet sprayed with nonstick spray to medium heat. Cook and stir shrimp for 4 minutes, or until just cooked through.

Remove shrimp and set aside. If needed, clean skillet. Remove from heat, re-spray, and return to medium heat. Add noodles, sauce, and cheese wedge, breaking the wedge into pieces. Cook and stir until cheese has melted, mixed with sauce, and coated noodles, 2 to 3 minutes.

Stir in shrimp and all remaining ingredients. Cook and stir until hot, 1 to 2 minutes. Eat!

MAKES 1 SERVING

FETTUCCINE HUNGRY CHICK-FREDO

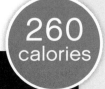
260 calories

You'll Need: strainer, skillet, nonstick spray
Prep: 10 minutes
Cook: 15 minutes

Entire recipe: 260 calories, 5g fat, 578mg sodium, 10.5g carbs, 4g fiber, 1.5g sugars, 38g protein

INGREDIENTS

1 bag House Foods Tofu Shirataki Fettuccine Shaped Noodle Substitute

One 5-ounce boneless skinless raw chicken breast cutlet, pounded to ½-inch thickness

Dash each salt and black pepper

1 teaspoon fat-free sour cream

2 teaspoons reduced-fat Parmesan-style grated topping

1 wedge The Laughing Cow Light Creamy Swiss cheese

Optional seasonings: garlic powder, paprika

DIRECTIONS

Use a strainer to rinse and drain noodles. Thoroughly pat dry. Roughly cut noodles.

Bring a skillet sprayed with nonstick spray to medium-high heat. Season chicken with a dash each salt and pepper and place in the skillet. Cook for 4 minutes.

Flip chicken and cook for 4 more minutes, or until cooked through.

Remove chicken and slice into strips. If needed, clean skillet. Remove from heat, re-spray, and bring to medium heat. Add noodles, sour cream, Parm-style topping, and cheese wedge, breaking the wedge into pieces. Cook and stir until cheese has melted, mixed with sour cream, and coated noodles, 2 to 3 minutes.

Stir in sliced chicken and cook and stir until hot, 1 to 2 minutes. Yum!

MAKES 1 SERVING

SUPER-SCHMANCY HUNGRY GIRLFREDO

299 calories

You'll Need: strainer, skillet, nonstick spray
Prep: 10 minutes
Cook: 15 minutes

Entire recipe: 299 calories, 5g fat, 762mg sodium, 23.5g carbs, 8g fiber, 8g sugars, 34.5g protein

INGREDIENTS

1 bag House Foods Tofu Shirataki Fettuccine Shaped Noodle Substitute
4 ounces raw boneless skinless chicken breast, cut into bite-sized pieces
2 dashes each salt and black pepper, or more to taste
1 teaspoon fat-free sour cream
2 teaspoons reduced-fat Parmesan-style grated topping
1 wedge The Laughing Cow Light Creamy Swiss cheese
⅓ cup frozen peas, thawed
2 tablespoons bagged sun-dried tomatoes (not packed in oil), chopped
¼ teaspoon garlic powder

DIRECTIONS

Use a strainer to rinse and drain noodles. Thoroughly pat dry. Roughly cut noodles.

Bring a skillet sprayed with nonstick spray to medium-high heat. Add chicken and season with a dash each salt and pepper. Cook and stir for 5 minutes, or until chicken is cooked through.

Remove chicken and set aside. If needed, clean skillet. Remove from heat, re-spray, and bring to medium heat. Add noodles, sour cream, Parm-style topping, and cheese wedge, breaking the wedge into pieces. Cook and stir until cheese has melted, mixed with sour cream, and coated noodles, 2 to 3 minutes.

Stir in chicken, peas, sun-dried tomatoes, garlic powder, and remaining dash each salt and black pepper. Cook and stir until hot, 1 to 2 minutes. EAT!

MAKES 1 SERVING

ITALIAN-STYLE BACON GIRLFREDO

266 calories

You'll Need: strainer, skillet, nonstick spray
Prep: 10 minutes
Cook: 15 minutes

Entire recipe: 266 calories, 7g fat, 901mg sodium, 15g carbs, 5.25g fiber, 4g sugars, 33.5g protein

INGREDIENTS

1 bag House Foods Tofu Shirataki Spaghetti Shaped Noodle Substitute
4 ounces raw boneless skinless chicken breast, cut into bite-sized pieces
1 tablespoon fat-free sour cream
1 wedge The Laughing Cow Light Creamy Swiss cheese
¼ cup roasted red peppers packed in water, drained and roughly chopped
¼ cup canned sliced mushrooms, drained
2 teaspoons reduced-fat Parmesan-style grated topping
1 tablespoon precooked real crumbled bacon

Optional seasonings: salt and black pepper

DIRECTIONS

Use a strainer to rinse and drain noodles. Thoroughly pat dry. Roughly cut noodles.

Bring a skillet sprayed with nonstick spray to medium-high heat. Cook and stir chicken for 5 minutes, or until cooked through.

Remove chicken and set aside. If needed, clean skillet. Remove from heat, re-spray, and bring to medium heat. Add noodles, sour cream, and cheese wedge, breaking the wedge into pieces. Cook and stir until cheese has melted, mixed with sour cream, and coated noodles, 2 to 3 minutes.

Stir in cooked chicken, peppers, mushrooms, and Parm-style topping. Cook and stir until hot, 1 to 2 minutes.

Serve topped with bacon and enjoy!

MAKES 1 SERVING

BUFFALO VEGGIE HUNGRY GIRLFREDO

215 calories

You'll Need: strainer, microwave-safe bowl, skillet, nonstick spray
Prep: 10 minutes
Cook: 10 minutes

Entire recipe: 215 calories, 5g fat, 625mg sodium, 27g carbs, 8g fiber, 7g sugars, 10.5g protein

INGREDIENTS

1 bag House Foods Tofu Shirataki Fettuccine Shaped Noodle Substitute

1 cup frozen mixed vegetables

2 teaspoons reduced-fat Parmesan-style grated topping

2 wedges The Laughing Cow Light Creamy Swiss cheese

5 splashes Frank's RedHot Original Cayenne Pepper Sauce

Optional seasonings: salt and black pepper

DIRECTIONS

Use a strainer to rinse and drain noodles. Thoroughly pat dry. Roughly cut noodles.

Microwave frozen veggies in a microwave-safe bowl for 2 minutes, or until thawed. Blot away excess moisture.

Bring a skillet sprayed with nonstick spray to medium heat. Add noodles, Parm-style topping, and cheese wedges, breaking the wedges into pieces. Cook and stir until cheese has melted and coated noodles, 2 to 3 minutes.

Stir in veggies and hot sauce. Cook and stir until hot, 1 to 2 minutes. Enjoy!

MAKES 1 SERVING

CREAMY SALMON GIRLFREDO

315 calories

You'll Need: strainer, skillet, nonstick spray
Prep: 10 minutes
Cook: 15 minutes

Entire recipe: 315 calories, 13g fat, 782mg sodium, 14.5g carbs, 6g fiber, 2.5g sugars, 31.5g protein

INGREDIENTS

1 bag House Foods Tofu Shirataki Fettuccine Shaped Noodle Substitute

One 4-ounce raw skinless salmon fillet

Dash each salt and black pepper

½ cup chopped asparagus

1 tablespoon Hellmann's/Best Foods Dijonnaise

¼ teaspoon chopped garlic

1 wedge The Laughing Cow Light Creamy Swiss cheese

1 cup chopped spinach leaves

2 teaspoons reduced-fat Parmesan-style grated topping

DIRECTIONS

Use a strainer to rinse and drain noodles. Thoroughly pat dry. Roughly cut noodles.

Bring a skillet sprayed with nonstick spray to medium-high heat. Add salmon and sprinkle with salt and pepper. Cook for 4 minutes.

Flip salmon and add asparagus. Cook for about 4 minutes, stirring asparagus, until salmon is just cooked through and asparagus has slightly softened.

Remove salmon and asparagus. If needed, clean skillet. Remove from heat, re-spray, and bring to medium heat. Add noodles, Dijonnaise, garlic, and cheese wedge, breaking the wedge into pieces. Cook and stir until cheese has melted, mixed with Dijonnaise, and coated noodles, 2 to 3 minutes.

Stir in spinach, Parm-style topping, and asparagus. Add salmon and break into pieces with a spatula. Cook and stir until spinach has wilted and dish is hot, 1 to 2 minutes. EAT!

MAKES 1 SERVING

CIN-SATIONAL CINCINNATI CHILI

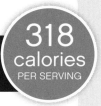

318 calories
PER SERVING

You'll Need: large pot with a lid, nonstick spray, strainer, large microwave-safe bowl
Prep: 15 minutes | **Cook:** 40 minutes

⅙th of recipe (about ⅔ cup noodles, 1 cup chili, and ¼ cup cheese):
318 calories, 4.5g fat, 894mg sodium, 35.5g carbs, 11g fiber, 11g sugars, 34g protein

INGREDIENTS

1 pound raw extra-lean ground beef
2 cups chopped onion
One 15-ounce can red kidney beans, drained and rinsed
One 14.5-ounce can crushed tomatoes
One 14.5-ounce can diced tomatoes (not drained)
One 6-ounce can tomato paste
1 tablespoon unsweetened cocoa powder
2 teaspoons chili powder
2 teaspoons chopped garlic
1½ teaspoons Worcestershire sauce
1 teaspoon cinnamon
½ teaspoon ground cumin
¼ teaspoon ground allspice
1 dried bay leaf
4 bags House Foods Tofu Shirataki Spaghetti Shaped
    Noodle Substitute
1½ cups shredded fat-free cheddar cheese

DIRECTIONS

Bring a large pot sprayed with nonstick spray to medium-high heat. Add beef and onion. Cook, stir, and crumble until beef is fully cooked and onion has softened, 7 to 8 minutes.

Drain excess liquid. Add all remaining ingredients *except* noodles and cheese. Mix in ½ cup water and bring to a boil.

Reduce to a simmer, cover, and cook for 20 minutes, or until thickened to your desired consistency.

Meanwhile, use a strainer to rinse and drain noodles well. Thoroughly pat dry. Roughly cut noodles. Place in a large microwave-safe bowl.

Remove chili from heat, and remove and discard bay leaf. Mix well.

Microwave noodles for 2½ minutes, or until hot. Drain excess liquid, and thoroughly pat dry. Serve noodles topped with chili and cheese!

MAKES 6 SERVINGS

HG ALTERNATIVE!

Wanna make and enjoy just the chili, minus the noodles 'n cheese? Go for it! A serving of the chili by itself (about 1 cup) has 253 calories, 4g fat, 599mg sodium, 31.5g carbs, 9g fiber, 10.5g sugars, and 24g protein. Three cheers for THAT!

BEEF STROGATAKI

291 calories

You'll Need: strainer, medium bowl, large skillet, nonstick spray
Prep: 10 minutes
Cook: 20 minutes

Entire recipe: 291 calories, 10g fat, 955mg sodium, 17g carbs, 5g fiber, 4g sugars, 31g protein

INGREDIENTS

1 bag House Foods Tofu Shirataki Fettuccine
    Shaped Noodle Substitute
1 teaspoon dry au jus gravy mix
4 ounces thinly sliced raw lean beefsteak filet
    (freeze slightly before slicing)
½ cup sliced mushrooms
½ cup thinly sliced onion
1 wedge The Laughing Cow Light Creamy Swiss cheese
1 teaspoon fat-free plain yogurt

Optional seasonings: salt and black pepper

DIRECTIONS

Use a strainer to rinse and drain noodles. Thoroughly pat dry. Roughly cut noodles.

In a medium bowl, combine gravy mix with 1 cup water and stir to dissolve.

Bring a large skillet sprayed with nonstick spray to medium-high heat. Cook beef for about 4 minutes per side, until fully cooked.

Remove beef and set aside. If needed, clean skillet. Remove from heat, re-spray, and return to medium-high heat. Add mushrooms, onion, and gravy mixture to the skillet. Cook and stir until veggies are tender and sauce has thickened, about 8 minutes.

Add cheese wedge, breaking it into pieces. Cook and stir until cheese has melted and mixed with sauce, about 1 minute. Stir in yogurt.

Add noodles and beef and cook and stir until hot and well mixed, 3 to 4 minutes. Eat up!

MAKES 1 SERVING

SIMPLY THE PESTO SPAGHETTI

177 calories
PER SERVING

You'll Need: small blender or food processor, strainer, skillet, nonstick spray
Prep: 10 minutes
Cook: 5 minutes

½ of recipe (about 1 cup): 177 calories, 10.75g fat, 490mg sodium, 13g carbs, 4.75g fiber, 1.5g sugars, 8g protein

INGREDIENTS

1 cup fresh basil leaves
¼ cup fat-free ricotta cheese
2 tablespoons reduced-fat Parmesan-style
    grated topping
2 tablespoons pine nuts
1 teaspoon olive oil
1 teaspoon chopped garlic
¼ teaspoon each salt and black pepper,
    or more to taste
2 bags House Foods Tofu Shirataki
    Spaghetti Shaped Noodle Substitute

DIRECTIONS

To make the sauce, place all ingredients *except* noodles in a small blender or food processor, and blend until a smooth paste forms.

Use a strainer to rinse and drain noodles. Thoroughly pat dry. Roughly cut noodles.

Bring a skillet sprayed with nonstick spray to medium-high heat. Cook and stir noodles until hot, about 2 minutes. Add sauce, stir to coat, and serve!

MAKES 2 SERVINGS

For more recipes, tips & tricks, sign up for FREE daily emails at hungry-girl.com!

CLAM-TASTIC SHIRATAKI PASTA

181 calories
PER SERVING

You'll Need: strainer, large skillet, nonstick spray
Prep: 15 minutes
Cook: 10 minutes

½ of recipe (about 1½ cups):
181 calories, 6.5g fat, 667mg sodium, 20g carbs, 5g fiber, 3.5g sugars, 10g protein

INGREDIENTS

2 bags House Foods Tofu Shirataki Fettuccine Shaped Noodle Substitute

1 cup chopped onion

2 teaspoons chopped garlic

One 6.5-ounce can chopped clams in clam juice (not drained)

2 tablespoons light whipped butter or light buttery spread

2 teaspoons lemon juice

¼ teaspoon red pepper flakes, or more to taste

¼ teaspoon dried oregano

2 teaspoons reduced-fat Parmesan-style grated topping

Optional seasonings: salt and black pepper
Optional topping: chopped fresh parsley

DIRECTIONS

Use a strainer to rinse and drain noodles. Thoroughly pat dry. Roughly cut noodles.

Bring a large skillet sprayed with nonstick spray to medium heat. Cook and stir onion and garlic until slightly softened, about 5 minutes.

Add noodles and all other ingredients *except* Parm-style topping. Cook and stir until hot and well mixed, about 3 minutes.

Serve sprinkled with Parm-style topping. Eat up!

MAKES 2 SERVINGS

CHICKEN CARBONARA A LA HUNGRY GIRL

313 calories

You'll Need: strainer, microwave-safe bowl, whisk, skillet, nonstick spray
Prep: 10 minutes
Cook: 10 minutes

Entire recipe: 313 calories, 8.5g fat, 990mg sodium, 17g carbs, 5.75g fiber, 3.5g sugars, 40g protein

INGREDIENTS

1 bag House Foods Tofu Shirataki Spaghetti Shaped Noodle Substitute

1 wedge The Laughing Cow Light Creamy Swiss cheese

¼ cup fat-free liquid egg substitute

1 tablespoon reduced-fat Parmesan-style grated topping

3 ounces raw boneless skinless chicken breast, chopped

½ cup sliced mushrooms

½ teaspoon chopped garlic

¼ cup frozen no-salt-added peas

2 tablespoons precooked real crumbled bacon

Optional seasonings: salt and black pepper

DIRECTIONS

Use a strainer to rinse and drain noodles. Thoroughly pat dry. Roughly cut noodles.

Place cheese wedge in a microwave-safe bowl, breaking it into pieces. Microwave for 15 seconds and stir until smooth. Add egg substitute, Parm-style topping, and 2 tablespoons water. Whisk until mixed and mostly smooth.

Bring a skillet sprayed with nonstick spray to medium-high heat. Add chicken, mushrooms, and garlic. Cook and stir until mushrooms begin to brown, about 2 minutes. Add peas and cook and stir until hot, about 2 more minutes.

Add noodles and bacon and cook and stir until noodles are hot and chicken is fully cooked, about 3 minutes.

Reduce heat to low. Add egg mixture and, stirring constantly, cook until it has thickened and coated noodles, at least 2 minutes. Now chew!

MAKES 1 SERVING

SPICY SOUTHERN SHRIMP FETTUCCINE

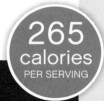

265 calories PER SERVING

You'll Need: strainer, skillet, nonstick spray
Prep: 10 minutes
Cook: 15 minutes

½ of recipe (about 2 cups): 265 calories, 7.5g fat, 523mg sodium, 18g carbs, 6g fiber, 5g sugars, 29g protein

INGREDIENTS

2 bags House Foods Tofu Shirataki Fettuccine Shaped Noodle Substitute
1 cup chopped bell pepper
½ cup chopped onion
1 teaspoon chopped garlic
8 ounces raw shrimp, peeled, tails removed, deveined
½ teaspoon Cajun seasoning, or more to taste
1 tablespoon light whipped butter or light buttery spread
2 wedges The Laughing Cow Light Creamy Swiss cheese
2 teaspoons reduced-fat Parmesan-style grated topping

Optional seasoning: salt

DIRECTIONS

Use a strainer to rinse and drain noodles. Thoroughly pat dry. Roughly cut noodles.

Bring a skillet sprayed with nonstick spray to medium-high heat. Add bell pepper, onion, and garlic. Cook and stir until softened, about 7 minutes.

Reduce heat to medium. Add shrimp and sprinkle with ¼ teaspoon Cajun seasoning. Cook and stir for 1 to 2 minutes, until cooked through.

Add noodles, butter, remaining ¼ teaspoon Cajun seasoning, and cheese wedges, breaking the wedges into pieces. Cook and stir until noodles are hot and cheese has melted, mixed with butter, and coated noodles, 2 to 3 minutes.

Serve sprinkled with Parm-style topping!

MAKES 2 SERVINGS

VODKA IMPASTA

181 calories

You'll Need: strainer, skillet, nonstick spray
Prep: 10 minutes
Cook: 10 minutes

Entire recipe: 181 calories, 5g fat, 786mg sodium, 25g carbs, 7g fiber, 9.5g sugars, 7.5g protein

INGREDIENTS

1 bag House Foods Tofu Shirataki Fettuccine Shaped Noodle Substitute
½ cup halved grape tomatoes or quartered cherry tomatoes
¼ cup chopped onion
½ teaspoon chopped garlic
Dash each salt and black pepper, or more to taste
⅓ cup low-fat marinara sauce
1 tablespoon chopped fresh basil
1 tablespoon reduced-fat Parmesan-style grated topping
1 wedge The Laughing Cow Light Creamy Swiss cheese

DIRECTIONS

Use a strainer to rinse and drain noodles. Thoroughly pat dry. Roughly cut noodles.

Bring a skillet sprayed with nonstick spray to medium heat. Add tomatoes, onion, garlic, salt, and pepper. Cook and stir until onion has softened, about 3 minutes.

Add noodles and all remaining ingredients, breaking the cheese wedge into pieces. Cook and stir until noodles are hot and cheese has melted, mixed with sauce, and coated noodles, about 3 minutes. EAT!

MAKES 1 SERVING

SUPER-DELICIOUS SHRIMP SCAMPI

 238 calories PER SERVING

You'll Need: strainer, small bowl, skillet, nonstick spray (butter flavored, optional)
Prep: 20 minutes
Cook: 10 minutes

½ of recipe (about 1¾ cups): 238 calories, 8.5g fat, 329mg sodium, 14g carbs, 5g fiber, 2g sugars, 26g protein

INGREDIENTS

1 small lemon
2 bags House Foods Tofu Shirataki Fettuccine Shaped Noodle Substitute
¼ cup chopped onion
1 teaspoon chopped garlic
8 ounces raw shrimp, peeled, tails removed, deveined
1 plum tomato, chopped
2 tablespoons light whipped butter or light buttery spread
2 teaspoons reduced-fat Parmesan-style grated topping

Optional seasonings: salt, black pepper, red pepper flakes, chopped parsley

DIRECTIONS

Cut lemon in half and, over a strainer, squeeze the juice from one half into a small bowl. Cut the other half into wedges.

Use a strainer to rinse and drain noodles. Thoroughly pat dry. Roughly cut noodles.

Bring a skillet sprayed with nonstick spray (butter flavored, if you've got it) to medium heat. Cook and stir onion and garlic until softened, 2 to 3 minutes.

Add shrimp and tomato. Cook and stir until shrimp are opaque, about 2 minutes. Add lemon juice and cook and stir for 1 minute.

Raise heat to medium high, add noodles, and mix well. Cook and stir until entire dish is hot and shrimp are cooked through, 1 to 2 minutes.

Stir in butter until melted. Serve sprinkled with Parm-style topping and garnished with lemon wedges!

MAKES 2 SERVINGS

CHICKEN FLORENTINE

 289 calories

You'll Need: strainer, skillet, nonstick spray
Prep: 15 minutes
Cook: 15 minutes

Entire recipe: 289 calories, 5.5g fat, 853mg sodium, 23.5g carbs, 6.5g fiber, 6g sugars, 34.5g protein

INGREDIENTS

1 bag House Foods Tofu Shirataki Fettuccine Shaped Noodle Substitute
4 ounces raw boneless skinless chicken breast, cut into bite-sized pieces
⅛ teaspoon each salt and black pepper
⅛ teaspoon garlic powder
½ cup sliced mushrooms
½ cup chopped onion
½ teaspoon chopped garlic
1 tablespoon fat-free mayonnaise
2 teaspoons reduced-fat Parmesan-style grated topping
1 wedge The Laughing Cow Light Creamy Swiss cheese
2 cups chopped spinach leaves

DIRECTIONS

Use a strainer to rinse and drain noodles. Thoroughly pat dry. Roughly cut noodles.

Bring a skillet sprayed with nonstick spray to medium-high heat. Add chicken and season with salt, pepper, and garlic powder. Add mushrooms, onion, and garlic. Cook and stir until veggies have softened and chicken is cooked through, about 5 minutes. Remove contents and set aside.

If needed, clean skillet. Remove from heat, re-spray, and bring to medium heat. Add noodles, mayo, Parm-style topping, and cheese wedge, breaking the wedge into pieces. Cook and stir until cheese has melted, mixed with mayo, and coated noodles, about 3 minutes.

Stir in spinach, chicken, and cooked veggies. Cook and stir until spinach has wilted and dish is hot, 2 to 3 minutes. EAT!

MAKES 1 SERVING

VAMPIRE-PROOF CHICKEN 'N VEGGIE PASTA

283 calories PER SERVING

You'll Need: strainer, skillet with a lid, nonstick spray | **Prep:** 10 minutes | **Cook:** 25 minutes

½ of recipe (about 2½ cups):
283 calories, 6g fat, 530mg sodium, 23g carbs, 9.5g fiber, 8g sugars, 34.5g protein

INGREDIENTS

2 bags House Foods Tofu Shirataki Spaghetti Shaped Noodle Substitute

8 ounces raw boneless skinless chicken breast cutlets

¼ teaspoon Italian seasoning

¼ teaspoon salt

⅛ teaspoon black pepper

2½ cups asparagus cut into 1-inch pieces (about 20 spears)

1 cup sliced brown mushrooms

¼ cup bagged sun-dried tomatoes (not packed in oil), thinly sliced

1 teaspoon chopped garlic

1 tablespoon light whipped butter or light buttery spread

1 tablespoon reduced-fat Parmesan-style grated topping

DIRECTIONS

Use a strainer to rinse and drain noodles. Thoroughly pat dry. Roughly cut noodles.

Bring a skillet sprayed with nonstick spray to medium-high heat. Add chicken and season with Italian seasoning, ⅛ teaspoon salt, and pepper. Cook for about 4 minutes per side, until fully cooked.

Remove chicken and set aside. If needed, clean skillet. Remove from heat, re-spray, and return to medium-high heat. Add asparagus and 2 tablespoons water. Cover and cook for 4 minutes. Meanwhile, slice chicken.

Uncover skillet and add mushrooms, tomatoes, and garlic. Cook and stir until tender, about 4 more minutes.

Add noodles and cook and stir until hot, about 2 minutes. Add butter, remaining ⅛ teaspoon salt, and sliced chicken. Cook and stir until butter has melted and ingredients are well mixed, about 1 minute.

Stir in Parm-style topping and serve!

MAKES 2 SERVINGS

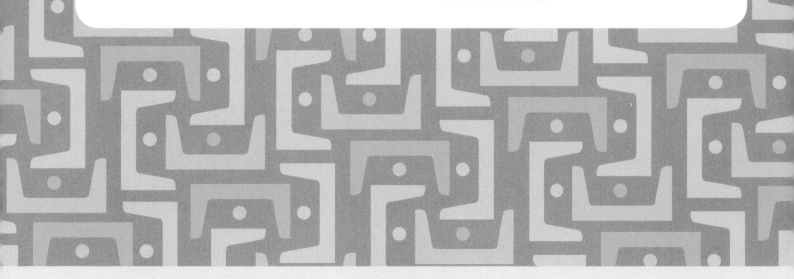

Pasta swappin' with **SPAGHETTI SQUASH** is a no-brainer! It's a fantastic and delicious pasta alternative that's 100 percent natural and SO low in calories . . .

SPAGHETTI SWAP & MEATBALLS

327 calories
PER SERVING

You'll Need: large baking pan, baking sheet, nonstick spray, 2 large bowls, strainer, medium pot
Prep: 20 minutes | **Cook:** 1 hour and 10 minutes

½ of recipe (2 cups squash with about ¾ cup sauce and 3 meatballs):
327 calories, 6g fat, 775mg sodium, 45g carbs, 9g fiber, 19g sugars, 26g protein

INGREDIENTS

Spaghetti
1 spaghetti squash (about 4½ pounds)

Meatballs
6 ounces raw extra-lean ground beef
2 tablespoons fat-free liquid egg substitute
1 teaspoon dried parsley
½ teaspoon chopped garlic
⅛ teaspoon each salt and black pepper

Sauce
½ cup finely diced onion
½ cup finely diced carrot
1 teaspoon chopped garlic
1½ cups canned crushed tomatoes
¼ cup chopped fresh basil
2 tablespoons tomato paste
1 teaspoon Italian seasoning
¼ teaspoon red pepper flakes, or more to taste
¼ teaspoon ground cumin
4 teaspoons reduced-fat Parmesan-style
    grated topping

DIRECTIONS

Preheat oven to 400 degrees.

Microwave squash for 3 to 4 minutes, until soft enough to cut. Halve lengthwise; scoop out and discard seeds. Fill a large baking pan with ½ inch water and place squash halves in the pan, cut sides down. Bake until tender, about 40 minutes.

Spray a baking sheet with nonstick spray.

Thoroughly mix meatball ingredients in a large bowl. Evenly form into 6 meatballs and place on the baking sheet, evenly spaced. Bake until just cooked through, about 10 minutes.

Use a fork to scrape out squash strands. Place in a strainer to drain excess moisture. Blot dry, if needed. Transfer to another large bowl and cover to keep warm.

Bring a medium pot sprayed with nonstick spray to medium-high heat. Cook and stir onion and carrot until slightly softened, 6 to 8 minutes. Add garlic and cook until fragrant, 1 to 2 minutes. Add all remaining sauce ingredients *except* Parm-style topping; stir to combine. Add meatballs and bring sauce to a low boil. Reduce heat to low. Gently stirring occasionally, simmer until veggies have softened and meatballs are hot, about 8 minutes.

Add sauce to spaghetti strands and stir to coat. Serve topped with meatballs and Parm-style topping!

MAKES 2 SERVINGS

HG ALTERNATIVE!

This recipe can also be made with 1½ cups of jarred low-fat marinara sauce . . . But our sauce is reeeeallly good!

CHEESY-PEASY SPAGHETTI SQUASH

171 calories
PER SERVING

You'll Need: large baking pan, blender or food processor (optional), strainer, large bowl, microwave-safe bowl, small microwave-safe dish
Prep: 10 minutes
Cook: 50 minutes

¼th of recipe (about 1½ cups): 171 calories, 3.5g fat, 429mg sodium, 25.5g carbs, 5g fiber, 10g sugars, 9g protein

INGREDIENTS

1 spaghetti squash (about 4½ pounds)
1 stick light string cheese
1½ cups frozen petite mixed vegetables
4 wedges The Laughing Cow Light Creamy Swiss cheese
¼ cup shredded fat-free cheddar cheese
1 tablespoon reduced-fat Parmesan-style grated topping

DIRECTIONS

Preheat oven to 400 degrees.

Microwave whole squash for 3 to 4 minutes, until soft enough to cut. Halve lengthwise; scoop out and discard seeds. Fill a large baking pan with ½ inch water and place squash halves in the pan, cut sides down. Bake until tender, about 40 minutes.

Meanwhile, break string cheese into thirds and place in a blender or food processor—blend at high speed until shredded. (Or pull into shreds and roughly chop.)

Use a fork to scrape out squash strands. Place in a strainer to drain excess moisture. Blot dry, if needed. Transfer to a large bowl and cover to keep warm.

Microwave frozen veggies in a microwave-safe bowl for 2 minutes. Stir well. Microwave for 1 minute, or until hot. Drain any excess water, and transfer veggies to the bowl with the squash strands.

In a small microwave-safe dish, microwave cheese wedges for 20 seconds, or until hot. Add to the large bowl along with shredded string cheese and cheddar cheese. Stir until cheeses have melted and are well mixed.

Serve sprinkled with Parm-style topping. Eat up!

MAKES 4 SERVINGS

SPAGHETTI SQUASH 'N SHRIMP ARRABBIATA

243 calories
PER SERVING

You'll Need: large baking pan, medium pot with a lid, nonstick spray, strainer, large bowl
Prep: 10 minutes
Cook: 50 minutes

¼th of recipe (about 1⅓ cups squash with 1 heaping cup shrimp and sauce): 243 calories, 2g fat, 838mg sodium, 37g carbs, 8.5g fiber, 15g sugars, 21g protein

INGREDIENTS

1 spaghetti squash (about 4½ pounds)
1 cup chopped onion
2 teaspoons chopped garlic
1 teaspoon red pepper flakes, or more to taste
One 28-ounce can crushed tomatoes (about 3 cups)
1 teaspoon Italian seasoning
12 ounces raw shrimp, peeled, tails removed, deveined
½ cup chopped fresh basil
¼ teaspoon each salt and black pepper

DIRECTIONS

Preheat oven to 400 degrees.

Microwave whole squash for 3 to 4 minutes, until soft enough to cut. Halve lengthwise; scoop out and discard seeds. Fill a large baking pan with ½ inch water and place squash halves in the pan, cut sides down. Bake until tender, about 40 minutes.

About 20 minutes before squash is done baking, bring a medium pot sprayed with nonstick spray to medium-high heat. Add onion, garlic, and red pepper flakes. Cook and stir until onion has softened and slightly browned, about 5 minutes.

Add tomatoes and Italian seasoning to the pot. Cook and stir until hot, 1 to 2 minutes. Reduce heat to medium low. Add shrimp and cook for about 5 minutes, until cooked through.

Remove pot from heat, stir in basil, and cover to keep warm.

Use a fork to scrape out squash strands. Place in a strainer to drain excess moisture. Blot dry, if needed. Transfer to a large bowl and season with salt and black pepper.

Top each serving of squash (about 1⅓ cups) with ¼th of the saucy shrimp mixture (1 heaping cup). Dig in!

MAKES 4 SERVINGS

BUTTERY GARLIC SPAGHETTI SQUASH

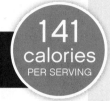

141 calories
PER SERVING

You'll Need: large baking pan, strainer, large bowl | **Prep:** 15 minutes | **Cook:** 45 minutes

¼th of recipe (about 1⅓ cups):
141 calories, 6.5g fat, 343mg sodium, 20g carbs, 4g fiber, 7.5g sugars, 2.5g protein

INGREDIENTS

1 spaghetti squash (about 4½ pounds)

¼ cup light whipped butter or light buttery spread

2 tablespoons reduced-fat Parmesan-style grated topping

1 teaspoon garlic powder

¼ teaspoon salt, or more to taste

Optional seasoning: black pepper

DIRECTIONS

Preheat oven to 400 degrees.

Microwave squash for 3 to 4 minutes, until soft enough to cut. Halve lengthwise; scoop out and discard seeds. Fill a large baking pan with ½ inch water and place squash halves in the pan, cut sides down. Bake until tender, about 40 minutes.

Use a fork to scrape out squash strands. Place in a strainer to drain excess moisture. Blot dry, if needed. Transfer to a large bowl.

Stir in remaining ingredients, until butter has melted, and enjoy!

MAKES 4 SERVINGS

PEPPERONI SPAGHETTI SQUASH

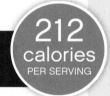

212 calories
PER SERVING

You'll Need: large baking pan, strainer, large bowl, large skillet, nonstick spray | **Prep:** 10 minutes | **Cook:** 1 hour

¼th of recipe (about 1¾ cups):
212 calories, 4g fat, 729mg sodium, 36.5g carbs, 5.5g fiber, 17g sugars, 10.5g protein

INGREDIENTS

1 spaghetti squash (about 4½ pounds)

2 cups sliced mushrooms

1 cup chopped onion

1 teaspoon chopped garlic

One 14.5-ounce can creamy tomato soup with 4g fat or less per serving

½ cup fat-free sour cream

30 slices turkey pepperoni, chopped

¼ cup chopped fresh basil

Optional seasonings: salt, black pepper, red pepper flakes

DIRECTIONS

Preheat oven to 400 degrees.

Microwave squash for 3 to 4 minutes, until soft enough to cut. Halve lengthwise; scoop out and discard seeds. Fill a large baking pan with ½ inch water and place squash halves in the pan, cut sides down. Bake until tender, about 40 minutes.

Use a fork to scrape out squash strands. Place in a strainer to drain excess moisture. Blot dry, if needed. Transfer to a large bowl and cover to keep warm.

Bring a large skillet sprayed with nonstick spray to medium-high heat. Add mushrooms, onion, and garlic, and cook and stir until softened, about 8 minutes. Stir in soup, sour cream, pepperoni, and basil. Cook and stir until hot and well mixed, about 2 minutes.

Add contents of the skillet to the bowl of squash strands and mix well. Serve it up!

MAKES 4 SERVINGS

MEDITERRANEAN SPAGHETTI SQUASH

332 calories
PER SERVING

You'll Need: large baking pan, strainer, large bowl, large skillet, nonstick spray
Prep: 15 minutes
Cook: 55 minutes

½ of recipe (about 3 cups): 332 calories, 15g fat, 843mg sodium, 44.5g carbs, 10.5g fiber, 17g sugars, 12.5g protein

INGREDIENTS

1 spaghetti squash (about 4½ pounds)
1 teaspoon chopped garlic
4 cups chopped spinach leaves
1 cup chopped tomato
½ cup crumbled reduced-fat feta cheese
2 tablespoons chopped fresh basil
2 tablespoons sliced black olives
1 tablespoon olive oil
¼ teaspoon each salt and black pepper

DIRECTIONS

Preheat oven to 400 degrees.

Microwave squash for 3 to 4 minutes, until soft enough to cut. Halve lengthwise; scoop out and discard seeds. Fill a large baking pan with ½ inch water and place squash halves in the pan, cut sides down. Bake until tender, about 40 minutes.

Use a fork to scrape out squash strands. Place in a strainer to drain excess moisture. Blot dry, if needed. Transfer to a large bowl and cover to keep warm.

Bring a large skillet sprayed with nonstick spray to medium-high heat. Cook and stir garlic until fragrant, about 1 minute. Add spinach and cook and stir until just wilted, 1 to 2 minutes.

Remove skillet from heat and blot away excess moisture. Add garlic spinach to the bowl of squash strands. Add remaining ingredients and thoroughly mix. Enjoy!

MAKES 2 SERVINGS

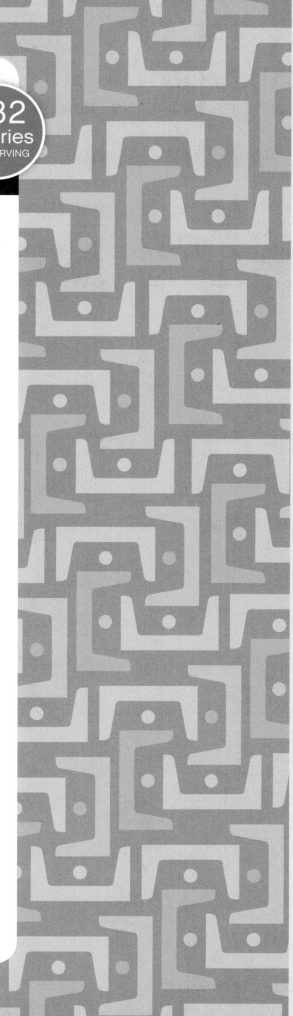

LA-LA-LA-LA-LASAGNA! Layers and layers of unconventional fun! We use eggplant to supersize our lasagna without adding many calories at all!

EZ CHEESY LASAGNA FOR TWO

238 calories PER SERVING

You'll Need: baking sheet, loaf pan, nonstick spray, 2 medium bowls, skillet
Prep: 15 minutes | **Cook:** 50 minutes

½ of lasagna:
238 calories, 4g fat, 845mg sodium, 31.5g carbs, 5g fiber, 10g sugars, 17.5g protein

INGREDIENTS

Two ¼-inch-thick eggplant slices
    (cut lengthwise from a long eggplant),
    patted dry
2 tablespoons liquid egg whites (about
    1 egg white)
½ cup fat-free ricotta cheese
1 tablespoon chopped fresh basil
½ teaspoon chopped garlic
¼ teaspoon salt
Dash ground nutmeg
1 cup chopped mushrooms
1 cup canned crushed tomatoes
½ tablespoon Italian seasoning
2 sheets oven-ready lasagna noodles
¼ cup shredded part-skim mozzarella cheese
1 tablespoon reduced-fat Parmesan-style
    grated topping

Optional seasoning: black pepper

DIRECTIONS

Preheat oven to 425 degrees. Spray a baking sheet and a loaf pan with nonstick spray.

Lay eggplant on the baking sheet and spray with nonstick spray. Bake for 10 minutes. Flip eggplant and bake until browned and softened, about 10 more minutes.

Meanwhile, in a medium bowl, thoroughly mix egg whites, ricotta cheese, basil, garlic, salt, and nutmeg.

Bring a skillet sprayed with nonstick spray to medium-high heat. Cook and stir mushrooms until softened, about 4 minutes. Stir mushrooms into ricotta mixture.

In another medium bowl, mix crushed tomatoes with Italian seasoning.

Evenly layer ingredients in the loaf pan: ¼ cup seasoned tomatoes, 1 lasagna sheet, half of the mushroom-ricotta mixture, ¼ cup seasoned tomatoes, 1 eggplant slice. Repeat layering with remaining ingredients.

Sprinkle with mozzarella cheese and grated topping. Bake until cheese is lightly browned, 20 to 25 minutes. Serve and enjoy!

MAKES 2 SERVINGS

Flip to the photo inserts to see over 100 recipe pics! And for photos of ALL the recipes, go to hungry-girl.com/books.

HUNGRY GIRLFREDO WHITE LASAGNA

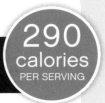
290 calories
PER SERVING

You'll Need: 8-inch by 8-inch baking pan, nonstick spray, medium bowl, large skillet, microwave-safe bowl
Prep: 15 minutes | **Cook:** 45 minutes

¼th of lasagna:
290 calories, 6.5g fat, 726mg sodium, 33g carbs, 3g fiber, 10g sugars, 21.5g protein

INGREDIENTS

1 cup fat-free ricotta cheese

¼ cup liquid egg whites (about 2 egg whites)

1 teaspoon chopped garlic

¼ teaspoon dried oregano

¼ teaspoon dried basil

¼ teaspoon each salt and black pepper

1½ cups chopped mushrooms

2 cups chopped spinach leaves

3 medium zucchini, ends removed, halved widthwise, cut lengthwise into ¼-inch-thick strips

¾ cup fat-free sour cream

4 wedges The Laughing Cow Light Creamy Swiss cheese

¼ cup reduced-fat Parmesan-style grated topping

4 sheets oven-ready lasagna noodles

½ cup shredded part-skim mozzarella cheese

Optional seasonings: additional salt and black pepper

DIRECTIONS

Preheat oven to 425 degrees. Spray an 8-inch by 8-inch baking pan with nonstick spray.

In a medium bowl, thoroughly mix ricotta cheese, egg whites, garlic, oregano, basil, ⅛ teaspoon salt, and ⅛ teaspoon black pepper.

Bring a large skillet sprayed with nonstick spray to medium-high heat. Cook and stir mushrooms until softened, about 4 minutes. Add spinach and cook and stir until wilted, about 2 minutes.

Remove skillet from heat and blot away excess moisture. Stir cooked veggies into ricotta mixture.

Remove skillet from heat, re-spray, and return to medium-high heat. Working in batches, as needed, cook zucchini until softened, about 2 minutes per side.

To make the sauce, in a microwave-safe bowl, mix sour cream with cheese wedges, breaking the wedges into pieces as you add them. Stir in 2 tablespoons Parm-style topping and remaining ⅛ teaspoon each salt and black pepper. Microwave for 45 seconds, or until very warm. Stir until smooth.

Evenly layer ingredients in the baking pan: ⅓rd of zucchini strips, half of the ricotta-veggie mixture, 2 lasagna sheets, and ⅓rd of the sauce.

Repeat layering step. Top with remaining zucchini and sauce. Sprinkle with mozzarella cheese and remaining 2 tablespoons Parm-style topping.

Bake until cheese has lightly browned, 25 to 30 minutes. Enjoy!

MAKES 4 SERVINGS

VEGGIE-RIFIC NOODLE-FREE LASAGNA

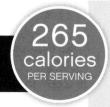
265 calories
PER SERVING

You'll Need: 8-inch by 8-inch baking pan, nonstick spray, grill pan, 2 large bowls
Prep: 20 minutes | **Cook:** 1 hour

¼th of lasagna:
265 calories, 4.5g fat, 926mg sodium, 32.5g carbs, 11g fiber, 13.5g sugars, 24g protein

INGREDIENTS

3 medium zucchini, ends removed,
    sliced lengthwise
1 large portabella mushroom, sliced into strips
1 large eggplant, ends removed, sliced lengthwise
2 cups canned crushed tomatoes
¼ teaspoon garlic powder
¼ teaspoon onion powder
¼ teaspoon Italian seasoning
One 16-ounce package frozen chopped spinach,
    thawed and squeezed dry
1 cup fat-free ricotta cheese
2 tablespoons fat-free liquid egg substitute
1 tablespoon chopped fresh basil
¼ teaspoon salt
Dash ground nutmeg
1 cup frozen ground-beef-style soy
    crumbles, thawed
½ cup shredded part-skim mozzarella cheese
1 tablespoon reduced-fat Parmesan-style
    grated topping

DIRECTIONS

Preheat oven to 425 degrees. Spray an 8-inch by 8-inch baking pan with nonstick spray.

Lay paper towels next to the stove, to drain veggies during the next step.

Bring a grill pan sprayed with nonstick spray to medium-high heat. Working in batches as needed, lay zucchini, mushroom, and eggplant slices in the pan and cook until softened, about 2 minutes per side. Transfer cooked veggies to the paper towels.

In a large bowl, mix crushed tomatoes, garlic powder, onion powder, and Italian seasoning.

In another large bowl, mix spinach, ricotta cheese, egg substitute, basil, salt, and nutmeg.

Evenly layer ingredients in the baking pan: half of the seasoned tomatoes, half of the sliced veggies, half of the spinach mixture, and all of the soy crumbles.

Evenly layer remaining veggies, in the opposite direction of the first layer, followed by remaining spinach mixture and remaining seasoned tomatoes. Top with mozzarella cheese and Parm-style topping.

Bake until cheese has lightly browned, about 30 minutes. Mmmmm!

MAKES 4 SERVINGS

PUMPKIN LASAGNA

343 calories
PER SERVING

You'll Need: 8-inch by 8-inch baking pan, nonstick spray, large skillet, medium bowl
Prep: 15 minutes | **Cook:** 45 minutes

¼th of lasagna:
343 calories, 9.5g fat, 803mg sodium, 32.5g carbs, 5.5g fiber, 8g sugars, 27.5g protein

INGREDIENTS

Four ¼-inch-thick eggplant slices (cut lengthwise from a long eggplant), patted dry
10 ounces raw extra-lean ground beef
1 tablespoon dried minced onion
½ teaspoon each salt and black pepper
½ cup fat-free sour cream
4 wedges The Laughing Cow Light Creamy Swiss cheese
One 15-ounce can pure pumpkin
¼ cup light plain soymilk
1 teaspoon chopped garlic
½ teaspoon ground nutmeg
4 sheets oven-ready lasagna noodles
½ cup shredded part-skim mozzarella cheese
¼ cup reduced-fat Parmesan-style grated topping

DIRECTIONS

Preheat oven to 425 degrees. Spray an 8-inch by 8-inch baking pan with nonstick spray.

Bring a large skillet sprayed with nonstick spray to medium-high heat. Cook eggplant until softened, about 2 minutes per side. (Work in batches as needed.)

Remove eggplant and blot away excess moisture. Remove skillet from heat, re-spray, and return to medium-high heat. Add beef and sprinkle with minced onion and ¼ teaspoon each salt and pepper. Cook and crumble for 5 minutes, or until fully cooked.

Add sour cream and cheese wedges, breaking wedges into pieces. Cook and stir until cheese has melted, mixed with sour cream, and coated beef, 2 to 3 minutes. Remove from heat.

In a medium bowl, mix pumpkin, soymilk, garlic, nutmeg, and remaining ¼ teaspoon each salt and black pepper.

Spread ⅓rd of the pumpkin mixture (about ⅔ cup) into the baking pan. Evenly layer with half of each ingredient: lasagna sheets, beef mixture, eggplant slices, remaining pumpkin mixture.

Repeat layering with remaining ingredients. Sprinkle with mozzarella cheese and Parm-style topping.

Bake until cheese has lightly browned, 25 to 30 minutes. Enjoy!

MAKES 4 SERVINGS

Perhaps the most surprising of all pasta swaps,
BROCCOLI COLE SLAW will shock you in the best way possible . . .

SLAW AND ORDER

148 calories PER SERVING

You'll Need: large skillet with a lid, nonstick spray
Prep: 5 minutes
Cook: 20 minutes

½ of recipe (1 heaping cup): 148 calories, 3g fat, 610mg sodium, 24.5g carbs, 6g fiber, 10g sugars, 8g protein

INGREDIENTS

One 12-ounce bag (4 cups) broccoli cole slaw
1 cup creamy tomato soup with 4g fat or less per serving or canned crushed tomatoes
1 teaspoon chopped garlic, or more to taste
Dash onion powder, or more to taste
Dash each salt and black pepper, or more to taste
Dash red pepper flakes, or more to taste
3 tablespoons reduced-fat Parmesan-style grated topping

DIRECTIONS

Bring a large skillet sprayed with nonstick spray to medium-high heat. Add broccoli slaw and ½ cup water. Cover and cook until fully softened, 10 to 12 minutes. Uncover and, if needed, cook and stir until water has evaporated, 2 to 3 minutes.

Add soup/tomatoes, garlic, seasonings, and 2 tablespoons Parm-style topping. Cook and stir until hot, 3 to 4 minutes.

Serve topped with remaining 1 tablespoon Parm-style topping!

MAKES 2 SERVINGS

CHICKEN AMORE PASTA SWAP

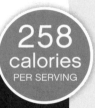

258 calories PER SERVING

You'll Need: medium bowl, large skillet with a lid, nonstick spray, large bowl
Prep: 10 minutes
Cook: 25 minutes

½ of recipe (about 2 cups): 258 calories, 3g fat, 705mg sodium, 29g carbs, 6.5g fiber, 15g sugars, 29g protein

INGREDIENTS

1 cup creamy tomato soup with 4g fat or less per serving
½ cup fat-free sour cream
2 tablespoons chopped fresh basil
¼ teaspoon Italian seasoning
One 12-ounce bag (4 cups) broccoli cole slaw
6 ounces raw boneless skinless chicken breast, cut into bite-sized pieces
⅛ teaspoon each salt and black pepper
1 cup portabella mushrooms cut into bite-sized pieces

DIRECTIONS

In a medium bowl, thoroughly mix soup with sour cream. Stir in basil and Italian seasoning.

Bring a large skillet sprayed with nonstick spray to medium-high heat. Add broccoli slaw and ½ cup water. Cover and cook until fully softened, 10 to 12 minutes. Uncover and, if needed, cook and stir until water has evaporated, 2 to 3 minutes.

Transfer slaw to a large bowl and blot away excess moisture. Remove skillet from heat, re-spray, and return to medium-high heat. Add chicken and season with salt and pepper. Add mushrooms and cook and stir until chicken is cooked through and mushrooms have softened, about 5 minutes.

Add soup mixture and slaw to the skillet. Cook and stir until hot and well mixed, 1 to 2 minutes. Chew!

MAKES 2 SERVINGS

BROCCOLI SLAW TURKEY BOLOGNESE

298 calories PER SERVING

You'll Need: 2 medium bowls, large skillet with a lid, nonstick spray
Prep: 10 minutes
Cook: 30 minutes

½ **of recipe (about 2 cups):** 298 calories, 7.5g fat, 638mg sodium, 27.5g carbs, 9g fiber, 12.5g sugars, 30.5g protein

INGREDIENTS

1¼ cups canned crushed tomatoes
¼ cup tomato paste
1 teaspoon chopped garlic
1 teaspoon balsamic vinegar
½ teaspoon Worcestershire sauce
½ teaspoon dried oregano
½ teaspoon dried basil
One 12-ounce bag (4 cups) broccoli cole slaw
8 ounces raw lean ground turkey
⅛ teaspoon each salt and black pepper

DIRECTIONS

In a medium bowl, mix all ingredients *except* broccoli slaw, turkey, salt, and pepper.

Bring a large skillet sprayed with nonstick spray to medium-high heat. Add broccoli slaw and ½ cup water. Cover and cook until fully softened, 10 to 12 minutes. Uncover and, if needed, cook and stir until water has evaporated, 2 to 3 minutes.

Transfer slaw to another medium bowl and blot away excess moisture. Remove skillet from heat, re-spray, and return to medium-high heat. Add turkey and season with salt and pepper. Cook and crumble for 4 to 5 minutes, until fully cooked.

Add tomato mixture and slaw to the skillet and cook and stir until hot, 2 to 3 minutes. Enjoy!

MAKES 2 SERVINGS

HG ALTERNATIVE!

Swap out the turkey for extra-lean ground beef. Mmmmm . . .

Sometimes you just gotta have the real thing. So why not start with HIGH-FIBER PASTA, and get super-sized portions (and even more fiber) by including lots of delicious veggies?!

TAKES-THE-CAKE ZITI BAKE

286 calories PER SERVING

You'll Need: large pot, large bowl, extra-large skillet, nonstick spray, 8-inch by 8-inch baking pan
Prep: 10 minutes | **Cook:** 40 minutes

¼th of ziti bake:
286 calories, 7g fat, 455mg sodium, 41g carbs, 5g fiber, 7g sugars, 16.5g protein

INGREDIENTS

5 ounces (about 1½ cups) uncooked high-fiber
   ziti or penne pasta
1 cup thinly sliced onion
2 cups chopped brown mushrooms
1 tablespoon chopped garlic
2 cups spinach leaves
¾ cup light or low-fat ricotta cheese
2 tablespoons chopped fresh basil
1½ cups canned crushed tomatoes
½ cup plus 2 tablespoons shredded part-skim
   mozzarella cheese
2 tablespoons reduced-fat Parmesan-style
   grated topping

DIRECTIONS

Preheat oven to 375 degrees.

In a large pot, cook pasta al dente according to package directions. Drain and transfer to a large bowl.

Meanwhile, bring an extra-large skillet sprayed with nonstick spray to medium heat. Cook and stir onion until slightly softened, about 3 minutes. Add mushrooms and garlic, and raise temperature to medium high. Cook and stir until mushrooms are soft, about 3 more minutes.

Add spinach to the skillet and cook and stir until it has wilted and excess moisture has evaporated, about 8 minutes. Remove from heat, pat dry, and stir in the ricotta cheese and basil.

Transfer contents of the skillet to the bowl of cooked pasta. Add tomatoes and 1/2 cup mozzarella cheese, and toss to mix.

Spray an 8-inch by 8-inch baking pan with nonstick spray. Evenly place pasta mixture in the pan. Top with Parm-style topping and remaining 2 tablespoons mozzarella cheese.

Bake until entire dish is hot and cheese on top has melted, about 15 minutes. Eat up!

MAKES 4 SERVINGS

SOY-CRUMBLE SWAPPING: THE MEATY 411

Using frozen soy crumbles in place of ground meat saves you calories, fat grams, and time. But if you prefer ground meat, you can use that too. For every cup of frozen crumbles called for in a recipe, use 4 ounces of raw ground meat. Just cook and crumble it in a skillet sprayed with nonstick spray before adding to the recipe.

FUNKADELIC CHILI MAC

297 calories PER SERVING

You'll Need: 2 large pots with lids, nonstick spray
Prep: 10 minutes | **Cook:** 15 minutes

¼th of recipe (about 1¾ cups):
297 calories, 2g fat, 637mg sodium, 55.5g carbs, 9.75g fiber, 11.5g sugars, 19g protein

INGREDIENTS

One 14.5-ounce can stewed tomatoes,
    roughly chopped, juice reserved
1 cup canned red kidney beans, drained
    and rinsed
1 cup frozen ground-beef-style soy crumbles
1 onion, chopped
1 bell pepper, stem removed, seeded, chopped
1 cup chopped portabella mushrooms
⅓ cup tomato paste
1 teaspoon chili powder, or more to taste
½ teaspoon chopped garlic
¼ teaspoon ground cumin, or more to taste
5 ounces (about 1⅓ cups) uncooked
    high-fiber elbow macaroni
¼ cup shredded fat-free cheddar cheese

Optional seasoning: cayenne pepper

DIRECTIONS

To make the chili, bring a large pot sprayed with nonstick spray to medium heat. Add all ingredients—including the reserved tomato juice—*except* the macaroni and cheese. Thoroughly stir. Cover and cook until veggies are tender, about 15 minutes, occasionally uncovering to stir.

Meanwhile, in another large pot, prepare macaroni according to package instructions, about 7 minutes. Drain and cover to keep warm.

Mix pasta into chili and serve topped with cheese

MAKES 4 SERVINGS

GROUND-FOR-GROUND CHART OF HG'S FAVORITE CRUMBLES

Frozen Ground-Beef-Style Soy Crumbles (1 cup) =
125 calories, 2.5g fat, 380mg sodium, 11g carbs, 6.5g fiber, 0.5g sugars, 20g protein

Extra-Lean Ground Beef (4 ounces uncooked) =
140 calories, 4.5g fat, 80mg sodium, 0g carbs, 0g fiber, 0g sugars, 24g protein

Lean Ground Turkey (4 ounces uncooked) =
160 calories, 8g fat, 90mg sodium, 0g carbs, 0g fiber, 0g sugars, 22g protein

SUPER-SIZED PESTO PASTA

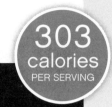
303 calories
PER SERVING

You'll Need: small blender or food processor, medium-large pot, 2 large microwave-safe bowls, vegetable peeler
Prep: 20 minutes
Cook: 25 minutes

½ of recipe (about 1½ cups): 303 calories, 7.5g fat, 689mg sodium, 51.5g carbs, 8g fiber, 7g sugars, 13g protein

INGREDIENTS

Sauce
¾ cup fresh basil leaves
2 tablespoons light or low-fat ricotta cheese
1 tablespoon reduced-fat Parmesan-style grated topping
1 tablespoon pine nuts
1 teaspoon chopped garlic
½ teaspoon olive oil
½ teaspoon salt, or more to taste
¼ teaspoon black pepper, or more to taste

Pasta
4 ounces uncooked high-fiber fettuccine
2 medium zucchini, ends removed

DIRECTIONS

Place all sauce ingredients in a small blender or food processor, and blend until a smooth paste forms. Cover and refrigerate.

In a medium-large pot, cook pasta per package instructions, about 8 minutes. Drain pasta, transfer to a large microwave-safe bowl, and cover to keep warm.

Use a veggie peeler to peel zucchini into super-thin strips; rotate zucchini after each strip to yield a width similar to fettuccine. Place in another large microwave-safe bowl. Cover and microwave for 2 to 3 minutes, until soft. Drain and blot away excess moisture.

Thoroughly mix squash into pasta. Top with sauce and toss to coat. Microwave for 1 minute, or until hot. Eat up!

MAKES 2 SERVINGS

ROASTED VEGGIE FETTUCCINE

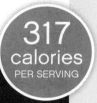
317 calories
PER SERVING

You'll Need: baking sheet, nonstick spray, medium-large pot, large microwave-safe bowl
Prep: 15 minutes
Cook: 45 minutes

½ of recipe (about 2 cups): 317 calories, 5g fat, 419mg sodium, 62.5g carbs, 10g fiber, 9g sugars, 11g protein

INGREDIENTS

4 ounces uncooked high-fiber fettuccine
1 tablespoon light whipped butter or light buttery spread
1 tablespoon chopped fresh basil
1 tablespoon reduced-fat Parmesan-style grated topping
1 teaspoon lemon juice
¼ teaspoon each salt and black pepper
1 cup cubed butternut squash
½ cup grape or cherry tomatoes
½ medium red onion, quartered
1 zucchini, halved lengthwise and cut into 1-inch pieces
1 cup eggplant cut into 1-inch cubes
1 tablespoon chopped garlic

DIRECTIONS

Preheat oven to 450 degrees. Spray a baking sheet with nonstick spray.

In medium-large pot, cook pasta per package instructions, about 8 minutes. Drain and transfer to a large microwave-safe bowl. Top and toss with butter, basil, Parm-style topping, lemon juice, and ⅛ teaspoon each salt and pepper. Cover to keep warm.

Distribute veggies onto the baking sheet in an even layer and spray with nonstick spray. Season with remaining ⅛ teaspoon each salt and pepper. Bake until slightly blackened, 25 to 30 minutes.

Sprinkle garlic over veggies and bake until garlic has browned, about 5 minutes.

Stir roasted veggies into pasta. Microwave until hot, if needed. Enjoy!

MAKES 2 SERVINGS

CHUNKY EGGPLANT PENNE FOR TWO

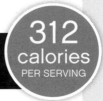

312 calories
PER SERVING

You'll Need: baking sheet, nonstick spray, medium pot with a lid, small pot
Prep: 10 minutes | **Cook:** 50 minutes

½ of recipe (2 heaping cups):
312 calories, 4.5g fat, 579mg sodium, 60g carbs, 16.5g fiber, 15g sugars, 14g protein

INGREDIENTS

1 eggplant, ends removed, cut into 1-inch cubes

1 cup cherry tomatoes

⅛ teaspoon each salt and black pepper

3 ounces (about 1 cup) uncooked high-fiber penne pasta

¼ cup finely chopped onion

1 teaspoon chopped garlic

1 cup canned crushed tomatoes

¼ teaspoon red pepper flakes

¼ cup chopped fresh basil

¼ cup crumbled reduced-fat feta cheese

Optional seasonings: additional salt and black pepper

DIRECTIONS

Preheat oven to 450 degrees. Spray a baking sheet with nonstick spray.

Evenly place eggplant and cherry tomatoes on the sheet. Spray with nonstick spray, and sprinkle with salt and black pepper. Bake until eggplant is tender and tomatoes are soft and slightly blackened, 25 to 30 minutes.

Meanwhile, cook pasta in a medium pot per package instructions, about 8 minutes. Drain and cover to keep warm.

To make the sauce, bring a small pot sprayed with nonstick spray to medium heat. Cook and stir onion and garlic until slightly softened, about 2 minutes. Stir in crushed tomatoes and red pepper flakes. Cook and stir until onion has fully softened, about 5 minutes.

Gently stir sauce and baked veggies into the cooked pasta. Sprinkle each serving with basil and feta. EAT!

MAKES 2 SERVINGS

✳ Flip to the photo inserts to see over 100 recipe pics! And for photos of ALL the recipes, go to hungry-girl.com/books.

SUPER-SIZED SPINACH FETTUCCINE GIRLFREDO

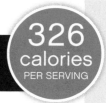

326 calories PER SERVING

You'll Need: medium-large pot, 2 large microwave-safe bowls, vegetable peeler, medium microwave-safe bowl
Prep: 20 minutes | **Cook:** 15 minutes

½ of recipe (about 1¾ cups):
326 calories, 4.5g fat, 582mg sodium, 54.5g carbs, 4.5g fiber, 9g sugars, 14.5g protein

INGREDIENTS

Pasta
4 ounces uncooked spinach fettuccine
2 medium zucchini, ends removed

Sauce
3 tablespoons fat-free sour cream
1 tablespoon reduced-fat Parmesan-style grated topping
3 wedges The Laughing Cow Light Creamy Swiss cheese
¼ teaspoon garlic powder
⅛ teaspoon salt
Dash black pepper

DIRECTIONS

In a medium-large pot, cook pasta per package instructions, about 8 minutes. Drain pasta, transfer to a large microwave-safe bowl, and cover to keep warm.

Use a veggie peeler to peel zucchini into super-thin strips; rotate zucchini after each strip to yield a width similar to fettuccine. Place in another large microwave-safe bowl. Cover and microwave for 2 to 3 minutes, until soft. Drain and blot away excess moisture.

Thoroughly mix zucchini into fettuccine. Cover to keep warm.

In a medium microwave-safe bowl, mix all sauce ingredients, breaking cheese wedges into pieces. Stir in 2 tablespoons water. Microwave at 50 percent power for 1 minute. Stir and microwave at 50 percent power for 30 seconds, or until melted.

Spoon sauce over pasta and toss to coat. Microwave for 1 minute, or until hot. Eat up!

MAKES 2 SERVINGS

Hungry for More Pasta?

Flip to the Comfortably Yum chapter for NINE Mac & Cheese recipes!

CHAPTER 10

PIZZA

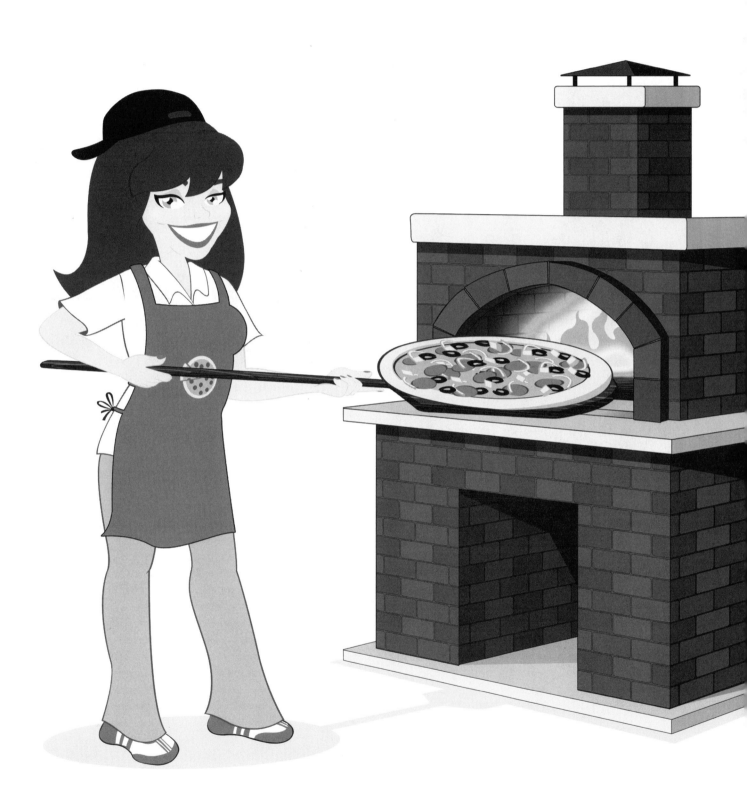

PIZZA

EZ Thin-Crust Pizza

Crispy White Pizza

Thin-Crust Enchilada Pizza

The HG Special Pizza

Thin-Crust Pepperoni & Mushroom Pizza

Garlic Chicken Pizza

Best BBQ Chicken Pizza

The Great Greek Pizza

American Buffalo Chicken Pizza

Mediterranean Pizza

Veggie & Ricotta Pizza

Sloppy Joe Pizza

Garlic-Bread White Pizza

Salad-Topped Pita Pizza

Sausage-Topped Pizza Swap

Bring on the Breakfast Pizza

Breakfast Pizza Mexicali

Pepperoni Breakfast Pizza

White-Cheese Breakfast Pizza

Meat Lover's Breakfast Pizza

Easy Caprese Breakfast Pizzas

Perfect Pepperoni Pizzas

Chicken Girlfredo Pizza

Pizza Luau

Purple Pizza Eaters

Pesto Pizzas

Pizza-bellas

White Pizza-bellas

Sausage-Loaded Pizza-bellas

Greek Pizza-bellas

Potato-Skin Pepperoni Pizza

Mini Deep Dish Spinach Pizzas

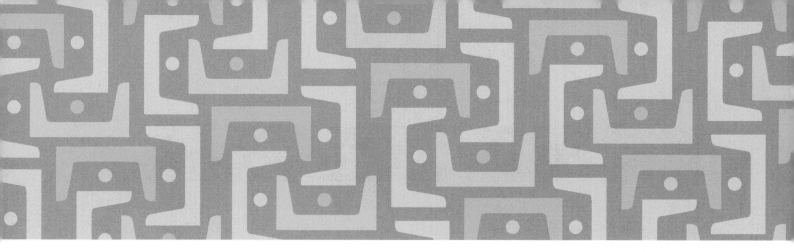

Wow . . . 94 percent of Americans regularly eat pizza, and yet it's typically loaded with fatty calories. Hungry Girl pizza recipes are unique, satisfying, and 100 percent guilt-free, thanks in part to some creative crusts!

A QUICK GUIDE TO SYMBOLS:

15 Minutes or Less

This symbol lets you know a recipe should take you no more than fifteen minutes from start to finish! That includes prep and cook time.

30 Minutes or Less

Just like the 15-minute version, this one points out recipes that take 30 minutes or less to whip up.

Meatless

You guessed it—no meat here! That includes beef, poultry, and fish. Some recipes give the option of a meatless ingredient. If you want your meal without meat, go with the meatless choice.

Single Serving

Pretty straightforward. These are recipes for one.

5 Ingredients or Less

Fans of HG know that we like to keep things simple. And these recipes contain just five ingredients or less!

Photos

These recipes can be seen in one of the book's photo inserts. The number in the symbol tells you which insert. Find photos of all the recipes at hungry-girl.com/books!

223

EZ THIN-CRUST PIZZA

181 calories

You'll Need: baking sheet, nonstick spray, blender or food processor (optional) | **Prep:** 5 minutes | **Cook:** 10 minutes

Entire recipe:
181 calories, 5g fat, 657mg sodium, 27g carbs, 6.5g fiber, 2.5g sugars, 12.5g protein

INGREDIENTS

1 medium-large high-fiber flour tortilla with 110 calories or less
1 stick light string cheese
2 tablespoons pizza sauce
Dash Italian seasoning
Dash garlic powder
Dash onion powder

DIRECTIONS

Preheat oven to 375 degrees. Spray a baking sheet with nonstick spray.

Lay tortilla on the sheet and bake until slightly crispy, about 5 minutes.

Break string cheese into thirds and place in a blender or food processor—blend at high speed until shredded. (Or pull into shreds and roughly chop.)

Flip tortilla and spread with sauce, leaving a ½-inch border. Sprinkle with spices and top with cheese.

Bake until cheese has melted and tortilla is crisp, about 5 minutes. Slice and eat!

MAKES 1 SERVING

CRISPY WHITE PIZZA

232 calories

You'll Need: baking sheet, nonstick spray, small bowl, skillet | **Prep:** 10 minutes | **Cook:** 15 minutes

Entire recipe:
232 calories, 7g fat, 765mg sodium, 34g carbs, 7.5g fiber, 8g sugars, 16g protein

INGREDIENTS

⅓ cup light or low-fat ricotta cheese
1 tablespoon shredded part-skim mozzarella cheese
¼ cup thinly sliced onion
¼ teaspoon garlic powder
⅛ teaspoon salt
Dash black pepper
1 medium-large high-fiber flour tortilla with 110 calories or less
4 thin slices plum tomato
4 fresh basil leaves

DIRECTIONS

Preheat oven to 375 degrees. Spray a baking sheet with nonstick spray.

In a small bowl, mix ricotta cheese with mozzarella cheese.

Bring a skillet sprayed with nonstick spray to medium heat. Cook and stir onion until softened and slightly browned, about 5 minutes.

Stir onion into cheese mixture. Mix in garlic powder, salt, and pepper.

Lay tortilla on the baking sheet and bake until slightly crispy, about 5 minutes.

Flip tortilla and spread with cheese-onion mixture, leaving a ½-inch border. Top with tomato and basil.

Bake until hot, about 5 minutes. Pizza for one!

MAKES 1 SERVING

THIN-CRUST ENCHILADA PIZZA

296 calories

You'll Need: baking sheet, nonstick spray
Prep: 10 minutes
Cook: 10 minutes

Entire recipe: 296 calories, 9g fat, 877mg sodium, 31.5g carbs, 7.5g fiber, 2g sugars, 29g protein

INGREDIENTS

1 medium-large high-fiber flour tortilla with 110 calories or less
2 tablespoons red enchilada sauce
Dash cayenne pepper
Dash ground cumin
2 ounces cooked and shredded (or finely chopped) skinless chicken breast
2 tablespoons canned black beans, drained and rinsed
¼ cup shredded reduced-fat Mexican-blend cheese
1 tablespoon chopped scallions
1 tablespoon chopped cilantro

Optional topping: fat-free sour cream

DIRECTIONS

Preheat oven to 375 degrees. Spray a baking sheet with nonstick spray.

Lay tortilla on the sheet and bake until slightly crispy, about 5 minutes.

Flip tortilla and spread with enchilada sauce, leaving a ½-inch border. Sprinkle with cayenne pepper and cumin. Top sauce with chicken, beans, and cheese.

Bake until toppings are hot and cheese has melted, about 5 minutes.

Sprinkle with scallions and cilantro!

MAKES 1 SERVING

THE HG SPECIAL PIZZA

285 calories

You'll Need: baking sheet, nonstick spray
Prep: 5 minutes
Cook: 10 minutes

Entire recipe: 285 calories, 8.5g fat, 930mg sodium, 37.5g carbs, 8.5g fiber, 7g sugars, 20.5g protein

INGREDIENTS

1 medium-large high-fiber flour tortilla with 110 calories or less
1 wedge The Laughing Cow Light Creamy Swiss cheese
¼ cup reduced-sodium creamy tomato soup with 4g fat or less per serving
¼ cup frozen ground-beef-style soy crumbles, thawed
3 tablespoons chopped red onion
½ tablespoon reduced-fat Parmesan-style grated topping
¼ teaspoon garlic powder
1 piece Mini Babybel Light cheese, chopped

DIRECTIONS

Preheat oven to 375 degrees. Spray a baking sheet with nonstick spray.

Lay tortilla on the sheet and bake until slightly crispy, about 5 minutes.

Flip tortilla and spread with cheese wedge, leaving a ½-inch border. Cover cheese with soup, soy crumbles, and onion. Sprinkle with Parm-style topping and garlic powder, and top with chopped cheese.

Bake until chopped cheese has melted and tortilla is crispy, about 5 minutes. Slice and eat!

MAKES 1 SERVING

FLOUR-TORTILLA ALTERNATIVE!

These recipes call for high-fiber tortillas with 110 calories or less. We love La Tortilla Factory Smart & Delicious Low Carb High Fiber Large Tortillas—only 80 calories each! Use one of these, and you can subtract 30 calories from your recipe's calorie count.

THIN-CRUST PEPPERONI & MUSHROOM PIZZA

212 calories

You'll Need: baking sheet, nonstick spray, blender or food processor (optional)
Prep: 5 minutes
Cook: 10 minutes

Entire recipe: 212 calories, 6.5g fat, 942mg sodium, 28.5g carbs, 6.5g fiber, 3g sugars, 16g protein

INGREDIENTS

1 stick light string cheese
1 medium-large high-fiber flour tortilla with 110 calories or less
2 tablespoons pizza sauce
5 slices turkey pepperoni
2 tablespoons canned sliced mushrooms, drained

Optional seasonings: Italian seasoning, garlic powder, onion powder

DIRECTIONS

Preheat oven to 375 degrees. Spray a baking sheet with nonstick spray.

Break string cheese into thirds and place in a blender or food processor—blend at high speed until shredded. (Or pull into shreds and roughly chop.)

Lay tortilla on the sheet and bake until slightly crispy, about 5 minutes.

Flip tortilla and spread with sauce, leaving a ½-inch border. Sprinkle with cheese, and top with pepperoni and mushrooms.

Bake until cheese has melted and tortilla is crisp, about 5 minutes. Slice and eat!

MAKES 1 SERVING

GARLIC CHICKEN PIZZA

320 calories

You'll Need: baking sheet, nonstick spray, blender or food processor (optional), small bowl
Prep: 10 minutes
Cook: 15 minutes

Entire recipe: 320 calories, 7.5g fat, 902mg sodium, 34g carbs, 6.5g fiber, 2.5g sugars, 32g protein

INGREDIENTS

1 stick light string cheese
1 wedge The Laughing Cow Light Creamy Swiss cheese
2 teaspoons reduced-fat Parmesan-style grated topping
¼ teaspoon chopped garlic
¼ teaspoon garlic powder
Dash black pepper
1 high-fiber pita
2 ounces cooked and shredded (or finely chopped) skinless chicken breast
2 tablespoons diced tomato
2 tablespoons chopped fresh basil

Optional topping: red pepper flakes

DIRECTIONS

Preheat oven to 375 degrees. Spray a baking sheet with nonstick spray.

Break string cheese into thirds and place in a blender or food processor—blend at high speed until shredded. (Or pull into shreds and roughly chop.)

In a small bowl, mix cheese wedge, 1 teaspoon Parm-style topping, chopped garlic, ⅛ teaspoon garlic powder, and black pepper.

Lay pita on the baking sheet. Evenly spread with cheese-wedge mixture and sprinkle with shredded string cheese, leaving a ½-inch border.

Top with chicken and sprinkle with remaining ⅛ teaspoon garlic powder. Top with tomato, basil, and remaining 1 teaspoon Parm-style topping.

Bake until hot and lightly browned, 10 to 12 minutes. Enjoy!

MAKES 1 SERVING

BEST BBQ CHICKEN PIZZA

340 calories

You'll Need: baking sheet, nonstick spray, blender or food processor (optional), small bowl
Prep: 10 minutes
Cook: 15 minutes

Entire recipe: 340 calories, 5g fat, 925mg sodium, 39g carbs, 6g fiber, 10g sugars, 36.5g protein

INGREDIENTS

1 stick light string cheese
3 ounces cooked and chopped skinless chicken breast
2 tablespoons BBQ sauce with 45 calories or less per 2-tablespoon serving
1 high-fiber pita
1½ tablespoons finely chopped red onion
1 teaspoon chopped cilantro

DIRECTIONS

Preheat oven to 375 degrees. Spray a baking sheet with nonstick spray.

Break string cheese into thirds and place in a blender or food processor—blend at high speed until shredded. (Or pull into shreds and roughly chop.)

In a small bowl, toss chopped chicken with 1 tablespoon BBQ sauce.

Lay pita on the baking sheet and spread with remaining 1 tablespoon BBQ sauce, leaving a ½-inch border. Sprinkle with cheese, top with saucy chicken, and sprinkle with onion.

Bake until hot and lightly browned, 10 to 12 minutes.

Top with cilantro. YUMMMM!

MAKES 1 SERVING

THE GREAT GREEK PIZZA

277 calories

You'll Need: baking sheet, nonstick spray, blender or food processor (optional), medium bowl
Prep: 10 minutes
Cook: 15 minutes

Entire recipe: 277 calories, 4.75g fat, 990mg sodium, 38g carbs, 8.5g fiber, 4.5g sugars, 19g protein

INGREDIENTS

1 stick light string cheese
½ cup thawed-from-frozen chopped spinach, squeezed dry
2 tablespoons crumbled fat-free feta cheese
½ teaspoon crushed garlic
1 high-fiber pita
3 tablespoons canned crushed tomatoes
2 thin slices red onion, rings separated and halved
1 tablespoon sliced black olives
4 slices plum tomato
Dash dried oregano *or* ¼ teaspoon fresh oregano

Optional seasonings: salt and black pepper

DIRECTIONS

Preheat oven to 375 degrees. Spray a baking sheet with nonstick spray.

Break string cheese into thirds and place in a blender or food processor—blend at high speed until shredded. (Or pull into shreds and roughly chop.)

In a medium bowl, mix spinach, feta cheese, and garlic.

Lay pita on the baking sheet and spread with crushed tomatoes, leaving a ½-inch border. Top with spinach-feta mixture and sprinkle with shredded string cheese.

Top with onion, olives, and tomato, and sprinkle with oregano.

Bake until hot and lightly browned, 10 to 12 minutes. Enjoy!

MAKES 1 SERVING

AMERICAN BUFFALO CHICKEN PIZZA

245 calories

You'll Need: baking sheet, nonstick spray, small bowl | **Prep:** 5 minutes | **Cook:** 15 minutes

Entire recipe:
245 calories, 4g fat, 864mg sodium, 31g carbs, 6g fiber, 2g sugars, 24g protein

INGREDIENTS

2 ounces cooked and chopped skinless chicken breast

1 teaspoon Frank's RedHot Original Cayenne Pepper Sauce, or more to taste

1 high-fiber pita

1 wedge The Laughing Cow Light Creamy Swiss cheese

1 teaspoon reduced-fat Parmesan-style grated topping

1 tablespoon chopped scallions

DIRECTIONS

Preheat oven to 375 degrees. Spray a baking sheet with nonstick spray.

In a small bowl, toss chicken with hot sauce.

Lay pita on the baking sheet. Spread with cheese, leaving a ½-inch border. Top with saucy chicken and sprinkle with Parm-style topping.

Bake until hot and lightly browned, 10 to 12 minutes.

Sprinkle with scallions. Yum time!

MAKES 1 SERVING

MEDITERRANEAN PIZZA

226 calories

You'll Need: baking sheet, nonstick spray, skillet | **Prep:** 5 minutes | **Cook:** 15 minutes

Entire recipe:
226 calories, 5.5g fat, 924mg sodium, 37.5g carbs, 9g fiber, 4.5g sugars, 12g protein

INGREDIENTS

½ cup roughly chopped spinach leaves

1 high-fiber pita

2 tablespoons pizza sauce

2 tablespoons crumbled reduced-fat feta cheese

4 cherry tomatoes, halved

1 artichoke heart packed in water, drained and chopped

1 tablespoon chopped fresh basil

1 tablespoon sliced black olives

DIRECTIONS

Preheat oven to 375 degrees. Spray a baking sheet with nonstick spray.

Bring a skillet sprayed with nonstick spray to medium heat. Cook and stir spinach until slightly wilted, about 2 minutes. Remove from heat and pat dry.

Lay pita on the baking sheet and spread with sauce, leaving a ½-inch border. Top with spinach and remaining ingredients.

Bake until hot and lightly browned, 10 to 12 minutes. Yum!

MAKES 1 SERVING

VEGGIE & RICOTTA PIZZA

255 calories

You'll Need: baking sheet, nonstick spray, skillet, medium bowl
Prep: 10 minutes
Cook: 20 minutes

Entire recipe: 255 calories, 5.5g fat, 826mg sodium, 42.5g carbs, 8.5g fiber, 7.5g sugars, 16g protein

INGREDIENTS

¼ cup sliced mushrooms
¼ cup chopped onion
1 cup chopped spinach leaves
¼ cup light or low-fat ricotta cheese
1 tablespoon finely chopped fresh basil
⅛ teaspoon garlic powder
⅛ teaspoon black pepper
Dash salt
1 high-fiber pita
2 tablespoons pizza sauce
2 teaspoons reduced-fat Parmesan-style grated topping

Optional topping: red pepper flakes

DIRECTIONS

Preheat oven to 375 degrees. Spray a baking sheet with nonstick spray.

Bring a skillet sprayed with nonstick spray to medium-high heat. Cook and stir mushrooms and onion until softened, about 5 minutes. Add spinach and cook and stir until wilted, 1 to 2 minutes. Remove from heat and blot away excess moisture.

In a medium bowl, thoroughly mix ricotta cheese, basil, and seasonings.

Lay pita on the baking sheet. Evenly spread with pizza sauce, leaving a ½-inch border. Top with cooked veggies. Drop ricotta mixture in evenly sized mounds over the veggie layer and sprinkle with Parm-style topping.

Bake until hot and lightly browned, 10 to 12 minutes. Enjoy!

MAKES 1 SERVING

SLOPPY JOE PIZZA

306 calories

You'll Need: baking sheet, nonstick spray, blender or food processor (optional), skillet
Prep: 5 minutes
Cook: 20 minutes

Entire recipe: 306 calories, 8g fat, 914mg sodium, 38g carbs, 7g fiber, 6g sugars, 26g protein

INGREDIENTS

1 stick light string cheese
2 ounces raw lean ground turkey
3 tablespoons canned sloppy joe sauce
2 tablespoons diced onion
1 high-fiber pita

DIRECTIONS

Preheat oven to 375 degrees. Spray a baking sheet with nonstick spray.

Break string cheese into thirds and place in a blender or food processor—blend at high speed until shredded. (Or pull into shreds and roughly chop.)

Bring a skillet sprayed with nonstick spray to medium heat. Cook and crumble turkey for 4 minutes, or until fully cooked. Add sauce and onion. Cook and stir until warm, about 1 minute.

Lay pita on the baking sheet. Evenly spread turkey mixture onto the pita, leaving a ½-inch border, and sprinkle with cheese.

Bake until hot and lightly browned at the edges, 10 to 12 minutes. Enjoy!

MAKES 1 SERVING

GARLIC-BREAD WHITE PIZZA

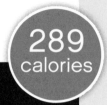
289 calories

You'll Need: baking sheet, nonstick spray, blender or food processor (optional), very small bowl, small bowl
Prep: 10 minutes
Cook: 15 minutes

Entire recipe: 289 calories, 9.5g fat, 834mg sodium, 35.5g carbs, 6.5g fiber, 4.5g sugars, 20.5g protein

INGREDIENTS

1 stick light string cheese
½ tablespoon light whipped butter or light buttery spread
1 teaspoon garlic powder
1 high-fiber pita
¼ cup light or low-fat ricotta cheese
Dash each salt and black pepper
1 teaspoon reduced-fat Parmesan-style topping

DIRECTIONS

Preheat oven to 375 degrees. Spray a baking sheet with nonstick spray.

Break string cheese into thirds and place in a blender or food processor—blend at high speed until shredded. (Or pull into shreds and roughly chop.)

In a very small bowl, mix butter with garlic powder. Lay pita on the baking sheet and spread with butter mixture, leaving a ½-inch border. Bake until butter has melted, 1 to 2 minutes.

In a small bowl, mix ricotta cheese, shredded string cheese, salt, pepper, and Parm-style topping. Spread mixture over the pita, leaving a ½-inch border.

Bake until hot and lightly browned at the edges, 10 to 12 minutes. Enjoy!

MAKES 1 SERVING

SALAD-TOPPED PITA PIZZA

271 calories

You'll Need: baking sheet, nonstick spray, blender or food processor (optional), large bowl
Prep: 10 minutes
Cook: 10 minutes

Entire recipe: 271 calories, 6.5g fat, 705mg sodium, 43.5g carbs, 9g fiber, 9g sugars, 16g protein

INGREDIENTS

1 stick light string cheese
1 high-fiber pita
Dash Italian seasoning
2 cups finely chopped romaine lettuce
¼ cup chopped tomato
¼ cup thinly sliced red onion
2 tablespoons fat-free or low-fat balsamic or red wine vinaigrette
1 teaspoon reduced-fat Parmesan-style grated topping

DIRECTIONS

Preheat oven to 375 degrees. Spray a baking sheet with nonstick spray.

Break string cheese into thirds and place in a blender or food processor—blend at high speed until shredded. (Or pull into shreds and roughly chop.)

Lay pita on the baking sheet, and sprinkle with shredded string cheese and Italian seasoning. Bake until hot and lightly browned, 8 to 10 minutes.

Let cheese-topped pita cool, about 10 minutes. To make the salad, mix romaine, tomato, and onion in a large bowl. Toss with vinaigrette.

Top pita with salad and Parm-style topping. Grab a fork and knife, and dig in!

MAKES 1 SERVING

SAUSAGE-TOPPED PIZZA SWAP

290 calories

You'll Need: baking sheet, nonstick spray, blender or food processor (optional), skillet
Prep: 10 minutes
Cook: 20 minutes

Entire recipe: 290 calories, 8g fat, 834mg sodium, 33g carbs, 7g fiber, 3g sugars, 19g protein

INGREDIENTS

1 stick light string cheese
1 frozen meatless or turkey sausage patty
with 80 calories or less
2 tablespoons diced bell pepper
2 tablespoons diced onion
1 high-fiber pita
2 tablespoons pizza sauce

Optional toppings: garlic powder, red pepper flakes

DIRECTIONS

Preheat oven to 375 degrees. Spray a baking sheet with nonstick spray.

Break string cheese into thirds and place in a blender or food processor—blend at high speed until shredded. (Or pull into shreds and roughly chop.)

Bring a skillet sprayed with nonstick spray to medium heat. Cook sausage patty for 4 minutes. Flip patty and cook for 2 minutes.

Add veggies to the skillet with the sausage and cook for 2 minutes, or until sausage is hot and cooked through and veggies have slightly softened and lightly browned.

Lay pita on the baking sheet and evenly spread with pizza sauce, leaving a ½-inch border. Sprinkle with cheese.

Roughly chop sausage and sprinkle over cheese, along with veggies. Bake until hot and lightly browned, 10 to 12 minutes. Enjoy!

MAKES 1 SERVING

BRING ON THE BREAKFAST PIZZA

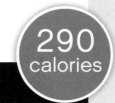

148 calories

You'll Need: blender or food processor (optional), small skillet with a lid, nonstick spray
Prep: 5 minutes
Cook: 10 minutes

Entire recipe: 148 calories, 3.5g fat, 652mg sodium, 7.5g carbs, 1g fiber, 3.5g sugars, 20g protein

INGREDIENTS

1 stick light string cheese
2 tablespoons chopped green bell pepper
2 tablespoons chopped mushrooms
½ cup fat-free liquid egg substitute
3 tablespoons pizza sauce

Optional toppings: salt, black pepper, oregano, garlic powder, onion powder, red pepper flakes

DIRECTIONS

Break string cheese into thirds and place in a blender or food processor—blend at high speed until shredded. (Or pull into shreds and roughly chop.)

Bring a small skillet sprayed with nonstick spray to medium-high heat. Cook and stir pepper and mushrooms until slightly softened, about 5 minutes. Remove from skillet and set aside.

Reduce heat to medium. Add egg substitute and let it coat the skillet bottom. Cover and cook until solid enough to flip, about 3 minutes.

Carefully flip egg "crust." Evenly top with sauce, leaving a ½-inch border. Sprinkle with cheese and cooked veggies.

Cover and cook until cheese has melted, 1 to 2 minutes. Chew!

MAKES 1 SERVING

BREAKFAST PIZZA MEXICALI

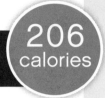

206 calories

You'll Need: small skillet with a lid, nonstick spray | **Prep:** 5 minutes | **Cook:** 10 minutes

Entire recipe:
206 calories, 8.5g fat, 841mg sodium, 8g carbs, 2g fiber, 3.5g sugars, 23.5g protein

INGREDIENTS

1 ounce soy chorizo
½ cup fat-free liquid egg substitute
¼ cup canned fire-roasted diced tomatoes, lightly drained
¼ cup shredded reduced-fat Mexican-blend cheese

DIRECTIONS

Bring a small skillet sprayed with nonstick spray to medium heat. Cook and crumble soy chorizo until browned, about 3 minutes. Remove chorizo and set aside.

If needed, clean skillet. Remove skillet from heat, re-spray, and bring to medium heat. Add egg substitute and let it coat the skillet bottom. Cover and cook until solid enough to flip, about 3 minutes.

Carefully flip egg "crust." Evenly top with tomatoes, leaving a ½-inch border. Sprinkle with cheese and cooked chorizo. Cover and cook until cheese has melted, 1 to 2 minutes. Enjoy!

MAKES 1 SERVING

PEPPERONI BREAKFAST PIZZA

172 calories

You'll Need: blender or food processor (optional), small skillet with a lid, nonstick spray
Prep: 5 minutes | **Cook:** 10 minutes

Entire recipe:
172 calories, 4.5g fat, 882mg sodium, 7g carbs, 0.5g fiber, 3g sugars, 23g protein

INGREDIENTS

1 stick light string cheese
½ cup fat-free liquid egg substitute
2 dashes garlic powder
2 dashes onion powder
3 tablespoons pizza sauce
6 slices turkey pepperoni

Optional topping: red pepper flakes

DIRECTIONS

Break string cheese into thirds and place in a blender or food processor—blend at high speed until shredded. (Or pull into shreds and roughly chop.)

Bring a small skillet sprayed with nonstick spray to medium heat. Add egg substitute and let it coat the skillet bottom. Sprinkle with a dash each garlic powder and onion powder. Cover and cook until solid enough to flip, about 3 minutes.

Carefully flip egg "crust." Top with sauce, leaving a ¼-inch border. Sprinkle with remaining dash each garlic powder and onion powder. Top sauce with cheese and pepperoni. Cover and cook until cheese has melted and pepperoni is hot, 1 to 2 minutes. Enjoy!

MAKES 1 SERVING

WHITE-CHEESE BREAKFAST PIZZA

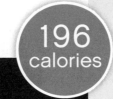
196 calories

You'll Need: blender or food processor (optional), small bowl, small skillet with a lid, nonstick spray
Prep: 5 minutes
Cook: 10 minutes

Entire recipe: 196 calories, 6g fat, 853mg sodium, 9g carbs, 1g fiber, 4.5g sugars, 26g protein

INGREDIENTS

1 stick light string cheese
¼ cup light or low-fat ricotta cheese
1 cup roughly chopped spinach leaves
¼ teaspoon garlic powder
⅛ teaspoon each salt and black pepper
½ cup fat-free liquid egg substitute
1 teaspoon reduced-fat Parmesan-style grated topping

DIRECTIONS

Break string cheese into thirds and place in a blender or food processor—blend at high speed until shredded. (Or pull into shreds and roughly chop.)

In a small bowl, mix ricotta cheese with shredded string cheese.

Bring a small skillet sprayed with nonstick spray to medium heat. Cook and stir spinach until wilted, about 1 minute.

Remove from heat and blot away excess moisture. Stir spinach into cheese mixture. Mix in garlic powder, salt, and pepper.

Re-spray skillet and return to medium heat. Add egg substitute and let it coat the skillet bottom. Cover and cook until solid enough to flip, about 3 minutes.

Carefully flip egg "crust." Evenly top with spinach-cheese mixture, leaving a ½-inch border. Sprinkle with Parm-style topping. Cover and cook until cheese topping is hot, 1 to 2 minutes. Enjoy!

MAKES 1 SERVING

MEAT LOVER'S BREAKFAST PIZZA

255 calories

You'll Need: blender or food processor (optional), small bowl, small skillet with a lid, microwave-safe plate (optional), nonstick spray
Prep: 5 minutes
Cook: 25 minutes

Entire recipe: 255 calories, 8.5g fat, 950mg sodium, 8.5g carbs, 1g fiber, 2g sugars, 31g protein

INGREDIENTS

1 stick light string cheese
2 tablespoons canned crushed tomatoes
⅛ teaspoon Italian seasoning
1 frozen meatless or turkey sausage patty with 80 calories or less
1 slice center-cut bacon or turkey bacon
½ cup fat-free liquid egg substitute
3 slices turkey pepperoni, chopped

DIRECTIONS

Break string cheese into thirds and place in a blender or food processor—blend at high speed until shredded. (Or pull into shreds and roughly chop.)

In a small bowl, combine crushed tomatoes with Italian seasoning.

One at a time, prepare sausage patty and bacon in a small skillet or on a microwave-safe plate in the microwave. (See packages for cook times and temperature.) Chop or crumble.

Bring a small skillet sprayed with nonstick spray to medium heat. Add egg substitute and let it coat the skillet bottom. Cover and cook until solid enough to flip, about 3 minutes.

Carefully flip egg "crust." Top with seasoned crushed tomatoes, cheese, sausage, bacon, and chopped pepperoni. Cover and cook until cheese has melted and toppings are hot, 1 to 2 minutes. Enjoy!

MAKES 1 SERVING

EASY CAPRESE BREAKFAST PIZZAS

185 calories

You'll Need: baking sheet, nonstick spray, blender or food processor (optional), small bowl, skillet
Prep: 5 minutes | **Cook:** 10 minutes

Entire recipe:
185 calories, 5g fat, 430mg sodium, 23.5g carbs, 6g fiber, 1.5g sugars, 14g protein

INGREDIENTS

1 stick light string cheese

1 teaspoon light whipped butter or light buttery spread

½ teaspoon crushed garlic

1 light English muffin

6 fresh basil leaves

2 thick slices plum tomato

Optional seasonings: salt and black pepper

DIRECTIONS

Preheat oven to 375 degrees. Spray a baking sheet with nonstick spray.

Break string cheese into thirds and place in a blender or food processor—blend at high speed until shredded. (Or pull into shreds and roughly chop.)

In a small bowl, mix butter with garlic. Split English muffin into halves and place on the baking sheet. Spread with butter mixture, sprinkle with cheese, and top with basil.

Bring a skillet sprayed with nonstick spray to medium-high heat. Cook tomato slices until lightly blackened, 1 to 2 minutes per side.

Place a tomato slice on each muffin half. Bake until hot and lightly browned, about 5 minutes. Devour!

MAKES 1 SERVING

PERFECT PEPPERONI PIZZAS

211 calories

You'll Need: baking sheet, nonstick spray, blender or food processor (optional)
Prep: 5 minutes | **Cook:** 15 minutes

Entire recipe:
211 calories, 6g fat, 823mg sodium, 29g carbs, 6.5g fiber, 2.5g sugars, 16.5g protein

INGREDIENTS

1 stick light string cheese

1 light English muffin

2 tablespoons pizza sauce

8 slices turkey pepperoni

Optional seasonings: salt, black pepper, oregano, garlic powder, onion powder, red pepper flakes

DIRECTIONS

Preheat oven to 350 degrees. Spray a baking sheet with nonstick spray.

Break string cheese into thirds and place in a blender or food processor—blend at high speed until shredded. (Or pull into shreds and roughly chop.)

Split English muffin into halves and place on the baking sheet. Spread with pizza sauce, sprinkle with cheese, and top with pepperoni.

Bake until hot and lightly browned, 10 to 12 minutes. Dig in!

MAKES 1 SERVING

CHICKEN GIRLFREDO PIZZA

233 calories

You'll Need: baking sheet, nonstick spray, blender or food processor (optional), small bowl
Prep: 10 minutes
Cook: 15 minutes

Entire recipe: 233 calories, 5.5g fat, 782mg sodium, 27.5g carbs, 6g fiber, 2.5g sugars, 21g protein

INGREDIENTS

1 stick light string cheese
1 wedge The Laughing Cow Light Creamy Swiss cheese
1 teaspoon fat-free sour cream
¼ teaspoon crushed garlic
Dash each salt and black pepper, or more to taste
1 light English muffin
1 ounce cooked and chopped skinless chicken breast

DIRECTIONS

Preheat oven to 375 degrees. Spray a baking sheet with nonstick spray.

Break string cheese into thirds and place in a blender or food processor—blend at high speed until shredded. (Or pull into shreds and roughly chop.)

In a small bowl, combine cheese wedge, sour cream, garlic, salt, and pepper. Stir until smooth.

Split English muffin into halves and place on the baking sheet. Spread both halves with cheese-wedge mixture. Top with chicken and shredded string cheese.

Bake until hot and lightly browned, 10 to 12 minutes. Dig in!

MAKES 1 SERVING

PIZZA LUAU

230 calories

You'll Need: baking sheet, nonstick spray, blender or food processor (optional)
Prep: 5 minutes
Cook: 15 minutes

Entire recipe: 230 calories, 4.5g fat, 808mg sodium, 34g carbs, 6.5g fiber, 9.5g sugars, 17g protein

INGREDIENTS

1 stick light string cheese
1 light English muffin
2 tablespoons low-fat marinara sauce
½ ounce shaved deli ham (about 2 slices), chopped
1 pineapple ring packed in juice, drained, chopped
1 tablespoon chopped red onion

DIRECTIONS

Preheat oven to 350 degrees. Spray a baking sheet with nonstick spray.

Break string cheese into thirds and place in a blender or food processor—blend at high speed until shredded. (Or pull into shreds and roughly chop.)

Split English muffin into halves and place on the baking sheet. Spread with sauce, sprinkle with cheese, and top with remaining ingredients.

Bake until hot and lightly browned, 10 to 12 minutes. YUM!

MAKES 1 SERVING

✳ Flip to the photo inserts to see over 100 recipe pics! And for photos of ALL the recipes, go to hungry-girl.com/books.

PURPLE PIZZA EATERS

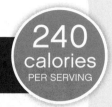

240 calories
PER SERVING

You'll Need: baking sheet, nonstick spray, blender or food processor (optional), microwave-safe bowl, small bowl
Prep: 10 minutes | **Cook:** 15 minutes

½ of recipe (2 mini pizzas):
240 calories, 5g fat, 812mg sodium, 32g carbs, 6.75g fiber, 2g sugars, 20.5g protein

INGREDIENTS

2 sticks light string cheese

3 ounces purple potato, thinly sliced

¼ cup fat-free ricotta cheese

2 drops purple food coloring (or a drop each of red and blue)

⅛ teaspoon garlic powder

2 dashes salt, or more to taste

2 tablespoons finely chopped red onion

2 light English muffins

2 tablespoons precooked real crumbled bacon

Optional seasoning: black pepper

DIRECTIONS

Preheat oven to 375 degrees. Spray a baking sheet with nonstick spray.

Break each string cheese stick into thirds and place in a blender or food processor—blend at high speed until shredded. (Or pull into shreds and roughly chop.)

Place potato slices in a microwave-safe bowl with 2 tablespoons water. Cover and microwave for 2 minutes, or until slightly softened. Drain and chop into bite-sized pieces.

In a small bowl, thoroughly mix ricotta cheese, food coloring, garlic powder, and salt. Stir in onion.

Split English muffins into halves and place on the baking sheet. Evenly spread with ricotta mixture. Top with chopped potato and sprinkle with shredded string cheese and bacon.

Bake until hot and lightly browned, 10 to 12 minutes. Chew, you crazy thing!

MAKES 2 SERVINGS

HG ALTERNATIVE!
If you can't find purple spuds, grab a small red-skinned potato!

PESTO PIZZAS

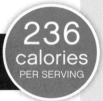
**236
calories
PER SERVING**

You'll Need: baking sheet, nonstick spray, small blender or food processor | **Prep:** 10 minutes | **Cook:** 15 minutes

½ of recipe (2 mini pizzas):
236 calories, 9g fat, 590mg sodium, 31g carbs, 7.5g fiber, 3g sugars, 15g protein

INGREDIENTS

2 sticks light string cheese

½ cup fresh basil leaves

2 tablespoons light or low-fat ricotta cheese

1 tablespoon reduced-fat Parmesan-style grated topping

1 tablespoon pine nuts

½ teaspoon olive oil

½ teaspoon chopped garlic

¼ teaspoon black pepper

⅛ teaspoon salt

2 light English muffins

4 cherry tomatoes, quartered

DIRECTIONS

Preheat oven to 375 degrees. Spray a baking sheet with nonstick spray.

Break each string cheese stick into thirds and place in a small blender or food processor—blend at high speed until shredded. (Or pull into shreds and roughly chop.)

In a small blender or food processor, combine basil, ricotta cheese, Parm-style topping, pine nuts, olive oil, garlic, pepper, and salt. Blend or process to a smooth paste.

Split English muffins into halves and place on the baking sheet. Evenly spread with basil mixture. Sprinkle with shredded string cheese and top with tomatoes.

Bake until hot and lightly browned, 12 to 14 minutes. Dig in!

MAKES 2 SERVINGS

HG TIP:

If you're noshing solo, bake only two of the mini pizzas. Wrap the others in plastic wrap and freeze for another time—then just thaw, bake, and eat!

PIZZA-BELLAS

 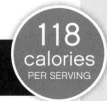

118 calories PER SERVING

You'll Need: baking sheet, nonstick spray, blender or food processor (optional), small bowl
Prep: 10 minutes
Cook: 20 minutes

½ of recipe (1 pizza-bella): 118 calories, 4.75g fat, 487mg sodium, 7.5g carbs, 1.75g fiber, 3g sugars, 11.5g protein

INGREDIENTS

2 sticks light string cheese
2 large portabella mushrooms, stems chopped and reserved
¼ cup canned crushed tomatoes
½ teaspoon chopped garlic
Dash Italian seasoning
8 slices turkey pepperoni, chopped
2 tablespoons sliced black olives

DIRECTIONS

Preheat oven to 400 degrees. Spray a baking sheet with nonstick spray.

Break each string cheese stick into thirds and place in a blender or food processor—blend at high speed until shredded. (Or pull into shreds and roughly chop.)

Place mushroom caps on the sheet, rounded sides down. Bake until slightly tender, about 8 minutes.

Remove sheet, but leave oven on. Blot away excess moisture from mushroom caps.

In a small bowl, mix crushed tomatoes, garlic, and Italian seasoning. Divide mixture between mushroom caps, and sprinkle with cheese. Top with chopped mushroom stems, pepperoni, and olives.

Bake until mushrooms are tender, filling is hot, and cheese has melted, 8 to 10 minutes. Enjoy!

MAKES 2 SERVINGS

WHITE PIZZA-BELLAS

130 calories PER SERVING

You'll Need: baking sheet, nonstick spray, blender or food processor (optional), skillet, medium bowl
Prep: 10 minutes
Cook: 20 minutes

½ of recipe (1 pizza-bella): 130 calories, 4.5g fat, 395mg sodium, 11g carbs, 2g fiber, 5g sugars, 13.5g protein

INGREDIENTS

2 sticks light string cheese
2 large portabella mushrooms, stems chopped and reserved
¼ cup diced onion
⅓ cup light or low-fat ricotta cheese
⅛ teaspoon garlic powder
⅛ teaspoon salt
Dash black pepper
4 cherry tomatoes, quartered
5 basil leaves, chopped

Optional topping: red pepper flakes

DIRECTIONS

Preheat oven to 400 degrees. Spray a baking sheet with nonstick spray.

Break each string cheese stick into thirds and place in a blender or food processor—blend at high speed until shredded. (Or pull into shreds and roughly chop.)

Place mushroom caps on the sheet, rounded sides down. Bake until slightly tender, about 8 minutes. Remove sheet, but leave oven on.

Meanwhile, bring a skillet sprayed with nonstick spray to medium-high heat. Cook and stir onion and mushroom stems until slightly softened and lightly browned, about 3 minutes.

Transfer onion and mushroom stems to a medium bowl and blot away excess moisture. Stir in ricotta cheese, garlic powder, salt, and pepper.

Blot away excess moisture from mushroom caps. Divide ricotta mixture between the caps and sprinkle with shredded string cheese. Top with tomatoes and basil.

Bake until mushrooms are tender, filling is hot, and string cheese has melted, 8 to 10 minutes. Enjoy!

MAKES 2 SERVINGS

SAUSAGE-LOADED PIZZA-BELLAS

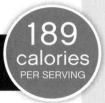

189 calories
PER SERVING

You'll Need: baking sheet, nonstick spray, blender or food processor (optional), skillet, medium bowl
Prep: 10 minutes | **Cook:** 20 minutes

½ of recipe (1 pizza-bella):
189 calories, 6.5g fat, 565mg sodium, 14g carbs, 3g fiber, 4.5g sugars, 17g protein

INGREDIENTS

2 sticks light string cheese

2 large portabella mushrooms, stems chopped and reserved

2 frozen meatless or turkey sausage patties with 80 calories or less each

¼ cup diced bell pepper

¼ cup diced onion

¼ cup pizza sauce

Optional toppings: garlic powder, red pepper flakes

DIRECTIONS

Preheat oven to 400 degrees. Spray a baking sheet with nonstick spray.

Break each string cheese stick into thirds and place in a blender or food processor—blend at high speed until shredded. (Or pull into shreds and roughly chop.)

Place mushroom caps on the sheet, rounded sides down. Bake until slightly tender, about 8 minutes. Remove sheet, but leave oven on.

Meanwhile, bring a skillet sprayed with nonstick spray to medium heat. Cook sausage patties for 4 minutes. Flip patties and add pepper, onion, and mushroom stems. Cook, stirring veggies, until sausage patties are cooked through and veggies are slightly softened and lightly browned, about 5 minutes.

Transfer cooked chopped veggies to a medium bowl and blot away excess moisture. Chop or crumble sausage.

Blot away excess moisture from mushroom caps. Spread with pizza sauce, sprinkle with shredded string cheese, and top with cooked veggies and sausage.

Bake until mushrooms are tender, filling is hot, and string cheese has melted, 8 to 10 minutes. Enjoy!

MAKES 2 SERVINGS

GREEK PIZZA-BELLAS

154 calories
PER SERVING

You'll Need: baking sheet, nonstick spray, blender or food processor (optional), skillet, medium bowl, small bowl
Prep: 10 minutes | **Cook:** 20 minutes

½ of recipe (1 pizza-bella):
154 calories, 6.5g fat, 494mg sodium, 11.5g carbs, 2.5g fiber, 4g sugars, 13.5g protein

INGREDIENTS

2 sticks light string cheese

2 large portabella mushrooms, stems chopped and reserved

1 cup chopped spinach leaves

¼ cup crumbled reduced-fat feta cheese

¼ teaspoon garlic powder

¼ cup canned crushed tomatoes

Dash dried oregano

2 tablespoons diced red onion

4 cherry tomatoes, quartered

2 tablespoons sliced black olives

DIRECTIONS

Preheat oven to 400 degrees. Spray a baking sheet with nonstick spray.

Break each string cheese stick into thirds and place in a blender or food processor—blend at high speed until shredded. (Or pull into shreds and roughly chop.)

Place mushroom caps on the sheet, rounded sides down. Bake until slightly tender, about 8 minutes. Remove sheet, but leave oven on.

Meanwhile, bring a skillet sprayed with nonstick spray to medium-high heat. Cook and stir mushroom stems until slightly softened, about 2 minutes. Add spinach and cook and stir until mushroom stems are lightly browned and spinach has wilted, about 1 minute.

Transfer cooked mushroom stems and spinach to a medium bowl and blot away excess moisture. Stir in feta cheese and garlic powder.

Blot away excess moisture from mushroom caps. In a small bowl, mix crushed tomatoes with oregano. Spread onto mushroom caps. Divide spinach-feta mixture between the caps and sprinkle with shredded string cheese.

Top with onion, tomatoes, and olives. Bake until mushrooms are tender, filling is hot, and string cheese has melted, 8 to 10 minutes. Eat up!

MAKES 2 SERVINGS

For more recipes, tips & tricks, sign up for FREE daily emails at **hungry-girl.com!**

POTATO-SKIN PEPPERONI PIZZA

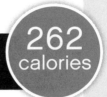
262 calories

You'll Need: baking sheet, nonstick spray, microwave-safe plate, blender or food processor (optional), skillet, medium bowl
Prep: 10 minutes | **Cook:** 35 minutes

Entire recipe:
262 calories, 6.5g fat, 805mg sodium, 36g carbs, 4.5g fiber, 7.5g sugars, 16g protein

INGREDIENTS

One 10-ounce russet potato
1 stick light string cheese
¼ cup chopped bell pepper
¼ cup chopped onion
¼ cup chopped mushrooms
¼ cup pizza sauce
6 slices turkey pepperoni, chopped
2 teaspoons reduced-fat Parmesan-style
    grated topping

DIRECTIONS

Preheat oven to 375 degrees. Spray a baking sheet with nonstick spray.

Pierce potato several times with a fork. On a microwave-safe plate, microwave for 5 minutes, or until slightly softened.

Flip potato over and microwave for 5 more minutes, or until soft.

Break string cheese into thirds and place in a blender or food processor—blend at high speed until shredded. (Or pull into shreds and roughly chop.)

Cut potato in half lengthwise and gently scoop out and discard most of the flesh, leaving about ¼ inch on the skins.

Place skins on the baking sheet and bake until crispy, 10 to 12 minutes. Remove sheet, but leave oven on.

Meanwhile, bring a skillet sprayed with nonstick spray to medium-high heat. Add pepper, onion, and mushrooms. Cook and stir until mostly softened, about 5 minutes.

Transfer veggies to a medium bowl and mix with pizza sauce. Evenly divide mixture among potato skins.

Top skins with shredded string cheese and pepperoni. Bake until sauce is hot and cheese has melted, about 4 minutes.

Sprinkle with Parm-style topping and dig in!

MAKES 1 SERVING

MINI DEEP DISH SPINACH PIZZAS

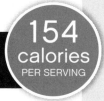

154 calories
PER SERVING

You'll Need: 12-cup muffin pan, nonstick spray, large bowl, medium bowl, rolling pin (optional)
Prep: 25 minutes | **Cook:** 15 minutes

⅟₁₂th of recipe (1 mini pizza):
154 calories, 4g fat, 578mg sodium, 20g carbs, 1.5g fiber, 3g sugars, 8g protein

INGREDIENTS

Two 10-ounce packages frozen chopped
    spinach, thawed and squeezed dry

1½ cups shredded part-skim mozzarella cheese

1 tablespoon chopped garlic

½ teaspoon salt

1 cup canned crushed tomatoes

¼ teaspoon Italian seasoning

¼ teaspoon garlic powder

¼ teaspoon onion power

1 package Pillsbury Classic Pizza
    Crust refrigerated dough

¼ cup reduced-fat Parmesan-style grated topping

DIRECTIONS

Preheat oven to 375 degrees. Spray a 12-cup muffin pan with nonstick spray.

In a large bowl, thoroughly mix spinach, shredded cheese, garlic, and salt. In a medium bowl, mix crushed tomatoes with remaining seasonings.

Roll or stretch out dough into a large rectangle of even thickness, at least 12 inches by 9 inches. Evenly cut dough into 12 squares. Place each square in a muffin cup, and press it into the bottom and up along the sides.

Evenly distribute spinach-cheese mixture among the cups, about 3 tablespoons each, and firmly pack it in.

Evenly top with seasoned crushed tomatoes, about 1 tablespoon per cup, and sprinkle with Parm-style topping, 1 teaspoon per cup.

Bake until dough is firm and golden brown and filling is hot, about 15 minutes. Enjoy!

MAKES 12 SERVINGS

Hungry for More Italian Eats?

There are MANY baked-not-fried Parmesan dishes in the Faux-Frys chapter. *Mangia!*

CHAPTER 11

MEXICAN

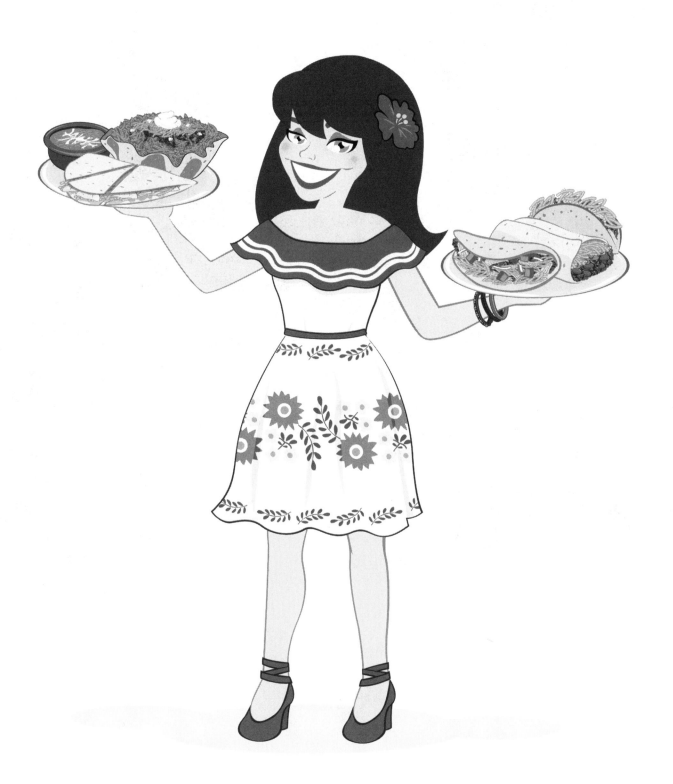

MEXICAN

Shrimp Cocktail Tacos
Mega-Meaty Meatless Tacos
Cool 'n Crunchy Salmon Tacos
Crunchy BBQ Chicken Tacos
iHungry Spaghetti Tacos
Cheeseburger Tacos
Breakfast Fiesta Crunchy Tacos
Saucy-Q Chicken Soft Tacos
Peach-BBQ Soft Fish Tacos
Amazing Ate-Layer Tostada
7-Layer Burrito Blitz
Snazzy Smothered Veggie Burritos
Chicken Fajita Burrito
Cheesy Chicken Quesadilla
Caramelized Onion Cheese Quesadilla
Tropical Shrimp Quesadilla

Clubhouse Chicken Quesadilla
SW BBQ Chicken Quesadilla
Buffalo Chicken Quesadilla
Cheeseburger Quesadilla
Cheesy Pizza Quesadilla
Lean 'n Green Shrimp-chilada
Cheesy Chicken Enchiladas
Lean Bean 'n Cheese Enchiladas
Pizza-ladas
Spinach Enchiladas
Surprise, It's Pumpkin! Enchiladas
Exploding Chicken Taquitos
Buffalo Chicken Taquitos
Jalapeño Cheese Taquitos
'Bella Asada Fajitas

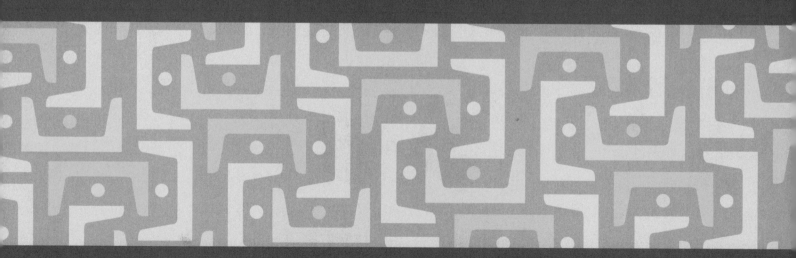

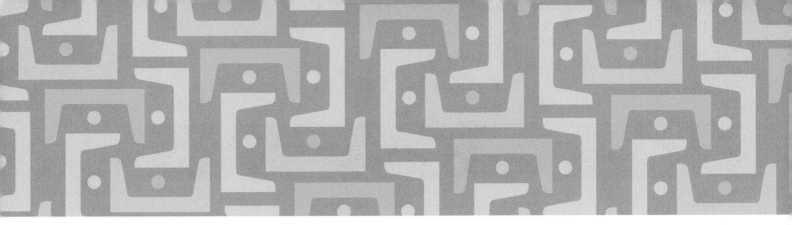

Mexican food typically clocks in with WAY too many calories and fat grams, (no) thanks to full-fat cheeses, sour cream, and fried tortillas. Not here, humans! HG Mexican fare has all the flavor of the originals—only with lighter nutritional stats. Fiesta time!!!

A QUICK GUIDE TO SYMBOLS:

15 Minutes or Less

This symbol lets you know a recipe should take you no more than fifteen minutes from start to finish! That includes prep and cook time.

30 Minutes or Less

Just like the 15-minute version, this one points out recipes that take 30 minutes or less to whip up.

Meatless

You guessed it—no meat here! That includes beef, poultry, and fish. Some recipes give the option of a meatless ingredient. If you want your meal without meat, go with the meatless choice.

Single Serving

Pretty straightforward. These are recipes for one.

5 Ingredients or Less

Fans of HG know that we like to keep things simple. And these recipes contain just five ingredients or less!

Photos

These recipes can be seen in one of the book's photo inserts. The number in the symbol tells you which insert. Find photos of all the recipes at hungry-girl.com/books!

SHRIMP COCKTAIL TACOS

243 calories

You'll Need: medium bowl | **Prep:** 5 minutes | **Chill:** 15 minutes

Entire recipe (2 tacos):
243 calories, 5g fat, 638mg sodium, 26.5g carbs, 3.5g fiber, 4g sugars, 21g protein

INGREDIENTS

3 ounces cooked ready-to-eat shrimp, chopped if large

¼ cup plus 2 tablespoons black bean and corn salsa

¼ cup shredded lettuce

2 corn taco shells

Optional toppings: fresh cilantro, fat-free sour cream

DIRECTIONS

In a medium bowl, mix shrimp with salsa. Cover and refrigerate for 15 minutes.

Divide lettuce and shrimp-salsa mixture between taco shells. Now chew!

MAKES 1 SERVING

MEGA-MEATY MEATLESS TACOS

197 calories PER SERVING

You'll Need: skillet, nonstick spray | **Prep:** 5 minutes | **Cook:** 10 minutes

⅓rd of recipe (2 tacos):
197 calories, 6g fat, 617mg sodium, 26.5g carbs, 3.5g fiber, 3.5g sugars, 11.5g protein

INGREDIENTS

2 cups finely chopped brown mushrooms

½ cup chopped onion

½ cup frozen ground-beef-style soy crumbles

2 teaspoons taco seasoning mix

6 corn taco shells

6 tablespoons shredded fat-free cheddar cheese

6 tablespoons pico de gallo (or chunky salsa)

Optional toppings: shredded lettuce, fresh cilantro

DIRECTIONS

Bring a skillet sprayed with nonstick spray to medium-high heat. Cook and stir mushrooms and onion until softened, about 6 minutes.

Reduce heat to medium. Add soy crumbles to veggies and sprinkle with taco seasoning. Cook and stir until hot, about 2 minutes.

Evenly distribute veggie-crumbles mixture among the taco shells, about 3 tablespoons each. Top each taco with a tablespoon of cheese and a tablespoon of pico de gallo. CHOMP!

MAKES 3 SERVINGS

COOL 'N CRUNCHY SALMON TACOS

263 calories

You'll Need: medium bowl
Prep: 10 minutes

Entire recipe (2 tacos): 263 calories,
8.5g fat, 737mg sodium, 27g carbs,
3g fiber, 5g sugars, 19.5g protein

INGREDIENTS

2 tablespoons fat-free sour cream

1 teaspoon ranch dressing/dip seasoning mix

One 2.6-ounce pouch boneless skinless
    pink salmon, roughly flaked
    (about ½ cup)

2 tablespoons finely chopped onion

¼ cup peeled and finely chopped cucumber

½ tablespoon chopped fresh dill

2 corn taco shells

¼ cup shredded lettuce

¼ cup diced tomato

DIRECTIONS

In a medium bowl, thoroughly mix sour
cream with ranch seasoning. Add salmon,
onion, cucumber, and dill, and stir to coat.

Divide salmon mixture between taco shells.
Top with lettuce and tomato and EAT!

MAKES 1 SERVING

CRUNCHY BBQ CHICKEN TACOS

366 calories

You'll Need: skillet, nonstick spray, medium bowl
Prep: 10 minutes
Cook: 20 minutes

Entire recipe (2 tacos): 366 calories,
7.5g fat, 761mg sodium, 44.5g carbs, 4g fiber,
14g sugars, 31g protein

INGREDIENTS

One 4-ounce raw boneless skinless chicken breast cutlet

3 tablespoons BBQ sauce with 45 calories or less per
    2-tablespoon serving

2 corn taco shells

2 tablespoons shredded lettuce

2 tablespoons canned black beans, drained and rinsed

2 tablespoons frozen sweet corn kernels, thawed

2 tablespoons chopped red onion

2 tablespoons chopped fresh cilantro

Optional topping: fat-free ranch dressing

DIRECTIONS

Bring a skillet sprayed with nonstick spray to
medium-high heat. Cook chicken for 6 to 8 minutes per
side, until cooked through.

Transfer chicken to a medium bowl and let slightly cool.
Shred with two forks—one to hold chicken in place and the
other to scrape across and shred it. Add BBQ sauce and stir
to coat.

Divide saucy chicken between taco shells, followed by
remaining ingredients. Enjoy!

MAKES 1 SERVING

TACO SHELL TIP:

Look for flat-bottomed shells. They're easier to work with.

iHUNGRY SPAGHETTI TACOS

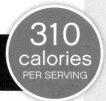
310 calories
PER SERVING

You'll Need: medium-large pot, large skillet, nonstick spray | **Prep:** 10 minutes | **Cook:** 15 minutes

⅙th of recipe (2 tacos):
310 calories, 7.5g fat, 728mg sodium, 41.5g carbs, 6.5g fiber, 4.5g sugars, 22g protein

INGREDIENTS

4 ounces uncooked high-fiber spaghetti

2 cups frozen ground-beef-style soy crumbles

2 cups canned crushed tomatoes

½ tablespoon taco seasoning mix

12 corn taco shells

1½ cups shredded fat-free cheddar cheese

1 cup shredded lettuce

⅔ cup chopped onion

DIRECTIONS

Break pasta in half and, in a medium-large pot, cook per package instructions, about 8 minutes. Drain well.

Bring a large skillet sprayed with nonstick spray to medium-high heat. Add soy crumbles, crushed tomatoes, and taco seasoning, and mix well. Cook and stir until hot, 2 to 4 minutes.

Add pasta to the skillet, and mix well. Evenly distribute mixture among taco shells, about ⅓ cup per shell. Evenly top with remaining ingredients!

MAKES 6 SERVINGS

CHEESEBURGER TACOS

269 calories

You'll Need: skillet and nonstick spray or microwave-safe plate | **Prep:** 5 minutes | **Cook:** 10 minutes

Entire recipe (2 tacos):
269 calories, 8.5g fat, 989mg sodium, 30g carbs, 6.5g fiber, 4.5g sugars, 17.5g protein

INGREDIENTS

1 frozen meatless hamburger-style patty with 100 calories or less

2 corn taco shells

1 slice fat-free American cheese

¼ cup shredded lettuce

4 hamburger dill pickle chips

2 tablespoons diced tomato

2 tablespoons diced onion

Optional toppings: ketchup, mustard, fat-free mayonnaise

DIRECTIONS

Place burger patty in a skillet sprayed with nonstick spray or on a microwave-safe plate in the microwave. (See package for cook time and temperature.)

Chop patty into bite-sized pieces and evenly divide between taco shells. Tear cheese slice in half, and place a half in each shell. Evenly top with remaining ingredients and dig in!

MAKES 1 SERVING

BREAKFAST FIESTA CRUNCHY TACOS

290 calories

You'll Need: small bowl, skillet, nonstick spray
Prep: 5 minutes
Cook: 5 minutes

Entire recipe (2 tacos): 290 calories, 7.5g fat, 842mg sodium, 34g carbs, 4.5g fiber, 4g sugars, 20g protein

INGREDIENTS

¼ cup fat-free refried beans
1 wedge The Laughing Cow Light Creamy Swiss cheese
2 corn taco shells
¼ cup finely chopped onion
½ teaspoon chopped garlic
½ cup fat-free liquid egg substitute
¼ teaspoon taco seasoning mix

Optional toppings: salsa, fat-free sour cream

DIRECTIONS

In a small bowl, thoroughly mix beans with cheese. Evenly divide mixture between taco shells.

Bring a skillet sprayed with nonstick spray to medium-high heat. Cook and stir onion and garlic until softened, about 2 minutes.

Add egg substitute and sprinkle with taco seasoning. Scramble until fully cooked, about 3 minutes. Evenly divide between taco shells. Enjoy!

MAKES 1 SERVING

SAUCY-Q CHICKEN SOFT TACOS

336 calories PER SERVING

You'll Need: skillet with a lid, nonstick spray, large bowl, medium bowl, microwave-safe plate
Prep: 10 minutes
Cook: 10 minutes

½ of recipe (2 tacos): 336 calories, 3g fat, 712mg sodium, 47g carbs, 4g fiber, 20g sugars, 29g protein

INGREDIENTS

8 ounces raw boneless skinless chicken breast cutlets
⅛ teaspoon each salt and black pepper
⅓ cup BBQ sauce with 45 calories or less per 2-tablespoon serving
⅓ cup chopped mango
⅓ cup chopped red onion
1 jalapeño pepper, seeded, finely chopped
2 tablespoons chopped fresh cilantro
½ tablespoon seasoned rice vinegar
Four 6-inch corn tortillas

DIRECTIONS

Bring a skillet sprayed with nonstick spray to medium-high heat. Season chicken with salt and black pepper and place in the skillet. Cover and cook for 4 minutes per side, or until cooked through.

Transfer chicken to a large bowl. Shred with two forks—one to hold it in place and the other to scrape across and shred it. Add BBQ sauce and stir to coat.

In a medium bowl, mix mango, onion, jalapeño pepper, cilantro, and vinegar.

Microwave tortillas on a microwave-safe plate for 15 seconds, or until warm.

Evenly distribute BBQ chicken and mango-onion mixture among the tortillas. Fold 'n chew!

MAKES 2 SERVINGS

JALAPEÑO QUICK TIP!

When handling jalapeños, don't touch your eyes—that pepper juice can STING. And wash your hands well immediately afterward.

PEACH-BBQ SOFT FISH TACOS

321 calories PER SERVING

You'll Need: small blender or food processor, wide bowl, whisk, skillet, nonstick spray, microwave-safe plate
Prep: 10 minutes | **Marinate:** 15 minutes | **Cook:** 5 minutes

½ of recipe (2 tacos):
321 calories, 5.5g fat, 411mg sodium, 42.5g carbs, 5g fiber, 18g sugars, 26.5g protein

INGREDIENTS

⅓ cup sliced peaches packed in juice, drained (about 4 slices)

¼ cup canned tomato sauce

2 tablespoons ketchup

2 teaspoons brown sugar (not packed)

1 teaspoon molasses

1 teaspoon cider vinegar

½ teaspoon garlic powder

¼ cup diced tomato

8 ounces raw tilapia

Four 6-inch corn tortillas

1 cup shredded cabbage

1 ounce sliced avocado (about ¼ avocado)

2 tablespoons chopped cilantro

DIRECTIONS

Puree peaches in a small blender or food processor. Transfer to a wide bowl. Add tomato sauce, ketchup, sugar, molasses, vinegar, and garlic powder, and thoroughly whisk. Stir in diced tomato. Add fish and gently coat. Cover and marinate in the fridge for 15 minutes.

Bring a skillet sprayed with nonstick spray to medium heat. Add fish and marinade. Cook for 2 minutes. Gently flip fish. Cook for 2 more minutes, or until fish is cooked through and marinade has thickened to a sauce-like consistency.

Remove skillet from heat and flake fish with a spatula.

Microwave tortillas on a microwave-safe plate for 15 seconds, or until warm.

Evenly distribute fish and sauce among tortillas. Top with cabbage, avocado, and cilantro. Fold each tortilla around its filling and chew!

MAKES 2 SERVINGS

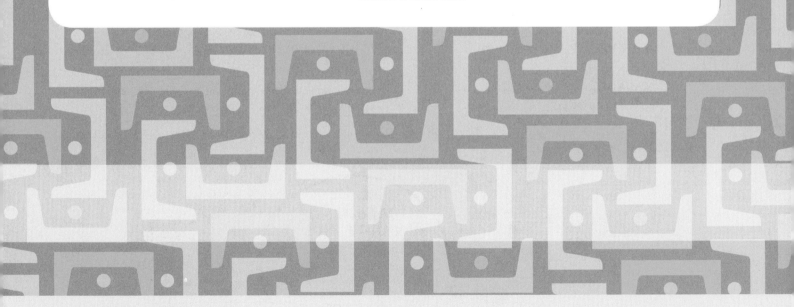

AMAZING ATE-LAYER TOSTADA

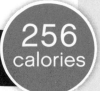

256 calories

You'll Need: baking sheet, nonstick spray, 2 microwave-safe bowls, plate | **Prep:** 15 minutes | **Cook:** 15 minutes

Entire recipe:
256 calories, 2.25g fat, 795mg sodium, 46.5g carbs, 8.75g fiber, 8.5g sugars, 17g protein

INGREDIENTS

1 medium-large corn tortilla
1 cup cubed butternut squash
½ teaspoon ground cumin
¼ teaspoon onion powder
¼ teaspoon garlic powder
Dash salt
Dash cayenne pepper
¼ cup frozen ground-beef-style soy crumbles
¼ teaspoon taco seasoning mix
½ cup shredded lettuce
2 tablespoons canned black beans, drained and rinsed
2 tablespoons shredded fat-free cheddar cheese
2 tablespoons salsa
2 tablespoons fat-free sour cream
1 tablespoon jarred jalapeño slices or mild banana
    pepper slices

DIRECTIONS

Preheat oven to 400 degrees. Spray a baking sheet with nonstick spray.

Lay tortilla on the sheet and mist with nonstick spray. Bake until crispy, about 8 minutes.

Place squash in a microwave-safe bowl with 1 tablespoon water. Cover and microwave for 6 minutes, or until soft.

Drain excess water from squash. Add cumin, onion powder, garlic powder, salt, and cayenne pepper. Mash well.

In another microwave-safe bowl, microwave soy crumbles for 25 seconds. Stir in taco seasoning, and microwave for another 25 seconds, or until hot.

Set crispy tortilla on a plate, and evenly layer with these ingredients: squash mixture, lettuce, black beans, seasoned soy crumbles, and cheese. Microwave for 30 seconds, or until hot.

Top with remaining ingredients and enjoy!

MAKES 1 SERVING

Flip to the photo inserts to see over 100 recipe pics! And for photos of ALL the recipes, go to hungry-girl.com/books.

7-LAYER BURRITO BLITZ

277 calories

You'll Need: microwave-safe bowl, microwave-safe plate
Prep: 5 minutes
Cook: 5 minutes

Entire recipe: 277 calories, 3g fat, 875mg sodium, 46g carbs, 14.5g fiber, 4g sugars, 22g protein

INGREDIENTS

¼ cup frozen ground-beef-style soy crumbles
1 medium-large high-fiber flour tortilla with 110 calories or less
⅓ cup canned black beans, drained and rinsed
2 tablespoons fat-free sour cream
½ cup chopped iceberg lettuce
2 tablespoons chopped onion
2 tablespoons shredded fat-free cheddar cheese
¼ cup chopped tomatoes

Optional seasonings: salt, black pepper, chili powder

DIRECTIONS

In a microwave-safe bowl, microwave soy crumbles for 45 seconds, or until hot. Season to taste.

Microwave tortilla on a microwave-safe plate for 10 seconds, or until warm. Layer these ingredients across the middle: black beans, soy crumbles, sour cream, lettuce, onion, cheese, and tomatoes.

Fold in the sides of the tortilla and tightly roll it up around the filling. Seven layers—all for you!

MAKES 1 SERVING

SNAZZY SMOTHERED VEGGIE BURRITOS

315 calories PER SERVING

You'll Need: baking sheet, nonstick spray, large skillet, microwave-safe bowl, microwave-safe plate
Prep: 15 minutes
Cook: 20 minutes

½ of recipe (1 burrito): 315 calories, 7g fat, 1,018mg sodium, 55.5g carbs, 13.5g fiber, 10g sugars, 17g protein

INGREDIENTS

1 cup chopped zucchini
1 cup chopped red bell pepper
1 cup chopped onion
⅔ cup fat-free refried beans
¼ teaspoon cumin
¼ teaspoon chili powder
¼ teaspoon garlic powder
2 medium-large high-fiber flour tortillas with 110 calories or less
⅓ cup red enchilada sauce
⅓ cup shredded reduced-fat Mexican-blend cheese

DIRECTIONS

Preheat oven to 400 degrees. Spray a baking sheet with nonstick spray.

Bring a large skillet sprayed with nonstick spray to medium-high heat. Add zucchini, pepper, and onion. Cook and stir until softened, 10 to 12 minutes.

In a microwave-safe bowl, thoroughly mix refried beans, cumin, chili powder, and garlic powder. Microwave for 1 minute, or until hot, and stir.

Microwave tortillas on a microwave-safe plate for 15 seconds, or until warm.

Lay tortillas flat and divide bean mixture between the bottom halves. Top with cooked veggies.

Fold in the sides of each tortilla and tightly roll it up around the filling. Place seam-side down on the baking sheet, side by side.

Top with sauce and cheese. Bake until cheese has melted and burritos are hot, 2 to 3 minutes. Eat up!

MAKES 2 SERVINGS

CHICKEN FAJITA BURRITO

You'll Need: medium bowl, skillet, nonstick spray, microwave-safe plate
Prep: 5 minutes | **Marinate:** 10 minutes | **Cook:** 10 minutes

Entire recipe:
304 calories, 3g fat, 850mg sodium, 39.5g carbs, 10g fiber, 4g sugars, 33.5g protein

INGREDIENTS

½ teaspoon fajita seasoning mix
3 ounces raw boneless skinless chicken breast,
    cut into bite-sized pieces
¼ cup thinly sliced onion
¼ cup thinly sliced bell pepper
1 medium-large high-fiber flour tortilla
    with 110 calories or less
¼ cup fat-free refried beans
2 tablespoons shredded fat-free cheddar cheese
1 tablespoon chopped fresh cilantro

DIRECTIONS

In a medium bowl, mix fajita seasoning with 2 teaspoons water. Add chicken, onion, and pepper, and toss to coat. Cover and marinate in the fridge for 10 minutes.

Bring a skillet sprayed with nonstick spray to medium-high heat. Add chicken mixture and excess marinade. Cook and stir until marinade has evaporated and chicken is fully cooked, about 5 minutes.

Microwave tortilla on a microwave-safe plate for 10 seconds, or until warm. Evenly spread with refried beans.

Distribute chicken mixture, cheese, and cilantro across the middle of the tortilla. Fold in the sides of the tortilla and tightly roll it up around the filling. Place burrito seam-side down on the plate, and microwave for 30 seconds, or until hot. Enjoy!

MAKES 1 SERVING

FLOUR-TORTILLA ALTERNATIVE!

These recipes call for high-fiber tortillas with 110 calories or less. Our top pick is La Tortilla Factory Smart & Delicious Low Carb High Fiber Large Tortillas—only 80 calories each! Use one of these, and you shave 30 calories off your recipe's calorie count.

CHEESY CHICKEN QUESADILLA

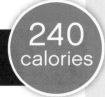

You'll Need: skillet, nonstick spray | **Prep:** 5 minutes | **Cook:** 5 minutes

Entire recipe:
240 calories, 3g fat, 705mg sodium, 24g carbs, 9g fiber, 1g sugars, 34g protein

INGREDIENTS

1 medium-large high-fiber flour tortilla with 110 calories or less

⅓ cup shredded fat-free cheddar cheese

2 ounces cooked and sliced skinless chicken breast

1 tablespoon diced scallions

Optional toppings: fat-free sour cream, salsa

DIRECTIONS

Bring a skillet sprayed with nonstick spray to medium-high heat. Lay tortilla in the skillet and evenly sprinkle with cheese. Top one half with chicken and scallions. Cook for 2 minutes.

Using a spatula, fold the cheese-only half over the chicken-topped half and press lightly to seal. Carefully flip and cook until crispy, about 3 minutes.

Slice and chew!

MAKES 1 SERVING

CARAMELIZED ONION CHEESE QUESADILLA

292 calories

You'll Need: skillet, nonstick spray, medium bowl | **Prep:** 5 minutes | **Cook:** 25 minutes

Entire recipe:
292 calories, 9.5g fat, 907mg sodium, 42g carbs, 8g fiber, 9g sugars, 16g protein

INGREDIENTS

1 cup diced sweet onion

Dash each salt and black pepper

¼ cup shredded reduced-fat Mexican-blend cheese

1 wedge The Laughing Cow Light Creamy Swiss cheese

1 medium-large high-fiber flour tortilla with 110 calories or less

DIRECTIONS

Bring a skillet sprayed with nonstick spray to medium-low heat. Add onion and sprinkle with salt and pepper. Stirring frequently, cook until caramelized, 15 to 20 minutes.

Transfer onion to a medium bowl. Add shredded cheese and cheese wedge, and thoroughly mix.

Lay tortilla flat and spread one half with onion-cheese mixture. Fold the bare half over and press gently to seal.

If needed, clean skillet. Re-spray and bring to medium-high heat. Cook quesadilla until hot and crispy, about 2 minutes per side. Slice into wedges and eat up!

MAKES 1 SERVING

TROPICAL SHRIMP QUESADILLA

287 calories

You'll Need: blender or food processor (optional), skillet, nonstick spray
Prep: 5 minutes
Cook: 5 minutes

Entire recipe: 287 calories, 7g fat, 841mg sodium, 33g carbs, 6.5g fiber, 8.5g sugars, 26.5g protein

INGREDIENTS

1 stick light string cheese
1 medium-large high-fiber flour tortilla with 110 calories or less
1 wedge The Laughing Cow Light Creamy Swiss cheese
¼ cup chopped mango
2 ounces cooked and chopped ready-to-eat shrimp
Dash cayenne pepper, or more to taste

DIRECTIONS

Break string cheese into thirds and place in a blender or food processor—blend at high speed until shredded. (Or pull into shreds and roughly chop.)

Lay tortilla flat, spread with cheese wedge, and sprinkle with shredded string cheese. Evenly top one half of the tortilla with mango and shrimp, and sprinkle with cayenne pepper. Fold the cheese-only half over the mango-and-shrimp-topped half and press lightly to seal.

Bring a skillet sprayed with nonstick spray to medium-high heat. Cook quesadilla until slightly crispy on the outside and hot on the inside, about 2 minutes per side. Cut into triangles and eat!

MAKES 1 SERVING

CLUBHOUSE CHICKEN QUESADILLA

309 calories

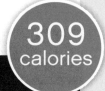

You'll Need: large skillet, nonstick spray, 2 small bowls
Prep: 10 minutes
Cook: 10 minutes

Entire recipe: 309 calories, 7g fat, 996mg sodium, 34g carbs, 8.5g fiber, 5g sugars, 32g protein

INGREDIENTS

¼ cup chopped onion
¼ cup chopped bell pepper
2 teaspoons fat-free ranch dressing
⅛ teaspoon hot sauce
½ ounce (about 1 tablespoon) mashed avocado
Dash each chili powder, ground cumin, and garlic powder
1 medium-large high-fiber flour tortilla with 110 calories or less
¼ cup shredded fat-free cheddar cheese
2 ounces cooked and chopped skinless chicken breast
1 tablespoon precooked real crumbled bacon

Optional toppings: fat-free sour cream, salsa

DIRECTIONS

Bring a large skillet sprayed with nonstick spray to medium-high heat. Cook and stir onion and pepper until softened, 3 to 5 minutes. Remove from skillet and set aside.

In a small bowl, mix ranch dressing with hot sauce. In another small bowl, mix avocado with chili powder, ground cumin, and garlic powder.

Lay tortilla flat and spread one half with avocado mixture. Evenly top avocado with 2 tablespoons cheese, followed by the chicken, bacon, and cooked veggies. Top with ranch mixture and remaining 2 tablespoons cheese.

If needed, clean skillet. Re-spray skillet and return to medium-high heat. Place the half-loaded tortilla flat in the skillet and cook for 2 minutes.

Fold the bare half of the tortilla over the filling with a spatula and press lightly to seal. Carefully flip and cook until crispy, about 3 minutes. Slice into wedges and chew!

MAKES 1 SERVING

SW BBQ CHICKEN QUESADILLA

299 calories

You'll Need: small bowl, grill or grill pan, nonstick spray | **Prep:** 10 minutes | **Cook:** 5 minutes

Entire recipe:
299 calories, 7.75g fat, 940mg sodium, 35g carbs, 7g fiber, 7g sugars, 27g protein

INGREDIENTS

1 tablespoon BBQ sauce with 45 calories or less per 2-tablespoon serving

1 wedge The Laughing Cow Light Creamy Swiss cheese

1 medium-large high-fiber flour tortilla with 110 calories or less

2 ounces cooked and shredded (or finely chopped) skinless chicken breast

2 tablespoons shredded reduced-fat Mexican-blend cheese

1 tablespoon canned black beans, drained and rinsed

1 tablespoon frozen sweet corn kernels, thawed

1 tablespoon chopped scallions

Optional toppings: salsa, fat-free ranch dressing, additional BBQ sauce

DIRECTIONS

In a small bowl, mix BBQ sauce with cheese wedge until blended. Lay tortilla flat and spread BBQ-cheese mixture on one half. Top mixture with remaining ingredients.

Spray a grill or grill pan with nonstick spray and bring to medium-high heat. Lay the half-loaded tortilla on the grill/grill pan, and cook for 2 minutes.

Using a spatula, fold the bare half of the tortilla over the filling and press lightly to seal. Carefully flip and cook until crispy, about 3 minutes. Slice into wedges and eat up!

MAKES 1 SERVING

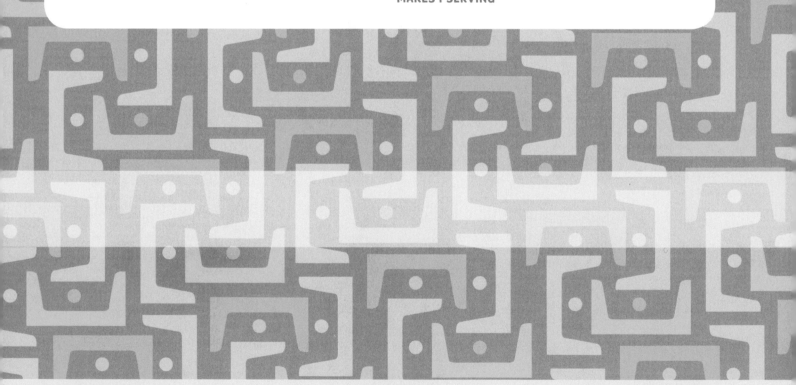

BUFFALO CHICKEN QUESADILLA

253 calories

You'll Need: small bowl, skillet, nonstick spray
Prep: 5 minutes
Cook: 5 minutes

Entire recipe: 253 calories, 7.5g fat, 927mg sodium, 26.5g carbs, 6g fiber, 2.5g sugars, 25.5g protein

INGREDIENTS

1 teaspoon Frank's RedHot Original Cayenne Pepper Sauce
1 wedge The Laughing Cow Light Blue Cheese (or Creamy Swiss) cheese
1 medium-large high-fiber flour tortilla with 110 calories or less
2 ounces cooked and shredded (or finely chopped) skinless chicken breast
2 tablespoons shredded part-skim mozzarella cheese

Optional dips: low-fat blue cheese dressing, additional hot sauce

DIRECTIONS

In a small bowl, mix hot sauce with cheese wedge until smooth. Lay tortilla flat and spread with cheese mixture.

Bring a skillet sprayed with nonstick spray to medium-high heat. Lay tortilla in the skillet and top one half with chicken and mozzarella cheese. Cook for 2 minutes.

Using a spatula, fold the cheese-only half of the tortilla over the filling and press down lightly to seal. Carefully flip and cook until crispy, about 3 minutes. Slice into wedges and enjoy!

MAKES 1 SERVING

CHEESEBURGER QUESADILLA

246 calories

You'll Need: microwave-safe plate, skillet, nonstick spray
Prep: 5 minutes
Cook: 15 minutes

Entire recipe: 246 calories, 5g fat, 1,044mg sodium, 35.5g carbs, 10g fiber, 4.5g sugars, 21g protein

INGREDIENTS

1 frozen meatless hamburger-style patty with 100 calories or less
2 tablespoons chopped onion
1 medium-large high-fiber flour tortilla with 110 calories or less
1 slice fat-free American cheese, chopped
1 tablespoon chopped pickles

Optional topping: ketchup

DIRECTIONS

On a microwave-safe plate, microwave burger patty for 1 minute, or until thawed. Chop into bite-sized pieces.

Bring a skillet sprayed with nonstick spray to medium-high heat. Cook and stir onion until softened, 3 to 5 minutes.

Lay tortilla flat and evenly top with chopped cheese. Top one half with onion, burger pieces, and pickles.

If needed, clean skillet. Re-spray skillet and return to medium-high heat. Place the half-loaded tortilla flat in the skillet and cook for 2 minutes.

Fold the cheese-only half over the filling and press lightly to seal. Carefully flip and cook until crispy, about 3 minutes. Slice into wedges and enjoy!

MAKES 1 SERVING

CHEESY PIZZA QUESADILLA

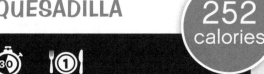

252 calories

You'll Need: blender or food processor (optional), small bowl, skillet, nonstick spray
Prep: 10 minutes
Cook: 10 minutes

Entire recipe: 252 calories, 7.25g fat, 979mg sodium, 31.5g carbs, 7.5g fiber, 5.5g sugars, 18g protein

INGREDIENTS

1 stick light string cheese
¼ cup canned crushed tomatoes
½ teaspoon Italian seasoning
¼ cup sliced mushrooms
¼ cup chopped green bell pepper
1 medium-large high-fiber flour tortilla with 110 calories or less
1 wedge The Laughing Cow Light Creamy Swiss cheese
4 slices turkey pepperoni, chopped

Optional dip: additional canned crushed tomatoes and Italian seasoning

DIRECTIONS

Break string cheese into thirds and place in a blender or food processor—blend at high speed until shredded. (Or pull into shreds and roughly chop.)

In a small bowl, mix tomatoes with Italian seasoning.

Bring a skillet sprayed with nonstick spray to medium-high heat. Cook and stir mushrooms and pepper until softened, about 4 minutes.

Remove veggies. Remove skillet from heat, re-spray, and return to medium heat. Spread one side of the tortilla with the cheese wedge and lay it in the skillet, cheese side up.

Evenly top one half of the tortilla with seasoned tomatoes, shredded string cheese, veggies, and pepperoni. Cook for 3 minutes.

Using a spatula, fold the cheese-only half of the tortilla over the filling and press lightly to seal. Carefully flip and cook until crispy, about 3 minutes.

Slice and devour!

MAKES 1 SERVING

LEAN 'N GREEN SHRIMP-CHILADA

184 calories
PER SERVING

You'll Need: 8-inch by 8-inch baking pan, nonstick spray, small bowl, microwave-safe plate
Prep: 5 minutes
Cook: 15 minutes

½ of recipe (1 enchilada): 184 calories, 3.5g fat, 510mg sodium, 18g carbs, 2g fiber, 3g sugars, 19g protein

INGREDIENTS

6 ounces raw shrimp, peeled, tails removed, deveined, chopped
½ cup plus 1 tablespoon green enchilada sauce
2 medium-large corn tortillas

DIRECTIONS

Preheat oven to 400 degrees. Spray an 8-inch by 8-inch baking pan with nonstick spray.

In a small bowl, combine shrimp with 1 tablespoon enchilada sauce and toss to coat.

Microwave tortillas on a microwave-safe plate for 15 seconds, or until warm.

Lay tortillas flat and divide shrimp mixture between the bottom halves. Tightly wrap up each tortilla and place in the baking pan, seam side down.

Top with remaining ½ cup enchilada sauce. Bake until hot, about 15 minutes. Serve 'em up!

MAKES 2 SERVINGS

CHEESY CHICKEN ENCHILADAS

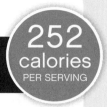
252 calories
PER SERVING

You'll Need: 8-inch by 8-inch baking pan, nonstick spray, skillet, medium bowl, microwave-safe plate
Prep: 10 minutes | **Cook:** 15 minutes

½ of recipe (1 enchilada):
252 calories, 3.5g fat, 840mg sodium, 20.5g carbs, 2.25g fiber, 4g sugars, 33g protein

INGREDIENTS

¼ cup chopped onion

6 ounces cooked and shredded skinless chicken breast

½ cup shredded fat-free cheddar cheese

½ cup plus 2 tablespoons green enchilada sauce

2 medium-large corn tortillas

Optional toppings: fat-free sour cream, chopped scallions

DIRECTIONS

Preheat oven to 400 degrees. Spray an 8-inch by 8-inch baking pan with nonstick spray.

Bring a skillet sprayed with nonstick spray to medium-high heat. Cook and stir onion until slightly browned, about 2 minutes.

Transfer onion to a medium bowl. Add chicken, ¼ cup cheese, and 2 tablespoons enchilada sauce. Mix well.

Microwave tortillas on a microwave-safe plate for 15 seconds, or until warm.

Lay tortillas flat and divide chicken mixture between the bottom halves. Tightly wrap up each tortilla and place in the baking pan, seam side down.

Top with remaining ½ cup enchilada sauce. Bake until hot, about 10 minutes.

Evenly sprinkle with remaining ¼ cup cheese. Bake until cheese has melted, about 2 minutes. Enjoy!

MAKES 2 SERVINGS

MASTER SHREDDER: THREE STEPS TO SHREDDED CHICKEN!

1. Fill a large pot about two-thirds of the way with water and bring to a boil on the stove.

2. Add raw boneless skinless chicken breast and boil until cooked through, about 10 minutes. Drain and transfer chicken to a bowl.

3. Once cool enough to handle, shred using two forks—one to hold the chicken in place and the other to scrape across the meat and shred it.

8 ounces of raw chicken = 6 ounces of cooked and shredded chicken

LEAN BEAN 'N CHEESE ENCHILADAS

187 calories PER SERVING

You'll Need: 8-inch by 8-inch baking pan, nonstick spray, skillet, small bowl, microwave-safe plate
Prep: 5 minutes
Cook: 20 minutes

½ of recipe (1 enchilada): 187 calories, 2g fat, 976mg sodium, 29g carbs, 4g fiber, 5g sugars, 12g protein

INGREDIENTS

¼ cup chopped onion
⅓ cup fat-free refried beans
1 tablespoon taco sauce
½ teaspoon taco seasoning mix
2 medium-large corn tortillas
1 slice fat-free cheddar cheese, halved
⅔ cup red enchilada sauce
¼ cup shredded fat-free cheddar cheese

Optional toppings: fat-free sour cream, chopped scallions

DIRECTIONS

Preheat oven to 400 degrees. Spray an 8-inch by 8-inch baking pan with nonstick spray.

Bring a skillet sprayed with nonstick spray to medium-high heat. Cook and stir onion until lightly browned, about 2 minutes.

Transfer onion to a small bowl. Add refried beans, taco sauce, and taco seasoning, and mix well.

Microwave tortillas on a microwave-safe plate for 15 seconds, or until warm.

Lay tortillas flat and place a half-slice of cheese on the bottom half of each tortilla. Divide bean mixture between the bottom halves of tortillas. Tightly wrap up each tortilla and place in the baking pan, seam side down.

Top with sauce and bake until hot, 10 to 12 minutes.

Sprinkle with shredded cheese and bake until cheese has melted, about 2 minutes. Mmmm!

MAKES 2 SERVINGS

PIZZA-LADAS

154 calories PER SERVING

You'll Need: 8-inch by 8-inch baking pan, nonstick spray, blender or food processor (optional), skillet, medium bowl, microwave-safe plate
Prep: 10 minutes
Cook: 20 minutes

½ of recipe (1 enchilada): 154 calories, 4g fat, 493mg sodium, 21.5g carbs, 3g fiber, 6g sugars, 8g protein

INGREDIENTS

1 stick light string cheese
½ cup diced bell pepper
½ cup diced onion
6 slices turkey pepperoni, chopped
¼ cup plus 2 tablespoons pizza sauce
Two 6-inch corn tortillas
2 teaspoons reduced-fat Parmesan-style grated topping

Optional topping: red pepper flakes

DIRECTIONS

Preheat oven to 400 degrees. Spray an 8-inch by 8-inch baking pan with nonstick spray.

Break string cheese into thirds and place in a blender or food processor—blend at high speed until shredded. (Or tear into shreds and roughly chop.)

Bring a skillet sprayed with nonstick spray to medium-high heat. Cook and stir bell pepper and onion until softened and slightly browned, about 5 minutes.

Transfer veggies to a medium bowl and mix in shredded string cheese, chopped pepperoni, and 2 tablespoons sauce.

Microwave tortillas on a microwave-safe plate for 15 seconds, or until warm.

Evenly distribute veggie-cheese mixture between tortillas. Tightly wrap up each tortilla and place in the baking pan, seam side down.

Top with remaining ¼ cup pizza sauce. Bake until hot, about 10 minutes. Sprinkle with Parm-style topping and enjoy!

MAKES 2 SERVINGS

SPINACH ENCHILADAS

197 calories PER SERVING

You'll Need: 8-inch by 8-inch baking pan, nonstick spray, small bowl, large bowl, microwave-safe plate
Prep: 10 minutes
Cook: 15 minutes

¼th of recipe (1 enchilada): 197 calories, 5.5g fat, 735mg sodium, 24g carbs, 2.5g fiber, 4g sugars, 9.5g protein

INGREDIENTS

2 wedges The Laughing Cow Light
    Creamy Swiss cheese
⅓ cup fat-free sour cream
1 tablespoon reduced-fat Parmesan-style
    grated topping
¼ teaspoon garlic powder
¼ teaspoon onion powder
⅛ teaspoon cayenne pepper
⅛ teaspoon each salt and black pepper
One 10-ounce package frozen chopped
    spinach, thawed and squeezed dry
4 medium-large corn tortillas
¾ cup green enchilada sauce
½ cup shredded reduced-fat
    Mexican-blend cheese

DIRECTIONS

Preheat oven to 400 degrees. Spray an 8-inch by 8-inch baking pan with nonstick spray.

In a small bowl, stir cheese wedges until smooth. Stir in sour cream, Parm-style topping, and spices.

In a large bowl, thoroughly mix spinach with cheese mixture.

Microwave tortillas on a microwave-safe plate for 15 seconds, or until warm.

Lay tortillas flat and evenly distribute spinach mixture among the bottom halves. Tightly wrap up each tortilla and place in the baking pan, seam side down.

Top with sauce and bake until hot, 10 to 12 minutes.

Sprinkle with shredded cheese and bake until cheese has melted, about 2 minutes. Mmmmm!

MAKES 4 SERVINGS

SURPRISE, IT'S PUMPKIN! ENCHILADAS

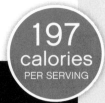

188 calories PER SERVING

You'll Need: 8-inch by 8-inch baking pan, nonstick spray, skillet, medium bowl, microwave-safe plate
Prep: 10 minutes
Cook: 20 minutes

½ of recipe (1 enchilada): 188 calories, 2g fat, 948mg sodium, 31g carbs, 5g fiber, 8g sugars, 10.5g protein

INGREDIENTS

⅓ cup chopped onion
⅔ cup canned pure pumpkin
1 ½ tablespoons taco sauce
1 teaspoon taco seasoning mix
2 medium-large corn tortillas
¾ cup red enchilada sauce
1 slice fat-free cheddar cheese, halved
¼ cup shredded fat-free cheddar cheese

Optional seasonings: salt and black pepper
Optional toppings: fat-free sour cream,
    chopped scallions

DIRECTIONS

Preheat oven to 400 degrees. Spray an 8-inch by 8-inch baking pan with nonstick spray.

Bring a skillet sprayed with nonstick spray to medium-high heat. Cook and stir onion until slightly browned, about 2 minutes.

Transfer onion to a medium bowl. Add pumpkin, taco sauce, and taco seasoning, and mix well.

Microwave tortillas on a microwave-safe plate for 15 seconds, or until warm.

Lay tortillas flat. Spread 2 tablespoons enchilada sauce onto the bottom half of each tortilla, and top each with a half-slice of cheese.

Divide the pumpkin mixture between the bottom halves of the tortillas. Tightly wrap up each tortilla and place in the baking pan, seam side down.

Top with remaining ½ cup enchilada sauce. Bake until hot, 10 to 12 minutes.

Sprinkle with cheese and bake until cheese has melted, about 2 minutes. Enjoy!

MAKES 2 SERVINGS

EXPLODING CHICKEN TAQUITOS

197 calories
PER SERVING

You'll Need: baking sheet, nonstick spray, medium bowl, toothpicks (optional)
Prep: 10 minutes | **Chill:** 15 minutes | **Cook:** 20 minutes

¼th of recipe (2 taquitos):
197 calories, 2.5g fat, 594mg sodium, 22.5g carbs, 3g fiber, 2g sugars, 20.5g protein

INGREDIENTS

10 ounces canned 98% fat-free chunk white
    chicken breast in water, drained and flaked

½ cup salsa

⅓ cup shredded fat-free cheddar cheese

¼ teaspoon taco seasoning mix

Eight 6-inch corn tortillas

Optional dips: red enchilada sauce,
    additional salsa, fat-free sour cream

DIRECTIONS

Preheat oven to 375 degrees. Spray a baking sheet with nonstick spray.

In a medium bowl, mix chicken with salsa. Cover and refrigerate for 15 minutes.

Drain any excess liquid from the chilled chicken mixture. Stir in cheese and taco seasoning.

Place tortillas between 2 damp paper towels. Microwave for 1 minute, or until warm and pliable.

One at a time, spread each tortilla with ⅛th of chicken mixture, about 2 tablespoons; tightly roll up into a tube, place on the baking sheet, seam side down, and secure with toothpicks if needed.

Bake until crispy, 14 to 16 minutes. (Don't worry if they crack and "explode" a little!) Eat up!

MAKES 4 SERVINGS

Flip to the photo inserts to see over 100 recipe pics! And for photos of ALL the recipes, go to hungry-girl.com/books.

BUFFALO CHICKEN TAQUITOS

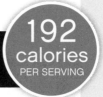

192 calories PER SERVING

You'll Need: baking sheet, nonstick spray, blender or food processor (optional), medium bowl, toothpicks (optional)
Prep: 10 minutes | **Cook:** 20 minutes

⅕th of recipe (2 taquitos):
192 calories, 4g fat, 731mg sodium, 21g carbs, 2g fiber, 1.5g sugars, 16g protein

INGREDIENTS

1 stick light string cheese

3 wedges The Laughing Cow Light Creamy Swiss cheese

3 tablespoons Frank's RedHot Original Cayenne Pepper Sauce

10 ounces canned 98% fat-free chunk white chicken breast in water, drained and flaked

Ten 6-inch corn tortillas

Optional dip: fat-free ranch dressing

DIRECTIONS

Preheat the oven to 375 degrees. Spray a baking sheet with nonstick spray.

Break string cheese into thirds and place in a blender or food processor; blend at high speed until shredded. (Or pull into shreds and roughly chop.)

In a medium bowl, mix cheese wedges with hot sauce until mostly smooth and uniform. Stir in chicken and shredded string cheese.

Place tortillas between 2 damp paper towels. Microwave for 1 minute, or until warm and pliable.

One at a time, spread each tortilla with ⅒th of chicken mixture, about 2 tablespoons; tightly roll up into a tube, place on the baking sheet, seam side down, and secure with toothpicks if needed.

Bake until crispy, 14 to 16 minutes. (Don't worry if they crack and "explode" a little!) Enjoy!

MAKES 5 SERVINGS

HG ALTERNATIVE!

If you're not into canned chicken, use 1½ cups of cooked and shredded skinless chicken breast instead. (But honestly, canned chicken rocks in these recipes.)

JALAPEÑO CHEESE TAQUITOS

200 calories PER SERVING

You'll Need: baking sheet, nonstick spray, medium bowl, toothpicks (optional)
Prep: 10 minutes
Cook: 20 minutes

¼th of recipe (2 taquitos): 200 calories, 7g fat, 474mg sodium, 22.5g carbs, 2.5g fiber, 2g sugars, 10g protein

INGREDIENTS

4 wedges The Laughing Cow Light Creamy Swiss cheese
¾ cup shredded part-skim mozzarella cheese
24 jarred jalapeño slices, drained, roughly chopped (about ¼ cup)
Eight 6-inch corn tortillas
Optional dip: fat-free ranch dressing

DIRECTIONS

Preheat the oven to 375 degrees. Spray a baking sheet with nonstick spray.

In a medium bowl, mix cheese wedges until smooth. Stir in mozzarella cheese and chopped jalapeños.

Place tortillas between 2 damp paper towels. Microwave for 1 minute, or until warm and pliable.

One at a time, spread each tortilla with ⅛th of cheese mixture, about 1½ tablespoons; tightly roll up into a tube, place on the baking sheet, seam side down, and secure with toothpicks if needed.

Bake until crispy, 14 to 16 minutes. (Don't worry if they crack and "explode" a little!) Enjoy!

MAKES 4 SERVINGS

'BELLA ASADA FAJITAS

275 calories PER SERVING

You'll Need: large skillet, small bowl, microwave-safe plate
Prep: 10 minutes
Cook: 10 minutes

½ of recipe (3 fajitas): 275 calories, 8g fat, 312mg sodium, 47g carbs, 8.5g fiber, 7.5g sugars, 7g protein

INGREDIENTS

1 teaspoon olive oil
2 large portabella mushroom caps, sliced
¾ cup sliced bell pepper
¾ cup sliced onion
¼ teaspoon garlic powder
¼ teaspoon salt
⅛ teaspoon chili powder, or more to taste
⅛ teaspoon ground cumin
Dash black pepper
½ cup chopped tomatoes
2 ounces (about ¼ cup) roughly mashed avocado
2 tablespoons chopped fresh cilantro
½ tablespoon lime juice
Six 6-inch corn tortillas

DIRECTIONS

Drizzle a large skillet with oil and bring to medium-high heat. Add mushrooms, bell pepper, and onion, and sprinkle with garlic powder, ⅛ teaspoon salt, chili powder, cumin, and black pepper. Cook and stir until veggies are tender, about 6 minutes.

In a small bowl, mix tomatoes, avocado, cilantro, lime juice, and remaining ⅛ teaspoon salt.

Microwave tortillas on a microwave-safe plate for 15 seconds, or until warm.

Top each tortilla with about ½ cup fajita veggies and a spoonful of the tomato-avocado mixture. Fold and chew!

MAKES 2 SERVINGS

CHAPTER 12

BURGERS & FRIES

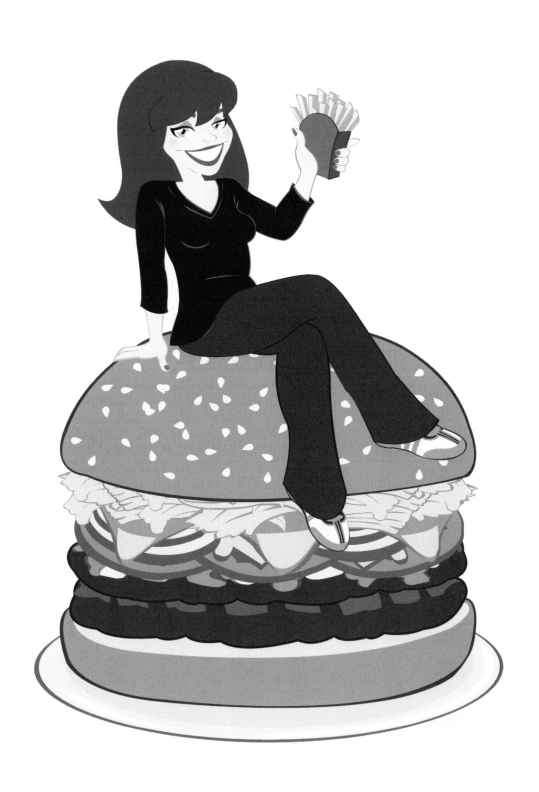

BURGERS & FRIES

BURGERS

Big Bopper Burger Stopper
A+ Avocado Burger
No-Buns-About-It
   Animal-Style Cheeseburger
Cobb Burger
Island Insanity Burger
Schmancy Steak-Style Burger
Philly-licious Cheesesteak Burger
Chili-rific Cheeseburger
Breakfast Burger
Spinach Arti-Cheeseburger
Chief of Beef Cheeseburger
Portabella Guac Burger
Hungry Mac 'Bella Stack Burger
HG's 100-Calorie Beef Patties
Spicy Cheese-Stuffed Burger Patties
Bacon Cheeseburger Patty
Outside-In Cheeseburger Patty
OMG! Onion Mushroom Goodness Burgers
Thanksgiving Burgers
Mamma Mia! Patties
Pizza Burgers a la HG
Tremendous Top-Shelf Turkey Burger
Red Hot & Blue Burger
Unique Greek Turkey Burgers
Cheesed-Up Taco Turkey Burgers
Philly Burgers
Bean 'n Veggie PattyCakes
Oatstanding Veggie Patties

FRIES

Bake-tastic Butternut Squash Fries
Mexican Butternut Fries
Ranch 'n Bacon Butternut Fries
Hungry Girlfredo Butternut Fries
Sweet Garlic Butternut Fries
Totally Turnip Fries
Turnip the Disco Fries
Bacon 'n Cheese Turnip Fries
Cheesy Beefy Turnip Fries
Grin 'n Carrot Fries & Dip

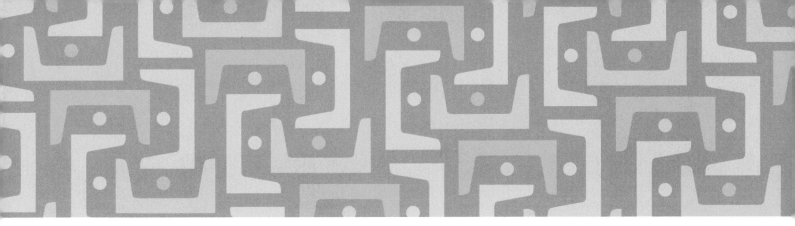

When you think of fast food, you probably think of burgers and fries. You probably also think of food that's off-limits due to sky-high stats. This section is packed with so many delicious fast-food swaps that you just might cry. Grab a tissue (and a fork!) . . .

A QUICK GUIDE TO SYMBOLS:

15 Minutes or Less

This symbol lets you know a recipe should take you no more than fifteen minutes from start to finish! That includes prep and cook time.

30 Minutes or Less

Just like the 15-minute version, this one points out recipes that take 30 minutes or less to whip up.

Meatless

You guessed it—no meat here! That includes beef, poultry, and fish. Some recipes give the option of a meatless ingredient. If you want your meal without meat, go with the meatless choice.

Single Serving

Pretty straightforward. These are recipes for one.

5 Ingredients or Less

Fans of HG know that we like to keep things simple. And these recipes contain just five ingredients or less!

Photos

These recipes can be seen in one of the book's photo inserts. The number in the symbol tells you which insert. Find photos of all the recipes at hungry-girl.com/books!

BURGERS

Everyone loves a burger every so often. This chapter gives a bazillion options for indulging in one of America's most beloved foods . . .

SOY-BURGER SWAPPIN'!

The next ten recipes call for 100-calorie hamburger-style meatless patties. Our favorites, Boca Original Vegan Meatless Burgers, have only 70 calories and 1 gram of fat. If you use Boca, feel free to slash 30 calories and 2 grams of fat from the recipe stats.

PREFER BEEF?

Just use one of our 100-Calorie Beef Patties . . . Recipe on page 280!

CAN'T FIND 100-CALORIE FLAT SANDWICH BUNS?

Go for the lowest-calorie hamburger buns you can find, preferably with some fiber. Just adjust the stats accordingly. Flip to the Recommended Products on page 5 for our bun picks!

BIG BOPPER BURGER STOPPER

228 calories

You'll Need: skillet, nonstick spray
Prep: 5 minutes
Cook: 10 minutes

Entire recipe: 228 calories, 4g fat, 860mg sodium, 35g carbs, 9.5g fiber, 6.5g sugars, 16g protein

INGREDIENTS

1 frozen meatless hamburger-style patty with 100 calories or less
One 100-calorie flat sandwich bun
1 slice tomato
1 slice onion
½ leaf romaine lettuce
3 hamburger dill pickle chips
1 teaspoon fat-free mayonnaise
1 teaspoon ketchup

DIRECTIONS

Bring a skillet sprayed with nonstick spray to medium heat. Cook patty for 4 minutes per side, or until cooked through.

Split bun into halves and place patty on the bottom half. Top with tomato, onion, lettuce, and pickle chips.

Spread the top of the bun with mayo and ketchup, and place it on top of the stack!

MAKES 1 SERVING

HG ALTERNATIVE!

Love cheese? Slap a slice of fat-free American on the bottom half of your bun. The cheesed-up version has just 253 calories!

A+ AVOCADO BURGER

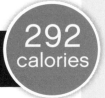
292
calories

You'll Need: skillet, nonstick spray | **Prep:** 5 minutes | **Cook:** 10 minutes

Entire recipe:
292 calories, 9.5g fat, 728mg sodium, 33.5g carbs, 11g fiber, 5g sugars, 19g protein

INGREDIENTS

One 100-calorie flat sandwich bun
1 wedge The Laughing Cow Light
    Creamy Swiss cheese
¼ cup shredded lettuce
1 slice tomato
1 slice red onion
1 frozen meatless hamburger-style patty
    with 100 calories or less
1 ounce sliced avocado (about ¼ avocado)

Optional toppings: yellow mustard, ketchup

DIRECTIONS

Split bun into halves and lightly toast. Spread bottom half with cheese and top with lettuce, tomato, and red onion.

Bring a skillet sprayed with nonstick spray to medium heat. Cook patty for 4 minutes per side, or until cooked through.

Place patty over the onion on the bun. Top with avocado and the top of the bun and enjoy!

MAKES 1 SERVING

NO-BUNS-ABOUT-IT ANIMAL-STYLE CHEESEBURGER

188
calories

You'll Need: plate, skillet, nonstick spray | **Prep:** 5 minutes | **Cook:** 10 minutes

Entire recipe:
188 calories, 3g fat, 862mg sodium, 23g carbs, 5g fiber, 9g sugars, 16g protein

INGREDIENTS

1 extra-large leaf iceberg or butter lettuce
1 frozen meatless hamburger-style patty with
    100 calories or less
1 teaspoon yellow mustard
⅓ cup chopped onion
1 slice fat-free cheddar cheese
1½ tablespoons fat-free Thousand Island dressing

Optional topping: hamburger dill pickle chips

DIRECTIONS

Place lettuce on a plate.

Bring a skillet sprayed with nonstick spray to medium heat. Cook patty for 4 minutes.

Flip patty and spread with mustard. Add onion to the skillet. Stirring onion occasionally, cook for 4 more minutes, or until patty is cooked through and onion is soft.

Top patty with cheese and cook until melted, about 45 seconds.

Place patty on the lettuce, and top with onion and dressing. Wrap lettuce up and around your burger and chew!

MAKES 1 SERVING

COBB BURGER

307 calories

You'll Need: skillet with a lid, nonstick spray | **Prep:** 5 minutes | **Cook:** 10 minutes

Entire recipe:
307 calories, 11.5g fat, 890mg sodium, 31.5g carbs, 10g fiber, 3.5g sugars, 22g protein

INGREDIENTS

One 100-calorie flat sandwich bun
½ leaf romaine lettuce
1 slice tomato
1 frozen meatless hamburger-style patty with 100 calories or less
2 tablespoons blue cheese crumbles
1 tablespoon precooked real crumbled bacon
½ ounce (about 1 tablespoon) diced avocado

DIRECTIONS

Split bun into halves. Top the bottom half with lettuce and tomato.

Bring a skillet sprayed with nonstick spray to medium heat. Cook patty for 4 minutes.

Flip patty and top with blue cheese and bacon. Cover and cook for 4 more minutes, or until patty is cooked through and toppings are hot.

Place loaded patty over the tomato on the bun. Top with avocado and the top of the bun. Dig in!

MAKES 1 SERVING

ISLAND INSANITY BURGER

264 calories

You'll Need: grill pan (or skillet), nonstick spray | **Prep:** 5 minutes | **Cook:** 15 minutes

Entire recipe:
264 calories, 4g fat, 976mg sodium, 44g carbs, 10g fiber, 14.5g sugars, 16.5g protein

INGREDIENTS

1 slice pineapple (fresh or packed in juice)
1 frozen meatless hamburger-style patty with 100 calories or less
One 100-calorie flat sandwich bun
1 tablespoon thick teriyaki marinade or sauce
2 thick slices tomato
1 lettuce leaf
½ tablespoon fat-free mayonnaise

DIRECTIONS

Bring a grill pan (or skillet) sprayed with nonstick spray to medium-high heat. Cook pineapple until slightly blackened and caramelized, about 3 minutes per side.

Remove pineapple and reduce heat to medium. Cook patty for 4 minutes per side, or until cooked through.

Split bun into halves and place the patty on the bottom half. Top with teriyaki marinade/sauce, pineapple, tomato, and lettuce. Spread the top half of the bun with mayo and finish off your burger with it. Now CHOMP!

MAKES 1 SERVING

HG ALTERNATIVE!

Top your patty with a slice of fat-free cheddar while it's still in the pan, and cook until melted, about 45 seconds. Your cheeseburger will have 290 calories.

SCHMANCY STEAK-STYLE BURGER

285 calories

You'll Need: skillet, nonstick spray
Prep: 5 minutes
Cook: 10 minutes

Entire recipe: 285 calories, 8g fat, 832mg sodium, 36g carbs, 10g fiber, 6.5g sugars, 19.5g protein

INGREDIENTS

One 100-calorie flat sandwich bun
½ leaf romaine lettuce
1 slice tomato
1 frozen meatless hamburger-style patty with 100 calories or less
One ½-inch-thick onion slice, rings intact
½ tablespoon steak sauce
2 tablespoons crumbled blue cheese

DIRECTIONS

Split bun into halves. Top the bottom half with lettuce and tomato.

Bring a skillet sprayed with nonstick spray to medium heat. Cook the patty and onion for 4 minutes.

Flip patty and onion. Cook for 4 minutes, or until patty is cooked through and onion is lightly browned.

Place patty over the tomato on the bun. Top with onion, steak sauce, blue cheese, and the top of the bun!

MAKES 1 SERVING

PHILLY-LICIOUS CHEESESTEAK BURGER

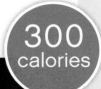

300 calories

You'll Need: large skillet (or grill pan), nonstick spray, small microwave-safe bowl
Prep: 5 minutes
Cook: 15 minutes

Entire recipe: 300 calories, 8.5g fat, 794mg sodium, 37g carbs, 9.5g fiber, 7.5g sugars, 21.5g protein

INGREDIENTS

One 100-calorie flat sandwich bun
⅓ cup sliced onion
⅓ cup sliced bell pepper
¼ cup sliced mushrooms
1 teaspoon olive oil
⅛ teaspoon black pepper, or more to taste
1 frozen meatless hamburger-style patty with 100 calories or less
2 teaspoons fat-free sour cream
1 slice fat-free American cheese

DIRECTIONS

Split bun into halves and lightly toast.

Bring a large skillet (or grill pan) sprayed with nonstick spray to medium-high heat. Add veggies, drizzle with oil, and sprinkle with black pepper. Cook and stir until slightly softened, about 3 minutes.

Reduce heat to medium. Move veggies to the sides of the skillet and place patty in the center. Stirring veggies occasionally, cook for 4 minutes.

Flip patty and, continuing to stir veggies, cook for 4 minutes, or until patty is cooked through and veggies are soft.

Place patty on the bottom half of the bun and top with veggies.

In a small microwave-safe bowl, mix sour cream with cheese, breaking cheese into small pieces as you add it. Microwave for 15 seconds, or until hot. Stir thoroughly. Microwave for another 10 seconds, or until cheese has fully melted. Mix well and spoon over veggies.

Finish off your burger with the top half of the bun. Now enjoy!

MAKES 1 SERVING

CHILI-RIFIC CHEESEBURGER

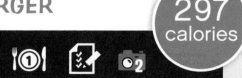

270 calories

You'll Need: skillet, nonstick spray, small microwave-safe bowl
Prep: 5 minutes
Cook: 10 minutes

Entire recipe: 270 calories, 4.5g fat, 973mg sodium, 38g carbs, 10.5g fiber, 6.5g sugars, 22.5g protein

INGREDIENTS

One 100-calorie flat sandwich bun
2 slices tomato
1 slice onion
1 frozen meatless hamburger-style patty with 100 calories or less
2 tablespoons low-fat veggie chili
1 slice fat-free American cheese
1 teaspoon yellow mustard
Optional topping: hamburger dill pickle chips

DIRECTIONS

Split bun in half and lightly toast. Top the bottom half with tomato and onion.

Bring a skillet sprayed with nonstick spray to medium heat. Cook patty for 4 minutes per side, or until cooked through. Place patty over onion on the bun.

In a small microwave-safe bowl, microwave chili for 45 seconds, or until hot.

Top patty with chili and cheese. Slap mustard onto the top half of the bun, and plop the bun top over the cheese. Now, the most important step of all . . .

Enjoy!

MAKES 1 SERVING

BREAKFAST BURGER

297 calories

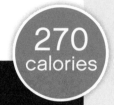

You'll Need: skillet, nonstick spray
Prep: 5 minutes
Cook: 10 minutes

Entire recipe: 297 calories, 10g fat, 773mg sodium, 29g carbs, 8.5g fiber, 3g sugars, 24.5g protein

INGREDIENTS

1 frozen meatless hamburger-style patty with 100 calories or less
One 100-calorie flat sandwich bun
1 large egg
1 tablespoon precooked real crumbled bacon
Optional seasonings: salt and black pepper

DIRECTIONS

Bring a skillet sprayed with nonstick spray to medium heat. Cook patty for 4 minutes per side, or until cooked through.

Split bun into halves and place patty on the bottom half.

If needed, clean skillet. Remove from heat, re-spray, and return to medium heat. Add egg and cook per your preference (we like it over medium), about 2 minutes.

Place egg over the patty on the bun. Sprinkle with bacon, and finish with the top of the bun!

MAKES 1 SERVING

SPINACH ARTI-CHEESEBURGER

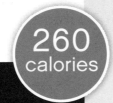
260 calories

You'll Need: skillet, nonstick spray, bowl
Prep: 5 minutes
Cook: 15 minutes

Entire recipe: 260 calories, 5g fat, 910mg sodium, 37g carbs, 12g fiber, 3.5g sugars, 19.5g protein

INGREDIENTS

⅓ cup chopped mushrooms
1 cup roughly chopped spinach leaves
1 artichoke heart packed in water, chopped
⅛ teaspoon garlic powder
⅛ teaspoon black pepper
1 wedge The Laughing Cow Light Creamy Swiss cheese
1 light English muffin
1 frozen meatless hamburger-style patty
    with 100 calories or less

DIRECTIONS

Bring a skillet sprayed with nonstick spray to medium-high heat. Cook and stir mushrooms until softened, about 5 minutes. Add spinach and cook and stir until wilted, about 1 minute.

Transfer mushroom-spinach mixture to a bowl, and pat dry. Add chopped artichoke heart, garlic powder, pepper, and cheese wedge, breaking the wedge into pieces. Thoroughly mix.

Split English muffin in half and lightly toast. Spread both halves with spinach-artichoke mixture.

Re-spray skillet and bring to medium heat. Cook patty for 4 minutes per side, or until cooked through.

Place patty on one muffin half and top with the other half. Eat up!

MAKES 1 SERVING

CHIEF OF BEEF CHEESEBURGER

289 calories

You'll Need: medium bowl, grill pan (or skillet), nonstick spray
Prep: 5 minutes
Cook: 10 minutes

Entire recipe: 289 calories, 6g fat, 724mg sodium, 26g carbs, 5.5g fiber, 4.5g sugars, 34.5g protein

INGREDIENTS

One 100-calorie flat sandwich bun
½ lettuce leaf
1 slice tomato
4 ounces raw extra-lean ground beef
1 tablespoon liquid egg whites (about half a large egg white)
Dash each salt and black pepper
Dash garlic powder
Dash onion powder
1 slice fat-free cheddar or American cheese
1 thin slice onion

Optional toppings: mustard, fat-free mayonnaise, ketchup, hamburger dill pickle chips

DIRECTIONS

Split bun into halves, and top the bottom half with lettuce and tomato.

In a medium bowl, thoroughly mix beef, egg whites, and seasonings. Evenly form into a patty about 4 inches wide.

Bring a grill pan (or skillet) sprayed with nonstick spray to medium-high heat. Cook patty for 3 to 4 minutes per side, or until cooked to your preference.

Top patty with cheese and cook until melted, about 45 seconds.

Transfer cheese-topped patty to the bottom half of the bun. Top with onion and the top half of the bun!

MAKES 1 SERVING

PORTABELLA MUSHROOM CAPS make GREAT burger swaps.

Don't believe it? Try these recipes, then get back to us. We'll wait . . .

PORTABELLA GUAC BURGER

216 calories

You'll Need: small bowl, skillet, microwave-safe plate (optional), nonstick spray
Prep: 5 minutes | **Cook:** 15 minutes

Entire recipe:
216 calories, 8g fat, 628mg sodium, 33g carbs, 8.5g fiber, 6.5g sugars, 10g protein

INGREDIENTS

One 100-calorie flat sandwich bun
½ leaf romaine lettuce
1 slice tomato
1 thin slice onion
1 ounce (about 2 tablespoons) mashed avocado
Dash each salt and black pepper, or more to taste
2 tablespoons pico de gallo (or chunky salsa)
1 slice center-cut bacon or turkey bacon
1 portabella mushroom cap

DIRECTIONS

Split bun into halves. Top the bottom half with lettuce, tomato, and onion.

To make the guacamole, in a small bowl, mix avocado, salt, and pepper. Stir in pico de gallo.

Cook bacon until crispy, either in a skillet over medium heat or on a microwave-safe plate in the microwave. (See package for cook time.)

Bring a skillet sprayed with nonstick spray to medium-high heat. Place mushroom cap in the skillet, rounded side down. Cover and cook until soft, about 4 minutes per side.

Place mushroom cap over onion on the bun. Break bacon in half and place over the mushroom cap. Top with guacamole and the top of the bun. Enjoy!

MAKES 1 SERVING

Flip to the photo inserts to see over 100 recipe pics! And for photos of ALL the recipes, go to hungry-girl.com/books.

HUNGRY MAC 'BELLA STACK BURGER

234 calories

You'll Need: small bowl, large skillet with lid, nonstick spray | **Prep:** 5 minutes | **Cook:** 10 minutes

Entire recipe:
234 calories, 2g fat, 946mg sodium, 45g carbs, 9.5g fiber, 12g sugars, 14.5g protein

INGREDIENTS

Sauce
1½ tablespoons fat-free Thousand Island dressing
1 teaspoon finely minced onion *or* ½ teaspoon dried minced onion
⅛ teaspoon granulated white sugar or Splenda No Calorie Sweetener (granulated)
⅛ teaspoon white wine vinegar

Sandwich
2 portabella mushroom caps
1½ small light hamburger buns (1 top and 2 bottoms)
¼ cup shredded lettuce
1 slice fat-free American cheese
1 tablespoon diced onion
3 hamburger dill pickle chips

DIRECTIONS

In a small bowl, thoroughly mix sauce ingredients.

Bring a large skillet sprayed with nonstick spray to medium-high heat. Place mushroom caps in the skillet, rounded sides down. Cover and cook until soft, about 4 minutes per side.

Spread one bottom bun with half of the sauce. Top with 2 tablespoons lettuce. Top with cheese and 1 mushroom cap, and sprinkle with ½ tablespoon diced onion.

Spread remaining half of the sauce on the other bun bottom, and place it on the sandwich, sauce side up. Top with pickle chips and remaining 2 tablespoons lettuce. Top with the remaining mushroom cap and remaining ½ tablespoon onion.

Add the bun top and open wide!

MAKES 1 SERVING

HG ALTERNATIVE!

Feel free to use 1 bun as opposed to 1½—just spread the 2nd half of the sauce on top of the 1st cooked mushroom (instead of the middle bun piece). Then your burger will have 194 calories, 1.5g fat, 854mg sodium, 38g carbs, 7.5g fiber, 12g sugars, and 12.5g protein.

HG'S 100-CALORIE BEEF PATTIES

103 calories PER SERVING

You'll Need: large bowl, grill pan (or large skillet), nonstick spray
Prep: 10 minutes
Cook: 20 minutes

⅙th of recipe (1 patty): 103 calories, 3g fat, 258mg sodium, <0.5g carbs, 0g fiber, <0.5g sugars, 16.5g protein

INGREDIENTS

1 pound raw extra-lean ground beef
¼ cup liquid egg whites (about 2 egg whites)
½ teaspoon each salt and black pepper
¼ teaspoon garlic powder
¼ teaspoon onion powder

DIRECTIONS

In a large bowl, thoroughly mix all ingredients. Evenly form into 6 patties, each about 3½ inches wide.

Bring a grill pan (or large skillet) sprayed with nonstick spray to medium-high heat. Cook patties for 4 minutes per side, or until cooked to your preference, working in batches as needed. Enjoy!

MAKES 6 SERVINGS

HG ALTERNATIVE!

These patties are the perfect size for HG recipes that call for hamburger-style meatless patties. Wanna SUPER-SIZE your patties? Make 4 instead of 6, and cook them for a few minutes longer. Each super-sized patty will have 150 calories and 5 grams of fat. Impressive!

SPICY CHEESE-STUFFED BURGER PATTIES

187 calories PER SERVING

You'll Need: medium bowl, large bowl, grill pan (or large skillet), nonstick spray
Prep: 15 minutes
Cook: 20 minutes

¼th of recipe (1 patty): 187 calories, 6g fat, 579mg sodium, 2.5g carbs, <0.5g fiber, 1g sugars, 25.5g protein

INGREDIENTS

4 wedges The Laughing Cow Light Creamy Swiss cheese
¼ cup jarred sliced jalapeño peppers, drained, patted dry, chopped
1 pound raw extra-lean ground beef
1 teaspoon Frank's RedHot Original Cayenne Pepper Sauce
½ teaspoon ground cumin
½ teaspoon garlic powder
½ teaspoon onion powder
¼ teaspoon each salt and black pepper

DIRECTIONS

In a medium bowl, thoroughly mix cheese wedges with chopped jalapeño peppers.

In a large bowl, thoroughly mix all other ingredients. Form a ball with ¼th of the mixture, and make a large hollow indentation with your thumb (past the center but not all the way through). Fill the hole with ¼th of cheese mixture and squeeze meat to seal, enclosing cheese. Flatten slightly into a thick patty. Repeat to make 3 more patties.

Bring a grill pan (or large skillet) sprayed with nonstick spray to medium-high heat. Cook patties for 4 to 8 minutes per side, until cooked to your preference. Enjoy!

MAKES 4 SERVINGS

BACON CHEESEBURGER PATTY

205 calories

You'll Need: grill pan (or skillet), nonstick spray
Prep: 5 minutes
Cook: 20 minutes

Entire recipe: 205 calories, 7.75g fat, 650mg sodium, 1g carbs, 0g fiber, 1g sugars, 28.5g protein

INGREDIENTS

4 ounces raw extra-lean ground beef
Dash each salt and black pepper
1 tablespoon precooked real crumbled bacon
1 wedge The Laughing Cow Light
    Creamy Swiss cheese

DIRECTIONS

Season beef with salt and pepper. Add bacon and knead to evenly distribute. Form into a ball, and make a large hollow indentation with your thumb (past the center but not all the way through).

Fill the hole with cheese and squeeze meat to seal, enclosing cheese. Flatten slightly into a thick patty.

Bring a grill pan (or skillet) sprayed with nonstick spray to medium-high heat. Cook patty for 4 to 8 minutes per side, until cooked to your preference. Enjoy!

MAKES 1 SERVING

OUTSIDE-IN CHEESEBURGER PATTY

179 calories

You'll Need: medium bowl, grill pan (or skillet), nonstick spray
Prep: 5 minutes
Cook: 20 minutes

Entire recipe: 179 calories, 6g fat, 452mg sodium, 1.5g carbs, 0g fiber, 1g sugars, 26g protein

INGREDIENTS

4 ounces raw extra-lean ground beef
⅛ teaspoon Worcestershire sauce
⅛ teaspoon garlic powder
⅛ teaspoon onion powder
Dash each salt and black pepper
1 wedge The Laughing Cow Light Creamy Swiss cheese

DIRECTIONS

In a medium bowl, thoroughly mix all ingredients *except* cheese.

Form into a ball, and make a large hollow indentation with your thumb (past the center but not all the way through).

Fill the hole with cheese and squeeze meat to seal, enclosing cheese. Flatten slightly into a thick patty.

Bring a grill pan (or skillet) sprayed with nonstick spray to medium-high heat. Cook patty for 4 to 8 minutes per side, until cooked to your preference. Enjoy!

MAKES 1 SERVING

STUFFED BURGER HEADS-UP:

Don't press on the patty with your spatula . . . your burger might ooze cheese—and flavor. Pressing patties is a bad idea in general . . .

OMG! ONION MUSHROOM GOODNESS BURGERS

185 calories PER SERVING

You'll Need: large skillet, nonstick spray, large bowl, grill pan (optional) | **Prep:** 10 minutes | **Cook:** 15 minutes

⅕th of recipe (1 patty):
185 calories, 8.25g fat, 535mg sodium, 4.5g carbs, 0.75g fiber, 1.5g sugars, 23.5g protein

INGREDIENTS

2 cups chopped mushrooms
1¼ pounds raw lean ground turkey
One 1-ounce packet onion soup/dip
    seasoning mix

DIRECTIONS

Bring a large skillet sprayed with nonstick spray to medium-high heat. Cook and stir mushrooms until softened, about 5 minutes.

Transfer mushrooms to a large bowl. Add turkey and sprinkle with onion soup/dip mix. Thoroughly mix. Evenly form into 5 patties.

Bring a grill pan (or large skillet) sprayed with nonstick spray to medium-high heat. Cook patties for 5 minutes per side, or until cooked through. Enjoy!

MAKES 5 SERVINGS

THANKSGIVING BURGERS

206 calories PER SERVING

You'll Need: large bowl, grill pan (or large skillet), nonstick spray | **Prep:** 10 minutes | **Cook:** 10 minutes

⅕th of recipe (1 patty):
206 calories, 8g fat, 322mg sodium, 11g carbs, 0.5g fiber, 7g sugars, 23g protein

INGREDIENTS

1¼ pounds raw lean ground turkey
3 tablespoons dried minced onion
1½ tablespoons (about ¼th of a 1-ounce packet)
    dry turkey or chicken gravy mix
¼ teaspoon ground dried sage
¼ teaspoon each salt and black pepper
⅓ cup sweetened dried cranberries, chopped

DIRECTIONS

In a large bowl, thoroughly mix all ingredients *except* cranberries. Mix in chopped cranberries, making sure they don't stick together. Evenly form into 5 patties.

Bring a grill pan (or large skillet) sprayed with nonstick spray to medium-high heat. Cook patties for 5 minutes per side, or until cooked through. Enjoy!

MAKES 5 SERVINGS

MAMMA MIA! PATTIES

168 calories
PER SERVING

You'll Need: large bowl, grill pan (or large skillet), nonstick spray
Prep: 10 minutes
Cook: 20 minutes

¼th of recipe (1 patty): 168 calories, 4.5g fat, 230mg sodium, 4.5g carbs, 1g fiber, 2.5g sugars, 24.5g protein

INGREDIENTS

1 pound raw extra-lean ground beef
¼ cup bagged sun-dried tomatoes (not packed in oil), finely chopped
1 teaspoon garlic powder
½ teaspoon onion powder
½ teaspoon Italian seasoning
¼ teaspoon each salt and black pepper

DIRECTIONS

In a large bowl, thoroughly mix all ingredients. Evenly form into 4 patties.

Bring a grill pan (or large skillet) sprayed with nonstick spray to medium-high heat. Cook patties for 4 to 8 minutes per side, until cooked to your preference. Enjoy!

MAKES 4 SERVINGS

PIZZA BURGERS A LA HG

223 calories
PER SERVING

You'll Need: blender or food processor (optional), large skillet, nonstick spray, large bowl, grill pan (optional)
Prep: 10 minutes
Cook: 25 minutes

¼th of recipe (1 patty with cheese and sauce): 223 calories, 7g fat, 559mg sodium, 9g carbs, 1.5g fiber, 5g sugars, 31g protein

INGREDIENTS

2 sticks light string cheese
1 cup chopped mushrooms
½ cup chopped green bell pepper
½ cup chopped onion
1 pound raw extra-lean ground beef
2 tablespoons ketchup
1 teaspoon garlic powder
½ teaspoon dried oregano
½ teaspoon dried basil
Dash each salt and black pepper
½ cup pizza sauce
12 slices turkey pepperoni

DIRECTIONS

Break each string cheese stick into thirds and place in a blender or food processor—blend at high speed until shredded. (Or pull into shreds and roughly chop.)

Bring a large skillet sprayed with nonstick spray to medium-high heat. Cook and stir veggies until softened, about 5 minutes.

Transfer veggies to a large bowl. Add beef, ketchup, and seasonings. Thoroughly mix. Evenly form into 4 patties.

Bring a grill pan (or large skillet) sprayed with nonstick spray to medium-high heat. Cook patties for 4 to 8 minutes per side, or until cooked to your preference. Reduce heat to medium low. Evenly top patties with sauce, cheese, and pepperoni. Cook until sauce is hot and cheese has melted, about 2 minutes. Dig in!

MAKES 4 SERVINGS

TREMENDOUS TOP-SHELF TURKEY BURGER

184 calories

You'll Need: small blender or food processor, medium bowl, grill pan (or skillet), nonstick spray
Prep: 10 minutes
Cook: 10 minutes

Entire recipe: 184 calories, 6.5g fat, 502mg sodium, 12g carbs, 2g fiber, 4g sugars, 20.5g protein

INGREDIENTS

½ slice light white bread
3 ounces raw lean ground turkey
¼ cup finely chopped mushrooms
3 tablespoons finely chopped onion
1 tablespoon fat-free liquid egg substitute
½ tablespoon finely chopped parsley
½ tablespoon Best Foods/Hellmann's Dijonnaise
½ tablespoon ketchup
¼ teaspoon crushed garlic
Dash salt

DIRECTIONS

Place bread in a small blender or food processor, and pulse into crumbs.

Transfer crumbs to a medium bowl. Add all remaining ingredients and thoroughly mix. Evenly form into a thick patty.

Bring a grill pan (or skillet) sprayed with nonstick spray to medium-high heat. Cook patty for 5 minutes per side, or until cooked through. Enjoy!

MAKES 1 SERVING

RED HOT & BLUE BURGER

183 calories
PER SERVING

You'll Need: large bowl, grill pan (or large skillet), nonstick spray
Prep: 10 minutes
Cook: 20 minutes

¼th of recipe (1 patty): 183 calories, 7g fat, 547mg sodium, 2g carbs, 0g fiber, 0.5g sugars, 26g protein

INGREDIENTS

1 pound raw extra-lean ground beef
⅓ cup chopped onion
¼ cup crumbled blue cheese
2 tablespoons Frank's RedHot
    Original Cayenne Pepper Sauce
2 tablespoons fat-free liquid egg substitute
¼ teaspoon garlic powder
⅛ teaspoon each salt and black pepper

DIRECTIONS

In a large bowl, thoroughly mix all ingredients. Evenly form into 4 patties.

Bring a grill pan (or large skillet) sprayed with nonstick spray to medium-high heat. Cook patties for 4 to 8 minutes per side, or until cooked to your preference. Enjoy!

MAKES 4 SERVINGS

HG GROCERY SHOPPING TIP: GROUND MEAT

Lean turkey
Look for labels that say at least 93% fat-free or no more than 7 percent fat. Or check out the nutritional facts: Each 4-ounce serving should have about 160 calories and 7 to 8 grams of fat.

Extra-lean ground beef
Look for labels that specify 96% to 99% fat-free or no more than 4 percent fat. The nutritional stats per 4-ounce serving should be about 145 calories and 5 grams of fat.

UNIQUE GREEK TURKEY BURGERS

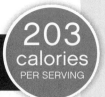

203 calories
PER SERVING

You'll Need: large skillet, nonstick spray, large bowl, grill pan (optional) | **Prep:** 10 minutes | **Cook:** 20 minutes

¼th of recipe (1 patty):
203 calories, 8g fat, 420mg sodium, 3g carbs, 1g fiber, 1g sugars, 29g protein

INGREDIENTS

¼ cup finely chopped onion
1 teaspoon chopped garlic
4 cups chopped spinach leaves
1 pound raw lean ground turkey
½ cup crumbled fat-free feta cheese
¼ cup liquid egg whites (about 2 egg whites)
½ teaspoon dried basil
½ teaspoon dried oregano
¼ teaspoon each salt and black pepper

DIRECTIONS

Bring a large skillet sprayed with nonstick spray to medium-high heat. Cook and stir onion and garlic until softened, about 4 minutes.

Add spinach to the skillet with onion and garlic. Cook and stir until spinach has wilted and excess moisture has evaporated, 3 to 5 minutes.

Transfer veggies to a large bowl and pat dry. Add all remaining ingredients and thoroughly mix. Evenly form into 4 patties.

Bring a grill pan (or skillet) sprayed with nonstick spray to medium-high heat. Cook patties for 5 minutes per side, or until cooked through. Chew!

MAKES 4 SERVINGS

CHEESED-UP TACO TURKEY BURGERS

219 calories
PER SERVING

You'll Need: large bowl, grill pan (or large skillet), nonstick spray | **Prep:** 10 minutes | **Cook:** 10 minutes

⅕th of recipe (1 patty):
219 calories, 10.5g fat, 379mg sodium, 4g carbs, 0g fiber, 1.5g sugars, 27g protein

INGREDIENTS

1¼ pounds raw lean ground turkey
¼ cup liquid egg whites (about 2 egg whites)
⅔ cup fresh pico de gallo, drained
1 tablespoon taco seasoning mix
½ cup plus 2 tablespoons shredded
    reduced-fat Mexican-blend cheese

DIRECTIONS

In a large bowl, thoroughly mix all ingredients *except* cheese. Evenly form into 5 patties.

Bring a grill pan (or large skillet) sprayed with nonstick spray to medium-high heat.

Cook patties for 5 minutes. Flip patties and cook for 3 minutes. Evenly distribute cheese among patties, 2 tablespoons each, and continue to cook until cheese has melted and patties are cooked through, 1 to 2 minutes. Enjoy!

MAKES 5 SERVINGS

PHILLY BURGERS

200 calories PER SERVING

You'll Need: large skillet, nonstick spray, large bowl, grill pan (optional)
Prep: 15 minutes
Cook: 40 minutes

¼th of recipe (1 patty): 200 calories, 5g fat, 507mg sodium, 8.5g carbs, 1g fiber, 4.5g sugars, 29g protein

INGREDIENTS

1 cup finely chopped onion
1 cup finely chopped mushrooms
1 cup finely chopped green bell pepper
1 pound raw extra-lean ground beef
¼ teaspoon each salt and black pepper
4 slices fat-free American cheese

DIRECTIONS

Bring a large skillet sprayed with nonstick spray to medium-high heat. Cook and stir onion, mushrooms, and bell pepper until slightly softened, 8 to 10 minutes.

Transfer veggies to a large bowl and pat dry. Add all remaining ingredients *except* cheese and thoroughly mix. Evenly form into 4 patties.

Bring a grill pan (or large skillet) sprayed with nonstick spray to medium-high heat. Working in batches as needed, cook patties for 4 to 8 minutes per side, or until cooked to your preference. Top each patty with a cheese slice and cook until cheese has melted, about 45 seconds. Enjoy!

MAKES 4 SERVINGS

BEAN 'N VEGGIE PATTYCAKES

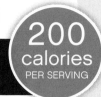

139 calories PER SERVING

You'll Need: large skillet, nonstick spray, large bowl, blender
Prep: 25 minutes
Chill: 1 hour
Cook: 30 minutes

⅙th of recipe (1 patty): 139 calories, 1g fat, 372mg sodium, 24.5g carbs, 5.5g fiber, 5g sugars, 9g protein

INGREDIENTS

5 cups chopped portabella mushrooms
1 cup finely chopped onion
1 teaspoon chopped garlic
¼ teaspoon each salt and black pepper
One 15-ounce can black beans, drained and rinsed
½ cup fat-free liquid egg substitute
¼ cup chopped fresh basil
¼ cup all-purpose flour
¼ cup finely chopped bagged sun-dried tomatoes (not packed in oil)
2 tablespoons reduced-fat Parmesan-style grated topping

DIRECTIONS

Bring a large skillet sprayed with nonstick spray to medium-high heat. Add mushrooms, onion, garlic, salt, and pepper. Cook and stir until softened, about 10 minutes. Transfer to a large bowl lined with paper towels.

Place beans, egg substitute, and basil in a blender, and puree until mostly smooth.

Remove paper towels from veggie bowl, and blot away excess moisture. Thoroughly mix in bean mixture and flour. Stir in sun-dried tomatoes and Parm-style topping. Cover and refrigerate until cool and set, at least 1 hour.

Evenly divide and form mixture into 6 patties, about ½ cup each. If needed, clean skillet. Re-spray and bring to medium heat. Working in batches, cook patties until firm and lightly browned, 3 to 4 minutes per side. (Flip gently so patties keep their shape.) Enjoy!

MAKES 6 SERVINGS

For more recipes, tips & tricks, sign up for FREE daily emails at hungry-girl.com!

OATSTANDING VEGGIE PATTIES

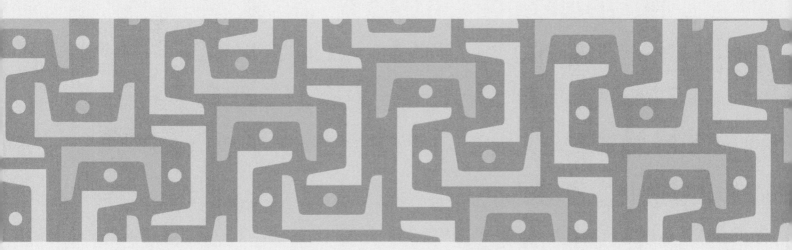

70 calories PER SERVING

You'll Need: blender or food processor, small nonstick pot, large skillet, nonstick spray, large bowl
Prep: 20 minutes | **Chill:** 1 hour 30 minutes | **Cook:** 35 minutes

⅕th of recipe (1 patty):
70 calories, 0.5g fat, 585mg sodium, 16g carbs, 5g fiber, 3g sugars, 4g protein

INGREDIENTS

½ cup Fiber One Original bran cereal
⅓ cup old-fashioned oats
1 cup diced onion
1 cup diced bell pepper
1 cup diced mushrooms
1 cup diced green beans
¼ cup fat-free liquid egg substitute
2 teaspoons reduced-sodium/lite soy sauce
1 teaspoon salt
¼ teaspoon black pepper
¼ teaspoon garlic powder

DIRECTIONS

In a blender or food processor, grind bran cereal to a breadcrumb-like consistency.

In a small nonstick pot, bring ⅓ cup water to a boil. Remove from heat and stir in oats.

Bring a large skillet sprayed with nonstick spray to medium-high heat. Cook and stir all the veggies until slightly softened, about 5 minutes.

Transfer veggies to a large bowl and let cool. Thoroughly pat dry. Add ground cereal, oat mixture, and remaining ingredients. Stir well. Cover and refrigerate until chilled, at least 1½ hours.

Evenly divide and form mixture into 5 patties. If needed, clean skillet. Re-spray skillet and bring to medium heat. Working in batches, cook patties until firm and lightly browned, about 7 minutes per side. (Flip gently so patties keep their shape.) Enjoy!

MAKES 5 SERVINGS

FRIES

Who says French fries HAVE to be made out of potatoes? Sad people who haven't experienced the joy of baked veggie fries, that's who. Fries made from squash, turnips, and carrots are life changing. So change your life!!!

BAKED-NOT-FRIED FRY TIPS

Cut your fries into similar sizes.
Otherwise some may burn while others are barely cooked.

Don't crowd your fries.
If you put too many on one sheet, they won't crisp up.

The thicker the fries, the longer the cook time.
That pretty much sums it up.

Try a crinkle cutter.
While your fries will taste delicious no matter how you slice 'em, authentic-looking crinkle cuts make them cuter and more fun to chew. Look for one with a handle for easy . . . handling.

BUTTERNUT SQUASH TIPS & TRICKS . . .

* Choose a squash that's mostly long and narrow with a short round section. The round part is hollow and full of seeds; the long section is solid squash, perfect for cutting into spears.

* If the squash is too firm to cut, pop it in the microwave for a minute to soften it.

* For the most accurate nutritional stats when making fries, weigh out and use 20 ounces of the peeled and sliced squash.

BAKE-TASTIC BUTTERNUT SQUASH FRIES

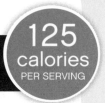
125 calories
PER SERVING

You'll Need: 2 baking sheets, nonstick spray, vegetable peeler | **Prep:** 25 minutes | **Cook:** 40 minutes

½ of recipe:
125 calories, <0.5g fat, 158mg sodium, 33g carbs, 5.5g fiber, 6g sugars, 3g protein

INGREDIENTS

One 2-pound or half of a 4-pound butternut squash (20 ounces once peeled and sliced)

⅛ teaspoon coarse salt, or more to taste

Optional dip: ketchup

DIRECTIONS

Preheat oven to 425 degrees. Spray 2 baking sheets with nonstick spray.

Peel squash and slice off the ends. Cut in half widthwise, just above the round section. Cut the round piece in half lengthwise and scoop out the seeds.

Cut squash into French-fry-shaped spears. Thoroughly pat dry. Lay spears on the sheets and sprinkle with salt. Bake for 20 minutes.

Flip spears and bake until mostly tender on the inside and crispy on the outside, about 15 minutes.

MAKES 2 SERVINGS

MEXICAN BUTTERNUT FRIES

210 calories
PER SERVING

You'll Need: 2 baking sheets, nonstick spray, vegetable peeler | **Prep:** 25 minutes | **Cook:** 40 minutes

½ of recipe:
210 calories, 3g fat, 426mg sodium, 42g carbs, 7.5g fiber, 7.5g sugars, 8g protein

INGREDIENTS

One 2-pound or half of a 4-pound butternut squash (20 ounces once peeled and sliced)

2 teaspoons taco seasoning mix

¼ cup canned black beans, drained and rinsed

¼ cup shredded reduced-fat Mexican-blend cheese

¼ cup chopped scallions

Optional toppings or dips: fat-free sour cream, salsa

DIRECTIONS

Preheat oven to 425 degrees. Spray 2 baking sheets with nonstick spray.

Peel squash and slice off the ends. Cut in half widthwise, just above the round section. Cut the round piece in half lengthwise and scoop out the seeds.

Cut squash into French-fry-shaped spears. Thoroughly pat dry. Lay spears on the sheets and sprinkle with taco seasoning. Bake for 20 minutes.

Flip spears and bake until mostly tender on the inside and crispy on the outside, about 15 minutes.

Closely arrange spears on the center of each sheet. Top with black beans and cheese. Bake until cheese has melted, about 3 minutes.

Sprinkle with scallions and enjoy!

MAKES 2 SERVINGS

RANCH 'N BACON BUTTERNUT FRIES

235 calories PER SERVING

You'll Need: 2 baking sheets, nonstick spray, small bowl, vegetable peeler, skillet or microwave-safe plate
Prep: 25 minutes
Cook: 40 minutes

½ of recipe: 235 calories, 5.5g fat, 880mg sodium, 39g carbs, 5.5g fiber, 10g sugars, 8.5g protein

INGREDIENTS

⅓ cup fat-free sour cream
½ tablespoon ranch dressing/dip seasoning mix
One 2-pound or half of a 4-pound butternut squash (20 ounces once peeled and sliced)
⅛ teaspoon coarse salt
4 slices turkey bacon

Optional topping: chopped scallions

DIRECTIONS

Preheat oven to 425 degrees. Spray 2 baking sheets with nonstick spray.

In a small bowl, thoroughly mix sour cream with ranch mix. Cover and refrigerate.

Peel squash and slice off the ends. Cut in half widthwise, just above the round section. Cut the round piece in half lengthwise and scoop out the seeds.

Cut squash into French-fry-shaped spears. Thoroughly pat dry. Lay spears on the sheets and sprinkle with salt. Bake for 20 minutes.

Flip spears and bake until mostly tender on the inside and crispy on the outside, about 15 minutes.

Meanwhile, cook bacon until crispy, either in a skillet over medium heat or on a microwave-safe plate in the microwave. (See package for cook time.) Cut into very thin strips.

Toss fries with bacon strips and drizzle or serve with ranch mixture. Eat up!

MAKES 2 SERVINGS

HUNGRY GIRLFREDO BUTTERNUT FRIES

213 calories PER SERVING

You'll Need: 2 baking sheets, nonstick spray, microwave-safe bowl
Prep: 25 minutes
Cook: 40 minutes

½ of recipe: 213 calories, 3.5g fat, 527mg sodium, 39g carbs, 5.5g fiber, 9g sugars, 7.5g protein

INGREDIENTS

One 2-pound or half of a 4-pound butternut squash (20 ounces once peeled and sliced)
⅛ teaspoon coarse salt, or more to taste
3 tablespoons fat-free sour cream
1 tablespoon reduced-fat Parmesan-style grated topping
⅛ teaspoon garlic powder
Dash black pepper
3 wedges The Laughing Cow Light Creamy Swiss cheese

DIRECTIONS

Preheat oven to 425 degrees. Spray 2 baking sheets with nonstick spray.

Peel squash and slice off the ends. Cut in half widthwise, just above the round section. Cut the round piece in half lengthwise and scoop out the seeds.

Cut squash into French-fry-shaped spears. Thoroughly pat dry. Lay spears on the sheets and sprinkle with salt. Bake for 20 minutes.

Flip spears and bake until mostly tender on the inside and crispy on the outside, about 15 minutes.

In a microwave-safe bowl, mix sour cream, Parm-style topping, garlic powder, black pepper, and cheese wedges, breaking wedges into pieces. Stir in 2 tablespoons water. Microwave at 50 percent power for 1 minute. Stir and microwave at 50 percent power for 30 seconds, or until melted.

Stir sour cream mixture, spoon over fries, and enjoy!

MAKES 2 SERVINGS

SWEET GARLIC BUTTERNUT FRIES

  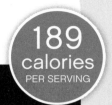

189 calories
PER SERVING

You'll Need: 2 baking sheets, nonstick spray, vegetable peeler, aluminum foil, small microwave-safe bowl
Prep: 25 minutes
Cook: 40 minutes

½ of recipe: 189 calories, 1.5g fat, 453mg sodium, 45g carbs, 6g fiber, 13g sugars, 3.5g protein

INGREDIENTS

One 2-pound or half of a 4-pound butternut squash (20 ounces once peeled and sliced)
¼ teaspoon coarse salt
½ head of garlic
½ teaspoon olive oil
2 tablespoons sweet Asian chili sauce

Optional seasoning: additional coarse salt

DIRECTIONS

Preheat oven to 425 degrees. Spray 2 baking sheets with nonstick spray.

Peel squash and slice off the ends. Cut in half widthwise, just above the round section. Cut the round piece in half lengthwise and scoop out the seeds.

Cut squash into French-fry-shaped spears. Thoroughly pat dry. Lay spears on the sheets and sprinkle with ⅛ teaspoon salt.

Remove outer layer of garlic, leaving the skins around the cloves intact. Slice ¼ inch off the top, exposing the cloves.

Place on a piece of foil, cut side up, and coat the top with oil. Tightly wrap foil around garlic, enclosing it completely.

Place foil-wrapped garlic on one of the baking sheets. Bake for 20 minutes.

Flip spears and bake until mostly tender on the inside and crispy on the outside, about 15 minutes.

Once cool, unwrap garlic and remove cloves; discard skin. Place cloves in a small microwave-safe bowl. Add remaining ⅛ teaspoon salt and mash with a fork until mostly smooth. Mix in chili sauce. Microwave for 10 seconds, or until softened.

Serve fries with garlic sauce on top or on the side!

MAKES 2 SERVINGS

TOTALLY TURNIP FRIES

96 calories
PER SERVING

You'll Need: 2 baking sheets, nonstick spray
Prep: 10 minutes
Cook: 30 minutes

½ of recipe: 96 calories, <0.5g fat, 373mg sodium, 22g carbs, 6g fiber, 13g sugars, 3g protein

INGREDIENTS

1½ pounds turnips (about 2 medium turnips)
⅛ teaspoon each salt and black pepper

Optional dip: ketchup

DIRECTIONS

Preheat oven to 425 degrees. Spray 2 baking sheets with nonstick spray.

Cut turnips into French-fry-shaped spears and lay them on the sheets. Sprinkle with salt and pepper. Bake for 15 minutes.

Flip spears. Bake until tender on the inside and crispy on the outside, about 15 more minutes. Chew, you!

MAKES 2 SERVINGS

 Flip to the photo inserts to see over 100 recipe pics! And for photos of ALL the recipes, go to **hungry-girl.com/books**.

TURNIP THE DISCO FRIES

284 calories PER SERVING

You'll Need: 2 baking sheets, nonstick spray, small nonstick pot
Prep: 10 minutes
Cook: 35 minutes

½ of recipe: 284 calories, 1g fat, 913mg sodium, 58g carbs, 9.5g fiber, 15.5g sugars, 13g protein

INGREDIENTS

1½ pounds turnips (about 2 medium turnips)
One 12-ounce russet potato
3 slices fat-free American cheese, torn into strips
½ cup jarred fat-free or nearly fat-free chicken gravy

Optional seasonings: salt and black pepper
Optional topping: chopped chives

DIRECTIONS

Preheat oven to 425 degrees. Spray 2 baking sheets with nonstick spray.

Cut turnips and potato into French-fry-shaped spears and lay them on the sheets. Bake for 15 minutes.

Flip spears. Bake until tender on the inside and crispy on the outside, about 15 more minutes. Closely arrange spears on the center of the sheets. Top with cheese and bake until melted, about 3 minutes.

Place gravy in a small nonstick pot, and set temperature to low. Cook and stir until hot, 1 to 2 minutes.

Serve fries with gravy. Enjoy!

MAKES 2 SERVINGS

BACON 'N CHEESE TURNIP FRIES

195 calories PER SERVING

You'll Need: 2 baking sheets, nonstick spray, skillet or microwave-safe plate, small nonstick pot
Prep: 10 minutes
Cook: 30 minutes

½ of recipe: 195 calories, 4.5g fat, 880mg sodium, 25.5g carbs, 6g fiber, 15.5g sugars, 12.5g protein

INGREDIENTS

1½ pounds turnips (about 2 medium turnips)
2 slices center-cut bacon or turkey bacon
¼ cup light plain soymilk
2 slices fat-free cheddar or American cheese
2 wedges The Laughing Cow Light Creamy Swiss cheese

Optional seasonings: salt and black pepper
Optional topping: chopped scallions

DIRECTIONS

Preheat oven to 425 degrees. Spray 2 baking sheets with nonstick spray.

Cut turnips into French-fry-shaped spears and lay them on the sheets. Bake for 15 minutes.

Flip spears. Bake until tender on the inside and crispy on the outside, about 15 more minutes.

Meanwhile, cook bacon until crispy, either in a skillet over medium heat or on a microwave-safe plate in the microwave. (See package for cook time.) Chop or crumble.

Pour soymilk into a small nonstick pot. Add cheese slices and wedges, breaking them into pieces. Bring to medium-low heat. Cook and stir until sauce is hot and uniform, 5 to 8 minutes.

Top fries with cheese sauce and chopped or crumbled bacon. Dig in!

MAKES 2 SERVINGS

CHEESY BEEFY TURNIP FRIES

229 calories PER SERVING

You'll Need: 2 baking sheets, nonstick spray, skillet, medium bowl
Prep: 10 minutes
Cook: 40 minutes

½ of recipe: 229 calories, 3.5g fat, 796mg sodium, 28.5g carbs, 6.5g fiber, 16.5g sugars, 20.5g protein

INGREDIENTS

1½ pounds turnips (about 2 medium turnips)
½ cup finely chopped onion
4 ounces raw extra-lean ground beef
⅛ teaspoon each salt and black pepper
2 slices fat-free cheddar or American cheese
1 wedge The Laughing Cow Light Creamy Swiss cheese, room temperature

DIRECTIONS

Preheat oven to 425 degrees. Spray 2 baking sheets with nonstick spray.

Cut turnips into French-fry-shaped spears and lay them on the sheets. Bake for 15 minutes.

Flip spears. Bake until tender on the inside and crispy on the outside, about 15 more minutes.

Bring a skillet sprayed with nonstick spray to medium-high heat. Add onion and beef and sprinkle with salt and black pepper. Cook, stir, and crumble until beef is fully cooked and onion has softened, about 5 minutes. Transfer to a medium bowl and immediately add cheese slices and cheese wedge, breaking them into small pieces, and stir until melted and well mixed.

Serve fries topped with beef mixture and enjoy!

MAKES 2 SERVINGS

GRIN 'N CARROT FRIES & DIP

201 calories PER SERVING

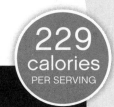

You'll Need: 2 baking sheets, nonstick spray, small bowl
Prep: 15 minutes
Cook: 30 minutes

½ of recipe: 201 calories, 2g fat, 733mg sodium, 40g carbs, 9.5g fiber, 19.5g sugars, 7.5g protein

INGREDIENTS

½ cup fat-free sour cream
1 teaspoon ranch dressing/dip seasoning mix
1 tablespoon precooked crumbled bacon
1½ pounds carrots (about 8 large carrots), tops removed, peeled
¼ teaspoon coarse salt, or more to taste

DIRECTIONS

Preheat oven to 425 degrees. Spray 2 baking sheets with nonstick spray.

In a small bowl, mix sour cream with ranch mix. Stir in crumbled bacon. Cover and refrigerate.

Cut carrots into French-fry-shaped spears and lay them on the sheets. Sprinkle with salt. Bake for 15 minutes.

Flip spears. Bake until tender on the inside and slightly crispy on the outside, about 15 more minutes.

Serve fries with sour cream mixture for dipping!

MAKES 2 SERVINGS

CHAPTER 13

CHINESE

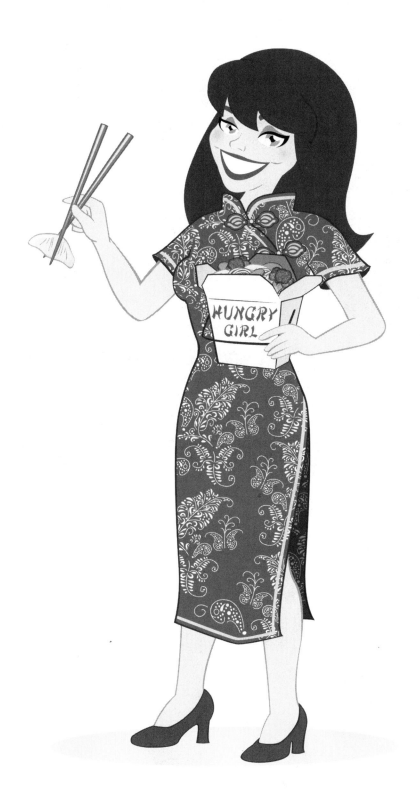

CHINESE

Sassy Veggie Egg Rolls

Shrimpylicious Egg Rolls

Fully Loaded Egg Rolls

Hot & Hungry Szechuan Shrimp

Asian-Style Honey BBQ Chicken

So Low Mein with Chicken

Veggie So Low Mein

Eggplant Stir-Fry

Veggie-Friendly Asian Lettuce Wraps

Turbo Tofu Stir-Fry

Veggie-rific Fried Rice

Chop-Chop Beef Stir-Fry

Egg-cellent Foo Young

Sweet & Sticky Sesame Chicken

Veggie-Loaded Cashew Chicken

Mmmmm Moo Shu Chicken

Oh Honey! Walnut Shrimp

Sweet & Sticky Orange Chicken

Orange Beef Stir-Fry

WOWOWOW! Kung Pao

Sweet & Sour Chicken 1-2-3

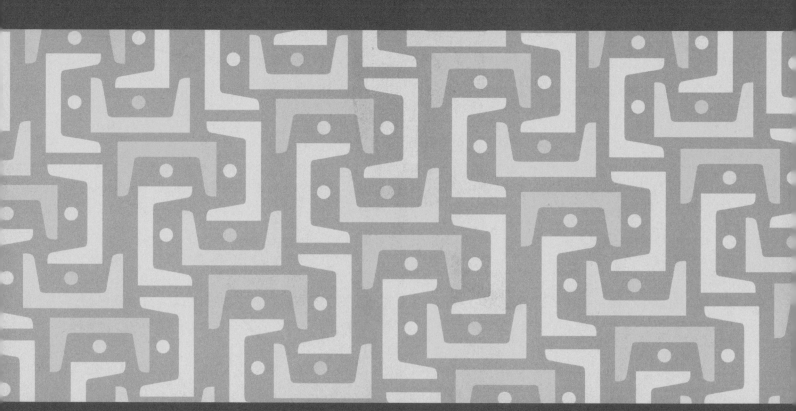

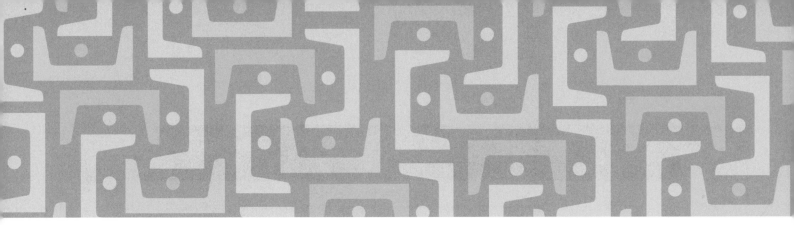

HG-ified stir-frys, egg rolls, moo shu, low mein, egg foo young, and MORE . . . all here for your chewing pleasure.

A QUICK GUIDE TO SYMBOLS:

15 Minutes or Less

This symbol lets you know a recipe should take you no more than fifteen minutes from start to finish! That includes prep and cook time.

30 Minutes or Less

Just like the 15-minute version, this one points out recipes that take 30 minutes or less to whip up.

Meatless

You guessed it—no meat here! That includes beef, poultry, and fish. Some recipes give the option of a meatless ingredient. If you want your meal without meat, go with the meatless choice.

Single Serving

Pretty straightforward. These are recipes for one.

5 Ingredients or Less

Fans of HG know that we like to keep things simple. And these recipes contain just five ingredients or less!

Photos

These recipes can be seen in one of the book's photo inserts. The number in the symbol tells you which insert. Find photos of all the recipes at hungry-girl.com/books!

SASSY VEGGIE EGG ROLLS

82 calories PER SERVING

You'll Need: baking sheet, nonstick spray, large microwave-safe bowl | **Prep:** 20 minutes | **Cook:** 35 minutes

1/12th of recipe (1 egg roll):
82 calories, <0.5g fat, 211mg sodium, 18g carbs, 1.5g fiber, 3g sugars, 3g protein

INGREDIENTS

2½ cups bagged coleslaw mix

1 cup chopped onion

½ cup chopped bean sprouts

½ cup chopped celery

½ cup pineapple chunks packed in juice, drained and chopped

½ cup canned sliced water chestnuts, drained and chopped

2 tablespoons reduced-sodium/lite soy sauce

1½ tablespoons chopped garlic

12 large square egg roll wrappers

Optional seasonings: salt and black pepper

DIRECTIONS

Preheat oven to 375 degrees. Spray a baking sheet with nonstick spray.

Place coleslaw mix in a large microwave-safe bowl with 2 tablespoons water. Cover and microwave for 3 minutes, or until softened.

Drain any excess water and blot away excess moisture. Add all other ingredients *except* wrappers and mix well. If you like, season to taste with salt and pepper.

Lay an egg roll wrapper flat on a dry surface. Evenly distribute 2 heaping tablespoons slaw mixture (1/12th of mixture) in a row a little below the center of the wrapper. Moisten all four edges by dabbing your fingers in water and going over the edges smoothly. Fold the sides about ¾ inch toward the middle, to keep mixture from falling out. Roll up the wrapper around the mixture and continue to the top. Seal with a dab of water.

Place on the baking sheet, and repeat with remaining mixture and wrappers.

Spray egg rolls with nonstick spray. Bake until golden brown, 25 to 30 minutes. Enjoy!

MAKES 12 SERVINGS

QUICK Q&A WITH HG:

Where can I find egg roll wrappers?

With the tofu and other refrigerated Asian products.

SHRIMPYLICIOUS EGG ROLLS

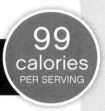

99 calories
PER SERVING

You'll Need: baking sheet, nonstick spray, large microwave-safe bowl
Prep: 30 minutes | **Marinate:** 20 minutes (optional) | **Cook:** 35 minutes

⅙th of recipe (1 egg roll):
99 calories, 0.5g fat, 380mg sodium, 16.5g carbs, 1.5g fiber, 2g sugars, 7g protein

INGREDIENTS

4 cups bagged coleslaw mix
4 oz. cooked and chopped ready-to-eat shrimp
½ cup canned sliced water chestnuts, drained
    and cut into strips
¼ cup chopped bean sprouts
¼ cup chopped scallions
1 stalk celery, thinly sliced widthwise
2 tablespoons reduced-sodium/lite soy sauce
1 teaspoon crushed garlic
¼ teaspoon ground ginger
⅛ teaspoon salt
Dash black pepper
6 large square egg roll wrappers

Optional dip: sweet & sour sauce

DIRECTIONS

Preheat oven to 375 degrees. Spray a baking sheet with nonstick spray.

Place coleslaw mix in a large microwave-safe bowl with 2 tablespoons water. Cover and microwave for 3 minutes, or until softened.

Drain any excess water. Add all other ingredients *except* wrappers and mix well. For added flavor intensity, cover and marinate in the fridge for 20 minutes (optional).

Lay an egg roll wrapper flat on a dry surface. Evenly distribute about ½ cup slaw mixture (⅙th of mixture) in a row a little below the center of the wrapper.

Moisten all four edges by dabbing your fingers in water and going over the edges smoothly. Fold the sides about ¾ inch toward the middle, to keep mixture from falling out. Roll up the wrapper around the mixture and continue to the top. Seal with a dab of water.

Place on the baking sheet, and repeat with remaining mixture and wrappers.

Spray egg rolls with nonstick spray. Bake until golden brown, 25 to 30 minutes. Enjoy!

MAKES 6 SERVINGS

✳ Flip to the photo inserts to see over 100 recipe pics! And for photos of ALL the recipes, go to **hungry-girl.com/books**.

FULLY LOADED EGG ROLLS

109 calories PER SERVING

You'll Need: baking sheet, nonstick spray, small bowl, skillet, large bowl
Prep: 30 minutes | **Marinate:** 10 minutes, plus 20 minutes (optional) | **Cook:** 35 minutes

⅛th of recipe (1 egg roll):
109 calories, 1.5g fat, 380mg sodium, 15g carbs, 1g fiber, 2g sugars, 9g protein

INGREDIENTS

2½ tablespoons reduced-sodium/lite
    soy sauce

½ teaspoon granulated white sugar or
    Splenda No Calorie Sweetener (granulated)

4 ounces raw boneless pork tenderloin,
    finely chopped

3 cups bagged coleslaw mix

One 6-ounce can (4 ounces drained)
    tiny shrimp, drained

¼ cup chopped bean sprouts

¼ cup chopped scallions

1 stalk celery, thinly sliced widthwise

2 teaspoons crushed garlic

1 teaspoon sesame oil

½ teaspoon ground ginger

⅛ teaspoon black pepper

8 large square egg roll wrappers

Optional dip: sweet & sour sauce

DIRECTIONS

Preheat oven to 375 degrees. Spray a baking sheet with nonstick spray.

In a small bowl, mix ½ tablespoon soy sauce with sugar or Splenda. Add pork and coat well. Cover and marinate in the fridge for 10 minutes.

Bring a skillet sprayed with nonstick spray to medium-high heat. Add coleslaw mix, pork, and any excess marinade. Cook and stir for 3 to 5 minutes, until pork is cooked through.

Transfer mixture to a large bowl. Add remaining 2 tablespoons soy sauce and all other remaining ingredients *except* wrappers. Mix well. For added flavor intensity, cover and marinate in the fridge for 20 minutes (optional).

Lay an egg roll wrapper flat on a dry surface. Evenly distribute about ⅓ cup slaw mixture (⅛th of mixture) in a row a little below the center of the wrapper.

Moisten all four edges by dabbing your fingers in water and going over the edges smoothly. Fold the sides about ¾ inch toward the middle, to keep mixture from falling out. Roll the wrapper up around the mixture and continue to the top. Seal with a dab of water.

Place on the baking sheet, and repeat with remaining mixture and wrappers.

Spray egg rolls with nonstick spray. Bake until golden brown, 25 to 30 minutes. Enjoy!

MAKES 8 SERVINGS

HOT & HUNGRY SZECHUAN SHRIMP

245 calories
PER SERVING

You'll Need: medium bowl, wok (or large skillet), nonstick spray
Prep: 15 minutes
Cook: 10 minutes

½ of recipe (about 2 cups): 245 calories, 1.5g fat, 987mg sodium, 32.5g carbs, 4.5g fiber, 12.5g sugars, 24.5g protein

INGREDIENTS

1 tablespoon cornstarch

1½ tablespoons ketchup

1½ tablespoons reduced-sodium/lite soy sauce

½ tablespoon Sriracha chili sauce (shelf-stable Asian hot sauce)

1 teaspoon granulated white sugar or Splenda No Calorie Sweetener (granulated)

¼ teaspoon red pepper flakes, or more to taste

1 cup chopped green beans

1 cup chopped green bell pepper

1 cup chopped onion

1 teaspoon chopped garlic

1 teaspoon chopped ginger

8 ounces (about 14) raw large shrimp, peeled, tails removed, deveined

½ cup sliced water chestnuts, drained

DIRECTIONS

In a medium bowl, mix cornstarch with ⅓ cup water until dissolved. Thoroughly mix in ketchup, soy sauce, chili sauce, sugar or Splenda, and red pepper flakes.

Bring a wok (or large skillet) sprayed with nonstick spray to medium-high heat. Add green beans, bell pepper, onion, garlic, and ginger. Cook and stir until slightly softened, about 5 minutes.

Add shrimp and water chestnuts. Stir sauce and add as well. Cook and stir until sauce has thickened and shrimp are cooked through, about 3 minutes. Enjoy!

MAKES 2 SERVINGS

ASIAN-STYLE HONEY BBQ CHICKEN

291 calories
PER SERVING

You'll Need: small bowl, large sealable bag, baking pan, nonstick spray, pastry brush
Prep: 15 minutes
Marinate: 30 minutes
Cook: 20 minutes

½ of recipe (about 7 pieces): 291 calories, 3.5g fat, 1,061mg sodium, 28g carbs, 0.5g fiber, 25g sugars, 35g protein

INGREDIENTS

2 tablespoons hoisin sauce

2 tablespoons honey

2 tablespoons reduced-sodium/lite soy sauce

½ teaspoon ground ginger

⅛ teaspoon cayenne pepper

10 ounces raw boneless skinless chicken breast, cut into about fourteen ½-inch-wide strips

⅛ teaspoon each salt and black pepper

2 teaspoons toasted sesame seeds

2 tablespoons chopped scallions

DIRECTIONS

In a small bowl, thoroughly mix hoisin sauce, honey, soy sauce, ginger, and cayenne pepper.

Season chicken with salt and pepper and place in a large sealable bag. Add 3 tablespoons of the sauce mixture and seal. Set remaining sauce aside. Marinate chicken in the fridge for 30 minutes.

Preheat oven to 375 degrees. Spray a baking pan with nonstick spray.

Place chicken in the pan and discard the bag of excess marinade. Bake for 8 minutes.

Flip chicken and brush with remaining sauce. Bake until chicken is cooked through, about 8 more minutes.

Serve topped with sesame seeds and scallions!

MAKES 2 SERVINGS

SO LOW MEIN WITH CHICKEN

177 calories
PER SERVING

You'll Need: strainer, medium bowl, wok (or large skillet), nonstick spray | **Prep:** 15 minutes | **Cook:** 15 minutes

¼th of recipe (about 1½ cups):
177 calories, 1.5g fat, 925mg sodium, 21.5g carbs, 6g fiber, 7g sugars, 18g protein

INGREDIENTS

3 bags House Foods Tofu Shirataki Spaghetti Shaped Noodle Substitute

¼ cup reduced-sodium/lite soy sauce

1 tablespoon cornstarch

1 tablespoon granulated white sugar

2 teaspoons chicken-flavored powdered consommé

One 12-ounce bag frozen stir-fry vegetables

8 ounces raw boneless skinless chicken breast, cut into strips

1 cup bean sprouts

½ cup chopped mushrooms

½ cup thinly sliced zucchini

½ cup chopped scallions

¼ cup shredded carrots

DIRECTIONS

Use a strainer to rinse and drain noodles. Thoroughly pat dry. Roughly cut noodles.

To make the sauce, in a medium bowl, combine soy sauce, cornstarch, sugar, and consommé. Add ½ cup hot water and stir until cornstarch dissolves.

Bring a wok (or large skillet) sprayed with nonstick spray to medium-high heat. Add all ingredients *except* noodles and sauce. Cook and stir for 5 to 7 minutes, until chicken is cooked through and all veggies are hot.

Add sauce and cook and stir until thickened, about 3 to 4 minutes.

Add noodles and cook and stir until well mixed and hot, about 2 minutes. Serve and enjoy!

MAKES 4 SERVINGS

HG SWEET ALTERNATIVE!

If made with an equal amount of Splenda No Calorie Sweetener (granulated) in place of the sugar, each serving will have 167 calories, 19g carbs, and 4g sugars.

For more recipes, tips & tricks, sign up for FREE daily emails at **hungry-girl.com!**

VEGGIE SO LOW MEIN

128 calories PER SERVING

You'll Need: strainer, medium bowl, wok (or large skillet), nonstick spray | **Prep:** 15 minutes | **Cook:** 15 minutes

¼th of recipe (about 1½ cups):
128 calories, 1.5g fat, 940mg sodium, 23g carbs, 6g fiber, 9g sugars, 6g protein

INGREDIENTS

3 bags House Foods Tofu Shirataki Spaghetti Shaped Noodle Substitute
½ cube vegetable bouillon
¼ cup reduced-sodium/lite soy sauce
1 tablespoon cornstarch
1 tablespoon granulated white sugar
One 12-ounce bag frozen stir-fry vegetables
1 cup sliced mushrooms
1 cup thinly sliced zucchini
1 cup bean sprouts
½ cup chopped scallions
¼ cup shredded carrots

HG SWEET ALTERNATIVE!

If made with an equal amount of Splenda No Calorie Sweetener (granulated) in place of the sugar, each serving will have 120 calories, 20g carbs, and 6g sugars.

DIRECTIONS

Use a strainer to rinse and drain noodles. Thoroughly pat dry. Roughly cut noodles.

To make the sauce, in a medium bowl, stir to dissolve bouillon in ½ cup hot water. Add soy sauce, cornstarch, and sugar, and stir until cornstarch dissolves.

Bring a wok (or large skillet) sprayed with nonstick spray to medium-high heat. Add all ingredients *except* noodles and sauce. Cook and stir until all veggies are hot, 5 to 7 minutes.

Add sauce and cook and stir until thickened, about 3 to 4 minutes.

Add noodles and cook and stir until well mixed and hot, about 2 minutes. Serve and enjoy!

MAKES 4 SERVINGS

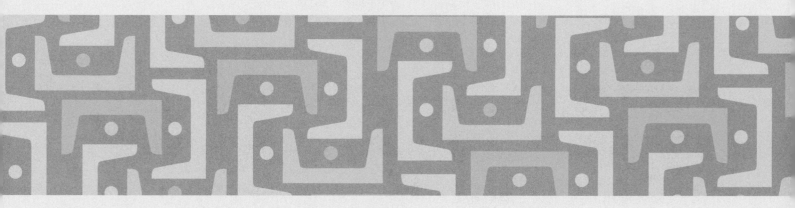

EGGPLANT STIR-FRY

 155 calories PER SERVING

You'll Need: small bowl, wok (or large skillet), nonstick spray
Prep: 15 minutes
Cook: 20 minutes

½ of recipe (about 1⅔ cups): 155 calories, 0.5g fat, 593mg sodium, 34.5g carbs, 11.5g fiber, 17.5g sugars, 5g protein

INGREDIENTS

1 tablespoon reduced-sodium/lite
    soy sauce
1 tablespoon sweet Asian chili sauce
½ tablespoon vegetarian-friendly
    oyster sauce
⅛ teaspoon ground ginger
1 medium eggplant, ends removed,
    cut widthwise into ½-inch slices
1 cup onion sliced into 1-inch strips
1 jalapeño pepper, stem removed, seeded,
    sliced into rings
1 teaspoon chopped garlic
1 cup chopped tomatoes

DIRECTIONS

In a small bowl, mix soy sauce, chili sauce, oyster sauce, ginger, and 2 tablespoons water.

Cut eggplant slices into quarters. Bring a wok (or large skillet) sprayed with nonstick spray to medium-high heat. Add eggplant, onion, jalapeño pepper, and garlic. Cook and stir until softened, 13 to 15 minutes.

Add sauce mixture and tomatoes. Cook and stir until tomatoes are hot, about 1 minute. Mmmmm!

MAKES 2 SERVINGS

VEGGIE-FRIENDLY ASIAN LETTUCE WRAPS

 220 calories PER SERVING

You'll Need: medium bowl, skillet, nonstick spray
Prep: 5 minutes
Cook: 10 minutes

½ of recipe (3 wraps): 220 calories, 3.5g fat, 971mg sodium, 30g carbs, 8g fiber, 10g sugars, 21g protein

INGREDIENTS

2 tablespoons reduced-sodium/lite soy sauce
1 tablespoon brown sugar (not packed)
2 teaspoons Asian-style chili garlic sauce
½ teaspoon sesame oil
1¾ cups frozen ground-beef-style soy crumbles
1 cup canned sliced water chestnuts, drained
    and chopped
¾ cup chopped shiitake mushrooms
1 cup bean sprouts
½ cup chopped scallions
6 medium iceberg lettuce leaves (or leaves from
    another round, firm head of lettuce)

DIRECTIONS

In a medium bowl, thoroughly mix soy sauce, brown sugar, garlic sauce, and sesame oil.

Bring a skillet sprayed with nonstick spray to medium heat. Cook and stir soy crumbles until thawed, about 3 minutes.

Add chopped water chestnuts, mushrooms, bean sprouts, and sauce mixture. Cook and stir until veggies have softened, 2 to 3 minutes.

Add scallions and cook and stir until hot, about 1 minute. Let slightly cool and then divide among lettuce leaves!

MAKES 2 SERVINGS

JALAPEÑO QUICK TIP!

When handling jalapeños, don't touch your eyes—that pepper juice can STING. And wash your hands well immediately afterward.

TURBO TOFU STIR-FRY

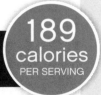

189 calories PER SERVING

You'll Need: medium bowl, whisk, skillet with a lid, nonstick spray, large bowl
Prep: 10 minutes | **Cook:** 15 minutes

¼th of recipe (about 1⅓ cups):
189 calories, 6.5g fat, 768mg sodium, 16.5g carbs, 4g fiber, 7g sugars, 13g protein

INGREDIENTS

One 12-ounce package block-style
  extra-firm tofu, drained
2 tablespoons reduced-sodium/lite soy sauce
2 tablespoons vegetarian-friendly oyster sauce
2 teaspoons cornstarch
1 teaspoon sesame oil
Dash ground ginger
Dash red pepper flakes
⅛ teaspoon salt
4 cups frozen stir-fry vegetables
3 cups frozen broccoli florets
½ teaspoon chopped garlic

HG FYI:

Tofu also comes in
14-ounce to 16-ounce
packages. If you can't find a
12-ounce package, go for one
of these larger packages and
just use 12 ounces
(about ¾ths of it).

DIRECTIONS

Lay tofu block on a dry surface with the shorter sides on the left and right. Vertically cut into ½-inch-wide pieces. Horizontally cut each piece into 4 smaller pieces.

In a medium bowl, combine soy sauce, oyster sauce, cornstarch, sesame oil, ginger, and red pepper flakes. Whisk until cornstarch has dissolved.

Bring a skillet sprayed with nonstick spray to high heat. Add tofu and sprinkle with salt. Cook until golden brown, about 6 minutes, gently flipping to evenly brown.

Transfer tofu to a large bowl and cover to keep warm.

To the skillet, add stir-fry veggies, broccoli, and garlic. Cover and cook until hot, about 5 minutes.

Give the sauce mixture a stir and add to the skillet, along with the tofu. Cook and stir until sauce has thickened slightly and tofu is hot, about 3 minutes. Dig in!

MAKES 4 SERVINGS

VEGGIE-RIFIC FRIED RICE

167 calories
PER SERVING

You'll Need: medium bowl, wok (or large skillet), nonstick spray, large bowl
Prep: 10 minutes
Cook: 15 minutes

⅕th of recipe (about 1 cup): 167 calories, 0.5g fat, 630mg sodium, 30g carbs, 4g fiber, 4g sugars, 8.5g protein

INGREDIENTS

One 1-ounce packet fried rice seasoning mix
⅛ teaspoon garlic powder
⅛ teaspoon ground ginger
1 tablespoon reduced-sodium/lite soy sauce
¾ cup fat-free liquid egg substitute
2 cups frozen diced carrots and peas
1 cup chopped mushrooms
2 cups cooked brown rice, chilled
1 cup chopped bean sprouts
¼ cup chopped scallions

Optional seasonings: salt and black pepper

DIRECTIONS

In a medium bowl, combine seasoning mix, garlic powder, and ground ginger. Add soy sauce and 3 tablespoons hot water, and stir until seasoning mix has dissolved.

Bring a wok (or large skillet) sprayed with nonstick spray to medium heat. Scramble egg substitute until fully cooked, 3 to 4 minutes, using a spatula to break it up into bite-sized pieces.

Transfer cooked egg substitute to a large bowl. If needed, clean wok. Remove from heat, re-spray, and return to medium heat. Add frozen vegetables and mushrooms, and cook and stir until frozen veggies are hot and mushrooms have softened, 5 to 7 minutes.

Transfer veggies to the large bowl. Remove wok from heat, re-spray, and bring to high heat. Add rice and seasoning mixture, and thoroughly stir. Add bean sprouts, scallions, and the contents of the large bowl. Cook and stir until liquid has evaporated and contents are well mixed and hot, about 1 minute. Enjoy!

MAKES 5 SERVINGS

CHOP-CHOP BEEF STIR-FRY

293 calories

You'll Need: medium bowl, whisk, skillet, nonstick spray
Prep: 15 minutes
Marinate: 15 minutes
Cook: 10 minutes

Entire recipe: 293 calories, 6.5g fat, 914mg sodium, 26g carbs, 7.5g fiber, 7g sugars, 35g protein

INGREDIENTS

½ cup fat-free beef broth
½ tablespoon cornstarch
½ tablespoon reduced-sodium/lite soy sauce
½ tablespoon chopped garlic
¼ teaspoon red pepper flakes
4 ounces raw lean beefsteak filet
Dash salt
2 cups broccoli florets
1 cup sliced mushrooms
1 cup sugar snap peas
2 tablespoons chopped scallions

DIRECTIONS

In a medium bowl, combine beef broth, cornstarch, soy sauce, garlic, and red pepper. Whisk until cornstarch dissolves.

Season beef with salt and thinly slice. Add to the bowl and coat well. Cover and marinate in the fridge for 10 to 15 minutes.

Bring a skillet sprayed with nonstick spray to medium-high heat. Add broccoli, mushrooms, sugar snap peas, scallions, and ¼ cup of the marinade. Cook and stir until broccoli has softened, about 3 minutes.

Add beef and remaining marinade. Cook and stir for about 3 more minutes, until beef is fully cooked. Enjoy!

MAKES 1 SERVING

EGG-CELLENT FOO YOUNG

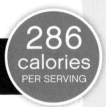

You'll Need: small nonstick pot with a lid, whisk, large bowl, large skillet, nonstick spray, plate
Prep: 15 minutes | **Cook:** 20 minutes

½ of recipe (about 5 pancakes with sauce):
286 calories, 2g fat, 1,026mg sodium, 21.5g carbs, 2.5g fiber, 7g sugars, 45g protein

INGREDIENTS

1½ cups fat-free chicken broth

1½ tablespoons cornstarch

1 tablespoon reduced-sodium/lite soy sauce

1 cup fat-free liquid egg substitute

1 cup finely chopped onion

1 cup chopped bean sprouts

½ cup chopped mushrooms

½ teaspoon chopped garlic

4 ounces raw bay shrimp, peeled, tails removed, deveined

4 ounces cooked and shredded (or finely chopped) skinless chicken breast

¼ cup chopped scallions

HG FYI:

If you can't find bay shrimp, go for medium-sized shrimp and chop before cooking.

HG ALTERNATIVE!

Save about 230mg sodium per serving by using low-sodium chicken broth.

DIRECTIONS

To make the sauce, in a small nonstick pot, whisk broth, cornstarch, and 2 teaspoons soy sauce until cornstarch has dissolved. Bring to a boil, stirring often.

Set heat to low. Cook and stir until thickened, about 4 minutes. Remove from heat and cover to keep warm.

In a large bowl, whisk egg substitute with remaining 1 teaspoon soy sauce until well mixed.

Bring a large skillet sprayed with nonstick spray to medium heat. Add onion, bean sprouts, mushrooms, and garlic. Cook and stir until slightly softened, about 3 minutes.

Add shrimp and cook and stir until veggies are soft and shrimp are cooked through, about 2 minutes.

Transfer contents of the skillet to the large bowl. Add chicken and scallions and stir well.

If needed, clean skillet. Remove from heat, re-spray, and bring to medium-high heat. Add half of the mixture in heaping ¼-cup portions to form about 5 small pancakes, using a spatula to help pancakes take shape. Cook for 1 to 2 minutes per side, until golden brown and cooked through.

Plate pancakes, and repeat with remaining mixture to make about 5 more pancakes.

Serve pancakes smothered with sauce. Mmmmm!

MAKES 2 SERVINGS

SWEET & STICKY SESAME CHICKEN

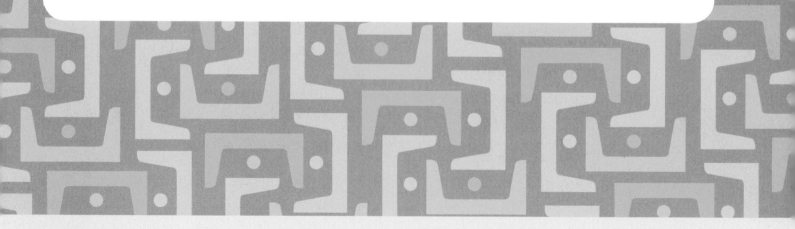

301 calories PER SERVING

You'll Need: baking sheet, nonstick spray, wide bowl, large bowl, medium bowl, whisk, skillet
Prep: 20 minutes | **Cook:** 15 minutes

½ of recipe (about 1 cup):
301 calories, 4g fat, 859mg sodium, 26.5g carbs, 2g fiber, 7g sugars, 38g protein

INGREDIENTS

¼ cup whole-wheat flour

10 ounces raw boneless skinless chicken breast, cut into nuggets

¼ cup fat-free liquid egg substitute

¼ cup fat-free chicken broth

1 tablespoon cornstarch

2 tablespoons sugar-free pancake syrup

2 tablespoons seasoned rice vinegar

1 tablespoon ketchup

½ tablespoon reduced-sodium/lite soy sauce

½ teaspoon sesame oil

½ teaspoon crushed garlic

1 teaspoon sesame seeds

2 tablespoons thinly sliced scallions

Optional seasoning: red pepper flakes

DIRECTIONS

Preheat oven to 375 degrees. Spray a baking sheet with nonstick spray.

Place flour in a wide bowl.

Place chicken in a large bowl, top with egg substitute, and toss to coat.

One at a time, shake nuggets to remove excess egg and coat with flour. Evenly lay on the baking sheet.

Bake until chicken is cooked through, about 10 minutes.

In a medium bowl, combine broth, cornstarch, syrup, vinegar, ketchup, soy sauce, sesame oil, and garlic. Whisk until cornstarch has dissolved.

Bring a skillet sprayed with nonstick spray to medium heat. Cook and stir broth mixture until thickened, 1 to 2 minutes.

Remove skillet from heat, add chicken, and toss to coat. Serve topped with sesame seeds and scallions!

MAKES 2 SERVINGS

VEGGIE-LOADED CASHEW CHICKEN

318 calories PER SERVING

You'll Need: medium bowl, wok (or large skillet), nonstick spray
Prep: 15 minutes
Cook: 15 minutes

½ of recipe (about 1½ cups): 318 calories, 9.5g fat, 863mg sodium, 25g carbs, 3g fiber, 10g sugars, 33.5g protein

INGREDIENTS

½ cup fat-free chicken broth
½ tablespoon cornstarch
1 tablespoon reduced-sodium/lite soy sauce
1 tablespoon seasoned rice vinegar
¼ teaspoon ground ginger
2 cups quartered mushrooms
1 cup chopped onion
1 teaspoon chopped garlic
8 ounces raw boneless skinless chicken breast, cut into bite-sized pieces
⅛ teaspoon each salt and black pepper
1 cup snow peas
¼ cup unsalted roasted cashews
2 tablespoons chopped scallions

DIRECTIONS

In a medium bowl, stir cornstarch into broth until dissolved. Mix in soy sauce, vinegar, and ginger.

Bring a wok (or large skillet) sprayed with nonstick spray to medium-high heat. Add mushrooms, onion, and garlic. Cook and stir until slightly softened, 5 to 6 minutes.

Season chicken with salt and pepper and add to the wok. Add snow peas and cashews. Cook and stir for about 4 minutes, until chicken is fully cooked.

Stir sauce mixture and add to the wok. Cook and stir until sauce has slightly thickened, about 2 minutes.

Top with scallions and dig in!

MAKES 2 SERVINGS

MMMMM MOO SHU CHICKEN

121 calories PER SERVING

You'll Need: medium bowl, wok (or large skillet), nonstick spray
Prep: 10 minutes
Cook: 10 minutes

⅕th of recipe (1 heaping cup): 121 calories, 1g fat, 835mg sodium, 15g carbs, 4.5g fiber, 6.5g sugars, 12.5g protein

INGREDIENTS

3 tablespoons reduced-sodium/lite soy sauce
3 tablespoons seasoned rice vinegar
1 teaspoon crushed garlic
½ teaspoon cornstarch
Dash black pepper
6 ounces raw boneless skinless chicken breast, cut into thin strips
One 12-ounce bag (4 cups) broccoli cole slaw
One 8-ounce can straw mushrooms, drained
½ cup canned bamboo shoots, drained and cut into thin strips
1 cup bean sprouts
2 tablespoons plus 2 teaspoons hoisin sauce

DIRECTIONS

To make the moo shu sauce, in a medium bowl, combine soy sauce, vinegar, garlic, cornstarch, and pepper. Mix until cornstarch dissolves.

Bring a wok (or large skillet) sprayed with nonstick spray to medium-high heat. Cook and stir chicken until no longer pink, about 2 minutes. Add slaw and cook and stir until soft, 3 to 4 minutes.

Add mushrooms, bamboo shoots, bean sprouts, and moo shu sauce. Cook and stir until sauce has thickened and chicken is cooked through, 3 to 4 minutes.

Serve drizzled with hoisin sauce. Mmmm!!!

MAKES 5 SERVINGS

HG TIP!
Try our moo shu wrapped in warm high-fiber flour tortillas. SO GOOD!

OH HONEY! WALNUT SHRIMP

208 calories
PER SERVING

You'll Need: baking sheet, nonstick spray, 2 wide bowls, medium bowl, small microwave-safe bowl, whisk
Prep: 15 minutes | **Cook:** 15 minutes

½ of recipe (about 7 shrimp):
208 calories, 4g fat, 658mg sodium, 18.5g carbs, 1g fiber, 10g sugars, 24g protein

INGREDIENTS

2½ tablespoons whole-wheat flour

2 dashes salt

Dash black pepper

8 ounces (about 14) raw large shrimp, peeled, tails removed, deveined

2 tablespoons fat-free liquid egg substitute

2 tablespoons fat-free mayonnaise

1 tablespoon honey

1 drop lemon juice

Dash chili powder

1 tablespoon chopped walnuts

DIRECTIONS

Preheat oven to 375 degrees. Spray a baking sheet with nonstick spray.

In a wide bowl, mix flour with a dash each salt and pepper.

Place shrimp in another wide bowl and pat dry. Top with egg substitute and toss to coat.

One at a time, gently shake shrimp to remove excess egg substitute and transfer to the seasoned flour; flip to evenly coat. Place on the baking sheet, evenly spaced.

Lightly mist shrimp with nonstick spray. Bake for 5 minutes. Flip shrimp. Bake until cooked through and slightly crispy, about 5 more minutes. Transfer to a medium bowl.

Meanwhile, in a small microwave-safe bowl, combine mayo, honey, lemon juice, chili powder, and remaining dash salt. Whisk until smooth.

Just before serving, microwave mayo mixture for 20 seconds, or until hot. Stir until smooth. Add to the shrimp bowl and toss to coat. Serve topped with walnuts. Enjoy!

MAKES 2 SERVINGS

HG HEADS UP:
Consume immediately! (This recipe does not refrigerate well.)

SWEET & STICKY ORANGE CHICKEN

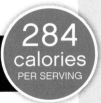

284 calories PER SERVING

You'll Need: baking sheet, nonstick spray, wide bowl, large bowl, medium bowl, whisk, skillet
Prep: 35 minutes | **Cook:** 15 minutes

½ of recipe (about 1 cup):
284 calories, 2g fat, 765mg sodium, 26g carbs, 2g fiber, 8.5g sugars, 37g protein

INGREDIENTS

¼ cup whole-wheat flour

10 ounces raw boneless skinless chicken breast, cut into bite-sized pieces

¼ cup fat-free liquid egg substitute

¼ cup fat-free chicken broth

1 tablespoon cornstarch

1½ tablespoons low-sugar orange marmalade

1½ tablespoons seasoned rice vinegar

1 tablespoon Splenda No Calorie Sweetener (granulated)

1 tablespoon reduced-sodium/lite soy sauce

1 teaspoon chopped garlic

1 teaspoon chopped ginger

Dash red pepper flakes

2 tablespoons chopped scallions

DIRECTIONS

Preheat oven to 375 degrees. Spray a baking sheet with nonstick spray.

Place flour in a wide bowl.

Place chicken in a large bowl, top with egg substitute, and toss to coat.

One at a time, shake chicken pieces to remove excess egg and coat with flour. Evenly lay on the baking sheet.

Bake until chicken is cooked through, about 10 minutes.

In a medium bowl, whisk broth with cornstarch until cornstarch has dissolved. Add marmalade, vinegar, sweetener, and soy sauce, and thoroughly whisk.

Bring a skillet sprayed with nonstick spray to medium heat. Cook and stir garlic and ginger until slightly softened and fragrant, about 1 minute.

Add broth mixture and red pepper flakes. Cook and stir until well mixed and slightly thickened, 1 to 2 minutes.

Remove skillet from heat, add chicken, and toss to coat. Serve topped with scallions and enjoy!

MAKES 2 SERVINGS

HG SWEET ALTERNATIVE!

Swap out the Splenda for the same amount of granulated white sugar, and each serving will have 305 calories, 31.5g carbs, and 14.5g sugars.

For more recipes, tips & tricks, sign up for FREE daily emails at hungry-girl.com!

ORANGE BEEF STIR-FRY

359 calories

You'll Need: medium bowl, whisk, large skillet, nonstick spray
Prep: 15 minutes
Marinate: 10 minutes
Cook: 10 minutes

Entire recipe: 359 calories, 9g fat, 784mg sodium, 40g carbs, 9.5g fiber, 20g sugars, 33g protein

INGREDIENTS

1 tablespoon low-sugar orange marmalade
½ tablespoon reduced-sodium/lite soy sauce
½ tablespoon seasoned rice vinegar
½ tablespoon cornstarch
¼ teaspoon ground ginger
⅛ teaspoon garlic powder
4 ounces raw lean beefsteak filet
Dash salt
2 cups broccoli florets
1 cup chopped red bell pepper
½ cup shredded carrots

Optional seasonings: salt, black pepper, red pepper flakes

DIRECTIONS

In a medium bowl, thoroughly mix marmalade with soy sauce. Add vinegar, cornstarch, ginger, and garlic powder. Add ⅓ cup water and whisk until cornstarch dissolves.

Season beef with salt and thinly slice. Add to the bowl and coat well. Cover and marinate in the fridge for 10 minutes.

Bring a large skillet sprayed with nonstick spray to medium-high heat. Add broccoli, bell pepper, carrots, and ¼ cup of the marinade. Cook and stir until slightly softened, about 5 minutes.

Add beef and remaining marinade. Cook and stir until veggies are tender and beef is cooked through, about 3 minutes. Eat!

MAKES 1 SERVING

WOWOWOW! KUNG PAO

245 calories
PER SERVING

You'll Need: medium bowl, wok (or large skillet), nonstick spray
Prep: 10 minutes
Cook: 10 minutes

½ of recipe (about 1½ cups): 245 calories, 4g fat, 720mg sodium, 21g carbs, 3g fiber, 11g sugars, 30g protein

INGREDIENTS

2 tablespoons reduced-sodium/lite soy sauce
1½ tablespoons rice vinegar
2 teaspoons granulated white sugar
½ tablespoon cornstarch
1 teaspoon Asian chili sauce, or more to taste
8 ounces raw boneless skinless chicken breast, cubed
⅛ teaspoon each salt and black pepper
¾ cup roughly chopped mushrooms
¾ cup roughly chopped bell pepper
½ cup chopped celery
½ cup chopped onion
1 teaspoon minced garlic
¼ cup canned sliced water chestnuts, drained and halved
1 tablespoon chopped dry-roasted unsalted peanuts

Optional seasoning: red pepper flakes

DIRECTIONS

To make the sauce, in a medium bowl, combine soy sauce, vinegar, sugar, cornstarch, and chili sauce. Add 2 tablespoons cold water and stir until cornstarch has dissolved.

Bring a wok (or large skillet) sprayed with nonstick spray to medium-high heat. Add chicken and season with salt and black pepper. Add mushrooms, bell pepper, celery, onion, garlic, and 2 tablespoons water. Cook and stir for about 7 minutes, until chicken is fully cooked.

Add water chestnuts and peanuts and raise heat to high. Stir sauce and add to wok. Cook and stir until sauce has thickened, 1 to 2 minutes. Enjoy!

MAKES 2 SERVINGS

HG SWEET ALTERNATIVE!

If made with an equal amount of Splenda No Calorie Sweetener (granulated) in place of the sugar, each serving will have 231 calories, 17g carbs, and 7g sugars.

SWEET & SOUR CHICKEN 1-2-3

295 calories PER SERVING

You'll Need: wok (or large skillet) with a lid, nonstick spray, small nonstick pot
Prep: 15 minutes | **Cook:** 20 minutes

⅓rd of recipe (about 2 cups):
295 calories, 2g fat, 730mg sodium, 37g carbs, 5.25g fiber, 27g sugars, 30g protein

INGREDIENTS

12 ounces raw boneless skinless chicken breast,
    cut into bite-sized pieces

⅛ teaspoon each salt and black pepper

1½ cups broccoli florets

1 cup chopped red bell pepper

1 cup chopped celery

16 ounces pineapple chunks packed in juice
    (not drained)

1 tablespoon cornstarch

3 tablespoons seasoned rice vinegar

1 tablespoon ketchup

1 tablespoon reduced-sodium/lite soy sauce

½ teaspoon chopped garlic

¼ teaspoon red pepper flakes

⅛ teaspoon ground ginger

2 cups bean sprouts

DIRECTIONS

Bring a wok (or large skillet) sprayed with nonstick spray to medium-high heat. Add chicken and season with salt and black pepper. Cook and stir until no longer pink, about 3 minutes.

Add broccoli, bell pepper, celery, and 2 tablespoons water. Cover and cook until veggies are tender, about 8 minutes.

Meanwhile, to make the sauce, drain the juice from the canned pineapple into a small nonstick pot. Add cornstarch and stir to dissolve. Add vinegar, ketchup, soy sauce, garlic, red pepper flakes, and ginger. Mix thoroughly. Bring to medium-high heat. Cook and stir until thickened, about 3 minutes.

Add pineapple chunks, bean sprouts, and sauce to the wok. Cook and stir until sprouts have softened and chicken is fully cooked, about 4 minutes. Enjoy!

MAKES 3 SERVINGS

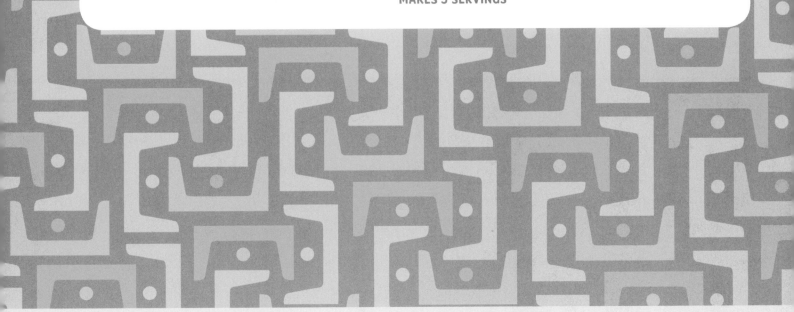

CHAPTER 14

COMFORTABLY YUM

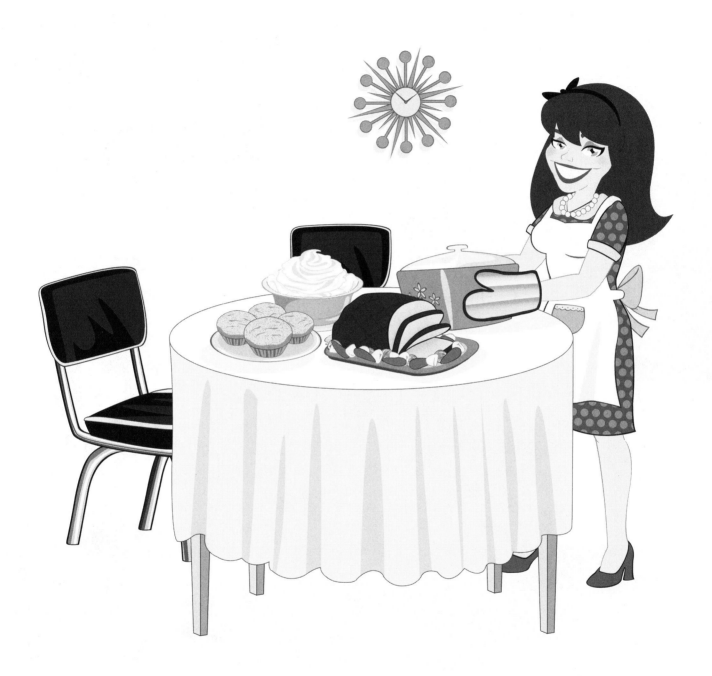

COMFORTABLY YUM

Corn MegaMuffins
Cheery Cherry Corn Muffins
Corndog Millionaire Muffins
Hungry Chick 'n Dumpling Surprise
BLT Hash Browns
Spaghetti Squash Hash Browns
Dan-Good Chili
Crazy Glazy Roast Pork Tenderloin
Crazy-Good Turkey Taco Meatloaf
Sweet & Sour Meatloaf
Southwestern Meatloaf
Big Beef 'n Bacon Meatloaf
Turkey & Veggie Meatloaf Minis
Big Southern-Style B-fast Trifle
Floosh's Stuffed Cabbage
Hungry Swirl Butternut Casserole
Loaded Hot Dog Casserole
Not-Your-Mom's Tater Tot Casserole
Rockin' Tuna Noodle Casserole
Shrimp & Tomato Faux-sotto
Creamy Pumpkin Faux-sotto
2-Good Twice-Baked Potato
Super-Sized Kickin' Chicken Pot Pie
Baked Chili Surprise
Twice-Baked Spaghetti Squash
Miracle Mashies
Great Garlic Miracle Mashies

Caramelized Onion Mashies
3-Cheese Miracle Mashies
Cheesy Scalloped Potatoes 'n Turnips
Super Stuffed Eggplant
Sloppy Janes
Chicken Pot Pockets
Hungry-licious Chicken Marsala
Shrimp & Grits for Hungry Chicks
Apple 'n Jack Grilled Cheese
Jalapeño Popper Grilled Cheese
BBQ Chicken Grilled Cheese
Grilled Cheese Dunkin' Duo
Greek Grilled Cheese
Hungry Grilled Graceland Special
Squash-tastic Shepherd's Pie
Hungry Chick Shepherd's Pie
Petite Wonton-Bottomed Shepherd's Pies
Too-EZ Mac 'n Cheese
Mega Mac & Cheese
BLT-rific Mac 'n Cheese
Buffalo Chicken Mac & Cheese
Bolognese-y Mac & Cheesy
Baked Pumpkin Mac & Cheese
Hot-Diggity Dog Cheesy Mac
BBQ Chicken Mac & Cheese
Sun-Dried Tomato Mac & Cheese

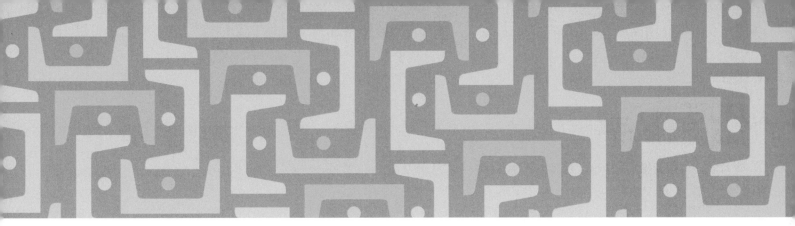

Comfort food makes us feel all warm and squishy inside. Everything about it is AWESOME—except the high calorie and fat counts associated with it. So we HG-ified TONS of favorites just for you—zapped 'em of their embarrassing stats. We don't blame you for tearing up. Go ahead, hug the book. Just do it—you know you want to!

A QUICK GUIDE TO SYMBOLS:

15 Minutes or Less

This symbol lets you know a recipe should take you no more than fifteen minutes from start to finish! That includes prep and cook time.

30 Minutes or Less

Just like the 15-minute version, this one points out recipes that take 30 minutes or less to whip up.

Meatless

You guessed it—no meat here! That includes beef, poultry, and fish. Some recipes give the option of a meatless ingredient. If you want your meal without meat, go with the meatless choice.

Single Serving

Pretty straightforward. These are recipes for one.

5 Ingredients or Less

Fans of HG know that we like to keep things simple. And these recipes contain just five ingredients or less!

Photos

These recipes can be seen in one of the book's photo inserts. The number in the symbol tells you which insert. Find photos of all the recipes at hungry-girl.com/books!

MUFFINS . . .
MADE OF CORN . . .
with various surprises inside. Yay!

CORN MEGAMUFFINS

158 calories PER SERVING

You'll Need: 12-cup muffin pan, foil baking cups or nonstick spray, large bowl, medium bowl
Prep: 10 minutes | **Cook:** 20 minutes

⅑th of recipe (1 muffin):
158 calories, 0.5g fat, 358mg sodium, 32g carbs, 1.5g fiber, 9g sugars, 6g protein

INGREDIENTS

1 cup all-purpose flour
¾ cup yellow cornmeal
¼ cup Splenda No Calorie Sweetener (granulated)
¼ cup granulated white sugar
1 tablespoon baking powder
¼ teaspoon salt
1 ½ cups canned cream-style corn
¾ cup fat-free liquid egg substitute
¾ cup fat-free plain Greek yogurt

DIRECTIONS

Preheat oven to 375 degrees. Line 9 cups of a 12-cup muffin pan with foil baking cups, or spray them with nonstick spray.

In a large bowl, mix flour, cornmeal, Splenda, sugar, baking powder, and salt.

In a medium bowl, thoroughly mix cream-style corn, egg substitute, and yogurt. Transfer contents to the large bowl and stir well.

Evenly distribute batter among the 9 lined or sprayed cups—cups will be FULL to the brims.

Bake until a toothpick inserted into the center of a muffin comes out clean, 15 to 20 minutes. Eat up!

MAKES 9 SERVINGS

HG SWEET ALTERNATIVE!

Skip the Splenda in this recipe and double the granulated white sugar; each muffin will have 177 calories, 37g carbs, and 14.5g sugars. Or double the Splenda and leave out the sugar; then each muffin will have 139 calories, 27g carbs, and 3.5g sugars. Swell!

CHEERY CHERRY CORN MUFFINS

You'll Need: 12-cup muffin pan, foil baking cups or nonstick spray, microwave-safe bowl, blender or large food processor, large bowl, medium bowl
Prep: 10 minutes
Cook: 35 minutes

1/12th of recipe (1 muffin): 158 calories, 0.5g fat, 267mg sodium, 33g carbs, 1.5g fiber, 15g sugars, 5g protein

INGREDIENTS

2 cups frozen unsweetened pitted dark sweet cherries
½ cup plus 1 tablespoon granulated white sugar
1 cup all-purpose flour
¾ cup yellow cornmeal
1 tablespoon baking powder
¼ teaspoon salt
One 14.75-ounce can cream-style corn
¾ cup fat-free liquid egg substitute
⅔ cup fat-free plain Greek yogurt

DIRECTIONS

Preheat oven to 375 degrees. Line a 12-cup muffin pan with foil baking cups, or spray it with nonstick spray.

Microwave cherries in a microwave-safe bowl for 1 to 2 minutes, until completely thawed. Do not drain.

Transfer cherries and excess liquid to a blender or large food processor. Add 1 tablespoon sugar. Pulse briefly, just until cherries reach a roughly chopped consistency.

In a large bowl, mix flour, cornmeal, baking powder, salt, and remaining ½ cup sugar.

In a medium bowl, thoroughly mix cream-style corn, egg substitute, and yogurt. Transfer contents to the large bowl and stir well.

Add cherry mixture to the large bowl and stir. Evenly distribute batter among the muffin cups—cups will be FULL to the brims.

Bake until a toothpick inserted into the center of a muffin comes out clean, 25 to 30 minutes. Enjoy!

MAKES 12 SERVINGS

HG SWEET ALTERNATIVE!

If made with an equal amount of Splenda No Calorie Sweetener (granulated) in place of the sugar, each muffin will have 127 calories, 24.5g carbs, and 5.5g sugars.

CORNDOG MILLIONAIRE MUFFINS

You'll Need: 12-cup muffin pan, foil baking cups or nonstick spray, large bowl, medium bowl
Prep: 15 minutes
Cook: 20 minutes

1/8th of recipe (1 muffin): 160 calories, 2g fat, 636mg sodium, 27g carbs, 1g fiber, 6.5g sugars, 9g protein

INGREDIENTS

⅔ cup all-purpose flour
½ cup yellow cornmeal
2½ tablespoons Splenda No Calorie Sweetener (granulated)
2½ tablespoons granulated white sugar
1½ teaspoons baking powder
¼ teaspoon salt
1 cup canned cream-style corn
½ cup fat-free liquid egg substitute
½ cup fat-free sour cream
7 hot dogs with about 40 calories and 1g fat or less each

DIRECTIONS

Preheat oven to 375 degrees. Line 8 cups of a 12-cup muffin pan with foil baking cups, or spray them with nonstick spray.

In a large bowl, mix flour, cornmeal, Splenda, sugar, baking powder, and salt.

In a medium bowl, thoroughly mix cream-style corn, egg substitute, and sour cream. Transfer contents to the large bowl and stir well.

Finely chop 5 hot dogs and stir into the contents of the large bowl. Evenly distribute batter among the 8 lined or sprayed cups.

Cut remaining 2 hot dogs into a total of 24 coins. Place 3 coins on top of each muffin cup.

Bake until a toothpick inserted into the center of a muffin comes out clean, 15 to 20 minutes. Dig in!

MAKES 8 SERVINGS

HG SWEET ALTERNATIVE!

Skip the Splenda in this recipe and double the granulated white sugar; each muffin will have 173 calories, 30.5g carbs, and 10.5g sugars. Or double the Splenda and leave out the sugar; then each muffin will have 147 calories, 23.5g carbs, and 2.5g sugars.

HUNGRY CHICK 'N DUMPLING SURPRISE

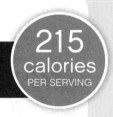
215 calories PER SERVING

You'll Need: extra-large pot with a lid, nonstick spray, 2 medium bowls
Prep: 20 minutes | **Cook:** 50 minutes

⅛th of recipe (about 1½ cups stew with 2 dumplings):
215 calories, 3g fat, 845mg sodium, 30g carbs, 4g fiber, 7.5g sugars, 16.5g protein

INGREDIENTS

Stew
3 large stalks celery, chopped

3 medium carrots, peeled and chopped

1 large onion, chopped

1 teaspoon chopped garlic

Two 14.5-ounce cans (about 3½ cups)
    fat-free chicken broth

12 ounces raw boneless skinless chicken breast

3 cups sliced mushrooms

½ teaspoon dried thyme

¼ teaspoon black pepper

1 dried bay leaf

One 10.75-ounce can 98% fat-free cream
    of chicken condensed soup

2 cups frozen peas

Dumplings
1½ cups Bisquick Heart Smart baking mix

⅔ cup fat-free milk

⅛ teaspoon each salt and black pepper

HG TIP:
Store leftover stew and dumplings separately to prevent soggy dumplings.

DIRECTIONS

Bring an extra-large pot sprayed with nonstick spray to medium-high heat. Add celery, carrots, onion, and garlic. Cook and stir until slightly softened, 6 to 8 minutes.

Add chicken broth, chicken breast, mushrooms, thyme, pepper, bay leaf, and 2 cups water. Stir well. Cover and bring to a boil.

Reduce to a simmer and cook for 25 minutes, or until chicken is cooked through.

Transfer chicken to a medium bowl. Re-cover pot, and let contents continue to simmer. Shred chicken with two forks—one to hold the chicken in place and the other to scrape across and shred it.

Add shredded chicken, condensed soup, and frozen peas to the pot. Stir thoroughly and return to a simmer.

Meanwhile, in a medium bowl, gently mix dumpling ingredients just until a soft dough forms; don't overmix.

Once stew is simmering, add dough in heaping tablespoons to form about 16 dumplings; add it slowly and evenly so dumplings don't stick together.

Cook for 5 minutes. Gently turn dumplings over and cook until firm, 5 to 7 minutes.

Remove and discard bay leaf, and serve it up!

MAKES 8 SERVINGS

BLT HASH BROWNS

220 calories PER SERVING

You'll Need: large skillet, nonstick spray
Prep: 10 minutes
Cook: 30 minutes

½ **of recipe:** 220 calories, 4g fat, 367mg sodium, 38g carbs, 4g fiber, 4g sugars, 9g protein

INGREDIENTS

3 slices center-cut bacon or turkey bacon
¼ cup chopped red onion
3 cups chopped spinach leaves
12 ounces shredded russet potato (about 2 cups), thoroughly patted dry
2 tablespoons bagged sun-dried tomatoes (not packed in oil), roughly chopped
Dash each salt and black pepper

Optional topping: fat-free sour cream

DIRECTIONS

Bring a large skillet sprayed with nonstick spray to medium heat. Cook bacon until crispy, about 4 minutes per side.

Chop or crumble bacon and set aside. If needed, clean skillet. Remove from heat, re-spray, and return to medium heat. Cook and stir onion until slightly softened, about 3 minutes.

Add spinach and cook and stir until wilted and free of excess moisture, about 3 minutes. Add bacon, shredded potato, tomatoes, salt, and pepper, and thoroughly mix. Evenly spread out mixture and gently press with a spatula.

Without stirring, cook until potato has browned, 5 to 7 minutes.

Flip mixture and cook for 3 to 4 minutes, until potato is fully cooked and browned. Enjoy!

MAKES 2 SERVINGS

SPAGHETTI SQUASH HASH BROWNS

96 calories PER SERVING

You'll Need: large microwave-safe bowl, strainer, large bowl, skillet, nonstick spray
Prep: 10 minutes
Cook: 15 minutes

½ **of recipe:** 96 calories, 0.5g fat, 342mg sodium, 23g carbs, 4.5g fiber, 9g sugars, 2g protein

INGREDIENTS

Half a spaghetti squash (about 2¼ pounds), seeds removed, halved
½ cup chopped onion
½ teaspoon chopped garlic
½ teaspoon onion powder
¼ teaspoon salt
⅛ teaspoon black pepper

DIRECTIONS

Place squash in a large microwave-safe bowl with 2 tablespoons water. Cover and microwave for 8 minutes, or until soft.

Scrape squash strands into a strainer, and let excess moisture drain. Thoroughly pat dry.

Transfer squash strands to a large bowl. Thoroughly mix in all remaining ingredients.

Bring a skillet sprayed with nonstick spray to high heat. Add squash mixture, spread into an even layer, and cook for 2 minutes.

Flip mixture and cook until lightly browned, about 2 more minutes. Serve it up!

MAKES 2 SERVINGS

DAN-GOOD CHILI

120 calories
PER SERVING

You'll Need: large nonstick pot, large skillet, nonstick spray, slotted spoon
Prep: 15 minutes | **Cook:** 2 hours 15 minutes

⅒th of recipe (about 1 cup):
120 calories, 1g fat, 820mg sodium, 26g carbs, 6g fiber, 10g sugars, 6g protein

INGREDIENTS

4¼ cups canned tomato sauce

1 cup canned diced tomatoes with green chiles

½ cup jarred jalapeño slices, drained and chopped

1½ tablespoons chili powder

1 teaspoon ground cumin

1¾ cups peeled and chopped carrots

2 teaspoons crushed garlic

1½ cups chopped onion

1½ cups chopped portabella mushrooms

1 large red bell pepper, stem removed, seeded, chopped

1 large green bell pepper, stem removed, seeded, chopped

1 cup canned sweet corn kernels, drained

¾ cup canned black beans, drained and rinsed

¾ cup canned red kidney beans, drained and rinsed

Optional seasoning: salt

WHO'S DAN?

The same person who created the Dan-Good Cioppino . . . My husband!

DIRECTIONS

In a large nonstick pot, mix tomato sauce, diced tomatoes with green chiles, jalapeños, chili powder, and cumin. Set heat to low.

Once mixture is hot, add carrots and garlic. Stir and continue to cook for about 5 minutes.

Meanwhile, bring a large skillet sprayed with nonstick spray to medium heat. Add onion, mushrooms, peppers, ½ cup water and, if you like, a few dashes of salt. Cook and stir until veggies have slightly softened, about 5 minutes.

Using a slotted spoon to drain any excess water, transfer veggies from the skillet to the large pot. Add corn and beans to the pot as well. Mix thoroughly.

Cook over low heat for about 2 hours, stirring every 20 minutes or so, until all veggies are tender.

Serve it up!

MAKES 10 SERVINGS

CRAZY GLAZY ROAST PORK TENDERLOIN

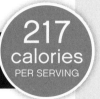

217 calories PER SERVING

You'll Need: small bowl, large sealable plastic bag, microwave-safe bowl, whisk, oven-safe skillet, nonstick spray
Prep: 15 minutes | **Marinate:** 1 hour | **Cook:** 25 minutes

¼th of recipe (about 3.25 ounces cooked pork with 2 tablespoons glaze):
217 calories, 4g fat, 560mg sodium, 18g carbs, <0.5g fiber, 14g sugars, 24g protein

INGREDIENTS

Marinade
2 tablespoons reduced-sodium/lite soy sauce

1 tablespoon Worcestershire sauce

1 tablespoon Dijon mustard

2 teaspoons brown sugar (not packed)

1 teaspoon crushed garlic

½ teaspoon ground ginger

Pork
One 1-pound raw pork tenderloin,
    trimmed of excess fat

Glaze
¼ cup jellied cranberry sauce

¼ cup low-sugar apricot preserves

2 tablespoons seasoned rice vinegar

1 tablespoon balsamic vinegar

DIRECTIONS

In a small bowl, mix marinade ingredients until sugar has mostly dissolved. Place pork and marinade in a large sealable plastic bag; remove air and seal. Gently knead marinade into meat through the bag. Marinate in the fridge for 1 hour.

Preheat oven to 425 degrees.

In a microwave-safe bowl, combine glaze ingredients. Whisk well.

Bring an oven-safe skillet sprayed with nonstick spray to high heat. Add pork and discard excess marinade. Evenly sear meat, rotating it occasionally, until dark on all sides, about 5 minutes total.

Place skillet in the oven and bake for 10 minutes. Spoon ⅓rd of the glaze (about ¼ cup) over the meat. Bake until pork center reaches 145 degrees, 5 to 10 minutes.

Remove pork from skillet and let rest for 10 minutes. Microwave remaining glaze for 30 seconds, or until warm.

Slice pork and serve with warm glaze, about 2 tablespoons per serving. YUM!

MAKES 4 SERVINGS

HG TIP:
If you're not sure if the skillet handle is oven-safe, wrap it in aluminum foil first.

For more recipes, tips & tricks, sign up for FREE daily emails at **hungry-girl.com!**

JUST LIKE MOM'S MEATLOAF . . .
only more interesting. And less fattening. Good stuff!

CRAZY-GOOD TURKEY TACO MEATLOAF

176 calories
PER SERVING

You'll Need: loaf pan, nonstick spray, skillet, large bowl | **Prep:** 10 minutes | **Cook:** 50 minutes

⅕th of loaf:
176 calories, 1.5g fat, 619mg sodium, 10.5g carbs, 1g fiber, 3g sugars, 29.5g protein

INGREDIENTS

¼ cup chopped green bell pepper

¼ cup chopped onion

1 pound raw extra-lean ground turkey

½ cup canned sweet corn kernels, drained

¼ cup fat-free liquid egg substitute

¼ cup quick-cooking oats

1 tablespoon taco seasoning mix

2 slices fat-free cheddar cheese

½ cup salsa

½ cup shredded fat-free cheddar cheese

DIRECTIONS

Preheat oven to 375 degrees. Spray a loaf pan with nonstick spray.

Bring a skillet sprayed with nonstick spray to medium heat. Cook and stir pepper and onion until slightly softened, about 3 minutes.

Transfer veggies to a large bowl. Add turkey, corn, egg substitute, oats, and taco seasoning, and thoroughly mix.

Evenly transfer half of the mixture to the loaf pan. Evenly top with cheese slices, followed by remaining meat mixture. Top with salsa.

Bake for 30 minutes.

Top loaf with shredded cheese. Bake until loaf is cooked through and shredded cheese has melted, about 15 minutes. Enjoy!

MAKES 5 SERVINGS

MEATLOAF TIP!

If needed, smooth out the surface of your loaf with the back of a spatula or spoon. Everyone likes an attractive loaf!

SWEET & SOUR MEATLOAF

227 calories
PER SERVING

You'll Need: loaf pan, nonstick spray, large bowl, small bowl
Prep: 20 minutes
Cook: 50 minutes

⅕th of loaf: 227 calories, 5g fat, 521mg sodium, 17.5g carbs, 0.5g fiber, 11g sugars, 25g protein

INGREDIENTS

Loaf
¼ cup chili sauce (the kind stocked near the ketchup)
¼ cup low-sugar grape jelly
1¼ pounds raw extra-lean ground beef
½ cup chopped onion
¼ cup quick-cooking oats
¼ cup fat-free liquid egg substitute
¼ teaspoon each salt and black pepper

Topping
2 tablespoons chili sauce (the kind stocked near the ketchup)
2 tablespoons low-sugar grape jelly

DIRECTIONS

Preheat oven to 400 degrees. Spray a loaf pan with nonstick spray.

To make the loaf, mix chili sauce with jelly in a large bowl. Add all other loaf ingredients and thoroughly mix. Transfer to the loaf pan.

In a small bowl, mix topping ingredients. Evenly spread topping over the loaf.

Bake until loaf is cooked through, about 50 minutes. Slice, serve, and enjoy!

MAKES 5 SERVINGS

SOUTHWESTERN MEATLOAF

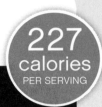
232 calories
PER SERVING

You'll Need: loaf pan, nonstick spray, skillet, large bowl
Prep: 10 minutes
Cook: 1 hour

⅕th of loaf: 232 calories, 6g fat, 565mg sodium, 14g carbs, 2.5g fiber, 5g sugars, 28.5g protein

INGREDIENTS

½ cup chopped red bell pepper
½ cup chopped onion
1¼ pounds raw extra-lean ground beef
¾ cup canned crushed tomatoes
¼ cup quick-cooking oats
¼ cup fat-free liquid egg substitute
¼ cup frozen sweet corn kernels, thawed
¼ cup canned black beans, drained and rinsed
½ teaspoon salt
¼ teaspoon black pepper
¼ teaspoon chili powder
2 tablespoons ketchup
¼ cup shredded reduced-fat Mexican-blend cheese

DIRECTIONS

Preheat oven to 400 degrees. Spray a loaf pan with nonstick spray.

Bring a skillet sprayed with nonstick spray to medium heat. Cook and stir bell pepper and onion until softened and lightly browned, 5 to 7 minutes.

Transfer pepper and onion to a large bowl, and pat dry. Add all remaining ingredients *except* ketchup and cheese. Mix thoroughly.

Transfer mixture to the loaf pan and evenly top with ketchup. Bake for 45 minutes.

Sprinkle meatloaf with cheese. Bake until loaf is cooked through and cheese has melted, about 5 minutes. Slice, serve, and eat!

MAKES 5 SERVINGS

BIG BEEF 'N BACON MEATLOAF

224 calories PER SERVING

You'll Need: loaf pan, nonstick spray, large skillet, microwave-safe plate (optional), large bowl, small bowl
Prep: 15 minutes
Cook: 1 hour 5 minutes

⅕th of loaf: 224 calories, 8g fat, 707mg sodium, 10g carbs, 1g fiber, 7g sugars, 26g protein

INGREDIENTS

6 slices center-cut bacon or turkey bacon
1 cup chopped mushrooms
½ cup chopped onion
1¼ pounds raw extra-lean ground beef
½ cup canned crushed tomatoes
3 tablespoons hickory-flavored BBQ sauce
½ teaspoon salt
¼ teaspoon black pepper
¼ teaspoon onion powder
¼ teaspoon garlic powder
2 tablespoons ketchup

DIRECTIONS

Preheat oven to 400 degrees. Spray a loaf pan with nonstick spray.

Cook bacon until crispy, either in a large skillet over medium heat or on a microwave-safe plate in the microwave. (See package for cook time.)

Bring a large skillet sprayed with nonstick spray to medium heat. Cook and stir mushrooms and onion until completely softened, 5 to 7 minutes.

Transfer veggies to a large bowl and pat dry. Chop or crumble 4 slices of bacon and add to the bowl. Add beef, tomatoes, 2 tablespoons BBQ sauce, salt, pepper, onion powder, and garlic powder. Mix thoroughly. Transfer to the loaf pan.

In a small bowl, mix ketchup with remaining 1 tablespoon BBQ sauce. Evenly spread mixture over the meatloaf.

Chop or crumble remaining 2 slices bacon and sprinkle over the loaf.

Bake until loaf is cooked through, about 50 minutes. Slice, serve, and enjoy!

MAKES 5 SERVINGS

TURKEY & VEGGIE MEATLOAF MINIS

142 calories PER SERVING

You'll Need: 12-cup muffin pan, foil baking cups or nonstick spray, box grater, large bowl
Prep: 15 minutes
Cook: 35 minutes

⅑th of recipe (1 mini meatloaf): 142 calories, 5.25g fat, 494mg sodium, 9g carbs, 1.5g fiber, 4g sugars, 14g protein

INGREDIENTS

1 small onion
¼ cup plus 3 tablespoons ketchup
1¼ pounds raw lean ground turkey
3 cups bagged broccoli cole slaw, roughly chopped
½ cup fat-free liquid egg substitute
½ cup quick-cooking oats
2 teaspoons garlic powder
1 teaspoon salt

DIRECTIONS

Preheat oven to 350 degrees. Line 9 cups of a 12-cup muffin pan with foil baking cups, or spray them with nonstick spray.

Grate onion into a large bowl. Add ¼ cup ketchup and all other ingredients. Thoroughly mix.

Evenly distribute turkey-veggie mixture among the muffin cups and top with ketchup, 1 teaspoon each.

Bake until firm with lightly browned edges, 30 to 35 minutes. Enjoy!

MAKES 9 SERVINGS

BIG SOUTHERN-STYLE B-FAST TRIFLE

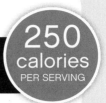

250 calories PER SERVING

You'll Need: medium pot, large serving bowl, skillet, nonstick spray | **Prep:** 10 minutes | **Cook:** 30 minutes

¼th of trifle (about 1¾ cups):
250 calories, 5g fat, 883mg sodium, 25g carbs, 3g fiber, 5g sugars, 24.5g protein

INGREDIENTS

½ cup quick-cooking grits

¼ teaspoon each salt and black pepper

2 wedges The Laughing Cow Light Creamy Swiss cheese

½ cup shredded fat-free cheddar cheese

1 cup chopped onion

1 cup chopped mushrooms

4 cups chopped spinach leaves

6 slices center-cut bacon or turkey bacon

2 cups fat-free liquid egg substitute

¼ teaspoon garlic powder

¼ teaspoon onion powder

1 cup diced tomatoes

Optional toppings: fat-free sour cream, chopped scallions

DIRECTIONS

In a medium pot, bring 2 cups water to a boil. Add grits and ⅛ teaspoon each salt and pepper.

Reduce heat to low. Cook and stir until water has fully absorbed, about 6 minutes.

Remove pot from heat. Thoroughly stir in cheese wedges, breaking them into pieces as you add them. Transfer to a large serving bowl. Sprinkle with cheddar cheese and cover to keep warm.

Bring a skillet sprayed with nonstick spray to medium-high heat. Add onion, mushrooms, and remaining ⅛ teaspoon each salt and pepper. Cook and stir until veggies have browned and softened, about 6 minutes. Add spinach and cook and stir until just wilted, about 1 minute.

Evenly layer veggies over cheesy grits, and re-cover to keep warm.

Remove skillet from heat, re-spray, and bring to medium heat. Cook bacon until crispy, about 4 minutes per side.

Remove bacon and set aside. If needed, clean skillet. Re-spray skillet and return to medium heat. Add egg substitute and sprinkle with garlic powder and onion powder. Scramble until fully cooked, about 5 minutes.

Evenly layer scrambled egg mixture over veggies. Chop or crumble bacon and sprinkle over eggs. Evenly top with tomatoes. Eat up!

MAKES 4 SERVINGS

FLOOSH'S STUFFED CABBAGE

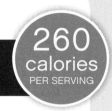

You'll Need: extra-large pot with a lid, large bowl, medium bowl, nonstick spray
Prep: 45 minutes | **Cook:** 1 hour 10 minutes

⅐th of recipe (2 cabbage rolls with sauce):
260 calories, 6.5g fat, 629mg sodium, 32.5g carbs, 3g fiber, 24g sugars, 18g protein

INGREDIENTS

Cabbage
1 extra-large head green cabbage (large enough to yield 14 large leaves), core carefully removed with a sharp knife

Filling
1¼ pounds raw lean ground turkey
¾ cup finely chopped onion
⅓ cup ketchup
1½ tablespoons tomato paste
1 tablespoon granulated white sugar or Splenda No Calorie Sweetener (granulated)
½ tablespoon chopped garlic

Sauce
2 cups low-fat marinara sauce
¾ cup jellied cranberry sauce
⅓ cup low-sugar grape jelly
⅓ teaspoon salt

DIRECTIONS

Place cored cabbage head in an extra-large pot and cover with water. Bring to a boil.

Cover and cook, rotating cabbage occasionally, until the leaves soften, loosen, and begin to fall off the head, 5 to 7 minutes. Remove pot from heat. Drain cabbage and set aside to cool.

Meanwhile, in a large bowl, thoroughly mix filling ingredients. In a medium bowl, mix sauce ingredients.

Gently remove 14 large leaves from cabbage head. (Refrigerate the rest for another use.)

Lay one cabbage leaf on a dry surface and top with 2 heaping tablespoons filling (¼th of filling). Spread out filling, fold in the sides of the cabbage, and roll up cabbage to enclose the filling.

Spray the extra-large pot with nonstick spray, and place cabbage roll in the pot, seam side down. Repeat with remaining 13 leaves and filling, gently stacking the rolls in the pot.

Cover cabbage rolls with prepared sauce. Cover the pot and set temperature to low. Cook for 1 hour, or until filling is cooked through. Enjoy!

MAKES 7 SERVINGS

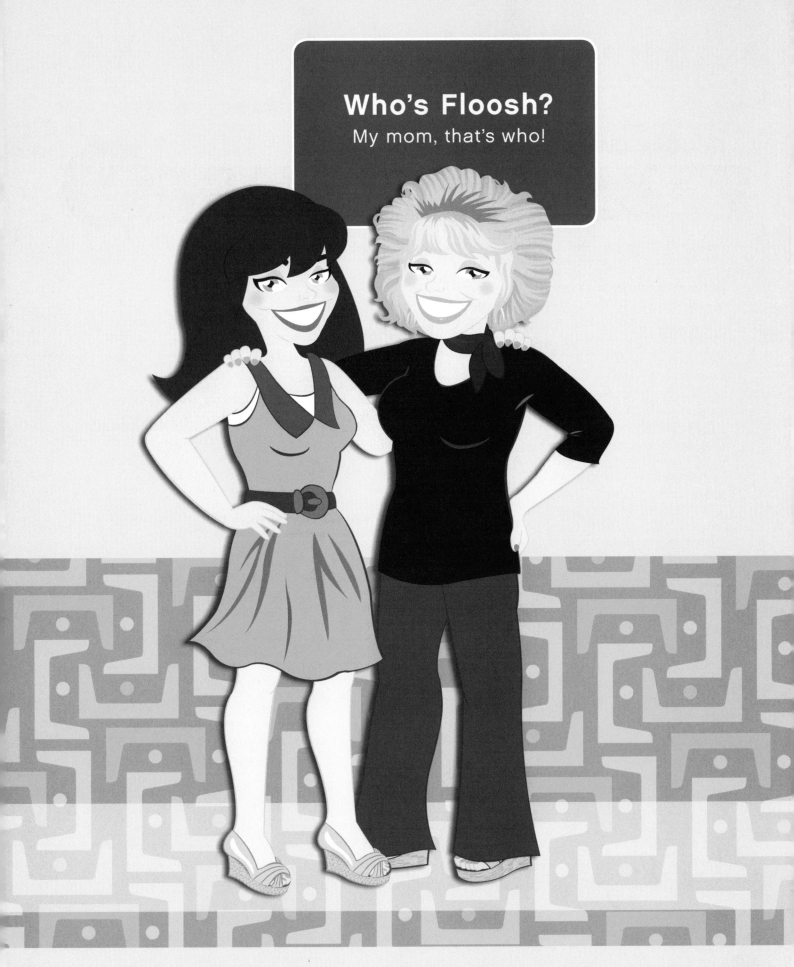

These CASSEROLES are baked and beautiful . . .

HUNGRY SWIRL BUTTERNUT CASSEROLE

146 calories PER SERVING

You'll Need: 2 large pots, 2 large bowls, potato masher, 8-inch by 8-inch baking pan, nonstick spray
Prep: 20 minutes | **Cook:** 35 minutes

⅙th of casserole (about 1 cup):
146 calories, 2g fat, 331mg sodium, 26g carbs, 4g fiber, 5g sugars, 6g protein

INGREDIENTS

4 cups cubed butternut squash

3 cups cauliflower florets

One 12-ounce russet potato, peeled and cubed

¼ cup shredded fat-free cheddar cheese

¼ teaspoon salt, or more to taste

4 wedges The Laughing Cow Light Creamy Swiss cheese

3 tablespoons fat-free half & half

1 tablespoon light whipped butter or light buttery spread

½ teaspoon chopped garlic

2 dashes black pepper, or more to taste

DIRECTIONS

Bring 2 large pots of water to a boil.

Add butternut squash to one pot; add cauliflower and potato to the other pot. Once returned to a boil, reduce heat to medium. Cook until veggies are very tender, 15 to 20 minutes.

Meanwhile, preheat broiler.

Drain and transfer cauliflower and potato to one large bowl. Drain and transfer squash to another large bowl.

Thoroughly mash squash. Add cheddar cheese, ⅛ teaspoon salt, and cheese wedges, breaking the wedges into pieces. Thoroughly stir.

To the bowl of cauliflower and potato, add half & half, butter, garlic, remaining ⅛ teaspoon salt, and pepper. Thoroughly mash.

Spray an 8-inch by 8-inch baking pan with nonstick spray. Spoon half of the squash mixture into one corner, and spoon the other half into the opposite corner. Evenly divide cauliflower-potato mixture between the two remaining corners.

Using a spoon, lightly swirl the mixtures together. Broil until top is crispy, about 8 to 10 minutes. Serve it up and enjoy!

MAKES 6 SERVINGS

LOADED HOT DOG CASSEROLE

179 calories PER SERVING

You'll Need: 8-inch by 8-inch baking pan, nonstick spray, large skillet, large bowl
Prep: 10 minutes
Cook: 50 minutes

⅙th of casserole (about 1½ cups):
179 calories, 2.5g fat, 806mg sodium, 24g carbs, 2g fiber, 6.5g sugars, 16g protein

INGREDIENTS

1 red bell pepper, stem removed, seeded, sliced into 2-inch strips
1 green bell pepper, stem removed, seeded, sliced into 2-inch strips
1 onion, sliced into 2-inch strips
7 hot dogs with about 40 calories and 1g fat or less each, cut into coins
4 hot dog buns, torn into pieces
1½ cups fat-free liquid egg substitute
¼ teaspoon garlic powder

Optional toppings: yellow mustard, ketchup

DIRECTIONS

Preheat oven to 350 degrees. Spray an 8-inch by 8-inch baking pan with nonstick spray.

Bring a large skillet sprayed with nonstick spray to high heat. Cook and stir peppers and onion until slightly blackened and softened, 8 to 10 minutes.

Transfer veggies to a large bowl. Add all remaining ingredients. Thoroughly stir.

Transfer mixture to the baking pan. Bake until firm and cooked through, 35 to 40 minutes. Mmmmmm!!!

MAKES 6 SERVINGS

NOT-YOUR-MOM'S TATER TOT CASSEROLE

273 calories PER SERVING

You'll Need: 8-inch by 8-inch baking pan, nonstick spray, large microwave-safe bowl, skillet
Prep: 10 minutes
Cook: 50 minutes

⅙th of casserole (about 1 cup): 273 calories, 7.5g fat, 880mg sodium, 35.5g carbs, 8g fiber, 5.5g sugars, 15.5g protein

INGREDIENTS

3 cups frozen chopped spinach
2 cups frozen petite mixed vegetables
2 cups frozen ground-beef-style soy crumbles
1 cup frozen shelled edamame
2 cups sliced mushrooms
1 cup chopped onion
1 teaspoon chopped garlic
One 10.75-ounce can 98% fat-free cream of mushroom condensed soup
36 frozen Ore-Ida Tater Tots (about 3 cups)

Optional seasonings: salt and black pepper

DIRECTIONS

Preheat oven to 375 degrees. Spray an 8-inch by 8-inch baking pan with nonstick spray.

Place frozen spinach, mixed veggies, soy crumbles, and edamame in a large microwave-safe bowl. Cover and microwave for 5 minutes. Stir well. Re-cover and microwave for 3 minutes, or until thawed.

Bring a skillet sprayed with nonstick spray to medium-high heat. Cook and stir mushrooms and onion until softened, about 6 minutes.

Drain any excess water from the large bowl. Stir in mushroom-onion mixture and garlic. Add condensed soup and stir to coat.

Evenly spoon mixture into the baking pan, and smooth out the surface. Place Tater Tots on top in a single layer.

Bake until inside is hot and Tater Tots are crispy, about 35 minutes. Serve it up!

MAKES 6 SERVINGS

ROCKIN' TUNA NOODLE CASSEROLE

167 calories PER SERVING

You'll Need: 8-inch by 8-inch baking pan, nonstick spray, strainer, large microwave-safe bowl
Prep: 10 minutes | **Cook:** 30 minutes

¼th of casserole:
167 calories, 5g fat, 882mg sodium, 14g carbs, 4g fiber, 2g sugars, 16.5g protein

INGREDIENTS

3 bags House Foods Tofu Shirataki Fettuccine Shaped Noodle Substitute

1 wedge The Laughing Cow Light Creamy Swiss cheese

6 ounces albacore tuna in water (two 3-ounce cans or about 1 large pouch), drained and flaked

½ cup frozen peas

One 10.75-ounce can 98% fat-free cream of mushroom condensed soup

3 tablespoons reduced-fat Parmesan-style grated topping

Optional seasonings: salt, black pepper, garlic powder, cayenne pepper

DIRECTIONS

Preheat oven to 375 degrees. Spray an 8-inch by 8-inch baking pan with nonstick spray.

Use a strainer to rinse and drain noodles. Thoroughly pat dry. Roughly cut noodles. In a large microwave-safe bowl, microwave noodles for 1 minute. Pat dry.

Add cheese wedge to noodles, breaking it into pieces. Microwave for 30 seconds, or until cheese has melted, and mix well.

Stir in tuna, peas, soup, and 1 tablespoon Parm-style topping. Transfer mixture to the baking pan.

Sprinkle with remaining 2 tablespoons Parm-style topping. Bake until hot and bubbly, 20 to 25 minutes. Enjoy!

MAKES 4 SERVINGS

Flip to the photo inserts to see over 100 recipe pics! And for photos of ALL the recipes, go to hungry-girl.com/books.

SHRIMP & TOMATO FAUX-SOTTO

407 calories PER SERVING

You'll Need: medium nonstick pot with a lid
Prep: 15 minutes
Cook: 45 minutes

½ of recipe (about 1¾ cups): 407 calories, 4.5g fat, 913mg sodium, 61.5g carbs, 7g fiber, 12.5g sugars, 27.5g protein

INGREDIENTS

1½ cups finely chopped cauliflower
1 cup diced onion
¾ cup fat-free chicken or vegetable broth
½ cup uncooked brown rice
¼ cup bagged sun-dried tomatoes
    (not packed in oil), chopped
1 teaspoon chopped garlic
⅛ teaspoon each salt and black pepper, or more to taste
6 ounces raw shrimp, peeled, tails removed, deveined
¼ cup chopped fresh basil
¼ cup fat-free sour cream
2 wedges The Laughing Cow Light Creamy Swiss cheese,
    room temperature

DIRECTIONS

In a medium nonstick pot, combine all ingredients *except* shrimp, basil, sour cream, and cheese wedges. Add 1 cup water and stir well. Bring to a boil.

Reduce to a simmer and cover. Cook for 30 minutes, or until rice is just cooked and veggies are tender.

Stir in shrimp. Re-cover and cook 5 minutes, or until shrimp are fully cooked.

Add basil, sour cream, and cheese wedges, breaking the wedges into pieces. Thoroughly stir. Cook and stir for 2 minutes to allow the basil flavor to develop. Enjoy!

MAKES 2 SERVINGS

CREAMY PUMPKIN FAUX-SOTTO

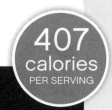

222 calories PER SERVING

You'll Need: large nonstick pot with a lid
Prep: 15 minutes
Cook: 45 minutes

¼th of recipe (about 1¼ cups): 222 calories, 2.75g fat, 464mg sodium, 41.5g carbs, 5.25g fiber, 6g sugars, 8g protein

INGREDIENTS

2 cups finely chopped cauliflower
1½ cups fat-free chicken or vegetable broth
1 cup diced onion
1 cup thinly sliced mushrooms
1 cup canned pure pumpkin
¾ cup uncooked brown rice
½ cup light plain soymilk
1 teaspoon chopped garlic
¼ teaspoon salt, or more to taste
⅛ teaspoon black pepper, or more to taste
1 tablespoon plus 1 teaspoon reduced-fat
    Parmesan-style grated topping
2 wedges The Laughing Cow Light
    Creamy Swiss cheese

DIRECTIONS

In a large nonstick pot, combine all ingredients *except* Parm-style topping and cheese wedges. Thoroughly stir. Bring to a boil.

Reduce to a simmer and cover. Cook for 35 minutes, or until rice is cooked and veggies are tender.

Add Parm-style topping and cheese wedges, breaking the wedges into pieces, and thoroughly stir. Serve it up!

MAKES 4 SERVINGS

2-GOOD TWICE-BAKED POTATO

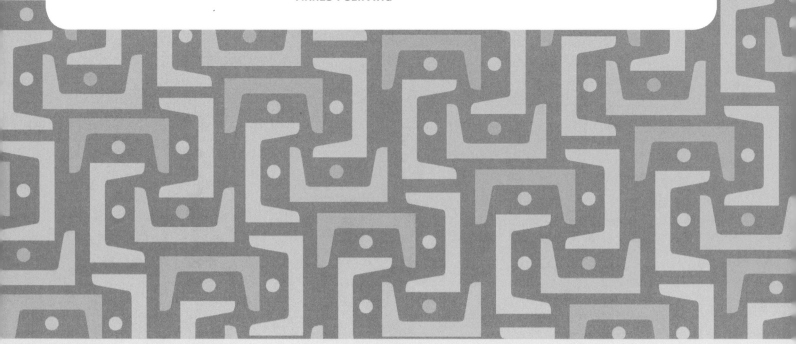

226 calories

You'll Need: 8-inch by 8-inch baking pan, nonstick spray, vegetable peeler, microwave-safe plate, small bowl
Prep: 5 minutes | **Cook:** 40 minutes

Entire recipe:
226 calories, 0.5g fat, 335mg sodium, 46g carbs, 5g fiber, 4g sugars, 9g protein

INGREDIENTS

One 8-ounce baking potato

2 tablespoons fat-free liquid non-dairy creamer

1 slice fat-free American cheese

Optional seasonings: salt, black pepper, paprika, parsley

DIRECTIONS

Preheat oven to 375 degrees. Spray an 8-inch by 8-inch baking pan with nonstick spray.

Puncture potato in several places with a fork. Peel the skin off the top and place potato on a microwave-safe plate. Microwave for 6 minutes, or until soft.

Scoop out the insides and transfer to a small bowl. Set the empty potato "shell" aside.

Add creamer and cheese to the bowl, breaking the cheese into pieces. Thoroughly mash. Spoon mixture into the potato shell.

Place potato in the baking pan and bake until top has lightly browned, 20 to 30 minutes. Time to eat!

MAKES 1 SERVING

SUPER-SIZED KICKIN' CHICKEN POT PIE

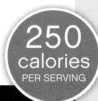

250 calories PER SERVING

You'll Need: 9-inch by 13-inch baking pan, nonstick spray, large skillet, large bowl
Prep: 5 minutes
Cook: 1 hour

⅛th of recipe: 250 calories, 6.5g fat, 623mg sodium, 27.5g carbs, 3.5g fiber, 6g sugars, 17g protein

INGREDIENTS

1 pound raw boneless skinless chicken breast, cut into bite-sized pieces
6 cups frozen mixed vegetables, thawed
Two 10.75-ounce cans 98% fat-free cream of celery condensed soup
1 package refrigerated Pillsbury Crescent Recipe Creations Seamless Dough Sheet

DIRECTIONS

Preheat oven to 350 degrees. Spray a 9-inch by 13-inch baking pan with nonstick spray.

Bring a large skillet sprayed with nonstick spray to medium-high heat. Cook and stir chicken for 10 to 15 minutes, until fully cooked.

Transfer chicken to a large bowl. Add thawed veggies and soup and mix well. Transfer to the baking pan.

Bake until hot and bubbly, about 30 minutes.

Place dough over the contents of the baking pan and carefully stretch to cover.

Bake until dough is fully cooked and golden brown, 12 to 15 minutes. Serve it up!

MAKES 8 SERVINGS

BAKED CHILI SURPRISE

215 calories PER SERVING

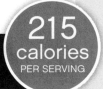

You'll Need: 8-inch by 8-inch baking pan, nonstick spray, skillet, medium bowl, whisk
Prep: 10 minutes
Cook: 30 minutes

¼th of recipe (about 1¼ cups): 215 calories, 3g fat, 581mg sodium, 39g carbs, 5.5g fiber, 9g sugars, 9.5g protein

INGREDIENTS

2 cups chopped mushrooms
1 cup chopped onion
½ cup frozen sweet corn kernels
1 cup chopped tomatoes
One 15-ounce can low-fat vegetarian chili
⅔ cup Bisquick Heart Smart baking mix
¼ cup fat-free milk
2 tablespoons fat-free liquid egg substitute

Optional seasonings: salt and black pepper
Optional topping: fat-free sour cream

DIRECTIONS

Preheat oven to 375 degrees. Spray an 8-inch by 8-inch baking pan with nonstick spray.

Bring a skillet sprayed with nonstick spray to medium heat. Add mushrooms, onion, and corn. Cook and stir until slightly softened, about 3 minutes. Add tomatoes and cook and stir until slightly softened, about 2 minutes.

Remove skillet from heat. Add chili and mix well. Evenly transfer mixture to the baking pan.

In a medium bowl, vigorously whisk baking mix, milk, and egg substitute until smooth. Evenly pour over the contents of the baking pan.

Bake until top is golden brown, about 25 minutes. Eat up!

MAKES 4 SERVINGS

TWICE-BAKED SPAGHETTI SQUASH

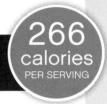

266 calories
PER SERVING

You'll Need: 9-inch by 13-inch baking pan, strainer, large bowl, medium bowl
Prep: 15 minutes | **Cook:** 1 hour 5 minutes

¼th of recipe:
266 calories, 8g fat, 810mg sodium, 33g carbs, 6g fiber, 14g sugars, 14.5g protein

INGREDIENTS

1 spaghetti squash (about 4½ pounds)

One 14.5-ounce can reduced-sodium creamy tomato soup with 4g fat or less per serving

½ tablespoon chopped garlic

½ tablespoon dried minced onion

1 teaspoon Italian seasoning

½ teaspoon black pepper

3 wedges The Laughing Cow Light Creamy Swiss cheese, room temperature

One 10-ounce package frozen chopped spinach, thawed and squeezed dry

One 7-ounce can sliced mushrooms, drained (about ⅔ cup)

¼ cup chopped fresh basil

1 cup shredded part-skim mozzarella cheese

DIRECTIONS

Preheat oven to 375 degrees.

Microwave squash for 3 to 4 minutes, until soft enough to cut. Halve lengthwise; scoop out and discard seeds.

Fill a 9-inch by 13-inch baking pan with ½ inch water and place squash halves in the pan, cut sides down. Bake until tender, about 40 minutes.

Remove pan, but leave oven on. Use a fork to scrape out squash strands. Place strands in a strainer to drain excess moisture. Pat dry, if needed. Transfer to a large bowl and cover to keep warm.

Drain water from the baking pan and place the hollow squash halves back in the pan.

In a medium bowl, thoroughly mix soup, garlic, minced onion, Italian seasoning, pepper, and cheese wedges, breaking the wedges into pieces as you add them.

Add soup mixture to the spaghetti squash strands. Add spinach, mushrooms, and basil, and thoroughly mix.

Evenly divide mixture between the hollow squash halves. Sprinkle with mozzarella cheese. Bake until filling is hot and mozzarella cheese has melted, 15 to 20 minutes.

Slice each piece in half, serve up, and enjoy!

MAKES 4 SERVINGS

MASHED POTATOES are almost TOO good. These HG'd-up versions are thru-the-roof delicious and have slashed calorie counts too, thanks to our BFF cauliflower.

MIRACLE MASHIES

82 calories PER SERVING

You'll Need: large pot, vegetable peeler, large bowl, potato masher | **Prep:** 10 minutes | **Cook:** 25 minutes

⅕th of recipe (about ⅔ cup):
82 calories, 1g fat, 168mg sodium, 16g carbs, 3g fiber, 2g sugars, 3g protein

INGREDIENTS

One 12-ounce russet potato

3 cups cauliflower florets

3 tablespoons fat-free half & half

1 tablespoon light whipped butter or light buttery spread

¼ teaspoon salt, or more to taste

Optional seasoning: black pepper

DIRECTIONS

Bring a large pot of water to a boil. Meanwhile, peel and cube potato.

Add cauliflower and cubed potato to boiling water. Once returned to a boil, reduce heat to medium. Cook until potatoes and cauliflower are very tender, 15 to 20 minutes.

Drain and transfer cauliflower and potato to a large bowl. Add half & half, butter, and salt. Thoroughly mash and mix. Enjoy!

MAKES 5 SERVINGS

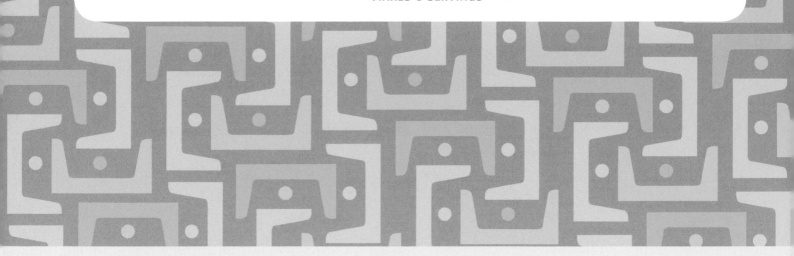

GREAT GARLIC MIRACLE MASHIES

120 calories PER SERVING

You'll Need: aluminum foil, baking pan, large pot, vegetable peeler, large bowl, potato masher
Prep: 15 minutes
Cook: 1 hour

⅕th of recipe (about ¾ cup): 120 calories, 3g fat, 315mg sodium, 20.5g carbs, 3.5g fiber, 3.5g sugars, 4g protein

INGREDIENTS

1 head of garlic
1 teaspoon olive oil
One 12-ounce russet potato
5 cups cauliflower florets (about 1 head)
3 tablespoons fat-free half & half
2 tablespoons light whipped butter
    or light buttery spread
½ teaspoon salt, or more to taste

Optional seasoning: black pepper
Optional topping: chopped chives

DIRECTIONS

Preheat oven to 425 degrees.

Remove papery outer layer from garlic, leaving skins around the cloves intact. Slice off the top of the garlic head, ¼ to ½ inch, exposing the tops of the cloves. Place garlic on a piece of foil, drizzle with oil, and use your fingers to coat.

Wrap foil tightly around garlic, enclosing it completely, and place in a baking pan. Bake for 40 minutes, or until soft enough to mash.

Meanwhile, bring a large pot of water to a boil. While waiting for water to boil, peel and cube the potato.

Add potato and cauliflower to boiling water. Once returned to a boil, reduce heat to medium. Cook until potato and cauliflower are very tender, 15 to 20 minutes.

Drain water and transfer potato and cauliflower to a large bowl. Unwrap garlic and remove cloves; discard skin. Add the soft cloves to the large bowl.

Add half & half, butter, and salt to the bowl. Thoroughly mash with a potato masher. Enjoy!

MAKES 5 SERVINGS

CARAMELIZED ONION MASHIES

133 calories PER SERVING

You'll Need: large skillet, large microwave-safe bowl
Prep: 15 minutes
Cook: 55 minutes

⅕th of recipe (about ¾ cup): 133 calories, 0.5g fat, 312mg sodium, 28g carbs, 2.5g fiber, 6.5g sugars, 3g protein

INGREDIENTS

½ tablespoon light whipped butter
    or light buttery spread
4 cups chopped sweet onions
2 teaspoons Dijon mustard
1⅓ cups instant mashed potato flakes
¼ teaspoon garlic powder
½ teaspoon salt
¼ cup fat-free sour cream

Optional seasonings: black pepper, additional salt

DIRECTIONS

Melt butter in a large skillet over medium-high heat. Cook and stir onions for 10 minutes.

Reduce heat to medium low. Stirring frequently, cook until caramelized, 35 to 40 minutes.

Stir in mustard and remove from heat.

In a large microwave-safe bowl, thoroughly mix potato flakes, garlic powder, salt, and 2⅓ cups water. Cover and microwave for 3 minutes, or until hot.

Stir in onions and sour cream. Enjoy!

MAKES 5 SERVINGS

3-CHEESE MIRACLE MASHIES

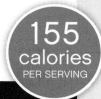

155 calories
PER SERVING

You'll Need: large pot, vegetable peeler, large bowl, potato masher, 5 microwave-safe bowls
Prep: 15 minutes
Cook: 30 minutes

⅕th of recipe (about ¾ cup):
155 calories, 4g fat, 483mg sodium, 20.5g carbs, 3.5g fiber, 4g sugars, 8g protein

INGREDIENTS

One 12-ounce russet potato
5 cups cauliflower florets (about 1 head)
3 tablespoons fat-free half & half
2 tablespoons light whipped butter
    or light buttery spread
2 tablespoons reduced-fat Parmesan-style
    grated topping
¼ teaspoon each salt and black pepper
4 wedges The Laughing Cow Light
    Creamy Swiss cheese
5 tablespoons shredded fat-free
    cheddar cheese

Optional topping: chopped chives

DIRECTIONS

Bring a large pot of water to a boil. Meanwhile, peel and cube potato.

Add potato and cauliflower to boiling water. Once returned to a boil, reduce heat to medium. Cook until very tender, 15 to 20 minutes.

Drain water and transfer potato and cauliflower to a large bowl. Add half & half, butter, Parm-style topping, salt, pepper, and cheese wedges, breaking the wedges into pieces. Mash thoroughly.

Place each serving (about ¾ cup) in a microwave-safe bowl and top with 1 tablespoon shredded cheese. Microwave for 30 seconds, or until shredded cheese has melted. Enjoy!

MAKES 5 SERVINGS

CHEESY SCALLOPED POTATOES 'N TURNIPS

208 calories
PER SERVING

You'll Need: 8-inch by 8-inch baking pan, nonstick spray, vegetable peeler, large bowl, large microwave-safe bowl, whisk
Prep: 15 minutes
Cook: 1 hour 15 minutes

¼th of recipe (about 1 cup): 208 calories, 3.5g fat, 665mg sodium, 33.5g carbs, 3g fiber, 10g sugars, 8g protein

INGREDIENTS

One 12-ounce russet potato
One 12-ounce turnip
1 cup fat-free sour cream
½ cup cheddar cheese condensed soup
¼ cup fat-free milk
1 teaspoon chopped garlic
¼ teaspoon each salt and black pepper, or more to taste
4 wedges The Laughing Cow Light Creamy Swiss cheese
½ cup chopped scallions

DIRECTIONS

Preheat oven to 350 degrees. Spray an 8-inch by 8-inch baking pan with nonstick spray.

Peel potato and turnip and thinly slice into half-moon slices. Place in a large bowl and toss gently to mix.

In a large microwave-safe bowl, combine sour cream, soup, milk, garlic, salt, and pepper. Add cheese wedges, breaking them into pieces, and mix well. Cover and microwave for 2 minutes, or until hot.

Whisk sour cream mixture until uniform in texture. Stir in ¼ cup scallions.

Place ⅓rd of the potato and turnip slices in an even layer along the bottom of the baking pan. Top with ⅓rd of the cheese mixture, about ⅔ cup.

Repeat layering twice, for a total of 3 potato-turnip layers and 3 cheese-mixture layers.

Bake until potatoes and turnips are tender, 60 to 70 minutes.

Sprinkle with remaining ¼ cup scallions. Enjoy!

MAKES 4 SERVINGS

SUPER STUFFED EGGPLANT

284
calories
PER SERVING

You'll Need: baking sheet, nonstick spray, large skillet, large bowl, blender or food processor (optional)
Prep: 25 minutes | **Cook:** 40 minutes

½ of recipe (1 eggplant half):
284 calories, 6.5g fat, 730mg sodium, 41g carbs, 13.5g fiber, 17g sugars, 21g protein

INGREDIENTS

1 large eggplant, stem end removed
1 cup chopped onion
1 cup chopped brown mushrooms
¾ cup chopped zucchini
¾ cup seeded and chopped tomato
¼ cup fat-free liquid egg substitute
¼ cup light or low-fat ricotta cheese
2 tablespoons tomato paste
2 teaspoons chopped garlic
½ teaspoon Italian seasoning
¼ teaspoon salt
2 sticks light string cheese
2 tablespoons reduced-fat Parmesan-style
    grated topping

DIRECTIONS

Preheat oven to 400 degrees. Spray a baking sheet with nonstick spray.

Halve the eggplant lengthwise. Carefully cut along the inside of each half, about ½ inch from the skin. Scoop out the insides and finely chop. Place the hollow eggplant shells on the baking sheet, cut sides up.

Bring a large skillet sprayed with nonstick spray to medium-high heat. Add chopped eggplant, onion, mushrooms, and zucchini. Cook and stir until mostly softened, about 6 minutes.

Transfer to a large bowl and blot away excess moisture. Thoroughly stir in all remaining ingredients *except* string cheese and Parm-style topping. Divide mixture between eggplant shells, lightly packing down until even.

Bake until shells have fully softened and tops have slightly browned, about 25 minutes. Leave oven on.

Meanwhile, break each stick of string cheese into thirds and place in a blender or food processor—blend at high speed until shredded. (Or pull into shreds and roughly chop.)

Sprinkle shredded string cheese and Parm-style topping over eggplant halves. Bake until shredded cheese has melted, about 5 minutes. Enjoy!

MAKES 2 SERVINGS

For more recipes, tips & tricks, sign up for FREE daily emails at **hungry-girl.com!**

SLOPPY JANES

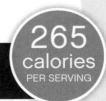

You'll Need: large skillet, nonstick spray
Prep: 15 minutes
Cook: 20 minutes

⅕th of recipe (1 sandwich): 265 calories, 7g fat, 717mg sodium, 30.5g carbs, 7g fiber, 11g sugars, 23g protein

INGREDIENTS

1 pound raw lean ground turkey
1 teaspoon dry steak seasoning blend
⅛ teaspoon salt
½ cup chopped onion
½ cup chopped red bell pepper
1 tablespoon Worcestershire sauce
1 tablespoon red wine vinegar
1 cup canned tomato sauce
¾ cup canned no-salt-added tomato sauce
2 tablespoons tomato paste
1 tablespoon granulated white sugar or Splenda No Calorie Sweetener (granulated)
5 light hamburger buns

DIRECTIONS

Spray a large skillet with nonstick spray and bring to medium-high heat. Add turkey and sprinkle with steak seasoning and salt. Cook and crumble for about 8 minutes, until mostly cooked.

Reduce heat to medium. Add onion, bell pepper, Worcestershire sauce, and vinegar. Mix well and cook and crumble for 5 minutes, or until meat is fully cooked.

Reduce heat to low. Add tomato sauces, tomato paste, and sugar or Splenda. Cook and stir until hot, about 5 minutes.

Toast buns, if desired. Evenly distribute the mixture among the bottom buns and then finish off with the tops of the buns. Enjoy!

MAKES 5 SERVINGS

HG ALTERNATIVE!

Can't find 80-calorie light buns? Just get the lowest-calorie buns you see and adjust the calorie count accordingly. Bonus points if they have fiber!

CHICKEN POT POCKETS

You'll Need: baking sheet, nonstick spray, small bowl, large bowl
Prep: 30 minutes
Cook: 20 minutes

1/12th of recipe (1 pocket): 119 calories, 1.25g fat, 280mg sodium, 17g carbs, 1g fiber, 1.5g sugars, 10g protein

INGREDIENTS

1 teaspoon cornstarch
One 10.75-ounce can 98% fat-free cream of celery condensed soup
2 cups frozen petite mixed vegetables
12 ounces cooked and finely chopped skinless chicken breast
12 large square egg roll wrappers

Optional seasonings: salt and black pepper

DIRECTIONS

Preheat oven to 350 degrees. Spray a baking sheet with nonstick spray.

In a small bowl, mix cornstarch with 1 teaspoon cold water until dissolved. Transfer mixture to a large bowl. Add soup and mix well. Stir in veggies and chicken.

Lay an egg roll wrapper flat on a dry surface. Moisten all four edges with water. Evenly distribute 1/12th of the chicken mixture (about ⅓ cup) on the bottom half of the wrapper. Fold the top half over the mixture so the top edge meets the bottom. Dab the edges with water and press firmly with the prongs of a fork to seal. Place on the baking sheet.

Repeat with remaining ingredients, for a total of 12 pockets, evenly spaced on the sheet.

Bake until edges begin to brown, 15 to 18 minutes. Dig in!

MAKES 12 SERVINGS

HUNGRY-LICIOUS CHICKEN MARSALA

240 calories PER SERVING

You'll Need: small microwave-safe bowl, medium bowl, whisk, large skillet, nonstick spray
Prep: 15 minutes
Cook: 20 minutes

½ of recipe (1 cutlet with sauce and mushrooms):
240 calories, 4g fat, 785mg sodium, 8.5g carbs, 0.5g fiber, 4.5g sugars, 34.5g protein

INGREDIENTS

1 tablespoon light whipped butter or light buttery spread
½ cup fat-free chicken broth
¼ cup marsala wine
1 teaspoon cornstarch
1½ cups sliced mushrooms
Two 5-ounce raw boneless skinless chicken breast cutlets, pounded to ½-inch thickness
¼ teaspoon each salt and black pepper
¼ teaspoon dried basil

DIRECTIONS

In a small microwave-safe bowl, microwave butter for 10 seconds, or until melted.

In a medium bowl, whisk melted butter, broth, wine, and cornstarch until cornstarch has dissolved.

Bring a large skillet sprayed with nonstick spray to medium-high heat. Cook and stir mushrooms until softened, 5 to 7 minutes.

Move mushrooms to the sides of the skillet. Season chicken with salt, pepper, and basil, and lay in the center of the skillet. Cook for 4 minutes, stirring mushrooms occasionally.

Flip chicken. Give broth mixture a stir and add to the skillet. Stirring mushrooms occasionally, cook until sauce has thickened and chicken is cooked through, about 5 minutes. Serve it and love it!

MAKES 2 SERVINGS

SHRIMP & GRITS FOR HUNGRY CHICKS

380 calories PER SERVING

You'll Need: medium pot with a lid, large skillet, nonstick spray
Prep: 15 minutes
Cook: 10 minutes

½ of recipe: 380 calories, 8g fat, 900mg sodium, 40g carbs, 2.5g fiber, 1g sugars, 40g protein

INGREDIENTS

½ cup quick-cooking grits
Dash salt
½ cup shredded fat-free cheddar cheese
1 tablespoon light whipped butter or light buttery spread
1 wedge The Laughing Cow Light Creamy Swiss cheese
8 ounces raw shrimp, peeled, tails removed, deveined
½ cup thinly sliced scallions
1 tablespoon chopped fresh parsley
1 teaspoon lemon juice
½ teaspoon chopped garlic
2 tablespoons precooked real crumbled bacon

Optional topping: hot sauce

DIRECTIONS

In a medium pot, bring 2 cups water to a boil. Add grits and salt and stir well. Reduce heat to lowest setting. Cook and stir until water has absorbed, 6 to 7 minutes.

Remove from heat and stir in shredded cheese, butter, and cheese wedge, breaking the wedge into pieces as you add it. Cover to keep warm.

Bring a large skillet sprayed with nonstick spray to medium heat. Cook shrimp for 2 minutes. Flip shrimp and cook until opaque, about 1 minute. Add scallions, parsley, lemon juice, and garlic. Stir well and remove from heat.

Serve grits topped with shrimp and bacon. Eat up, y'all!

MAKES 2 SERVINGS

Melty, toasty, cheesy goodness . . .
These **GRILLED CHEESE** recipes are MAGICAL.

APPLE 'N JACK GRILLED CHEESE

    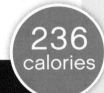

236 calories

You'll Need: skillet, nonstick spray
Prep: 5 minutes
Cook: 15 minutes

Entire recipe: 236 calories, 10g fat, 459mg sodium, 27g carbs, 6g fiber, 7g sugars, 13.5g protein

INGREDIENTS

¼ cup peeled and chopped apple
¼ cup chopped onion
2 slices light bread
1 ounce reduced-fat block-style Monterey Jack cheese, shredded (about ¼ cup)
2 teaspoons light whipped butter or light buttery spread

DIRECTIONS

Bring a skillet sprayed with nonstick spray to medium-high heat. Cook and stir apple and onion until slightly softened and browned, about 8 minutes.

Top one slice of bread with 2 tablespoons cheese, followed by cooked apple and onion. Sprinkle with remaining 2 tablespoons cheese and top with the remaining bread slice. Spread the top of the sandwich with 1 teaspoon butter.

Remove the skillet from heat, re-spray, and return to medium-high heat. Place sandwich in the skillet, buttered side down. Spread the top with remaining 1 teaspoon butter.

Cook until bread is lightly browned and cheese has melted, about 2 minutes per side, flipping carefully. Dig in!

MAKES 1 SERVING

JALAPEÑO POPPER GRILLED CHEESE

190 calories

You'll Need: skillet, nonstick spray
Prep: 5 minutes
Cook: 5 minutes

Entire recipe: 190 calories, 6g fat, 880mg sodium, 22g carbs, 5g fiber, 5g sugars, 12g protein

INGREDIENTS

2 slices light bread
1 wedge The Laughing Cow Light Creamy Swiss cheese
6 jarred jalapeño slices
1 slice fat-free American cheese
2 teaspoons light whipped butter or light buttery spread

DIRECTIONS

Lay bread slices flat and spread both with the cheese wedge. Top one slice with jalapeños and American cheese. Top with the other bread slice, cheesy side down. Spread the top of the sandwich with 1 teaspoon butter.

Bring a skillet sprayed with nonstick spray to medium-high heat. Place sandwich in the skillet, buttered side down. Spread the top with remaining 1 teaspoon butter.

Cook until bread is lightly browned and cheese has melted, about 2 minutes per side, flipping carefully. Dig in!

MAKES 1 SERVING

BBQ CHICKEN GRILLED CHEESE

282 calories

You'll Need: small bowl, skillet, nonstick spray
Prep: 10 minutes
Cook: 5 minutes

Entire recipe: 282 calories, 7g fat, 1,017mg sodium, 28g carbs, 5g fiber, 9g sugars, 26.5g protein

INGREDIENTS

2 ounces cooked and chopped skinless chicken breast
1 tablespoon BBQ sauce with 45 calories or less per 2-tablespoon serving
1½ tablespoons finely chopped red onion
1 teaspoon chopped cilantro
2 slices light bread
1 slice fat-free cheddar cheese
1 wedge The Laughing Cow Light Creamy Swiss cheese
2 teaspoons light whipped butter or light buttery spread

DIRECTIONS

In a small bowl, coat chicken with BBQ sauce. Stir in onion and cilantro.

Lay bread slices flat. Top one slice with cheddar cheese and chicken mixture. Spread the other slice with the cheese wedge and place over the chicken mixture, cheesy side down. Spread the top of the sandwich with 1 teaspoon butter.

Bring a skillet sprayed with nonstick spray to medium-high heat. Place sandwich in the skillet, buttered side down. Spread the top with remaining 1 teaspoon butter.

Cook until bread is lightly browned and cheese has melted, about 2 minutes per side, flipping carefully. Mmmm!

MAKES 1 SERVING

GRILLED CHEESE DUNKIN' DUO

257 calories

You'll Need: skillet, nonstick spray, microwave-safe bowl
Prep: 5 minutes
Cook: 5 minutes

Entire recipe: 257 calories, 8.5g fat, 989mg sodium, 30g carbs, 6g fiber, 10g sugars, 17.5g protein

INGREDIENTS

2 slices light bread
1 slice fat-free American cheese
1 piece Mini Babybel Light cheese, chopped
2 teaspoons light whipped butter or light buttery spread
½ cup reduced-sodium creamy tomato soup with 4g fat or less per serving

DIRECTIONS

Top one slice of bread with the cheese slice. Sprinkle with chopped cheese and top with remaining bread slice. Spread the top of the sandwich with 1 teaspoon butter.

Bring a skillet sprayed with nonstick spray to medium-high heat. Place sandwich in the skillet, buttered side down. Spread the top with remaining 1 teaspoon butter.

Cook until bread is lightly browned and cheese has melted, about 2 minutes per side, flipping carefully.

Microwave soup in a microwave-safe bowl for 1 minute, or until hot. Slice sandwich into 4 sticks and serve with the soup for dunking!

MAKES 1 SERVING

GREEK GRILLED CHEESE

   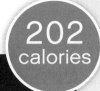

202 calories

You'll Need: skillet, nonstick spray
Prep: 5 minutes
Cook: 5 minutes

Entire recipe: 202 calories, 8.5g fat, 640mg sodium, 21g carbs, 5g fiber, 4g sugars, 11g protein

INGREDIENTS

2 slices light bread
1 wedge The Laughing Cow Light Creamy Swiss cheese
2 tablespoons crumbled reduced-fat feta cheese
1 tablespoon diced and seeded tomato
1 tablespoon diced red onion
1 tablespoon chopped basil
2 teaspoons light whipped butter or light buttery spread

DIRECTIONS

Lay bread slices flat and spread both with the cheese wedge. Top one slice with feta cheese, tomato, onion, and basil. Top with the other bread slice, cheesy side down. Spread the top of the sandwich with 1 teaspoon butter.

Bring a skillet sprayed with nonstick spray to medium-high heat. Place sandwich in the skillet, buttered side down. Spread the top with remaining 1 teaspoon butter.

Cook until bread is lightly browned and cheese has melted, about 2 minutes per side, flipping carefully. Dig in!

MAKES 1 SERVING

HUNGRY GRILLED GRACELAND SPECIAL

    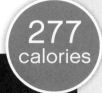

277 calories

You'll Need: skillet, nonstick spray
Prep: 5 minutes
Cook: 5 minutes

Entire recipe: 277 calories, 12g fat, 385mg sodium, 39g carbs, 7.5g fiber, 11g sugars, 9g protein

INGREDIENTS

1 tablespoon reduced-fat peanut butter, room temperature
2 slices light bread
½ medium banana, thinly sliced
1 tablespoon light whipped butter or light buttery spread

DIRECTIONS

Evenly spread peanut butter onto one slice of bread. Top with banana slices and the other bread slice. Spread the top of the sandwich with ½ tablespoon butter.

Bring a skillet sprayed with nonstick spray to medium-high heat. Place sandwich in the skillet with the buttered side down. Spread the top with remaining ½ tablespoon butter.

Cook until lightly browned on both sides, about 2 minutes per side. Serve and enjoy!

MAKES 1 SERVING

For more recipes, tips & tricks, sign up for FREE daily emails at hungry-girl.com!

SQUASH-TASTIC SHEPHERD'S PIE

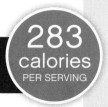

283 calories PER SERVING

You'll Need: 8-inch by 8-inch baking pan, nonstick spray, large microwave-safe bowl, skillet, potato masher
Prep: 15 minutes | **Cook:** 45 minutes

¼th of recipe:
283 calories, 9g fat, 650mg sodium, 25.5g carbs, 4g fiber, 5.5g sugars, 25g protein

INGREDIENTS

3½ cups cubed butternut squash
½ cup chopped onion
1 pound raw lean ground turkey
½ teaspoon chopped garlic
½ teaspoon salt
Dash garlic powder
Dash onion powder
Dash black pepper
¾ cup fat-free gravy
1½ cups frozen mixed vegetables, thawed
1 tablespoon light whipped butter
    or light buttery spread

DIRECTIONS

Preheat oven to 400 degrees. Spray an 8-inch by 8-inch baking pan with nonstick spray.

Place squash in a large microwave-safe bowl with 2 tablespoons water. Cover and microwave for 6 minutes, or until soft.

Meanwhile, bring a skillet sprayed with nonstick spray to medium-high heat. Cook and stir onion until slightly browned, 2 to 3 minutes.

Add turkey, chopped garlic, ¼ teaspoon salt, garlic powder, onion powder, and pepper. Cook and crumble for 10 minutes, or until turkey is fully cooked.

Drain any excess liquid and transfer turkey mixture to the baking pan. Evenly top with gravy, followed by thawed mixed veggies.

Drain excess water from squash and thoroughly mash. Mix in butter and remaining ¼ teaspoon salt. Evenly layer mixture over the veggies.

Bake until topping is firm, 20 to 25 minutes. Enjoy!

MAKES 4 SERVINGS

HUNGRY CHICK SHEPHERD'S PIE

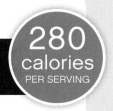

280 calories PER SERVING

You'll Need: 8-inch by 8-inch baking pan, nonstick spray, 2 large microwave-safe bowls, potato masher, large skillet
Prep: 30 minutes | **Cook:** 1 hour

¼th of pie:
280 calories, 1.75g fat, 576mg sodium, 36.5g carbs, 6g fiber, 7g sugars, 26.5g protein

INGREDIENTS

1 cup instant mashed potato flakes

3 cups frozen cauliflower florets

½ tablespoon light whipped butter or light buttery spread

2 dashes each salt and black pepper

12 ounces raw boneless skinless chicken breast cutlets

4 cups frozen mixed vegetables

One 8-ounce can sliced mushrooms, drained

½ cup fat-free chicken gravy

Optional seasonings: garlic powder, onion powder, paprika

DIRECTIONS

Preheat oven to 375 degrees. Spray an 8-inch by 8-inch baking pan with nonstick spray.

In a large microwave-safe bowl, thoroughly mix potato flakes with 1½ cups hot water. Add cauliflower and mix well. Cover and microwave for 3 minutes, or until potatoes have thickened and cauliflower is hot. Thoroughly mash. Mix in butter and a dash each salt and pepper.

Bring a large skillet sprayed with nonstick spray to medium-high heat. Add chicken and sprinkle with remaining dash each salt and pepper. Cook for 6 to 8 minutes per side, until cooked through. Set aside to cool.

Microwave frozen mixed veggies in a large microwave-safe bowl for 5 to 6 minutes, until thawed. Drain excess liquid and stir in mushrooms. Evenly transfer to the baking pan.

Chop chicken into bite-sized pieces. In the large bowl used to thaw the veggies, toss to coat chicken with gravy. Evenly distribute gravy-coated chicken over the veggies.

Evenly spoon potato-cauliflower mixture over the chicken, and smooth out the surface.

Bake until top is slightly browned, about 35 minutes. Dig in!

MAKES 4 SERVINGS

PETITE WONTON-BOTTOMED SHEPHERD'S PIES

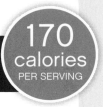
170
calories
PER SERVING

You'll Need: 12-cup muffin pan, nonstick spray, large bowl, skillet | **Prep:** 15 minutes | **Cook:** 25 minutes

⅙th of recipe (2 mini pies) :
170 calories, 3g fat, 450mg sodium, 24g carbs, 1.5g fiber, 2g sugars, 10g protein

INGREDIENTS

12 small square wonton wrappers

1 cup instant mashed potato flakes

½ tablespoon light whipped butter
    or light buttery spread

¼ teaspoon plus ⅛ teaspoon salt

¼ teaspoon black pepper

¼ cup chopped onion

8 ounces raw lean ground turkey

½ teaspoon garlic powder

¾ cup fat-free turkey gravy

1½ cups frozen petite mixed vegetables

DIRECTIONS

Preheat oven to 400 degrees. Spray a 12-cup muffin pan with nonstick spray.

Place a wonton wrapper in each cup of the muffin pan, and press it into the bottom and sides.

In a large bowl, thoroughly mix potato flakes with 1½ cups hot water. Mix in butter, ¼ teaspoon salt, and ⅛ teaspoon pepper.

Bring a skillet sprayed with nonstick spray to medium heat. Cook onion until softened, 3 to 4 minutes. Raise heat to medium high. Add turkey, garlic powder, remaining ⅛ teaspoon salt, and remaining ⅛ teaspoon pepper. Cook and crumble for 4 to 5 minutes, until turkey is fully cooked.

Drain any excess liquid from the skillet. Evenly distribute turkey mixture among the wontons in the muffin cups, about 1 tablespoon each. Evenly top with gravy, 1 tablespoon each.

Evenly distribute frozen veggies among the cups, about 2 tablespoons each, followed by the potato mixture, about 1 tablespoon each. Bake until the tops are slightly crispy and brown, about 15 minutes. Serve and enjoy!

MAKES 6 SERVINGS

Flip to the photo inserts to see over 100 recipe pics! And for photos of ALL the recipes, go to **hungry-girl.com/books.**

Everyone LOVES MAC & CHEESE—it's TOTAL comfort food. These decadent and fun cheesy-mac recipes are bulked up with veggies!

TOO-EZ MAC 'N CHEESE

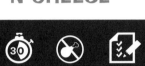

222 calories PER SERVING

You'll Need: large microwave-safe bowl, medium-large pot
Prep: 5 minutes
Cook: 20 minutes

¼th of recipe (1 heaping cup):
222 calories, 5.5g fat, 772mg sodium, 35g carbs, 6g fiber, 6g sugars, 8.5g protein

INGREDIENTS

24 ounces (about 6 cups) frozen Green Giant Broccoli & Cheese Sauce

4½ ounces (about 1¾ cups) uncooked high-fiber rotini pasta

3 wedges The Laughing Cow Light Creamy Swiss cheese

Optional seasonings: salt and black pepper

DIRECTIONS

Place broccoli & cheese sauce in a large microwave-safe bowl. Cover and microwave for 10 to 12 minutes, until sauce has melted and broccoli is hot.

In medium-large pot, cook pasta per package instructions, about 8 minutes. Drain pasta and stir into the broccoli & cheese sauce.

Add cheese wedges, breaking them into pieces. Mix thoroughly, until cheese has melted and is well mixed. Enjoy!

MAKES 4 SERVINGS

MEGA MAC & CHEESE

182 calories PER SERVING

You'll Need: large microwave-safe bowl, medium-large pot, medium microwave-safe bowl
Prep: 5 minutes
Cook: 15 minutes

¼th of recipe (1 heaping cup):
182 calories, 2.5g fat, 387mg sodium, 30g carbs, 4.5g fiber, 5.5g sugars, 10g protein

INGREDIENTS

3 cups frozen cauliflower florets

4½ ounces (about 1¼ cups) uncooked high-fiber elbow macaroni

2 tablespoons fat-free sour cream

2 slices fat-free American cheese

4 wedges The Laughing Cow Light Creamy Swiss cheese

Optional seasonings: salt and black pepper

DIRECTIONS

Place cauliflower in a large microwave-safe bowl; cover and microwave for 3 minutes. Uncover and stir. Re-cover and microwave for 2 to 3 minutes, until hot. Drain excess liquid. Roughly chop cauliflower, return to the bowl, and cover to keep warm.

In a medium-large pot, cook pasta per package instructions, about 8 minutes. Drain pasta and stir into cauliflower. Cover to keep warm.

In a medium microwave-safe bowl, mix sour cream, cheese slices, and cheese wedges, breaking slices and wedges into pieces. Microwave for 20 seconds. Stir well. Microwave for another 20 seconds, or until cheeses have melted. Stir well.

Add cheese mixture to the large bowl and thoroughly stir. Enjoy!

MAKES 4 SERVINGS

BLT-RIFIC MAC 'N CHEESE

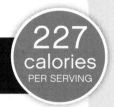

227 calories
PER SERVING

You'll Need: large skillet with a lid, microwave-safe plate (optional), medium-large pot with a lid, nonstick spray, microwave-safe bowl | **Prep:** 15 minutes | **Cook:** 25 minutes

¼th of recipe (about 1 cup):
227 calories, 5g fat, 491mg sodium, 33g carbs, 6g fiber, 4g sugars, 13g protein

INGREDIENTS

3 slices center-cut bacon or turkey bacon

4½ ounces (about 1½ cups) uncooked high-fiber penne pasta

2 large yellow summer squash

3 cups chopped spinach leaves

1 large tomato, chopped and seeded

2 tablespoons fat-free sour cream

2 slices fat-free cheddar cheese

4 wedges The Laughing Cow Light Creamy Swiss cheese

Optional seasonings: salt and black pepper

DIRECTIONS

Cook bacon until crispy, either in a large skillet over medium heat or on a microwave-safe plate in the microwave. (See package for cook time.) Crumble or chop.

In a medium-large pot, cook pasta per package instructions, about 8 minutes. Drain and cover to keep warm.

Meanwhile, cut squash into pieces similar in size to the penne, about 2 inches long and ½ inch thick.

Bring a large skillet sprayed with nonstick spray to medium heat. Add squash, cover, and cook for 5 minutes, occasionally uncovering to stir.

Add spinach and tomato to the skillet, re-cover, and continue to cook for 1 minute. Remove cover and cook and stir until spinach has wilted, tomato is soft, and most excess liquid has cooked off, about 3 minutes. Drain excess liquid, stir cooked veggies into pasta, and cover to keep warm.

In a microwave-safe bowl, mix sour cream, cheese slices, and cheese wedges, breaking slices and wedges into pieces as you add them. Microwave for 30 seconds, and stir thoroughly. Microwave for another 30 seconds, or until fully melted. Mix until smooth.

Add cheese mixture to veggies and pasta. Stir to coat. Top with bacon. Serve it up!

MAKES 4 SERVINGS

BUFFALO CHICKEN MAC & CHEESE

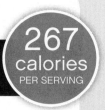

267 calories
PER SERVING

You'll Need: 8-inch by 8-inch baking pan, nonstick spray, medium-large pot, skillet, microwave-safe bowl
Prep: 15 minutes | **Cook:** 45 minutes

¼th of recipe:
267 calories, 3.5g fat, 924mg sodium, 35g carbs, 6.5g fiber, 5.5g sugars, 23g protein

INGREDIENTS

4½ ounces (about 1¼ cups) uncooked high-fiber elbow macaroni

2 stalks celery, chopped

2 medium carrots, chopped

1 small onion, chopped

8 ounces cooked and shredded skinless chicken breast

1 teaspoon chopped garlic

¼ cup Frank's RedHot Original Cayenne Pepper Sauce

½ cup fat-free sour cream

2 teaspoons yellow mustard

2 wedges The Laughing Cow Light Creamy Swiss cheese

1½ tablespoons reduced-fat Parmesan-style grated topping

1 tablespoon chopped fresh parsley

DIRECTIONS

Preheat oven to 350 degrees. Spray an 8-inch by 8-inch baking pan with nonstick spray.

In a medium-large pot, cook pasta per package instructions, about 8 minutes. Drain well.

Bring a skillet sprayed with nonstick spray to medium-high heat. Add celery, carrots, and onion. Cook and stir until slightly softened, about 5 minutes.

Add chicken, garlic, and 3 tablespoons hot sauce to the skillet. Mix thoroughly and remove from heat.

In a microwave-safe bowl, combine sour cream, mustard, remaining 1 tablespoon hot sauce, and cheese wedges, breaking the wedges into pieces. Mix well and microwave for 30 seconds, or until cheese has melted. Stir thoroughly.

Distribute half of the pasta into the baking pan. Evenly layer with the chicken-veggie mixture, remaining pasta, and sour cream mixture. Sprinkle with Parm-style topping and parsley.

Bake until hot and bubbly, about 30 minutes. Serve and enjoy!

MAKES 4 SERVINGS

BOLOGNESE-Y MAC & CHEESY

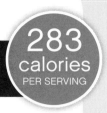

283 calories PER SERVING

You'll Need: large microwave-safe bowl, medium-large pot, large skillet, nonstick spray, medium microwave-safe bowl
Prep: 10 minutes | **Cook:** 30 minutes

¼th of recipe (about 1½ cups):
283 calories, 6g fat, 565mg sodium, 33.5g carbs, 5.5g fiber, 7g sugars, 22.5g protein

INGREDIENTS

3 cups frozen cauliflower florets

4½ ounces (about 1¾ cups) uncooked high-fiber rotini pasta

8 ounces raw lean ground turkey

⅛ teaspoon each salt and black pepper

¼ teaspoon garlic powder

¼ teaspoon onion powder

2 cups sliced mushrooms

1 teaspoon chopped garlic

½ cup canned crushed tomatoes

2 tablespoons fat-free sour cream

2 slices fat-free American cheese

4 wedges The Laughing Cow Light Creamy Swiss cheese

DIRECTIONS

Place cauliflower in a large microwave-safe bowl; cover and microwave for 3 minutes. Uncover and stir. Cover and microwave for another 3 minutes, or until hot. Drain excess liquid. Roughly chop cauliflower, return to the bowl, and cover to keep warm.

In a medium-large pot, cook pasta per package instructions, about 8 minutes. Drain pasta and stir into cauliflower. Cover to keep warm.

Bring a large skillet sprayed with nonstick spray to medium-high heat. Add turkey and season with salt, pepper, ⅛ teaspoon garlic powder, and ⅛ teaspoon onion powder. Add mushrooms and chopped garlic. Cook, crumble turkey, and stir for 6 to 8 minutes, until turkey is fully cooked and mushrooms are soft.

Add crushed tomatoes, remaining ⅛ teaspoon garlic powder, and remaining ⅛ teaspoon onion powder to the turkey mixture in the skillet. Cook and stir until hot, 1 to 2 minutes. Remove from heat.

In a medium microwave-safe bowl, mix sour cream, cheese slices, and cheese wedges, breaking slices and wedges into pieces. Microwave for 30 seconds. Stir well. Microwave for another 30 seconds, or until cheeses have melted. Stir until smooth.

Add cheese mixture to pasta and cauliflower and stir to coat. Stir in turkey mixture. If needed, microwave until hot. Enjoy!

MAKES 4 SERVINGS

BAKED PUMPKIN MAC & CHEESE

276 calories PER SERVING

You'll Need: 8-inch by 8-inch baking pan, nonstick spray, large microwave-safe bowl, medium-large pot, large skillet, microwave-safe bowl | **Prep:** 10 minutes | **Cook:** 1 hour and 5 minutes

¼th of recipe:
276 calories, 5g fat, 590mg sodium, 46.5g carbs, 8.5g fiber, 10.5g sugars, 11.5g protein

INGREDIENTS

3 cups frozen cauliflower florets

4½ ounces (about 1¼ cups) uncooked high-fiber elbow macaroni

1 tablespoon light whipped butter or light buttery spread

2 cups finely chopped onion

¼ teaspoon salt

Dash cayenne pepper

1 cup canned pure pumpkin

2 slices fat-free cheddar cheese

4 wedges The Laughing Cow Light Creamy Swiss cheese

1 ounce (about 15) reduced-fat sour cream & onion potato chips, crushed

DIRECTIONS

Preheat oven to 350 degrees. Spray an 8-inch by 8-inch baking pan with nonstick spray.

Place cauliflower in a large microwave-safe bowl; cover and microwave for 3 minutes. Uncover and stir. Cover and microwave for another 3 minutes, or until hot. Drain excess liquid. Roughly chop cauliflower and return to the bowl.

In a medium-large pot, cook pasta per package instructions, about 8 minutes. Drain pasta and stir into cauliflower.

Meanwhile, melt butter in a large skillet over medium-high heat. Add chopped onion, salt, and cayenne pepper. Cook and stir until softened, about 5 minutes. Reduce heat to medium low. Stirring frequently, cook until caramelized, 20 to 25 minutes.

Stir onion mixture into the cauliflower and pasta.

In a microwave-safe bowl, mix pumpkin, cheese slices, and cheese wedges, breaking slices and wedges into pieces. Microwave for 30 seconds. Stir well. Microwave for another 30 seconds, or until cheeses have melted. Stir well.

Add cheese mixture to the pasta, cauliflower, and onion mixture. Stir to coat. Transfer contents to the baking pan and cover with crushed chips.

Bake until lightly browned, about 20 minutes. Enjoy!

MAKES 4 SERVINGS

HOT-DIGGITY DOG CHEESY MAC

272 calories
PER SERVING

You'll Need: medium-large pot, large bowl, large skillet, nonstick spray, medium microwave-safe bowl
Prep: 15 minutes
Cook: 25 minutes

¼th of recipe (about 1⅓ cups):
272 calories, 3.5g fat, 976mg sodium, 44.5g carbs, 5g fiber, 11g sugars, 17g protein

INGREDIENTS

4½ ounces (about 1¼ cups) uncooked high-fiber elbow macaroni

1½ cups diced onion

1½ cups diced red bell pepper

7 hot dogs with about 40 calories and 1g fat or less each, chopped

½ cup fat-free sour cream

1 tablespoon yellow or spicy mustard

1 tablespoon ketchup

2 wedges The Laughing Cow Light Creamy Swiss cheese

DIRECTIONS

In a medium-large pot, cook pasta per package instructions, about 8 minutes. Drain, transfer to a large bowl, and cover to keep warm.

Bring a large skillet sprayed with nonstick spray to medium-high heat. Cook and stir onion and pepper until slightly softened, 6 to 7 minutes. Add chopped hot dogs and cook and stir until hot, about 2 minutes.

Remove skillet from heat. In a medium microwave-safe bowl, mix sour cream, mustard, ketchup, and cheese wedges, breaking wedges into pieces. Microwave for 30 seconds. Stir well. Microwave for another 30 seconds, or until cheese has melted. Stir until smooth.

Add sour cream mixture to pasta and stir to coat. Stir in hot dog mixture and enjoy!

MAKES 4 SERVINGS

BBQ CHICKEN MAC & CHEESE

365 calories
PER SERVING

You'll Need: 8-inch by 8-inch baking pan, nonstick spray, medium-large pot, large bowl, microwave-safe bowl, medium bowl
Prep: 10 minutes
Cook: 40 minutes

¼th of recipe: 365 calories, 6.5g fat, 798mg sodium, 45.5g carbs, 4g fiber, 14g sugars, 30g protein

INGREDIENTS

4½ ounces (about 1¼ cups) uncooked high-fiber elbow macaroni

½ cup fat-free sour cream

2 wedges The Laughing Cow Light Creamy Swiss cheese

2 cups frozen petite mixed vegetables, thawed

10 ounces cooked and shredded (or finely chopped) skinless chicken breast

½ cup BBQ sauce with 45 calories or less per 2-tablespoon serving

½ cup shredded reduced-fat Mexican-blend cheese

1½ tablespoons reduced-fat Parmesan-style grated topping

DIRECTIONS

Preheat oven to 350 degrees. Spray an 8-inch by 8-inch baking pan with nonstick spray.

In a medium-large pot, cook pasta per package instructions, about 8 minutes. Drain pasta and transfer to a large bowl.

In a microwave-safe bowl, mix sour cream with cheese wedges, breaking wedges into pieces. Microwave for 30 seconds, or until warm. Mix well, add to pasta, and stir to coat. Stir thawed veggies into pasta and transfer to the baking pan.

In a medium bowl, coat chicken with BBQ sauce. Evenly layer over veggie-pasta mixture in the pan. Sprinkle with shredded cheese and Parm-style topping.

Bake until hot, about 30 minutes. Eat!

MAKES 4 SERVINGS

SUN-DRIED TOMATO MAC & CHEESE

240 calories
PER SERVING

You'll Need: large microwave-safe bowl, medium-large pot, skillet, nonstick spray, medium microwave-safe bowl
Prep: 10 minutes | **Cook:** 25 minutes

¼th of recipe (about 1⅓ cups):
240 calories, 2.5g fat, 415mg sodium, 41.5g carbs, 7g fiber, 11.5g sugars, 11.5g protein

INGREDIENTS

3 cups frozen cauliflower florets

4½ ounces (about 1¼ cups) uncooked high-fiber elbow macaroni

1 cup chopped onion

½ cup bagged sun-dried tomatoes (not packed in oil), chopped

½ cup chopped fresh basil

2 tablespoons fat-free sour cream

2 slices fat-free American cheese

4 wedges The Laughing Cow Light Creamy Swiss cheese

SUN-DRIED TOMATO TIP:

If you can only find sun-dried tomatoes that are packed in oil, drain and rinse them really well, and then pat dry. This will get rid of excess fat.

DIRECTIONS

Place cauliflower in a large microwave-safe bowl; cover and microwave for 3 minutes. Uncover and stir. Re-cover and microwave for 2 to 3 minutes, until hot. Drain excess liquid. Roughly chop cauliflower, return to the bowl, and cover to keep warm.

In a medium-large pot, prepare pasta per package instructions, about 8 minutes. Drain pasta and stir into cauliflower. Cover to keep warm.

Bring a skillet sprayed with nonstick spray to medium-high heat. Cook and stir onion until softened and lightly browned, about 5 minutes. Add sun-dried tomatoes and basil and cook until basil has slightly wilted, about 2 minutes.

Stir onion mixture into the cauliflower and pasta. Cover to keep warm. In a medium microwave-safe bowl, mix sour cream, cheese slices, and cheese wedges, breaking slices and wedges into pieces. Microwave for 30 seconds. Stir well. Microwave for another 30 seconds, or until cheeses have melted. Stir well.

Add cheese mixture to the large bowl and thoroughly stir. Enjoy!

MAKES 4 SERVINGS

Hungry for More Coziness?
Check out the Crock Pots chapter for chilis, stews, soups & more!

CHAPTER 15

PARTY FOODS, COCKTAILS & HOLIDAY

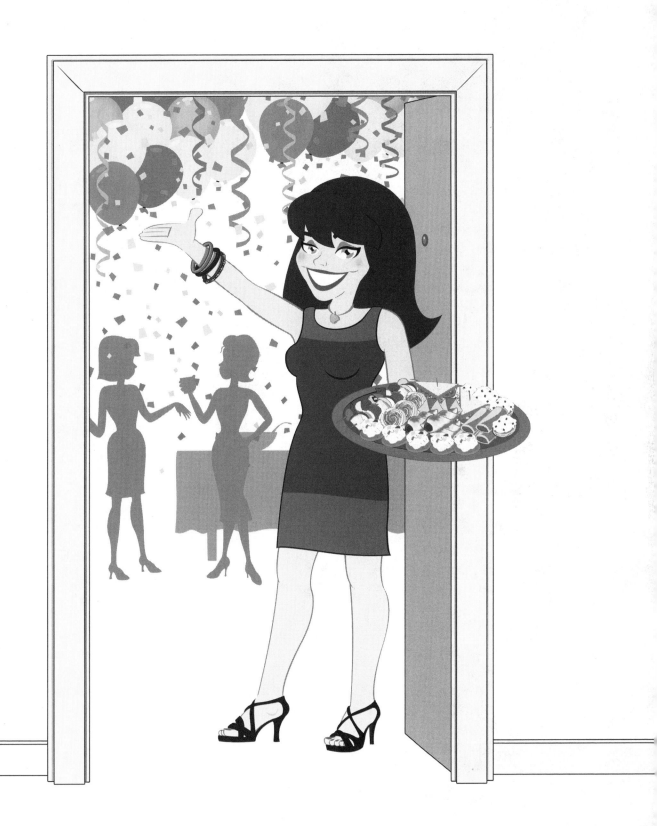

PARTY FOODS, COCKTAILS & HOLIDAY

PARTY FOODS

Hip-Hip-Hooray Chicken Satay
Bacon 'n Cheese Bell Pepper Skins
Portabella Skinny Skins
Best-Ever Potato Skins
Bacon-Wrapped Pepper Poppers
Bacon-Bundled BBQ Shrimp
Bacon-Wrapped Mango-BBQ Scallops
BLT Wonton Crunchies
Nacho Wonton Crunchies
Chinese Chicken Wonton Crunchies
Cobb Wonton Crunchies
Chicken Caesar Wonton Crunchies
Wonton 'Quitos
Tiny Taco Salads
Fiesta Wonton Crunchies
Mexi-licious Pot Stickers
The Crab Rangoonies
Cheesy Pepperoni Pizza Poppers
Spanako-pieces
Amazing Ate-Layer Dip
Buff Chick Hot Wing Dip
Rockin' Restaurant Spinach Dip
Roasted Veggie Spreaddip
Sweet Caramelized Onion Dip
Holy Moly Guacamole
Rockin' Roasted Corn Guac
Cheesy Chicken Egg Rolls
Sassy Southwestern Egg Rolls
De-Pudged Pigs in a Blanket
Garlic-Bread Pigs in a Blanket
Bacon-Wrapped Pigs in a Blanket
BB-Cutie Pigs in a Blanket
Honey Mustard & Swiss Pigs in a Blanket
Devilish Eggs
Mexi-Deviled Eggs
Four-Cheese Stuffed-Silly Mushrooms
Spicy Bacon-Stuffed Cheesy Mushrooms

Super-Stuffed Spinach-Feta Mushrooms
Ooey-Gooey Chili Cheese Nachos
Saucy Chick BBQ Nachos
Chili Cheese Dog Nachos
Pizza-Pied Nachos
Simply Sweet Meatballs
Cran-tastically Easy Meatballs

COCKTAILS

HG's Magical Low-Calorie Margarita
Freezy-Fresa Strawberry Margarita
Slammin' Strawberry Daiquiri
Piña Colada Freeze
Chilly Chocolate Mudslide
My Oh Mai Tai
Pineapple Frojitos
Mojito Madness
Super-Sour Lemon Drop
Kickin' Cranberry Cosmo
Apple Cinnamon Cosmo
Night & Day Nog-tinis
ChocoMint Martinis

HOLIDAY

Save-the-Day Stuffing
Cran-tastic Apple Cornbread Stuffing
Apple & Onion Stuffing
Rockin' Lean Bean Casserole
Kickin' Cranberry Sauce
Apple-licious Matzo Kugel
Peachy Cream Cinnamon Raisin Kugel
Love Ya Latkes
Crustless Pumpkin Quiche Supreme
I Can't Believe It's Not Sweet Potato Pie
No-Nonsense Nog
Cinn-fully Good Choco-Nog
Pumpkin-licious Nog

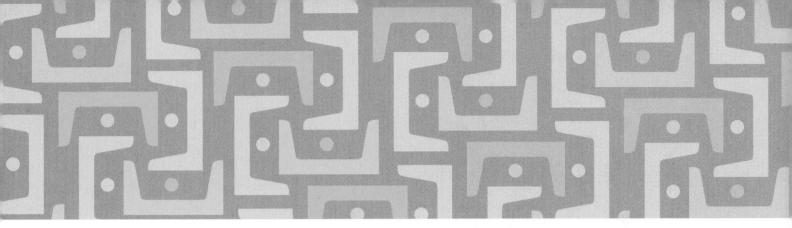

These are recipes that'll please the masses—masses who will have absolutely NO idea there's anything even remotely guilt-free about 'em . . .

A QUICK GUIDE TO SYMBOLS:

15 Minutes or Less

This symbol lets you know a recipe should take you no more than fifteen minutes from start to finish! That includes prep and cook time.

30 Minutes or Less

Just like the 15-minute version, this one points out recipes that take 30 minutes or less to whip up.

Meatless

You guessed it—no meat here! That includes beef, poultry, and fish. Some recipes give the option of a meatless ingredient. If you want your meal without meat, go with the meatless choice.

Single Serving

Pretty straightforward. These are recipes for one.

5 Ingredients or Less

Fans of HG know that we like to keep things simple. And these recipes contain just five ingredients or less!

Photos

These recipes can be seen in one of the book's photo inserts. The number in the symbol tells you which insert. Find photos of all the recipes at hungry-girl.com/books!

PARTY FOODS

These recipes are worth celebrating.
So party it up, HG-style . . .

HUNGRY FOR SWEET PARTY TREATS?

Flip forward to the
Sweet Stuff chapter for
cupcakes & MORE!

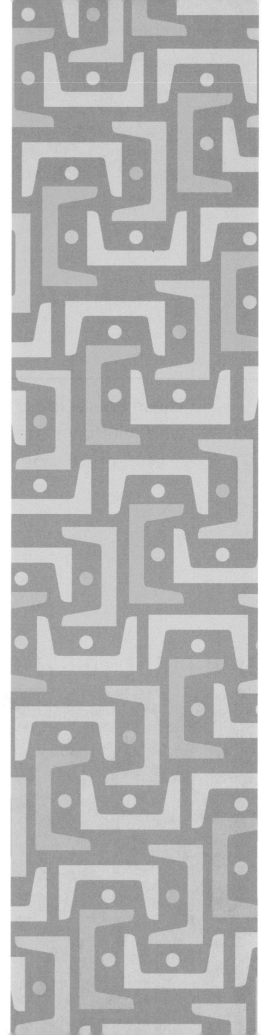

HIP-HIP-HOORAY CHICKEN SATAY

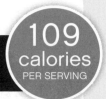

109 calories PER SERVING

You'll Need: baking sheet, nonstick spray, 12 skewers, small nonstick pot | **Prep:** 15 minutes | **Cook:** 10 minutes

⅙th of recipe (2 skewers with sauce):
109 calories, 2.75g fat, 269mg sodium, 4.5g carbs, 0.25g fiber, 2g sugars, 15.5g protein

INGREDIENTS

Chicken

12 ounces raw boneless skinless chicken breast, pounded to ½-inch thickness

⅛ teaspoon curry powder

⅛ teaspoon salt

2 dashes black pepper

Sauce

⅓ cup light plain soymilk

2 tablespoons reduced-fat peanut butter, room temperature

1½ tablespoons reduced-sodium/lite soy sauce

1 teaspoon granulated white sugar or Splenda No Calorie Sweetener (granulated)

¼ teaspoon crushed garlic

¼ teaspoon dried minced onion

⅛ teaspoon cayenne pepper

¼ cup fat-free plain yogurt

DIRECTIONS

Preheat oven to 375 degrees. Spray a baking sheet with nonstick spray.

Sprinkle chicken with seasonings. Evenly cut chicken into 12 strips, and thread each strip onto a skewer.

Place skewers on the baking sheet, and bake until chicken is cooked through, about 10 minutes.

Meanwhile, combine all sauce ingredients *except* yogurt in a small nonstick pot. Bring to medium-low heat. Stirring constantly, cook until hot and well mixed, about 5 minutes.

Remove sauce from heat and let cool slightly. Stir in yogurt until smooth and blended. Serve with chicken skewers, spoon it on, and enjoy!

MAKES 6 SERVINGS

HG ALTERNATIVE!

Wanna grill your chicken skewers? If using wooden skewers, presoak them in water for 30 minutes. Bring a grill or grill pan sprayed with nonstick spray to medium-high heat, and grill until chicken is cooked through, 1 to 2 minutes per side. If using a grill pan, remove from heat and re-spray between batches.

For more recipes, tips & tricks, sign up for FREE daily emails at hungry-girl.com!

BACON 'N CHEESE BELL PEPPER SKINS

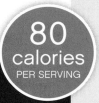

119 calories
PER SERVING

You'll Need: baking sheet, nonstick spray, large skillet or microwave-safe plate
Prep: 10 minutes
Cook: 40 minutes

¼th of recipe (2 pieces): 119 calories, 5.5g fat, 378mg sodium, 6.5g carbs, 1.25g fiber, 3.5g sugars, 11g protein

INGREDIENTS

2 red or yellow bell peppers
6 slices extra-lean turkey bacon
¾ cup shredded reduced-fat cheddar cheese
¼ cup chopped scallions
¼ cup fat-free sour cream

DIRECTIONS

Preheat oven to 350 degrees. Spray a baking sheet with nonstick spray.

Cut each pepper lengthwise into quarters, and remove stems and seeds. Place pepper pieces on the sheet, cut sides up. Bake until soft, about 20 minutes. Remove sheet, but leave oven on.

Meanwhile, cook bacon until crispy, either in a large skillet over medium heat or on a microwave-safe plate in the microwave. (See package for cook time.)

Chop or crumble bacon. Blot away excess moisture from pepper pieces. Evenly distribute cheese, scallions, and bacon among the pepper pieces.

Bake until cheese has melted, 5 to 10 minutes. Serve with sour cream and enjoy!

MAKES 4 SERVINGS

PORTABELLA SKINNY SKINS

80 calories
PER SERVING

You'll Need: baking sheet, nonstick spray, skillet or microwave-safe plate
Prep: 10 minutes
Cook: 25 minutes

¼th of recipe (1 portabella skin): 80 calories, 1.5g fat, 414mg sodium, 7g carbs, 1.5g fiber, 3g sugars, 10g protein

INGREDIENTS

2 slices center-cut bacon or turkey bacon
4 large portabella mushroom caps
¼ teaspoon salt
⅛ teaspoon black pepper
⅔ cup shredded fat-free cheddar cheese
½ cup chopped tomato
1 tablespoon chopped scallions

DIRECTIONS

Preheat oven to 450 degrees. Spray a baking sheet with nonstick spray.

Cook bacon until crispy, either in a skillet over medium heat or on a microwave-safe plate in the microwave. (See package for cook time.)

Place mushroom caps on the baking sheet, rounded sides down. Sprinkle with salt and pepper.

Distribute cheese among the mushroom caps. Bake until cheese has melted and mushroom caps are lightly browned, about 10 minutes.

Chop or crumble bacon and sprinkle over cheese. Distribute tomato and scallions among the mushroom caps.

Bake until toppings are hot, about 5 minutes. Mmmmm!

MAKES 4 SERVINGS

MEXICAN

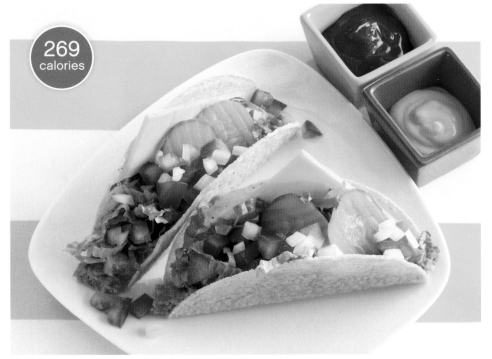

269 calories

Cheeseburger Tacos, p. 250

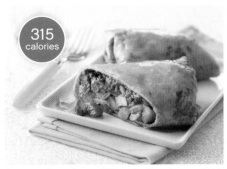

315 calories

Snazzy Smothered Veggie Burrito, p. 254

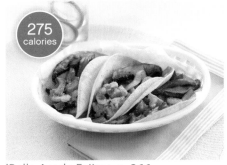

275 calories

'Bella Asada Fajitas, p. 266

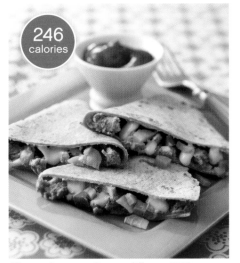

246 calories

Cheeseburger Quesadilla, p. 259

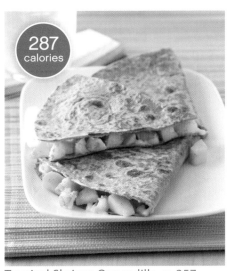

287 calories

Tropical Shrimp Quesadilla, p. 257

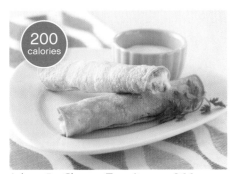

200 calories

Jalapeño Cheese Taquitos, p. 266

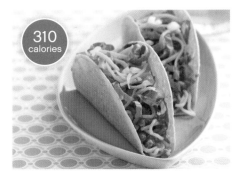

310 calories

iHungry Spaghetti Tacos, p. 250

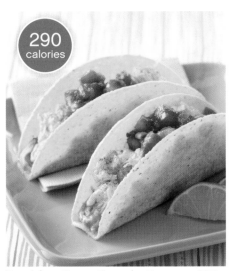

290 calories

Breakfast Fiesta Crunchy Tacos, p. 251

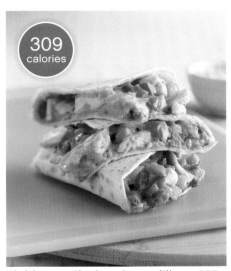

309 calories

Clubhouse Chicken Quesadilla, p. 257

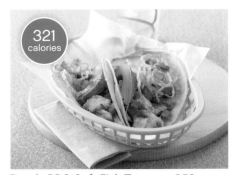

321 calories

Peach-BBQ Soft Fish Tacos, p. 252

BURGERS & FRIES

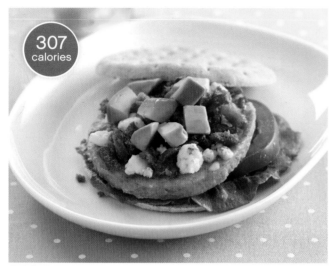

307 calories

Cobb Burger, p. 274

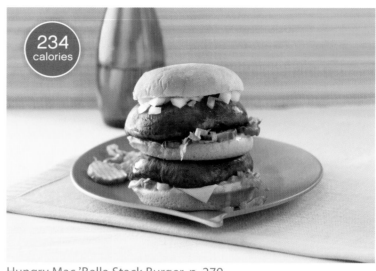

234 calories

Hungry Mac 'Bella Stack Burger, p. 279

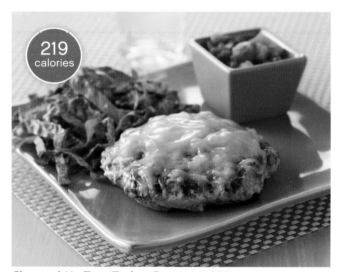

219 calories

Cheesed-Up Taco Turkey Burger, p. 285

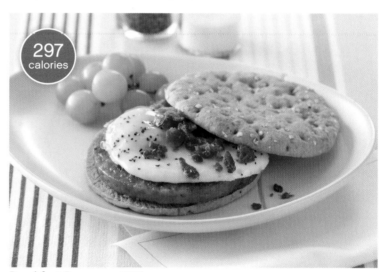

297 calories

Breakfast Burger, p. 276

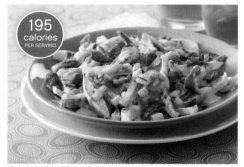

195 calories PER SERVING

Bacon 'n Cheese Turnip Fries, p. 292

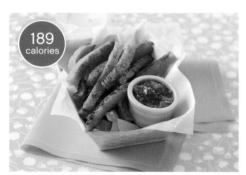

189 calories

Sweet Garlic Butternut Fries, p. 291

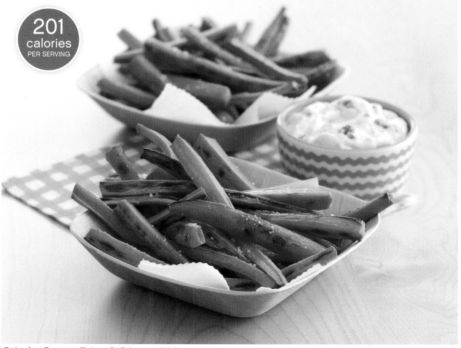

201 calories PER SERVING

Grin 'n Carrot Fries & Dip, p. 293

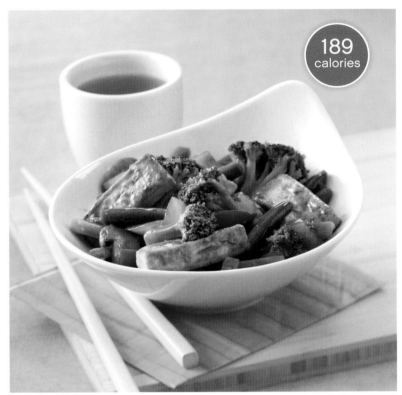

189 calories

Turbo Tofu Stir-Fry, p. 305

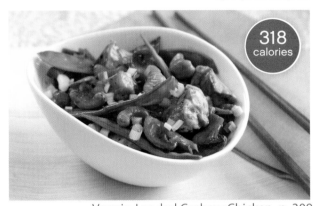

318 calories

Veggie-Loaded Cashew Chicken, p. 309

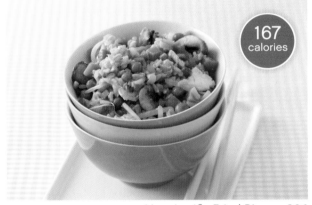

167 calories

Veggie-rific Fried Rice, p. 306

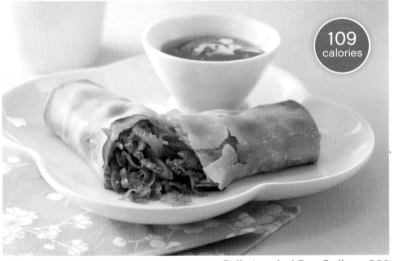

109 calories

Fully Loaded Egg Rolls, p. 300

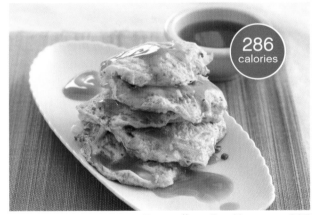

286 calories

Egg-cellent Foo Young, p. 307

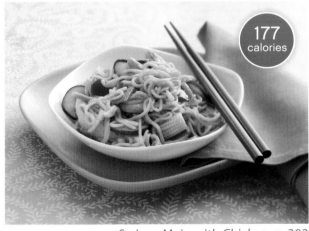

177 calories

So Low Mein with Chicken, p. 302

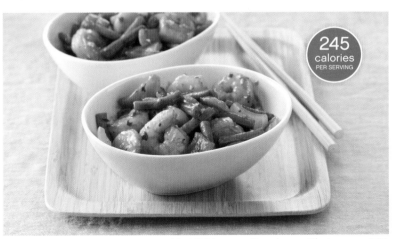

245 calories
PER SERVING

Hot & Hungry Szechuan Shrimp, p. 301

COMFORTABLY YUM

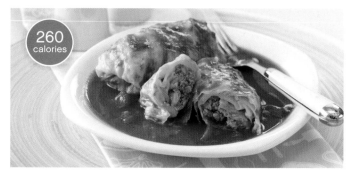

260 calories

Floosh's Stuffed Cabbage, p. 328

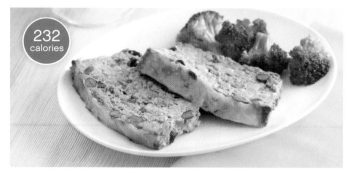

232 calories

Southwestern Meatloaf, p. 325

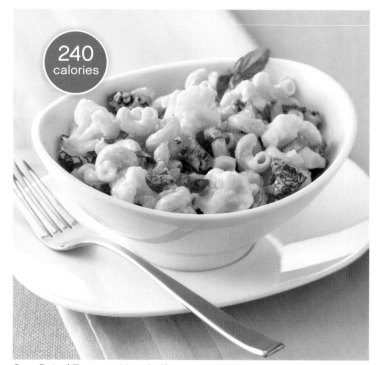

240 calories

Sun-Dried Tomato Mac & Cheese, p. 355

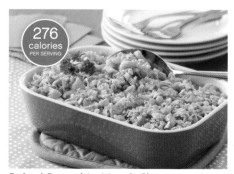

276 calories PER SERVING

Baked Pumpkin Mac & Cheese, p. 353

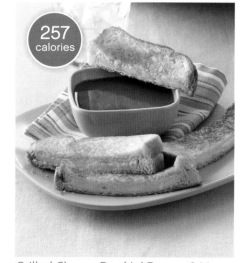

257 calories

Grilled Cheese Dunkin' Duo, p. 344

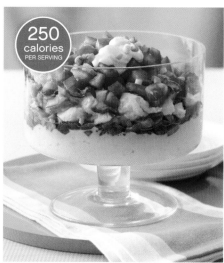

250 calories PER SERVING

Big Southern-Style B-fast Trifle, p. 327

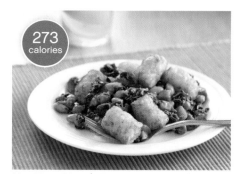

273 calories

Not-Your-Mom's Tater Tot Casserole, p. 331

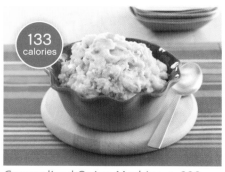

133 calories

Caramelized Onion Mashies, p. 338

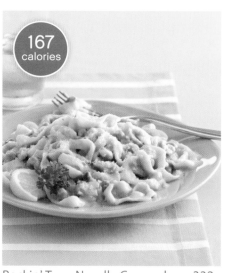

167 calories

Rockin' Tuna Noodle Casserole, p. 332

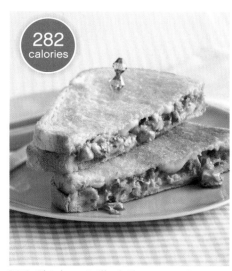

282 calories

BBQ Chicken Grilled Cheese, p. 344

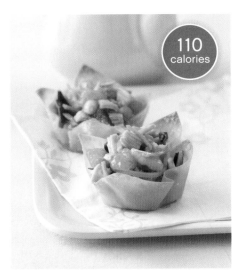

110 calories

Chinese Chicken Wonton Crunchies, p. 366

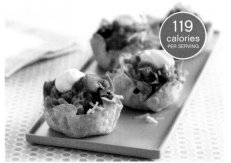

119 calories PER SERVING

Tiny Taco Salads, p. 368

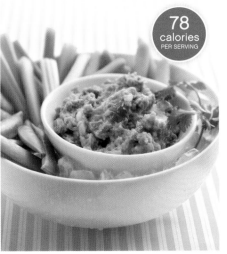

78 calories PER SERVING

Holy Moly Guacamole, p. 377

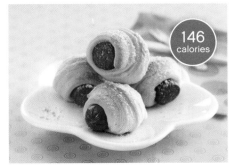

146 calories

Garlic-Bread Pigs in a Blanket, p. 380

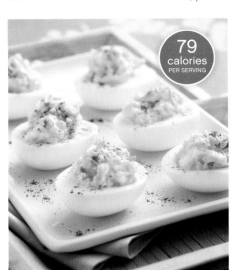

79 calories PER SERVING

Devilish Eggs, p. 382

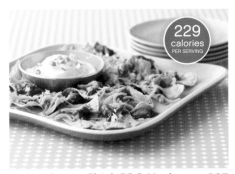

229 calories PER SERVING

Saucy Chick BBQ Nachos, p. 387

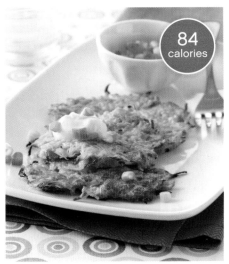

84 calories

Love Ya Latkes, p. 402

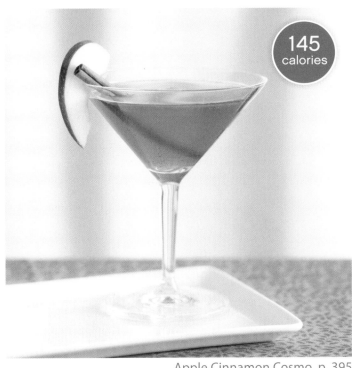

145 calories

Apple Cinnamon Cosmo, p. 395

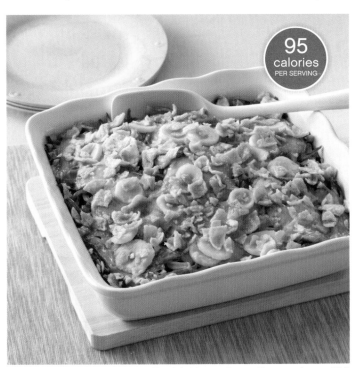

95 calories PER SERVING

Rockin' Lean Bean Casserole, p. 400

SWEET STUFF: FROM BROWNIES & FUDGE TO KRISPYMALLOWS

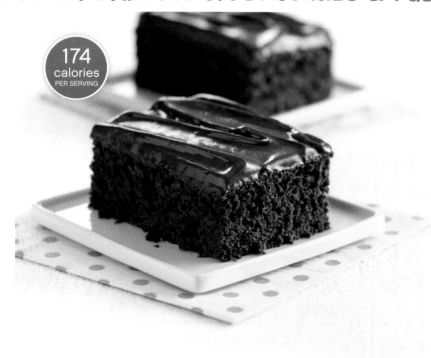

174 calories PER SERVING

Death-by-Chocolate Brownies, p. 414

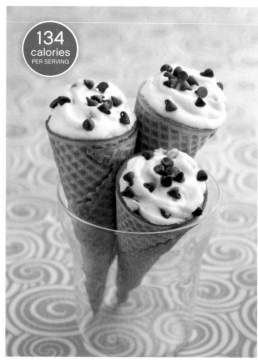

134 calories PER SERVING

Holy Moly Cannoli Cones, p. 418

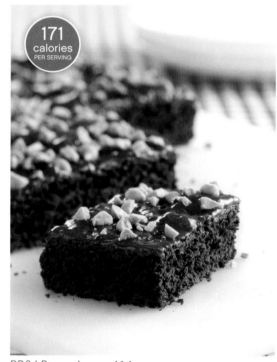

171 calories PER SERVING

PB&J Brownies, p. 414

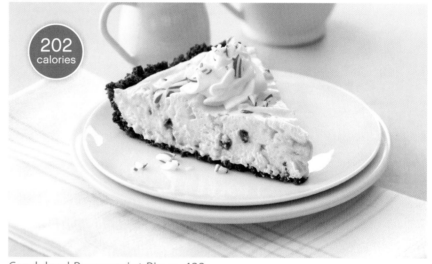

202 calories

Candyland Peppermint Pie, p. 423

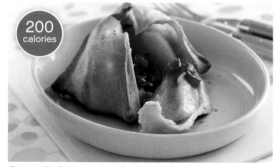

200 calories

Crazy-Delicious Apple Dumplings, p. 462

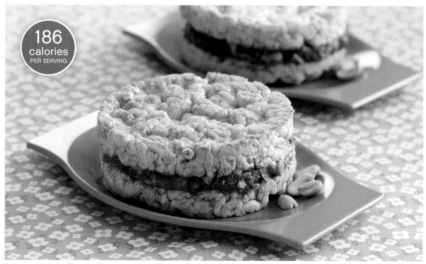

186 calories PER SERVING

Freezy-Cool Snickers Stackers, p. 486

SWEET STUFF: FROM BROWNIES & FUDGE TO KRISPYMALLOWS

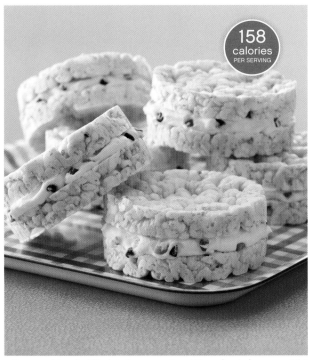

158 calories PER SERVING

Freezy Movie Night Concession Stand-wiches, p. 484

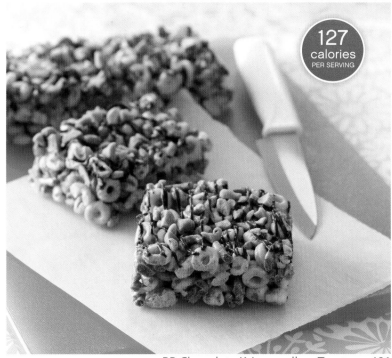

127 calories PER SERVING

PB Chocolate Krispymallow Treats, p. 491

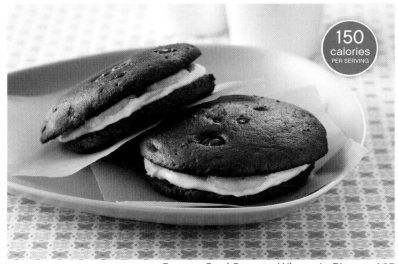

150 calories PER SERVING

Freezy-Cool Banana Whoopie Pies, p. 465

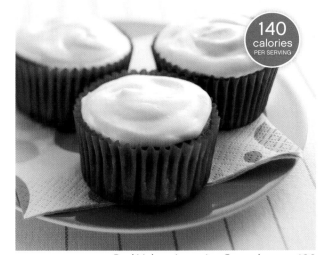

140 calories PER SERVING

Red Velvet Insanity Cupcakes, p. 429

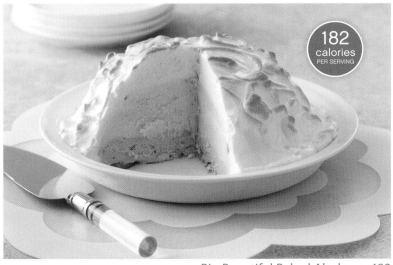

182 calories PER SERVING

Big Beautiful Baked Alaska, p. 482

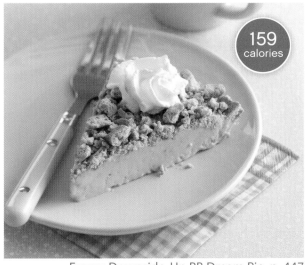

159 calories

Freezy Downside-Up PB Dream Pie, p. 447

SWEET STUFF: FROM BROWNIES & FUDGE TO KRISPYMALLOWS

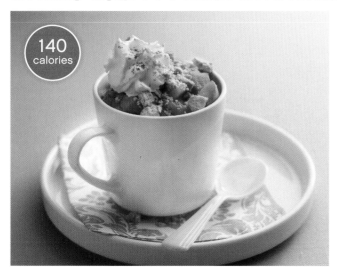

140 calories

Red Hot Apple Pie in a Cup, p. 432

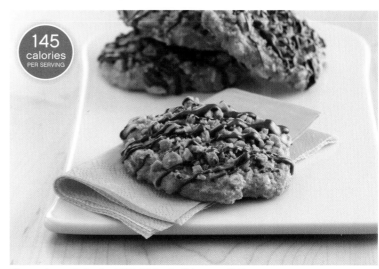

145 calories PER SERVING

Chocolate-Drizzled PB Chip Softies, p. 479

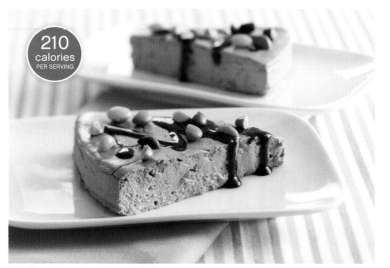

210 calories PER SERVING

PB Cup Cheesecake, p. 442

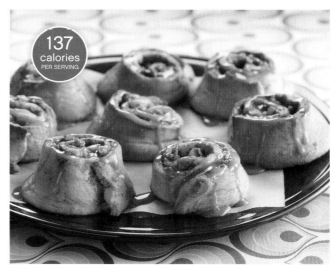

137 calories PER SERVING

Caramel Apple Cinnamon Buns, p. 469

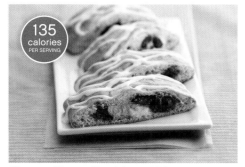

135 calories PER SERVING

Cheesy Cherry Danish, p. 459

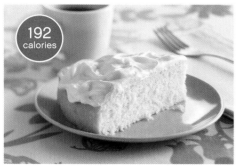

192 calories

Frosty the Vanilla Cake, p. 434

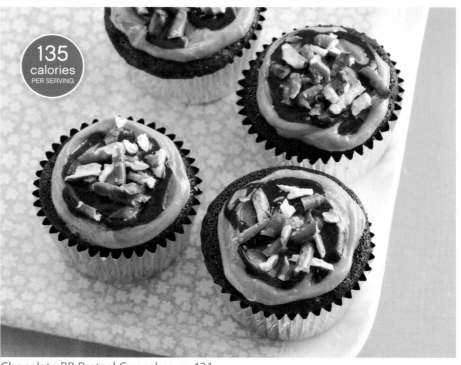

135 calories PER SERVING

Chocolate PB Pretzel Cupcakes, p. 431

BEST-EVER POTATO SKINS

202 calories PER SERVING

You'll Need: baking sheet, nonstick spray, microwave-safe plate, skillet (optional)
Prep: 10 minutes
Cook: 35 minutes

¼th of recipe (2 loaded potato skins): 202 calories, 7.5g fat, 295mg sodium, 23.5g carbs, 3.5g fiber, 2g sugars, 10g protein

INGREDIENTS

Four 10-ounce russet potatoes
3 slices center-cut bacon or turkey bacon
¾ cup shredded reduced-fat cheddar cheese
¼ cup chopped scallions
¼ cup reduced-fat/light sour cream

DIRECTIONS

Preheat oven to 375 degrees. Spray a baking sheet with nonstick spray.

Pierce potatoes several times with a fork, and place on a microwave-safe plate. Microwave for 5 minutes, or until they begin to soften.

Flip potatoes and microwave for 5 to 8 minutes, until soft on all sides.

Cut potatoes in half lengthwise. Scoop out and discard the inside flesh, leaving about ¼ inch inside the skin. Place the potato skins on the baking sheet.

Bake until crispy, 10 to 12 minutes. Remove sheet, but leave oven on.

Meanwhile, cook bacon until crispy, either in a skillet over medium heat or on a microwave-safe plate in the microwave. (See package for cook time.)

Chop or crumble bacon. Evenly distribute cheese and bacon among potato skins. Bake until cheese has melted, about 2 minutes.

Sprinkle with scallions and serve with sour cream for dipping. YUM!

MAKES 4 SERVINGS

BACON-WRAPPED PEPPER POPPERS

  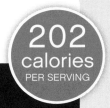

107 calories PER SERVING

You'll Need: baking sheet, nonstick spray, small bowl, toothpicks (optional)
Prep: 10 minutes
Cook: 20 minutes

¼th of recipe (3 poppers): 107 calories, 4.5g fat, 442mg sodium, 7.5g carbs, 1g fiber, 4.5g sugars, 8g protein

INGREDIENTS

¼ cup fat-free cream cheese, room temperature
2 wedges The Laughing Cow Light Creamy Swiss cheese
6 jalapeño peppers, halved lengthwise, seeds and stems removed
6 slices center-cut bacon or turkey bacon, halved widthwise

DIRECTIONS

Preheat oven to 375 degrees. Spray a baking sheet with nonstick spray.

In a small bowl, thoroughly mix cream cheese with cheese wedges until smooth. Evenly spoon and spread cheese mixture into the pepper halves.

Wrap a half-slice of bacon around each pepper half. Secure with a toothpick, if needed.

Evenly place pepper halves on the baking sheet. Bake until the bacon is just crispy, about 20 minutes. Serve and enjoy!

MAKES 4 SERVINGS

JALAPEÑO QUICK TIP!

Use a spoon to seed your jalapeños. When handling jalapeños, don't touch your eyes—that pepper juice can STING. And wash your hands well immediately afterward.

BACON-BUNDLED BBQ SHRIMP

154 calories PER SERVING

You'll Need: baking sheet, nonstick spray, medium bowl
Prep: 15 minutes
Cook: 15 minutes

¼th of recipe (4 shrimp): 154 calories, 5.5g fat, 612mg sodium, 6.5g carbs, <0.5g fiber, 5g sugars, 16.5g protein

INGREDIENTS

⅓ cup canned tomato sauce

3 tablespoons ketchup

1 tablespoon apple cider vinegar

1 tablespoon brown sugar (not packed)

½ teaspoon garlic powder

8 slices center-cut bacon or turkey bacon, halved widthwise

16 raw large (not jumbo) shrimp, peeled, tails removed, deveined

DIRECTIONS

Preheat oven to 425 degrees. Spray a baking sheet with nonstick spray.

In a medium bowl, thoroughly mix tomato sauce, ketchup, vinegar, sugar, and garlic powder.

Coat each half-slice of bacon in sauce mixture, wrap it around a shrimp, and place on the baking sheet, seam side down.

Bake until shrimp are cooked through, 10 to 15 minutes. So good!

MAKES 4 SERVINGS

BACON-WRAPPED MANGO-BBQ SCALLOPS

147 calories PER SERVING

You'll Need: baking sheet, nonstick spray, medium bowl, whisk, toothpicks
Prep: 15 minutes
Cook: 15 minutes

¼th of recipe (4 scallops): 147 calories, 5g fat, 534mg sodium, 9g carbs, <0.5g fiber, 6g sugars, 14.5g protein

INGREDIENTS

3 tablespoons canned tomato sauce

3 tablespoons mango nectar

2 tablespoons ketchup

2 teaspoons brown sugar (not packed)

2 teaspoons cider vinegar

1 teaspoon molasses

½ teaspoon garlic powder

8 slices center-cut bacon or turkey bacon, halved widthwise

16 raw large scallops

DIRECTIONS

Preheat oven to 425 degrees. Spray a baking sheet with nonstick spray.

To make the sauce, in a medium bowl, thoroughly whisk all ingredients *except* bacon and scallops.

Wrap a half-slice of bacon around each scallop and secure with a toothpick. Place scallops on the baking sheet.

Bake for 5 minutes. Flip scallops, and evenly top with sauce. Bake until the scallops are cooked through, 5 to 8 minutes. Yum!

MAKES 4 SERVINGS

Wonton wrappers are the Eli Manning of the HG kitchen. (He's a football player. A really good one who wins MVP awards constantly. Google him.) These recipes utilize their low-cal wonton-y magic . . .

BLT WONTON CRUNCHIES

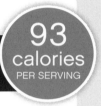

93 calories
PER SERVING

You'll Need: 12-cup muffin pan, nonstick spray, skillet or microwave-safe plate, large bowl, large plate
Prep: 15 minutes | **Cook:** 20 minutes

⅙th of recipe (2 wonton crunchies):
93 calories, 3g fat, 435mg sodium, 12g carbs, 1g fiber, 2g sugars, 3.5g protein

INGREDIENTS

6 slices center-cut bacon or turkey bacon

12 small square wonton wrappers

¼ cup fat-free mayonnaise

3 tablespoons Hellmann's/Best Foods Dijonnaise

Dash garlic powder

Dash each salt and black pepper

1 cup seeded and chopped plum tomatoes

2 cups finely chopped lettuce

DIRECTIONS

Preheat oven to 350 degrees. Spray a 12-cup muffin pan with nonstick spray.

Cook bacon until crispy, either in a skillet over medium heat or on a microwave-safe plate in the microwave. (See package for cook time.)

Place each wonton wrapper in a cup of the muffin pan, and press it into the bottom and sides. Lightly spray with nonstick spray. Bake until lightly browned, about 8 minutes.

Finely chop bacon. In a large bowl, mix mayo, Dijonnaise, garlic powder, salt, and pepper. Stir in tomatoes, lettuce, and bacon.

Once cool, transfer wonton shells to a large plate. Evenly distribute BLT mixture among the shells, about 3 tablespoons each. Enjoy!

MAKES 6 SERVINGS

QUICK Q&A WITH HG:

Where can I find wonton wrappers?
With the tofu and other refrigerated Asian products.

NACHO WONTON CRUNCHIES

130
calories
PER SERVING

You'll Need: 12-cup muffin pan, nonstick spray, medium bowl, large plate
Prep: 15 minutes
Cook: 10 minutes

⅙th of recipe (2 wonton crunchies): 130 calories, 3.5g fat, 375mg sodium, 13.5g carbs, 1.5g fiber, 1.5g sugars, 11g protein

INGREDIENTS

12 small square wonton wrappers
4 ounces cooked and finely chopped skinless chicken breast
¼ cup chunky salsa
¾ cup shredded reduced-fat Mexican-blend cheese
½ cup canned black beans, drained and rinsed
12 jarred jalapeño pepper slices, drained and chopped
¼ cup fat-free sour cream

DIRECTIONS

Preheat oven to 350 degrees. Spray a 12-cup muffin pan with nonstick spray.

Place a wonton wrapper in each cup of the muffin pan, and press it into the bottom and sides. Lightly spray with nonstick spray. Bake until very lightly browned, about 5 minutes. Remove pan, but leave oven on.

In a medium bowl, mix chicken with salsa.

Place ½ tablespoon cheese in the bottom of each wonton cup. Evenly distribute beans and chicken mixture among the cups. Top each cup with another ½ tablespoon cheese.

Bake until filling is hot and cheese has melted, about 5 minutes.

Transfer wonton cups to a large plate, and evenly distribute chopped jalapeño peppers and sour cream among them. Eat!

MAKES 6 SERVINGS

CHINESE CHICKEN WONTON CRUNCHIES

110
calories
PER SERVING

You'll Need: 12-cup muffin pan, nonstick spray, large bowl, large plate
Prep: 15 minutes
Cook: 10 minutes

⅙th of recipe (2 wonton crunchies): 110 calories, 1g fat, 304mg sodium, 15g carbs, 1g fiber, 4.5g sugars, 9g protein

INGREDIENTS

12 small square wonton wrappers
1½ cups bagged broccoli cole slaw, chopped
6 ounces cooked and finely chopped skinless chicken breast
½ cup mandarin orange segments packed in juice, drained and chopped
½ cup canned sliced water chestnuts, drained and chopped
⅓ cup low-fat sesame ginger dressing
¼ cup chopped scallions

DIRECTIONS

Preheat oven to 350 degrees. Spray a 12-cup muffin pan with nonstick spray.

Place each wonton wrapper into a cup of the muffin pan, and press it into the bottom and sides. Lightly spray with nonstick spray. Bake until lightly browned, about 8 minutes.

In a large bowl, mix together all remaining ingredients.

Once cool, transfer wonton shells to a large plate. Evenly distribute the mixture among the shells, about 3 tablespoons per shell. Enjoy!

MAKES 6 SERVINGS

COBB WONTON CRUNCHIES

128 calories PER SERVING

You'll Need: 12-cup muffin pan, nonstick spray, skillet or microwave-safe plate, large bowl, large plate
Prep: 15 minutes
Cook: 20 minutes

⅙th of recipe (2 wonton crunchies): 128 calories, 5g fat, 307mg sodium, 11.5g carbs, 1.5g fiber, 2g sugars, 9g protein

INGREDIENTS

5 slices center-cut bacon or turkey bacon

12 small square wonton wrappers

3 ounces cooked and finely chopped skinless chicken breast

1⅓ cups chopped plum tomatoes

1½ cups finely chopped romaine or iceberg lettuce

3 tablespoons light blue cheese dressing

2 ounces (about ¼ cup) chopped avocado

2 hard-boiled egg whites, chopped

DIRECTIONS

Preheat oven to 350 degrees. Spray a 12-cup muffin pan with nonstick spray.

Cook bacon until crispy, either in a skillet over medium heat or on a microwave-safe plate in the microwave. (See package for cook time.)

Place a wonton wrapper in each cup of the muffin pan, and press it into the bottom and sides. Lightly spray with nonstick spray. Bake until lightly browned, about 8 minutes.

In a large bowl, mix chicken, tomatoes, lettuce, and dressing. Finely chop bacon and add to the bowl. Gently stir in avocado and egg whites.

Once cool, transfer wonton shells to a large plate. Evenly distribute salad mixture among the shells, about 3 tablespoons each. Serve and devour!

MAKES 6 SERVINGS

CHICKEN CAESAR WONTON CRUNCHIES

109 calories PER SERVING

You'll Need: 12-cup muffin pan, nonstick spray, large bowl, large plate
Prep: 15 minutes
Cook: 10 minutes

⅙th of recipe (2 wonton crunchies): 109 calories, 3g fat, 274mg sodium, 10.5g carbs, 0.5g fiber, 1g sugars, 9g protein

INGREDIENTS

12 small square wonton wrappers

6 ounces cooked and finely chopped skinless chicken breast

2 cups finely chopped romaine or iceberg lettuce

¼ cup light/reduced-fat Caesar dressing

2 tablespoons reduced-fat Parmesan-style grated topping

DIRECTIONS

Preheat oven to 350 degrees. Spray a 12-cup muffin pan with nonstick spray.

Place a wonton wrapper in each cup of the muffin pan, and press it into the bottom and sides. Lightly spray with nonstick spray. Bake until lightly browned, about 8 minutes.

In a large bowl, thoroughly mix chicken, lettuce, and dressing.

Once cool, transfer wonton shells to a large plate. Evenly distribute salad mixture among the shells, about 3 tablespoons each. Top with Parm-style topping and eat up!

MAKES 6 SERVINGS

WONTON 'QUITOS

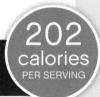

202 calories
PER SERVING

You'll Need: baking sheet, nonstick spray, medium bowl, toothpicks (optional)
Prep: 20 minutes
Chill: 15 minutes
Cook: 15 minutes

¼th of recipe (4 pieces): 202 calories, 2g fat, 759mg sodium, 20g carbs, 0.5g fiber, 2.5g sugars, 23g protein

INGREDIENTS

12½ ounces canned 98% fat-free chunk white chicken breast in water, drained and flaked
½ cup salsa verde (a.k.a. green salsa)
⅓ cup shredded fat-free cheddar cheese
¼ cup frozen sweet corn kernels, thawed
1 tablespoon chopped roasted red peppers
16 small square wonton wrappers

Optional dips: red enchilada sauce, additional salsa verde, fat-free sour cream

DIRECTIONS

Preheat oven to 375 degrees. Spray a baking sheet with nonstick spray.

In a medium bowl, mix chicken with salsa. Cover and refrigerate for 15 minutes.

Drain excess liquid from chicken mixture. Mix in cheese, corn, and roasted red peppers.

Lay a wonton wrapper flat on a dry surface. Place a heaping tablespoon of chicken mixture in the center, and evenly spread over the wonton. Roll the wonton up tightly into a cigar-shaped tube. If needed, secure with toothpicks.

Place on the baking sheet, seam side down. Repeat with remaining wrappers and chicken mixture.

Bake until crispy, about 15 minutes. Enjoy!

MAKES 4 SERVINGS

HG ALTERNATIVE!

If you're not into canned chicken, use 1½ cups of cooked & shredded skinless chicken breast instead. (But honestly, canned chicken rocks in this recipe.)

TINY TACO SALADS

119 calories
PER SERVING

You'll Need: 12-cup muffin pan, nonstick spray, microwave-safe bowl, large plate
Prep: 15 minutes
Cook: 10 minutes

⅙th of recipe (2 tiny salads): 119 calories, 2.5g fat, 446mg sodium, 15.5g carbs, 2.5g fiber, 1.5g sugars, 8.5g protein

INGREDIENTS

12 small square wonton wrappers
1 cup frozen ground-beef-style soy crumbles
½ cup fat-free refried beans
1 teaspoon taco seasoning mix
1½ cups shredded lettuce
½ cup shredded reduced-fat Mexican-blend cheese
1 tablespoon sliced black olives, chopped
6 tablespoons chunky salsa or pico de gallo
2 tablespoons fat-free sour cream

DIRECTIONS

Preheat oven to 350 degrees. Spray a 12-cup muffin pan with nonstick spray.

Place a wonton wrapper in each cup of the muffin pan, and press it into the bottom and sides. Lightly spray with nonstick spray. Bake until lightly browned, about 8 minutes.

In a microwave-safe bowl, mix soy crumbles, refried beans, and taco seasoning. Microwave for 1½ minutes, or until hot. Stir well.

Once cool, transfer wonton shells to a large plate. Evenly distribute shredded lettuce among shells, 2 tablespoons each. Top with soy-crumble mixture, about 1 tablespoon per shell. Evenly distribute cheese and chopped olives among the shells.

Finish off each mini taco salad with ½ tablespoon salsa or pico de gallo and ½ teaspoon sour cream. Serve and enjoy!

MAKES 6 SERVINGS

FIESTA WONTON CRUNCHIES

You'll Need: 12-cup muffin pan, nonstick spray, large bowl | **Prep:** 15 minutes | **Cook:** 15 minutes

1/12th of recipe (1 wonton crunchie):
55 calories, 0.5g fat, 190mg sodium, 6g carbs, 0.5g fiber, 0.5g sugars, 6g protein

55 calories PER SERVING

INGREDIENTS

12 small square wonton wrappers
2 tablespoons taco sauce
1 tablespoon fat-free cream cheese, room temperature
1 teaspoon taco seasoning mix
10 ounces canned 98% fat-free chunk white chicken breast in water, drained and flaked
¼ cup canned black beans, drained and rinsed
¼ cup frozen sweet corn kernels, thawed
¼ cup shredded fat-free cheddar cheese
½ cup chopped tomato
Optional seasonings: salt and black pepper

DIRECTIONS

Preheat oven to 350 degrees. Spray a 12-cup muffin pan with nonstick spray.

Place each wonton wrapper in a cup of the muffin pan, and press it into the bottom and sides. Lightly spray with nonstick spray. Bake until the corners just begin to brown, about 4 minutes.

Remove pan, but leave oven on.

In a large bowl, thoroughly mix taco sauce, cream cheese, and taco seasoning. Add chicken and stir to coat. Stir in beans, corn, and cheese.

Evenly distribute mixture among wonton shells, about 2 tablespoons each. Bake until filling is hot, about 8 minutes.

Serve topped with tomato and enjoy!

MAKES 12 SERVINGS

FUN WONTON-CRUNCHIE ALTERNATIVE!

When it comes to recipes with salad-style fillings, wider crunchie cups are fantastic! How do you do it? Spray the BOTTOM of the muffin pan with nonstick spray, and gently press wontons over the inverted cups. Then bake and fill as directed!

MEXI-LICIOUS POT STICKERS

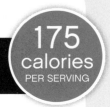
175 calories
PER SERVING

You'll Need: large skillet, nonstick spray, large bowl | **Prep:** 20 minutes | **Cook:** 30 minutes

⅙th of recipe (4 pot stickers):
175 calories, 3g fat, 459mg sodium, 21.5g carbs, 1.75g fiber, 1.5g sugars, 13.5g protein

INGREDIENTS

8 ounces raw lean ground turkey

½ tablespoon taco seasoning mix

1 small onion, chopped

¼ cup taco sauce

½ cup fat-free refried beans

½ cup shredded fat-free cheddar cheese

24 small square wonton wrappers

Optional toppings: salsa, fat-free sour cream

DIRECTIONS

Spray a large skillet with nonstick spray, and bring to medium-high heat. Cook and crumble turkey until browned and fully cooked, about 5 minutes.

Reduce heat to medium and sprinkle turkey with taco seasoning. Add onion and taco sauce. Cook and stir until onion has softened, about 5 minutes.

Transfer mixture to a large bowl. Stir in beans and cheese. Let cool completely. Meanwhile, wash skillet.

Lay a wonton wrapper flat on a dry surface. Place a heaping tablespoon filling (1⁄24th of filling) in the center. Moisten all four edges by dabbing your fingers in water and going over the edges smoothly. Fold the bottom left corner to meet the top right corner, forming a triangle and enclosing the filling. Press firmly on the edges to seal.

Repeat with remaining wrappers and filling.

Re-spray skillet with nonstick spray and return to medium-high heat. Working in batches and beginning with the flatter sides down, cook wontons until crispy, 3 to 4 minutes per side. (Between batches, remove skillet from heat and re-spray.) Enjoy!

MAKES 6 SERVINGS

Flip to the photo inserts to see over 100 recipe pics! And for photos of ALL the recipes, go to **hungry-girl.com/books.**

THE CRAB RANGOONIES

140 calories PER SERVING

You'll Need: baking sheet, nonstick spray, medium bowl | **Prep:** 20 minutes | **Cook:** 15 minutes

¼th of recipe (4 crab rangoonies):
140 calories, 1.25g fat, 593mg sodium, 20g carbs, 1g fiber, 2g sugars, 8.5g protein

INGREDIENTS

¼ cup fat-free cream cheese, room temperature

1 teaspoon reduced-sodium/lite soy sauce

2 wedges The Laughing Cow Light Creamy Swiss cheese

4 ounces (about ⅔ cup) flaked imitation crabmeat

¼ cup finely chopped scallions

½ teaspoon chopped garlic

16 small square wonton wrappers

Optional dips: sweet & sour sauce, Chinese-style hot mustard

DIRECTIONS

Preheat oven to 375 degrees. Spray a baking sheet with nonstick spray.

To make your filling, in a medium bowl, thoroughly mix cream cheese, soy sauce, and cheese wedges, breaking the wedges into pieces as you add them. Stir in crabmeat, scallions, and garlic.

Lay a wonton wrapper flat on a dry surface. Spoon a heaping ½ tablespoon filling (¹⁄₁₆th of filling) into the center. Moisten all four edges by dabbing your fingers in water and going over the edges smoothly. Fold the bottom left corner to meet the top right corner, forming a triangle and enclosing the filling. Press firmly on the edges to seal. Place on the baking sheet.

Repeat with remaining wrappers and filling. Spray the tops with nonstick spray.

Bake for 6 minutes. Flip stuffed wontons. Bake until golden brown, about 6 more minutes. Time to chew!

MAKES 4 SERVINGS

CHEESY PEPPERONI PIZZA POPPERS

135 calories
PER SERVING

You'll Need: baking sheet, nonstick spray, medium bowl, microwave-safe bowl
Prep: 20 minutes | **Cook:** 10 minutes

¼th of recipe (3 poppers):
135 calories, 3.5g fat, 496mg sodium, 16.5g carbs, 1g fiber, 3.5g sugars, 7g protein

INGREDIENTS

⅓ cup light or low-fat ricotta cheese

1½ teaspoons tomato paste

3 wedges The Laughing Cow Light Creamy Swiss cheese

12 slices turkey pepperoni, chopped

½ teaspoon dried minced onion

12 small square wonton wrappers

12 sprays I Can't Believe It's Not Butter! Spray

1 tablespoon reduced-fat Parmesan-style grated topping

⅛ teaspoon garlic powder

½ cup canned crushed tomatoes

⅛ teaspoon Italian seasoning

DIRECTIONS

Preheat oven to 375 degrees. Spray a baking sheet with nonstick spray.

In a medium bowl, thoroughly mix ricotta cheese, tomato paste, and cheese wedges, breaking the wedges into pieces as you add them. Stir in chopped pepperoni and minced onion.

Lay a wonton wrapper flat on a dry surface. Spoon a tablespoon filling (¹⁄₁₂th of filling) into the center. Moisten all four edges by dabbing your fingers in water and going over the edges smoothly. Fold the bottom left corner to meet the top right corner, forming a triangle and enclosing the filling. Press firmly on the edges to seal. Place on the baking sheet.

Repeat with remaining wrappers and filling. Spray the top of each "popper" with 1 spray of butter spray. Sprinkle with Parm-style topping and garlic powder.

Bake until golden brown, about 10 minutes.

Meanwhile, mix crushed tomatoes with Italian seasoning in a microwave-safe bowl. Microwave for 1 minute, or until hot. Stir and serve with poppers for dipping. YUM!

MAKES 4 SERVINGS

SPANAKO-PIECES

179 calories PER SERVING

You'll Need: baking sheet, nonstick spray, large bowl | **Prep:** 20 minutes | **Cook:** 15 minutes

¼th of recipe (4 pieces):
179 calories, 2g fat, 863mg sodium, 21.5g carbs, 1.5g fiber, 2.5g sugars, 12.5g protein

INGREDIENTS

One 10-ounce package frozen chopped spinach, thawed and squeezed dry
1 cup crumbled fat-free feta cheese
4 wedges The Laughing Cow Light Creamy Swiss cheese
⅓ cup diced onion
½ teaspoon chopped garlic
½ teaspoon dried parsley
⅛ teaspoon black pepper
⅛ teaspoon salt
16 small square wonton wrappers
16 sprays I Can't Believe It's Not Butter! Spray

DIRECTIONS

Preheat oven to 350 degrees. Spray a baking sheet with nonstick spray.

To make the filling, combine all ingredients *except* wonton wrappers and butter spray in a large bowl. Mix thoroughly.

Lay a wonton wrapper flat on a dry surface. Place a heaping tablespoon filling (1⁄16th of filling) in the upper-right portion, and slightly spread so it covers one triangular half of the wrapper. Fold the lower triangular half over the filling, and gently pat to adhere. (No need to seal the edges.) Place on the baking sheet. Repeat with remaining wrappers and filling.

Spritz the top of each piece with 1 spray of butter spray. Bake for 6 minutes. Carefully flip pieces. Bake until golden brown, 6 to 9 more minutes. Eat up!

MAKES 4 SERVINGS

Hungry for More Finger Foods?

Visit the Faux-Frys chapter for jalapeño poppers, boneless wings, and MORE.
And check out the taquitos in the Mexican chapter!

Don't get any kooky ideas and start using full-fat chips on these lightened-up dips. Stick with veggies, baked chips, and other no-guilt dippers. (Did you really need a reminder about that?)

AMAZING ATE-LAYER DIP

105 calories PER SERVING

You'll Need: medium bowl, 2 microwave-safe bowls (1 optional), potato masher, skillet, nonstick spray, deep flat-bottomed serving dish | **Prep:** 15 minutes | **Cook:** 15 minutes

⅛th of recipe (about 1 cup):
105 calories, 0.5g fat, 323mg sodium, 19g carbs, 4g fiber, 3g sugars, 7g protein

INGREDIENTS

1 cup diced onion

2 cups chopped cherry tomatoes

2½ cups cubed butternut squash

1 tablespoon taco seasoning mix

1 cup frozen ground-beef-style soy crumbles

1 cup canned black beans, drained and rinsed

4 cups shredded lettuce

½ cup fat-free sour cream

¼ cup shredded fat-free cheddar cheese

⅓ cup roasted red peppers packed in water, drained and chopped

Optional seasonings: salt, black pepper, lime juice

DIRECTIONS

In a medium bowl, mix onion with 1 cup tomatoes. If you like, season to taste with salt, black pepper, and lime juice.

Place squash in a microwave-safe bowl with 2 tablespoons water. Cover and microwave for 6 minutes, or until squash is tender enough to mash.

Sprinkle squash with 1 teaspoon taco seasoning. Thoroughly mash and mix.

Bring a skillet sprayed with nonstick spray to medium heat. Cook and stir soy crumbles until thawed, about 3 minutes.

Add remaining 1 cup tomatoes and remaining 2 teaspoons taco seasoning. Cook and stir until hot, about 3 more minutes.

If you like, microwave black beans in a microwave-safe bowl for 30 seconds, or until warm.

In a deep flat-bottomed serving dish, evenly layer ingredients: lettuce, mashed squash, onion-tomato mixture, sour cream, black beans, soy crumble mixture, cheese, and chopped red peppers. *Dip* in!

MAKES 8 SERVINGS

BUFF CHICK HOT WING DIP

68 calories PER SERVING

You'll Need: large microwave-safe bowl
Prep: 5 minutes
Cook: 5 minutes

¹⁄₁₅th of recipe (about ¼ cup):
68 calories, 1.5g fat, 616mg sodium,
2g carbs, 0g fiber, 1g sugars, 10g protein

INGREDIENTS

One 8-ounce tub fat-free cream cheese,
    room temperature
½ cup Frank's RedHot Original Cayenne
    Pepper Sauce
½ cup shredded part-skim mozzarella cheese
¼ cup fat-free ranch dressing
¼ cup fat-free plain Greek yogurt
20 ounces canned 98% fat-free
    chunk white chicken breast in water,
    drained and flaked

DIRECTIONS

Place cream cheese in a large microwave-safe
bowl and stir until smooth. Thoroughly mix in
hot sauce, cheese, dressing, and yogurt.

Stir in chicken. Microwave for 3 minutes.
Stir and microwave for 2 minutes, or until
hot. Enjoy!

MAKES 15 SERVINGS

ROCKIN' RESTAURANT SPINACH DIP

72 calories PER SERVING

You'll Need: loaf pan, nonstick spray,
medium nonstick pot, medium bowl, whisk
Prep: 10 minutes
Cook: 40 minutes

¹⁄₈th of recipe (3 heaping tablespoons):
72 calories, 1g fat, 310mg sodium, 9g carbs, 1g fiber,
4g sugars, 7g protein

INGREDIENTS

2 tablespoons minced shallots
1 teaspoon minced garlic
¼ cup plus 2 tablespoons fat-free mayonnaise
¼ cup fat-free sour cream
2 tablespoons light plain soymilk (or fat-free milk)
4 ounces fat-free firm block-style cheese
    (any kind), shredded
One 10-ounce package frozen chopped spinach,
    thawed and squeezed dry
½ cup canned sliced water chestnuts, drained and chopped
3 tablespoons plus 1 teaspoon reduced-fat
    Parmesan-style grated topping

Optional seasonings: salt and black pepper

DIRECTIONS

Preheat oven to 325 degrees. Spray a loaf pan with
nonstick spray.

Bring a medium nonstick pot to medium heat. Cook and
stir shallots and garlic until slightly softened, 1 to 2 minutes.

Remove shallot-garlic mixture from the pot.

In a medium bowl, whisk mayo, sour cream, and soymilk
until smooth. Transfer mixture to the pot. Bring to low heat.
Cook and stir until hot, about 3 minutes.

Add shredded cheese to the pot, and cook and stir
until melted, about 8 minutes. Add shallot-garlic
    mixture and all remaining ingredients.
        Thoroughly stir.

Transfer mixture to the loaf pan and bake until hot
and bubbly, 20 to 25 minutes. Voilà!

MAKES 8 SERVINGS

HG HEADS-UP:
Don't buy pre-shredded
fat-free cheese for this
recipe—it won't
melt as well!

ROASTED VEGGIE SPREADDIP

72 calories PER SERVING

You'll Need: baking sheet, nonstick spray, aluminum foil, large food processor or blender
Prep: 15 minutes | **Cook:** 40 minutes

⅛th of recipe (about ⅓ cup):
72 calories, 1g fat, 198mg sodium, 11.5g carbs, 3g fiber, 2g sugars, 5g protein

INGREDIENTS

1 head garlic
½ teaspoon olive oil
2 portabella mushrooms
1 red bell pepper, halved, seeded, stem removed
½ medium onion, halved
One 15-ounce can chickpeas/garbanzo beans, drained and rinsed
½ cup fat-free plain Greek yogurt
¼ cup chopped fresh basil
1 teaspoon lemon juice
¼ teaspoon salt
⅛ teaspoon black pepper

DIRECTIONS

Preheat oven to 425 degrees. Spray a baking sheet with nonstick spray.

Halve the head of garlic widthwise, exposing the cloves. Remove papery outer layer from the bottom half, leaving skins around cloves intact. (Discard or reserve the top half for another use.) Place bottom half on a piece of foil, cut side up, and coat the top with oil. Tightly wrap foil around garlic, enclosing it completely.

Place foil-wrapped garlic on the baking sheet, and bake for 20 minutes.

Remove sheet from the oven. Lay mushrooms, bell pepper, and onion on the sheet with the partly baked foil-wrapped garlic. Return sheet to the oven and bake until veggies are soft, about 20 minutes.

Once cool, unwrap garlic and remove cloves; discard skin. Add garlic cloves and veggies to a large food processor or blender. Add remaining ingredients and 3 tablespoons of water. Puree until smooth, stopping and stirring if processing/blending slows.

For best flavor, refrigerate for several hours. Serve and enjoy!

MAKES 8 SERVINGS

SWEET CARAMELIZED ONION DIP

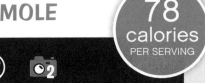

74 calories PER SERVING

You'll Need: large skillet, large bowl, whisk
Prep: 15 minutes
Cook: 45 minutes
Chill: overnight

⅙th of recipe (about ⅓ cup): 74 calories, 1.75g fat, 512mg sodium, 11g carbs, 0.5g fiber, 4.5g sugars, 3.5g protein

INGREDIENTS

1 tablespoon light whipped butter or light buttery spread
2 large sweet onions, chopped
½ teaspoon salt
¼ teaspoon cayenne pepper
1 teaspoon Dijon mustard
1 teaspoon balsamic vinegar
½ cup fat-free sour cream
½ cup fat-free mayonnaise
¼ cup plus 2 tablespoons fat-free cream cheese, room temperature

DIRECTIONS

Melt butter in a large skillet over medium-high heat. Add onions, salt, and cayenne pepper. Stirring frequently, cook for 10 minutes.

Reduce heat to medium low. Stirring frequently, cook until caramelized, 25 to 30 minutes.

Stir mustard and vinegar into the onions in the skillet. Cook and stir for 5 minutes. Remove from heat.

In a large bowl, whisk sour cream, mayo, and cream cheese until smooth. Thoroughly stir in onion mixture.

Cover and refrigerate overnight to allow flavors to combine. Serve and enjoy!

MAKES 6 SERVINGS

HOLY MOLY GUACAMOLE

78 calories PER SERVING

You'll Need: medium-large bowl, potato masher (or small blender or food processor)
Prep: 20 minutes

⅙th of recipe (about ⅓ cup): 78 calories, 3g fat, 320mg sodium, 10.5g carbs, 3.5g fiber, 4g sugars, 3.5g protein

INGREDIENTS

One 15-ounce can early/young peas, drained
4 ounces (about ½ cup) mashed avocado
¼ cup fat-free plain Greek yogurt
1 tablespoon plus 1 teaspoon lime juice
½ teaspoon minced garlic
¼ teaspoon salt, or more to taste
⅛ teaspoon black pepper, or more to taste
⅛ teaspoon ground cumin
⅛ teaspoon chili powder
⅓ cup chopped cherry or grape tomatoes
¼ cup finely chopped onion

Optional: chopped fresh cilantro, chopped jarred jalapeños

DIRECTIONS

Thoroughly mash peas in a medium-large bowl. (Or puree peas in a small blender or food processor and transfer to a medium-large bowl.)

Thoroughly mix in avocado, yogurt, lime juice, garlic, and seasonings.

Stir in tomatoes, onion and, if you like, optional ingredients. Enjoy!

MAKES 6 SERVINGS

ROCKIN' ROASTED CORN GUAC

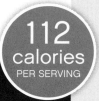

77
calories
PER SERVING

You'll Need: skillet, nonstick spray, medium-large bowl, potato masher (or small blender or food processor)
Prep: 20 minutes
Cook: 10 minutes

⅛th of recipe (about ⅓ cup):
77 calories, 2.5g fat, 294mg sodium, 11.5g carbs, 3g fiber, 4g sugars, 3g protein

INGREDIENTS

1 cup frozen sweet corn kernels

One 15-ounce can early/young peas, drained

4 ounces (about ½ cup) mashed avocado

¼ cup plain fat-free Greek yogurt

1 tablespoon plus 1 teaspoon lime juice

½ teaspoon chopped garlic

¼ teaspoon salt, or more to taste

⅛ teaspoon black pepper, or more to taste

⅛ teaspoon ground cumin

⅛ teaspoon chili powder

¾ cup chopped cherry or grape tomatoes

¼ cup finely chopped onion

Optional: chopped fresh cilantro, chopped jarred jalapeño slices

DIRECTIONS

Bring a skillet sprayed with nonstick spray to high heat. Cook and stir corn until thawed and slightly blackened, about 8 minutes.

Thoroughly mash peas in a medium-large bowl. (Or puree peas in a small blender or food processor and transfer to a medium-large bowl.) Thoroughly mix in avocado, yogurt, lime juice, garlic, and seasonings.

Stir in tomatoes, onion, cooked corn and, if you like, optional ingredients. Enjoy!

MAKES 8 SERVINGS

CHEESY CHICKEN EGG ROLLS

112
calories
PER SERVING

You'll Need: baking sheet, nonstick spray, large skillet, large bowl
Prep: 30 minutes
Cook: 55 minutes

⅙th of recipe (1 egg roll): 112 calories, 1.5g fat, 334mg sodium, 17g carbs, 1g fiber, 1.5g sugars, 8.5g protein

INGREDIENTS

½ tablespoon light whipped butter or light buttery spread

1 sweet onion, thinly sliced

¼ teaspoon salt

2 cups spinach leaves

½ tablespoon chopped garlic

4 ounces cooked and chopped skinless chicken breast

2 wedges The Laughing Cow Light Creamy Swiss cheese

6 large square egg roll wrappers

DIRECTIONS

Preheat oven to 375 degrees. Spray a baking sheet with nonstick spray.

Melt butter in a large skillet over medium-high heat. Add onion and salt. Stirring frequently, cook onion until softened and slightly browned, about 6 minutes.

Reduce heat to medium low. Stirring frequently, cook until caramelized, about 15 minutes.

Transfer onion to a large bowl. Remove skillet from heat, and wash if needed. Re-spray skillet and return to medium-high heat. Cook spinach and garlic until spinach has wilted, 1 to 2 minutes.

Transfer spinach and garlic to the large bowl. Add chicken and cheese wedges, breaking the wedges into pieces. Mix thoroughly.

Lay an egg roll wrapper flat on a dry surface. Evenly distribute about ⅓ cup chicken mixture (⅙th of mixture) in a row a little below the center of the wrapper.

Moisten all four edges by dabbing your fingers in water and going over the edges smoothly. Fold the sides about ¾ inch toward the middle, to keep mixture from falling out. Roll up the wrapper around the mixture and continue to the top. Seal with a dab of water.

Place on the baking sheet, and repeat with remaining chicken mixture and wrappers. Spray the tops with nonstick spray.

Bake until golden brown, 25 to 30 minutes. Dig in!

MAKES 6 SERVINGS

SASSY SOUTHWESTERN EGG ROLLS

181 calories PER SERVING

You'll Need: baking sheet, nonstick spray, medium microwave-safe bowl, microwave-safe plate, small bowl
Prep: 10 minutes | **Cook:** 15 minutes

½ of recipe (3 egg roll halves with sauce):
181 calories, 4.5g fat, 666mg sodium, 27g carbs, 14g fiber, 2g sugars, 19g protein

INGREDIENTS

Egg Rolls
¾ cup thawed-from-frozen chopped spinach, squeezed dry
1 ounce fat-free jalapeño jack cheese, shredded
     (about ¼ cup)
1 ounce cooked and shredded skinless chicken breast
2 tablespoons canned black beans, drained and rinsed
2 tablespoons canned sweet corn kernels, drained
1 tablespoon diced red chili pepper
Three 6-inch high-fiber flour tortillas with about
     50 calories each

Sauce
2 tablespoons fat-free sour cream
½ ounce (about 1 tablespoon) mashed avocado
½ teaspoon ranch dressing/dip seasoning mix
1 tablespoon diced tomato

Optional seasoning: black pepper

DIRECTIONS

Preheat oven to 400 degrees. Spray a baking sheet with nonstick spray.

In a medium microwave-safe bowl, mix spinach, cheese, chicken, beans, corn, and chili pepper. Microwave for 30 seconds, or until warm, and stir.

On a microwave-safe plate, microwave tortillas for 15 seconds, or until warm.

Lay one tortilla flat on a dry surface. Place one-third of the chicken-spinach mixture in the center. Fold in the sides of the tortilla, and roll up tortilla around the filling. Place on the baking sheet, seam side down. Repeat with remaining tortillas and chicken-spinach mixture.

Bake for 6 minutes. Flip egg rolls. Bake until crispy, about 6 more minutes.

Meanwhile, in a small bowl, thoroughly mix sour cream, avocado, and ranch mix until smooth. Top with tomato.

Slice egg rolls in half and serve with sauce for dipping!

MAKES 2 SERVINGS

DE-PUDGED PIGS IN A BLANKET

134 calories
PER SERVING

You'll Need: rolling pin (optional), baking sheet
Prep: 15 minutes
Cook: 15 minutes

⅛th of recipe (4 pigs in a blanket):
134 calories, 5g fat, 652mg sodium, 16g carbs, 0g fiber, 3g sugars, 8g protein

INGREDIENTS

8 hot dogs with about 40 calories and 1g fat or less each
1 package refrigerated Pillsbury Reduced Fat Crescent rolls

DIRECTIONS

Preheat oven to 375 degrees.

Cut each hot dog widthwise into 4 even pieces.

Place the 8 portions of dough on a dry surface. One at a time, slightly stretch or roll each piece into a larger triangle.

Cut each triangle into 4 long, narrow triangles. Beginning at the base of each narrow triangle, roll up 1 hot dog piece until the point of the triangle wraps around the center. Place your blanketed pigs on a baking sheet, evenly spaced.

Bake until dough is slightly browned and crispy, about 12 minutes. Enjoy!

MAKES 8 SERVINGS

PIGS IN A BLANKET HOT DOG TIP!

Do your franks come in a pack of seven? If you don't wanna buy another pack for just one dog, make seven servings instead of eight. Then bake up the extra portion of dough as a 90-calorie crescent roll . . .

GARLIC-BREAD PIGS IN A BLANKET

146 calories
PER SERVING

You'll Need: rolling pin (optional), baking sheet, microwave-safe bowl, pastry brush
Prep: 15 minutes
Cook: 15 minutes

⅛th of recipe (4 pigs in a blanket):
146 calories, 6g fat, 682mg sodium, 17.5g carbs, 0g fiber, 4g sugars, 7.5g protein

INGREDIENTS

8 hot dogs with about 40 calories and 1g fat or less each
1 package refrigerated Pillsbury Reduced Fat Crescent rolls
1 tablespoon light whipped butter or light buttery spread
1½ tablespoons reduced-fat Parmesan-style grated topping
1 teaspoon garlic powder

Optional dip: low-fat marinara sauce

DIRECTIONS

Preheat oven to 375 degrees.

Cut each hot dog widthwise into 4 even pieces.

Place the 8 portions of dough on a dry surface. One at a time, slightly stretch or roll each piece into a larger triangle.

Cut each triangle into 4 long, narrow triangles. Beginning at the base of each narrow triangle, roll up 1 hot dog piece until the point of the triangle wraps around the center. Place your blanketed pigs on a baking sheet, evenly spaced.

In a microwave-safe bowl, microwave butter for 15 seconds, or until just melted. Mix well. Brush melted butter on pigs in a blanket. Sprinkle with Parm-style topping and garlic powder.

Bake until dough is slightly browned and crispy, about 12 minutes. Enjoy!

MAKES 8 SERVINGS

BACON-WRAPPED PIGS IN A BLANKET

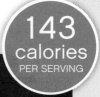
165 calories PER SERVING

You'll Need: toothpicks, grill pan (or large skillet), nonstick spray, rolling pin (optional), baking sheet
Prep: 15 minutes
Cook: 20 minutes

⅛th of recipe (4 pigs in a blanket):
165 calories, 7.5g fat, 795mg sodium, 17g carbs, 0g fiber, 4g sugars, 9.5g protein

INGREDIENTS

8 hot dogs with about 40 calories and 1g fat or less each
8 slices center-cut bacon or turkey bacon
1 package refrigerated Pillsbury Reduced Fat Crescent rolls

DIRECTIONS

Preheat oven to 375 degrees.

Break 8 toothpicks in half. Wrap each hot dog in a slice of bacon and secure each end with a toothpick half.

Bring a grill pan (or large skillet) sprayed with nonstick spray to medium heat. Cook bacon-wrapped hot dogs until bacon is crisp, about 6 minutes, rotating the hot dogs to evenly cook the bacon.

Place the 8 portions of dough on a dry surface. One at a time, slightly stretch or roll each piece into a larger triangle. Cut each triangle into 4 long, narrow triangles.

Blot away excess moisture from bacon-wrapped hot dogs. Evenly cut each hot dog into 4 pieces and remove toothpicks.

Beginning at the base of each narrow triangle, roll up 1 hot dog piece until the point of the triangle wraps around the center. Place your blanketed pigs on a baking sheet, evenly spaced.

Bake until dough is slightly browned and crispy, about 12 minutes. Enjoy!

MAKES 8 SERVINGS

BB-CUTIE PIGS IN A BLANKET

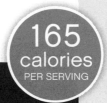
143 calories PER SERVING

You'll Need: rolling pin (optional), baking sheet
Prep: 15 minutes
Cook: 15 minutes

⅛th of recipe (4 pigs in a blanket):
143 calories, 5g fat, 693mg sodium, 19g carbs, 0g fiber, 5g sugars, 7g protein

INGREDIENTS

8 hot dogs with about 40 calories and 1g fat or less each
1 package refrigerated Pillsbury Reduced Fat Crescent rolls
2 tablespoons BBQ sauce with 45 calories or less per 2-tablespoon serving
1½ tablespoons dried minced onion

Optional dip: additional BBQ sauce

DIRECTIONS

Preheat oven to 375 degrees.

Cut each hot dog widthwise into 4 even pieces.

Place the 8 portions of dough on a dry surface. One at a time, slightly stretch or roll each piece into a larger triangle.

Cut each triangle into 4 long, narrow triangles. Beginning at the base of each narrow triangle, roll up 1 hot dog piece until the point of the triangle wraps around the center.

Place your blanketed pigs on a baking sheet, evenly spaced. Spread the tops with BBQ sauce. Sprinkle with minced onion and gently pat to adhere.

Bake until dough is slightly browned and crispy, about 12 minutes. Enjoy!

MAKES 8 SERVINGS

HONEY MUSTARD & SWISS PIGS IN A BLANKET

148 calories PER SERVING

You'll Need: small microwave-safe bowl, rolling pin (optional), baking sheet
Prep: 15 minutes
Cook: 15 minutes

⅛th of recipe (4 pigs in a blanket):
148 calories, 5.5g fat, 716mg sodium, 18g carbs, 0g fiber, 4.5g sugars, 7.5g protein

INGREDIENTS

2 wedges The Laughing Cow Light
    Creamy Swiss cheese
1½ tablespoons honey mustard
8 hot dogs with about 40 calories and
    1g fat or less each
1 package refrigerated Pillsbury
    Reduced Fat Crescent rolls

Optional dip: additional honey mustard

DIRECTIONS

Preheat oven to 375 degrees.

In a small microwave-safe bowl, microwave cheese wedges for 20 seconds, or until hot. Add mustard and stir until smooth.

Cut each hot dog widthwise into 4 even pieces.

Place the 8 portions of dough on a dry surface. One at a time, slightly stretch or roll each piece into a larger triangle.

Cut each triangle into 4 long, narrow triangles. Spread with cheese-mustard mixture. Beginning at the base of each narrow triangle, roll up 1 hot dog piece until the point of the triangle wraps around the center.

Place your blanketed pigs on a baking sheet, evenly spaced.

Bake until dough is slightly browned and crispy, about 12 minutes. Enjoy!

MAKES 8 SERVINGS

DEVILISH EGGS

79 calories PER SERVING

You'll Need: large microwave-safe bowl, potato masher, small blender or food processor, medium bowl
Prep: 15 minutes
Cook: 10 minutes
Chill: 1 hour

⅕th of recipe (4 egg halves): 79 calories, 1.5g fat, 373mg sodium, 6.25g carbs, 1g fiber, 2.5g sugars, 9g protein

INGREDIENTS

2 cups roughly chopped orange cauliflower
¼ cup fat-free mayonnaise
1 tablespoon sweet relish, patted dry
2 teaspoons minced shallots
1½ teaspoons yellow mustard
3 wedges The Laughing Cow Light Creamy Swiss cheese
10 hard-boiled eggs, peeled

Optional: salt, black pepper, paprika

DIRECTIONS

Place cauliflower in a large microwave-safe bowl with ⅓ cup water. Cover and microwave for 6 to 8 minutes, until soft.

Drain any excess water, and lightly mash cauliflower.

Transfer cauliflower to a small blender or food processor. Add mayo and briefly puree until just blended.

Transfer mixture to a medium bowl. Add relish, shallots, mustard, and cheese wedges, breaking the wedges into pieces. Thoroughly mix. If you like, season to taste with salt and pepper.

Cover and refrigerate until chilled, at least 1 hour.

Run a knife lengthwise along the circumference of each peeled egg to separate the white into halves (like cutting around the pit of an avocado). Discard yolks. Evenly distribute cauliflower mixture among egg-white halves. If you like, sprinkle with paprika. Party time!

MAKES 5 SERVINGS

HG TIP!

If you can't find orange cauliflower, use regular instead. But add a drop of yellow food coloring to the mixture if you want your Devilish Eggs to look like the real thing.

MEXI-DEVILED EGGS

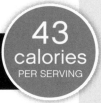

43 calories
PER SERVING

You'll Need: large plate, medium bowl | **Prep:** 30 minutes

¹⁄₁₂th of recipe (2 egg halves):
43 calories, 0.5g fat, 165mg sodium, 4.5g carbs, 1g fiber, 0.5g sugars, 5g protein

INGREDIENTS

12 hard-boiled eggs, peeled
1 cup fat-free refried beans
1 tablespoon salsa
¼ teaspoon ground cumin
⅛ teaspoon cayenne pepper
¼ cup fat-free sour cream
¼ teaspoon chili powder
2 tablespoons chopped cilantro
24 black olive slices

DIRECTIONS

Run a knife lengthwise along the circumference of each peeled egg to separate the white into halves (like cutting around the pit of an avocado). Discard yolks and set egg-white halves on a large plate, cut sides up.

In a medium bowl, mix refried beans, salsa, cumin, and cayenne pepper.

Evenly distribute bean mixture among egg-white halves, about 2 teaspoons each. Evenly distribute sour cream, ½ teaspoon per egg-white half.

Sprinkle with chili powder and cilantro, and top with olive slices. Serve 'em up! (Or refrigerate until you're ready.)

MAKES 12 SERVINGS

HARD-BOILING EGG WHITES: IT'S NOT THAT HARD . . .

Place the eggs in a pot and cover completely with water, leaving a few inches of the pot's inner edge above the water line. Bring to a boil, and then continue to cook for 10 minutes. Drain the water and fill the pot with very cold water. (Add ice if you've got it.) Once cool enough to handle, peel off the shells.

For more recipes, tips & tricks, sign up for FREE daily emails at **hungry-girl.com!**

Mushrooms on their own? Good. Mushrooms loaded up with delicious items?! BETTER!

FOUR-CHEESE STUFFED-SILLY MUSHROOMS

118 calories PER SERVING

You'll Need: baking sheet, nonstick spray, large skillet, medium bowl, small bowl
Prep: 20 minutes | **Cook:** 30 minutes

¼th of recipe (3 stuffed mushrooms):
118 calories, 1.5g fat, 359mg sodium, 16g carbs, 2.5g fiber, 6g sugars, 12g protein

INGREDIENTS

12 medium baby bella mushrooms (each about 2 inches wide), stems chopped and reserved
½ cup finely chopped onion
2 tablespoons chopped garlic
1½ cups roughly chopped spinach leaves
½ cup fat-free ricotta cheese
¼ cup fat-free cream cheese, room temperature
2 tablespoons shredded part-skim mozzarella cheese
¼ teaspoon ground nutmeg
¼ teaspoon salt
2 teaspoons reduced-fat Parmesan-style grated topping
1 teaspoon garlic powder

DIRECTIONS

Preheat oven to 375 degrees. Spray a baking sheet with nonstick spray.

Place mushroom caps on the sheet, rounded sides down. Bake until tender, 12 to 14 minutes. Leave oven on.

Meanwhile, bring a large skillet sprayed with nonstick spray to medium heat. Add chopped mushroom stems, onion, and chopped garlic. Cook and stir until softened, about 2 minutes. Add spinach and cook and stir until wilted, about 2 more minutes. Remove from heat and pat dry.

In a medium bowl, thoroughly mix ricotta cheese, cream cheese, mozzarella cheese, nutmeg, and salt. Stir in contents of the skillet.

Pat mushroom caps dry. Evenly distribute veggie-cheese mixture among the caps.

In a small bowl, mix Parm-style topping with garlic powder. Sprinkle over stuffed mushrooms.

Bake until topping begins to brown, 8 to 10 minutes. Enjoy!

MAKES 4 SERVINGS

SPICY BACON-STUFFED CHEESY MUSHROOMS

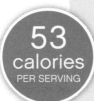

53 calories PER SERVING

You'll Need: baking sheet, nonstick spray, skillet, medium bowl
Prep: 20 minutes
Cook: 30 minutes

¼th of recipe (3 stuffed mushrooms):
53 calories, 2g fat, 306mg sodium, 4g carbs, 1g fiber, 1.5g sugars, 5g protein

INGREDIENTS

12 medium baby bella mushrooms (each about 2 inches wide), stems chopped and reserved
¼ cup diced red bell pepper
1 tablespoon diced jarred jalapeño slices (about 5 slices)
¼ teaspoon chopped garlic
3 tablespoons precooked real crumbled bacon
2 tablespoons shredded reduced-fat Monterey Jack cheese
2 tablespoons fat-free cream cheese, room temperature
⅛ teaspoon cayenne pepper
⅛ teaspoon each salt and black pepper

DIRECTIONS

Preheat oven to 375 degrees. Spray a baking sheet with nonstick spray.

Place mushroom caps on the sheet, rounded sides down. Bake until tender, 12 to 14 minutes. Leave oven on.

Meanwhile, bring a skillet sprayed with nonstick spray to medium heat. Add chopped mushroom stems, bell pepper, jalapeño, and garlic. Cook and stir until slightly softened, about 3 minutes.

Transfer contents of the skillet to a medium bowl and pat dry. Stir in all remaining ingredients.

Pat mushroom caps dry. Evenly distribute veggie-cheese mixture among the caps. Bake until filling is hot, 8 to 10 minutes. Eat up!

MAKES 4 SERVINGS

SUPER-STUFFED SPINACH-FETA MUSHROOMS

75 calories PER SERVING

You'll Need: baking sheet, nonstick spray, skillet, medium bowl
Prep: 20 minutes
Cook: 30 minutes

¼th of recipe (3 stuffed mushrooms):
75 calories, 2.5g fat, 480mg sodium, 6g carbs, 1.5g fiber, 1.5g sugars, 6.5g protein

INGREDIENTS

12 medium baby bella mushrooms (each about 2 inches wide), stems chopped and reserved
One 10-ounce package frozen chopped spinach, thawed and squeezed dry
½ cup crumbled reduced-fat feta cheese
½ teaspoon garlic powder
½ teaspoon onion powder
¼ teaspoon each salt and black pepper

DIRECTIONS

Preheat oven to 375 degrees. Spray a baking sheet with nonstick spray.

Place mushroom caps on the sheet, rounded sides down. Bake until tender, 12 to 14 minutes. Leave oven on.

Meanwhile, bring a skillet sprayed with nonstick spray to medium heat. Cook and stir chopped mushroom stems until soft, about 3 minutes.

Transfer mushroom stems to a medium bowl. Add all other ingredients and thoroughly mix.

Pat mushroom caps dry. Evenly distribute spinach mixture among the caps, about 2 tablespoons each. Bake until filling is hot, 8 to 10 minutes. Enjoy!

MAKES 4 SERVINGS

OOEY-GOOEY CHILI CHEESE NACHOS

234 calories PER SERVING

You'll Need: small nonstick pot, large microwave-safe bowl, large platter, medium microwave-safe bowl
Prep: 10 minutes | **Cook:** 10 minutes

⅙th of recipe (about 17 loaded chips):
234 calories, 5g fat, 897mg sodium, 34g carbs, 4.5g fiber, 4g sugars, 11g protein

INGREDIENTS

½ cup light plain soymilk

4 slices fat-free cheddar or American cheese

4 wedges The Laughing Cow Light
    Creamy Swiss cheese

One 7-ounce bag baked tortilla chips

1 cup low-fat turkey or veggie chili

¾ cup salsa

2 tablespoons fat-free sour cream

DIRECTIONS

Pour soymilk into a small nonstick pot. Add cheese slices and wedges, breaking them into pieces. Bring to medium-low heat. Cook and stir until sauce is hot and uniform, 5 to 8 minutes.

Microwave chips in a large microwave-safe bowl for 1 minute, or until warm. Spread them out on a large platter.

In a medium microwave-safe bowl, microwave chili for 1 minute, or until hot.

Pour cheese sauce over the chips. Top with chili, salsa, and sour cream. Time for nachos!

MAKES 6 SERVINGS

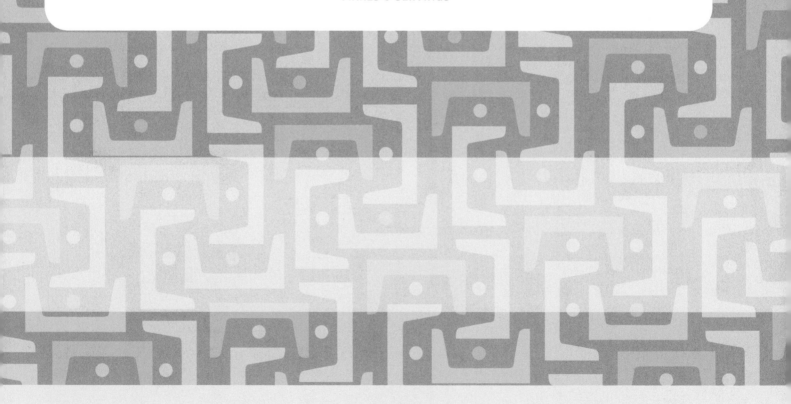

SAUCY CHICK BBQ NACHOS

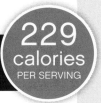

229 calories
PER SERVING

You'll Need: large ovenproof platter or baking sheet, nonstick spray, small bowl
Prep: 10 minutes | **Cook:** 10 minutes

⅕th of recipe (about 12 loaded chips):
229 calories, 3g fat, 875mg sodium, 26g carbs, 1.25g fiber, 7g sugars, 21g protein

INGREDIENTS

4 ounces (about 60) baked tortilla chips

10 ounces canned 98% fat-free chunk white chicken breast in water, drained and flaked

½ cup BBQ sauce with 45 calories or less per 2-tablespoon serving

1 cup shredded fat-free cheddar cheese

2 tablespoons chopped scallions

Optional topping: fat-free sour cream

DIRECTIONS

Preheat oven to 350 degrees. Spray a large ovenproof platter or baking sheet with nonstick spray.

Spread out tortilla chips on the platter or sheet.

In a small bowl, mix chicken with ¼ cup BBQ sauce. Evenly spoon over the chips.

Sprinkle chips with cheese and drizzle with remaining ¼ cup BBQ sauce.

Bake until toppings are hot, 8 to 10 minutes.

Sprinkle with scallions and enjoy!!!

MAKES 5 SERVINGS

CHILI CHEESE DOG NACHOS

218 calories
PER SERVING

You'll Need: large ovenproof platter or baking sheet, nonstick spray, skillet | **Prep:** 10 minutes | **Cook:** 5 minutes

⅟₇th of recipe (about 15 loaded chips):
218 calories, 3g fat, 674mg sodium, 36g carbs, 4.25g fiber, 4g sugars, 13g protein

INGREDIENTS

One 7-ounce bag baked tortilla chips

2 cups low-fat turkey or veggie chili

3 hot dogs with about 40 calories and 1g fat or less each, chopped

½ cup chopped white onion

3 slices fat-free American cheese, cut into thin strips

½ cup fat-free sour cream

DIRECTIONS

Preheat broiler. Spray a large ovenproof platter or baking sheet with nonstick spray.

Spread out tortilla chips on the platter or sheet.

Bring a skillet sprayed with nonstick spray to medium heat. Cook and stir chili and chopped hot dogs until hot, about 3 minutes.

Evenly spoon chili mixture over the chips. Top chips with onion and cheese strips.

Broil until cheese begins to melt and bubble, about 2 minutes.

Top or serve with sour cream!

MAKES 7 SERVINGS

PIZZA-PIED NACHOS

213 calories PER SERVING

You'll Need: baking sheet or ovenproof platter, nonstick spray, blender or food processor (optional), skillet
Prep: 10 minutes | **Cook:** 20 minutes

¼th of recipe (9 loaded chips):
213 calories, 5.5g fat, 744mg sodium, 28.5g carbs, 3.5g fiber, 4.5g sugars, 10.5g protein

INGREDIENTS

3 sticks light string cheese

Six 6-inch corn tortillas

2 dashes salt

½ cup chopped mushrooms

½ cup diced bell pepper

½ cup diced onion

1 cup pizza sauce

½ teaspoon garlic powder

2 tablespoons reduced-fat Parmesan-style grated topping

17 slices turkey pepperoni, chopped

DIRECTIONS

Preheat oven to 400 degrees. Spray a baking sheet or ovenproof platter with nonstick spray.

Break each string cheese stick into thirds and place in a blender or food processor—blend at high speed until shredded. (Or tear into pieces and roughly chop.)

To make the chips, stack tortillas and cut in half. Cut each stack of halves into 3 triangles, for a total of 36 pieces.

Evenly lay tortilla triangles flat on the sheet or platter, and cover with a generous mist of nonstick spray. Sprinkle with a dash of salt. Flip triangles and sprinkle with remaining dash of salt.

Bake for 5 minutes. Carefully flip triangles and bake until crispy, about 5 more minutes. Leave oven on.

Meanwhile, bring a skillet sprayed with nonstick spray to medium-high heat. Cook and stir veggies until slightly softened, about 5 minutes.

Reduce heat to low. Add pizza sauce and garlic powder. Mix well and continue to cook until hot.

Evenly top chips with sauce. Sprinkle with Parm-style topping and shredded string cheese. Top with pepperoni.

Bake until cheese has melted, about 5 minutes. Enjoy!

MAKES 4 SERVINGS

HG ALTERNATIVE!

For a meat-free option, feel free to swap the turkey pepperoni for some sliced black olives.

SIMPLY SWEET MEATBALLS

 199 calories PER SERVING

You'll Need: baking sheet, nonstick spray, large bowl
Prep: 5 minutes
Cook: 20 minutes

⅕th of recipe (4 meatballs):
199 calories, 8g fat, 390mg sodium, 8g carbs, 1g fiber, 6.5g sugars, 23g protein

INGREDIENTS

1¼ pounds raw lean ground turkey
One 8-ounce can pineapple tidbits packed in juice, drained
¾ cup canned crushed tomatoes
½ teaspoon salt
¼ teaspoon black pepper

DIRECTIONS

Preheat oven to 350 degrees. Spray a baking sheet with nonstick spray.

In a large bowl, thoroughly mix all ingredients. Firmly and evenly form into 20 meatballs and place on the baking sheet, evenly spaced.

Bake for 15 minutes. Flip meatballs. Bake until cooked through, about 5 minutes. Enjoy!

MAKES 5 SERVINGS

CRAN-TASTICALLY EASY MEATBALLS

 221 calories PER SERVING

You'll Need: baking sheet, nonstick spray, large bowl
Prep: 5 minutes
Cook: 15 minutes

⅕th of recipe (4 meatballs): 221 calories, 7.5g fat, 688mg sodium, 15g carbs, 0.5g fiber, 11g sugars, 22g protein

INGREDIENTS

1¼ pounds raw lean ground turkey
½ cup chili sauce (the kind stocked near the ketchup)
⅓ cup sweetened dried cranberries, roughly chopped
½ teaspoon salt
¼ teaspoon black pepper

DIRECTIONS

Preheat oven to 350 degrees. Spray a baking sheet with nonstick spray.

In a large bowl, thoroughly mix all ingredients. Firmly and evenly form into 20 balls and place on the baking sheet, evenly spaced.

Bake for 10 minutes. Gently flip meatballs. Bake until cooked through, about 5 minutes. Serve and enjoy!

MAKES 5 SERVINGS

Hungry for More Party Foods?

There are five kinds of jalapeño poppers starting on page 94, and three recipes for taquitos starting on page 264! Plus, check out the Crock Pots chapter for bean dip, cocktail weenies, and more!

COCKTAILS

Bottoms up!

GUILT-FREE MIXOLOGY TIPS

* For accurate nutritional info, use 80-proof (40% alcohol) rum, vodka, and tequila.

* Keep your ingredients cold, so they won't get watered down when you add ice.

* These recipes list fluid-ounce measurements. Using cups 'n spoons? Here's a handy conversion chart . . .

    1 ounce = 2 tablespoons
    1½ ounces = 3 tablespoons
    2 ounces = ¼ cup
    6 ounces = ¾ cup
    8 ounces = 1 cup

SHAKE THINGS UP . . .

* If your freezy beverage stops blending, turn off the machine, and remove the blender from the base. Stir it up and blend again.

* Ice is important, and pre-crushed ice is best. Make sure your ice isn't old or freezer-burned.

* When choosing a shaker, get one with a strainer attachment. Shakers without strainers are not nearly as effective . . .

HG'S MAGICAL LOW-CALORIE MARGARITA

115 calories

You'll Need: glass or shaker, margarita glass | **Prep:** 5 minutes

Entire recipe:
115 calories, 0g fat, 55mg sodium, 2g carbs, 0g fiber, <0.5g sugars, 0g protein

INGREDIENTS

6 ounces diet lemon-lime soda

1½ ounces tequila

1 ounce lime juice

One 2-serving packet (about 1 teaspoon) sugar-free lemonade powdered drink mix

1 cup crushed ice *or* 5 to 8 ice cubes

Optional garnish: lime slice

DIRECTIONS

In a glass or shaker, combine all ingredients *except* ice. Stir until drink mix has dissolved.

Fill a margarita glass with ice, pour, and enjoy!

MAKES 1 SERVING

FREEZY-FRESA STRAWBERRY MARGARITA

125 calories

You'll Need: glass, blender | **Prep:** 5 minutes

Entire recipe:
125 calories, 0g fat, 24mg sodium, 7g carbs, 1g fiber, 2g sugars, 0g protein

INGREDIENTS

Half a 2-serving packet (about ½ teaspoon) sugar-free strawberry powdered drink mix

6 ounces diet lemon-lime soda

1½ ounces tequila

1 ounce lime juice

4 frozen unsweetened strawberries, partially thawed

1 cup crushed ice *or* 5 to 8 ice cubes

Optional garnish: lime slice

DIRECTIONS

In a glass, combine powdered drink mix with soda and stir to dissolve.

Transfer mixture to a blender and add all other ingredients. Blend at high speed until smooth. Pour and drink up!

MAKES 1 SERVING

HG TIP!

Feel free to experiment with whatever strawberry-blend drink mixes you find on shelves. Strawberry kiwi, strawberry banana, strawberry tangerine . . .

SLAMMIN' STRAWBERRY DAIQUIRI

121 calories

You'll Need: glass, blender | **Prep:** 5 minutes

Entire recipe:
121 calories, 0g fat, 10mg sodium, 4g carbs, 0.5g fiber, 2g sugars, 0g protein

INGREDIENTS

One 2-serving packet (about 1 teaspoon)
    sugar-free strawberry powdered drink mix
1½ ounces white rum
½ ounce lime juice
3 frozen unsweetened strawberries,
    partially thawed
1 cup crushed ice *or* 5 to 8 ice cubes

DIRECTIONS

In a glass, combine drink mix with 4 ounces cold water and stir to dissolve.

Transfer mixture to a blender, and add all other ingredients. Blend at high speed until smooth.

Pour into the glass, and slurp that baby up!

MAKES 1 SERVING

PIÑA COLADA FREEZE

156 calories

You'll Need: blender, glass | **Prep:** 5 minutes

Entire recipe:
156 calories, <0.5g fat, 41mg sodium, 18g carbs, 0.5g fiber, 12g sugars, 2g protein

INGREDIENTS

1½ ounces coconut rum
1½ ounces sugar-free calorie-free coconut-flavored syrup
¼ cup fat-free vanilla ice cream
1 tablespoon crushed pineapple packed in juice
1 no-calorie sweetener packet
1 cup crushed ice *or* 5 to 8 ice cubes

Optional garnish: pineapple wedge

DIRECTIONS

Combine all ingredients in a blender, and blend at high speed until smooth.

Pour into a glass and enjoy!

MAKES 1 SERVING

CHILLY CHOCOLATE MUDSLIDE

156 calories

You'll Need: tall glass, blender
Prep: 5 minutes

Entire recipe: 156 calories, 0.5g fat, 177mg sodium, 10g carbs, 1g fiber, 6g sugars, 3g protein

INGREDIENTS

1 packet hot cocoa mix with 20 to 25 calories
2 no-calorie sweetener packets
2 ounces light vanilla soymilk
1½ ounces vodka
½ ounce sugar-free calorie-free vanilla-flavored syrup
1 teaspoon light chocolate syrup
1 cup crushed ice *or* 5 to 8 ice cubes

Optional topping: Fat Free Reddi-wip

DIRECTIONS

In a tall glass, combine cocoa mix with sweetener. Add ¼ cup hot water and stir to dissolve.

Transfer mixture to a blender, and add 2 tablespoons cold water. Add all other ingredients. Blend at high speed until smooth. Pour and enjoy!

MAKES 1 SERVING

MY OH MAI TAI

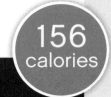
133 calories

You'll Need: glass or shaker, tall glass
Prep: 5 minutes

Entire recipe: 133 calories, 0g fat, 18mg sodium, 9g carbs, 0g fiber, 7g sugars, 0g protein

INGREDIENTS

2 ounces diet lemon-lime soda
2 ounces pineapple-orange juice
1 ounce rum
3 drops almond extract
1 no-calorie sweetener packet
1 cup crushed ice *or* 5 to 8 ice cubes
½ ounce dark spiced rum

Optional garnish: pineapple wedge

DIRECTIONS

In a glass or shaker, mix all ingredients *except* ice and dark spiced rum.

Fill a tall glass with ice and pour in the drink mixture. Top with dark spiced rum and enjoy!

MAKES 1 SERVING

SUGAR-FREE CALORIE-FREE SYRUP 411

Torani Sugar Free Syrups are the best, hands down. Find popular flavors like vanilla in the coffee aisle . . . Just make sure they're the zero-calorie, sugar-free ones (they make sugary versions too!). They can also be found at specialty stores like Cost Plus World Market and BevMo!

PINEAPPLE FROJITOS

 179 calories PER SERVING

You'll Need: 2 glasses, muddler, blender
Prep: 10 minutes

½ of recipe (1 drink): 179 calories, <0.5g fat, 11mg sodium, 21.5g carbs, 2g fiber, 14.5g sugars, 0.5g protein

INGREDIENTS

10 mint leaves
1 no-calorie sweetener packet
2 limes, each cut into 4 wedges
One 8-ounce can crushed pineapple packed in juice (not drained)
3 ounces rum
2 cups crushed ice *or* 10 to 16 ice cubes

DIRECTIONS

Evenly distribute mint and sweetener between 2 glasses. Add 2 lime wedges to each glass.

Squeeze the juice from the remaining lime wedges into the glasses. Discard these wedges.

Muddle (a.k.a. mash) the contents of each glass.

To a blender, add (undrained) pineapple, rum, and ice. Blend at high speed until smooth.

Evenly divide contents of the blender between the 2 glasses. Stir and drink up!

MAKES 2 SERVINGS

MOJITO MADNESS

 104 calories

You'll Need: glass, muddler
Prep: 5 minutes

Entire recipe: 104 calories, 0g fat, 19mg sodium, 2g carbs, 0.5g fiber, 0g sugars, 0g protein

INGREDIENTS

12 mint leaves
1 lime, cut into 4 wedges
1 cup crushed ice *or* 5 to 8 ice cubes
6 ounces diet lemon-lime soda
1½ ounces rum

Optional garnish: additional mint leaves

DIRECTIONS

Place the mint leaves and 3 lime wedges in a glass. Muddle (a.k.a. mash).

Add ice, soda, and rum to the glass. Stir well and garnish with the remaining 1 lime wedge. Enjoy!

MAKES 1 SERVING

MUDDLER ALTERNATIVE:

Don't have a muddler? Use one of the beaters from a handheld electric mixer to smush stuff!

SUPER-SOUR LEMON DROP

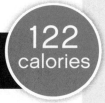

122 calories

You'll Need: shaker, glass | **Prep:** 5 minutes

Entire recipe:
122 calories, 0g fat, 10mg sodium, 7g carbs, <0.5g fiber, 1.5g sugars, <0.5g protein

INGREDIENTS

1 cup crushed ice *or* 5 to 8 ice cubes
2 ounces fresh-squeezed lemon juice
1 ½ ounces vodka
2 no-calorie sweetener packets
4 ounces diet lemon-lime soda

Optional garnish: lemon wedge

DIRECTIONS

Place ice in a shaker and add all other ingredients *except* soda. Shake vigorously and strain into a glass.

Top with soda, stir, and sip!

MAKES 1 SERVING

KICKIN' CRANBERRY COSMO

100 calories

   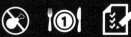

You'll Need: shaker, large martini glass
Prep: 5 minutes

Entire recipe: 100 calories, 0g fat, 32mg sodium, 2g carbs, 0g fiber, 1g sugars, 0g protein

INGREDIENTS

1 cup crushed ice *or* 5 to 8 ice cubes
5 ounces diet cranberry juice drink
1½ ounces vodka
1 teaspoon lime juice

Optional garnish: lime slice

DIRECTIONS

In a shaker filled with ice, combine juice drink, vodka, and lime juice. Shake it up and then strain into a large martini glass.

Enjoy!

MAKES 1 SERVING

APPLE CINNAMON COSMO

145 calories

You'll Need: shaker, large martini glass
Prep: 5 minutes

Entire recipe: 145 calories, 0g fat, 19mg sodium, 10g carbs, <0.5g fiber, 8g sugars, <0.5g protein

INGREDIENTS

1 cup crushed ice *or* 5 to 8 ice cubes
2 ounces diet cranberry juice drink
1½ ounces vodka
¼ teaspoon cinnamon
2 ounces sparkling apple cider

DIRECTIONS

In a shaker filled with ice, combine juice drink, vodka, and cinnamon. Shake and then strain it into a large martini glass. Top with cider and enjoy!

MAKES 1 SERVING

NIGHT & DAY NOG-TINIS

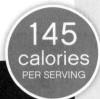

145 calories PER SERVING

You'll Need: shaker, 2 large martini glasses
Prep: 10 minutes

½ of recipe (1 nog-tini): 145 calories, 1g fat, 175mg sodium, 9g carbs, 0.5g fiber, 3g sugars, 3g protein

INGREDIENTS

1 tablespoon Jell-O Sugar Free Fat Free Vanilla Instant pudding mix
2 no-calorie sweetener packets
¼ teaspoon cinnamon
Dash ground nutmeg
8 ounces light vanilla soymilk
3 ounces vanilla vodka
1 cup crushed ice *or* 5 to 8 ice cubes

DIRECTIONS

Combine all dry ingredients in a shaker. Add soymilk and shake vigorously until pudding mix has mostly dissolved. Set aside to slightly thicken, about 5 minutes.

Add vodka and ice. Shake and strain into 2 large martini glasses. Sip!

MAKES 2 SERVINGS

CHOCOMINT MARTINIS

145 calories PER SERVING

You'll Need: tall glass, shaker, 2 martini glasses
Prep: 5 minutes

½ of recipe (1 martini): 145 calories, 0g fat, 90mg sodium, 7g carbs, 0.5g fiber, 4.5g sugars, 1g protein

INGREDIENTS

1 packet hot cocoa mix with 20 to 25 calories
1 no-calorie sweetener packet
2 tablespoons Cool Whip Free (thawed)
1 tablespoon light chocolate syrup
3 ounces vodka
2 drops peppermint extract
1 cup crushed ice *or* 5 to 8 ice cubes

Optional garnish: chocolate graham crackers

DIRECTIONS

In a tall glass, combine cocoa mix with sweetener. Add 2 ounces hot water and stir to dissolve. Add Cool Whip and syrup, and stir until smooth.

Add vodka, peppermint extract, and 2 ounces cold water. Sitr well, and transfer to a shaker filled with ice.

Shake vigorously and strain into 2 martini glasses. Enjoy!

MAKES 2 SERVINGS

Flip to the photo inserts to see over 100 recipe pics! And for photos of ALL the recipes, go to hungry-girl.com/books.

HOLIDAY

Seasonal favorites with an HG spin!

SAVE-THE-DAY STUFFING

89 calories PER SERVING

You'll Need: 8-inch by 8-inch baking pan, nonstick spray, large nonstick pot, aluminum foil
Prep: 15 minutes | **Cook:** 45 minutes

⅕th of recipe (about ¾ cup):
89 calories, 1.5g fat, 275mg sodium, 17g carbs, 4g fiber, 4g sugars, 5g protein

INGREDIENTS

6 slices light bread
1 cup fat-free chicken or vegetable broth
    (plus more if needed)
1 cup chopped celery
1 cup chopped onion
1 cup chopped mushrooms
2 teaspoons minced garlic
1 tablespoon light whipped butter or light buttery spread
¼ cup fat-free liquid egg substitute

Optional seasonings: salt, black pepper, rosemary, thyme

DIRECTIONS

Preheat oven to 350 degrees. Spray an 8-inch by 8-inch baking pan with nonstick spray.

Lightly toast bread slices. Cut them into cubes.

Place broth, celery, and onion in a large nonstick pot, and set heat to medium. Cook and stir for 10 minutes, until slightly softened.

Remove pot from heat and stir in mushrooms, garlic, and butter. Let broth mixture slightly cool.

Stir in egg substitute. Add bread cubes and stir to coat. Bread cubes should be moist, but not saturated. If needed, add a few extra tablespoons of broth to coat.

Transfer mixture to the baking pan. Cover with foil and bake for 20 minutes.

Remove foil. Fluff and rearrange stuffing. Bake uncovered until top has lightly browned, 10 to 15 minutes. Enjoy!

MAKES 5 SERVINGS

HG TIP!

Zazzle up your stuffing by adding any of the following to it before baking: 3 tablespoons raisins, 1 chopped medium pear, 2 tablespoons sliced almonds, 3 tablespoons sweetened dried cranberries, or 1 medium chopped Granny Smith apple. Each one adds less than 20 calories to each serving!

CRAN-TASTIC APPLE CORNBREAD STUFFING

159 calories PER SERVING

You'll Need: loaf pan, nonstick spray, medium bowl, whisk, 2 large bowls, 9-inch by 13-inch baking pan, large skillet
Prep: 20 minutes | **Cook:** 1 hour 30 minutes

⅛th of recipe (1 heaping cup):
159 calories, 0.5g fat, 375mg sodium, 34g carbs, 3.5g fiber, 15g sugars, 5g protein

INGREDIENTS

Cornbread
¾ cup canned cream-style corn
⅓ cup fat-free liquid egg substitute
⅓ cup fat-free plain Greek yogurt
½ cup all-purpose flour
⅓ cup yellow cornmeal
¼ cup granulated white sugar
½ tablespoon baking powder
⅛ teaspoon salt

Stuffing
4 slices light bread
¼ cup sweetened dried cranberries
1 large Fuji apple, cored and chopped
1 sweet onion, chopped
1½ cups chopped celery
1 teaspoon chopped garlic
2 cups fat-free chicken or vegetable broth
½ teaspoon dried sage
¼ teaspoon dried thyme
⅛ teaspoon each salt and black pepper

DIRECTIONS

To make the cornbread, preheat oven to 375 degrees. Spray a loaf pan with nonstick spray.

In a medium bowl, thoroughly whisk cream-style corn, egg substitute, and yogurt.

In a large bowl, mix all other cornbread ingredients. Add the mixture from the medium bowl and thoroughly stir.

Transfer mixture to the loaf pan. Bake until a toothpick inserted into the center comes out clean, about 25 minutes.

Let cornbread cool completely. For speedier cooling, remove it from the pan once slightly cooled.

To make the stuffing, bring oven to 350 degrees. Spray a 9-inch by 13-inch baking pan with nonstick spray.

Lightly toast bread slices. Meanwhile, chop cranberries and place in a large bowl. Cut bread into cubes and add to the bowl.

Bring a large skillet sprayed with nonstick spray to medium-high heat. Add chopped apple, onion, celery, and garlic. Cook and stir until softened, about 5 minutes.

Transfer apple mixture to the large bowl. Crumble cornbread into pieces and add to the bowl. Add all remaining ingredients and thoroughly mix.

Transfer mixture to the baking pan. Bake until firm, 35 to 40 minutes. Enjoy!

MAKES 8 SERVINGS

HG TIP!
Since the cornbread can take a while to cool, consider making it the night before (or a few hours before) you prepare the stuffing.

HG SWEET ALTERNATIVE!
If made with an equal amount of Splenda No Calorie Sweetener (granulated) in place of the sugar, each serving will have 138 calories, 28.5g carbs, and 8.5g sugars.

APPLE & ONION STUFFING

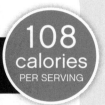

108 calories PER SERVING

You'll Need: 9-inch by 13-inch baking pan, nonstick spray, large nonstick pot, large bowl, aluminum foil
Prep: 15 minutes | **Cook:** 45 minutes

⅛th of recipe (about 1 cup):
108 calories, 1g fat, 206mg sodium, 24g carbs, 4.25g fiber, 12g sugars, 3g protein

INGREDIENTS

6 slices light bread

1 tablespoon light whipped butter or light buttery spread

2 cups chopped sweet onion

1 cup chopped celery

1 tablespoon minced shallots

½ tablespoon minced garlic

¼ teaspoon salt

4 cups chopped Fuji apples

¼ cup minced fresh parsley

¼ cup raisins (not packed)

⅓ cup fat-free chicken or vegetable broth (plus more if needed), room temperature

¼ cup fat-free liquid egg substitute

Optional seasoning: black pepper

DIRECTIONS

Preheat oven to 350 degrees. Spray a 9-inch by 13-inch baking pan with nonstick spray.

Lightly toast bread slices. Cut them into cubes.

Melt butter in a large nonstick pot over medium heat. Add onion, celery, shallots, garlic, and salt. Stirring frequently, cook veggies until softened, about 6 minutes.

Remove pot from heat and stir in apples, parsley, and raisins.

In a large bowl, thoroughly mix broth with egg substitute.

Add toasted bread cubes and stir to coat. Add veggie-apple mixture and gently stir. The bread cubes should be moist but not saturated. Add a few extra tablespoons of broth to coat, if needed.

Transfer stuffing mixture to the baking pan. Cover with foil and bake for 20 minutes.

Remove foil. Gently fluff and rearrange stuffing. Bake uncovered until the top is golden brown, 10 to 15 minutes. Devour!

MAKES 8 SERVINGS

ROCKIN' LEAN BEAN CASSEROLE

95 calories PER SERVING

You'll Need: 2- to 3-quart rectangular casserole dish, nonstick spray
Prep: 15 minutes
Cook: 55 minutes

⅛th of casserole: 95 calories, 2.5g fat, 539mg sodium, 16g carbs, 3.5g fiber, 5g sugars, 3.5g protein

INGREDIENTS

Two 16-ounce bags frozen French-style green beans, thawed, drained, dried

Two 10.75-ounce cans 98% fat-free cream of celery condensed soup

One 8-ounce can sliced water chestnuts, drained

1 ounce (about 15 pieces) onion-flavored soy crisps, crushed

DIRECTIONS

Preheat oven to 325 degrees. Spray a 2- to 3-quart rectangular casserole dish with nonstick spray.

Evenly layer ingredients in the casserole dish: half of the green beans, 1 can soup, and half of the water chestnuts. Repeat layering with remaining green beans, 1 can soup, and water chestnuts.

Bake for 45 minutes.

Top with crushed soy crisps. Bake until crisps are lightly browned, about 10 minutes. Enjoy!

MAKES 8 SERVINGS

KICKIN' CRANBERRY SAUCE

63 calories PER SERVING

You'll Need: medium nonstick pot with a lid, small bowl, large bowl
Prep: 10 minutes
Cook: 15 minutes
Chill: 5 hours

⅟₁₂th of recipe (about ⅓ cup): 63 calories, 1g fat, 20mg sodium, 13g carbs, 2g fiber, 8.5g sugars, 1g protein

INGREDIENTS

One 12-ounce bag whole cranberries
⅔ cup Splenda No Calorie Sweetener (granulated)
¼ cup granulated white sugar
One ¼-ounce envelope dry unflavored gelatin
1 cup peeled and finely chopped apple
⅛ teaspoon cinnamon
One 11-ounce can mandarin orange segments packed in juice
¼ cup thinly sliced roasted almonds, lightly crushed

DIRECTIONS

In a medium nonstick pot, combine cranberries, Splenda, sugar, and 1¾ cups water. Cover and bring to a boil.

Reduce to a simmer and cook for 10 minutes, occasionally uncovering to stir.

Meanwhile, in a small bowl, thoroughly mix gelatin with ¼ cup cold water.

Remove pot from heat and thoroughly mix in gelatin mixture. Stir in apple and cinnamon.

Transfer mixture to a large bowl and refrigerate until chilled and set, at least 5 hours.

Drain orange segments, roughly chop, and drain again. Stir chopped orange segments into the chilled cranberry mixture. Stir in crushed almonds and enjoy!

MAKES 12 SERVINGS

HG SWEET ALTERNATIVES!

Replace the Splenda with an equal amount of additional granulated white sugar; each serving will have 101 calories, 23g carbs, and 19.5g sugars. Or replace the sugar with the same amount of extra Splenda; then each serving will have 48 calories, 9g carbs, and 4g sugars. Cran-tastic!

APPLE-LICIOUS MATZO KUGEL

148 calories PER SERVING

You'll Need: 8-inch by 8-inch baking pan, nonstick spray, 2 large bowls, small microwave-safe bowl, whisk
Prep: 20 minutes | **Cook:** 45 minutes

⅛th of kugel:
148 calories, 2.5g fat, 253mg sodium, 26g carbs, 2g fiber, 11g sugars, 4.5g protein

INGREDIENTS

4 sheets matzo
¼ cup light whipped butter or light buttery spread
1 cup fat-free liquid egg substitute
¼ cup Splenda No Calorie Sweetener (granulated)
1 teaspoon vanilla extract
1 teaspoon cinnamon
½ teaspoon salt
3 cups finely chopped Fuji apples
½ cup sweetened dried cranberries, chopped

HG SWEET ALTERNATIVE!

If made with an equal amount of granulated white sugar in place of Splenda, each serving will have 170 calories, 32g carbs, and 17g sugars.

DIRECTIONS

Preheat oven to 350 degrees. Spray an 8-inch by 8-inch baking pan with nonstick spray.

Break matzo into small pieces and place in a large bowl. Add just enough warm water to cover, gently pressing down to wet any pieces that float.

Let soak until slightly softened, about 2 minutes. Drain well.

In a small microwave-safe bowl, microwave butter for 30 seconds, or until melted.

Transfer butter to another large bowl. Add egg substitute, Splenda, vanilla extract, cinnamon, and salt. Thoroughly whisk. Add matzo and gently stir. Fold in apples and chopped cranberries.

Transfer mixture to the baking pan. Bake until lightly browned and cooked through, about 45 minutes. Enjoy!

MAKES 8 SERVINGS

PEACHY CREAM CINNAMON RAISIN KUGEL

75 calories PER SERVING

You'll Need: loaf pan, nonstick spray, strainer, medium bowl, whisk, skillet
Prep: 10 minutes
Cook: 35 minutes

¼th of kugel: 75 calories, 0.5g fat, 202mg sodium, 11g carbs, 2g fiber, 7g sugars, 6g protein

INGREDIENTS

1 bag House Foods Tofu Shirataki Fettuccine
    Shaped Noodle Substitute
¼ cup fat-free liquid egg substitute
¼ cup fat-free cream cheese, room temperature
2 tablespoons Splenda No Calorie Sweetener (granulated)
¼ teaspoon vanilla extract
¼ teaspoon cinnamon
Dash salt
¼ cup fat-free cottage cheese
2 tablespoons raisins (not packed)
1 large firm peach, cut into bite-sized pieces

DIRECTIONS

Preheat oven to 425 degrees. Spray a loaf pan with nonstick spray.

Use a strainer to rinse and drain noodles. Thoroughly pat dry. Roughly cut noodles.

In a medium bowl, thoroughly whisk egg substitute, cream cheese, Splenda, vanilla extract, cinnamon, and salt. Stir in cottage cheese and raisins.

Bring a skillet sprayed with nonstick spray to medium heat. Cook and stir noodles to remove excess moisture, about 3 minutes.

Transfer noodles to the medium bowl. Add peach pieces and mix well. Transfer mixture to the baking pan.

Bake until firm, 25 to 30 minutes. Enjoy!

MAKES 4 SERVINGS

HG SWEET ALTERNATIVE!

Swap out the Splenda for the same amount of granulated white sugar, and each serving will have 96 calories, 16.5g carbs, and 13g sugars.

LOVE YA LATKES

84 calories PER SERVING

You'll Need: baking sheet, nonstick spray (olive oil variety, if available), large bowl
Prep: 20 minutes
Cook: 20 minutes

¼th of recipe (3 latkes): 84 calories, 1g fat, 324mg sodium, 16.5g carbs, 2.75g fiber, 3g sugars, 3g protein

INGREDIENTS

3 cups shredded butternut squash
½ cup shredded onion
¼ cup fat-free liquid egg substitute
2 tablespoons whole-wheat flour
½ teaspoon salt

Optional toppings: fat-free sour cream and chopped scallions *or* no-sugar-added applesauce and cinnamon

DIRECTIONS

Preheat oven to 450 degrees. Spray a baking sheet with a 3-second spray of nonstick spray (olive oil variety, if available).

Place shredded squash and onion between layers of paper towels, and press down firmly to remove all excess moisture. Repeat as needed.

In a large bowl, thoroughly mix squash, onion, egg substitute, flour, and salt.

Spoon squash mixture onto the sheet in 12 evenly spaced mounds. Use the back of a spoon to spread and flatten into 3-inch circles.

Bake for 8 minutes.

Remove sheet from oven and top latkes with another 3-second spray of nonstick spray. Flip latkes. Bake until crispy, about 10 minutes. Enjoy!

MAKES 4 SERVINGS

CRUSTLESS PUMPKIN QUICHE SUPREME

67 calories PER SERVING

You'll Need: 9-inch pie pan, nonstick spray, large skillet, large bowl | **Prep:** 10 minutes | **Cook:** 1 hour 15 minutes

⅛th of quiche:
67 calories, 1g fat, 332mg sodium, 8g carbs, 2g fiber, 3.5g sugars, 6g protein

INGREDIENTS

1 cup chopped sweet onion

1 cup chopped mushrooms

2 cups chopped spinach leaves

4 wedges The Laughing Cow Light Creamy Swiss cheese, room temperature

One 15-ounce can pure pumpkin

1¼ cups fat-free liquid egg substitute

2 teaspoons chopped garlic

½ teaspoon each salt and black pepper

⅛ teaspoon chili powder

DIRECTIONS

Preheat oven to 350 degrees. Spray a 9-inch pie pan with nonstick spray.

Bring a large skillet sprayed with nonstick spray to medium-high heat. Cook and stir onion until softened and slightly browned, about 6 minutes.

Transfer onion to a large bowl. Remove skillet from heat, re-spray, and return to medium-high heat. Cook and stir mushrooms until softened and lightly browned, about 4 minutes. Add spinach and cook until wilted and excess moisture has evaporated, about 2 minutes.

Transfer mushroom-spinach mixture to the large bowl. Add cheese wedges, breaking them into pieces, and thoroughly mix, until cheese has melted and is evenly distributed. Add all remaining ingredients and mix well.

Transfer mixture to the pie pan. Bake until firm and lightly browned, about 1 hour. Slice and enjoy!

MAKES 8 SERVINGS

✳ Flip to the photo inserts to see over 100 recipe pics! And for photos of ALL the recipes, go to **hungry-girl.com/books**.

I CAN'T BELIEVE IT'S NOT SWEET POTATO PIE

You'll Need: 8-inch by 8-inch baking pan, nonstick spray, large microwave-safe bowl, potato masher
Prep: 20 minutes | **Cook:** 1 hour 5 minutes

⅛th of pie:
142 calories, <0.5g fat, 263mg sodium, 33g carbs, 3g fiber, 12.5g sugars, 5g protein

INGREDIENTS

8 cups peeled and cubed butternut squash
⅔ cup light vanilla soymilk
⅔ cup sugar-free pancake syrup
½ cup Splenda No Calorie Sweetener (granulated)
2 teaspoons cinnamon
1 teaspoon vanilla extract
½ teaspoon salt
1 cup fat-free liquid egg substitute
2 cups miniature marshmallows

HG SWEET ALTERNATIVE!

Swap out the Splenda for the same amount of granulated white sugar, and each serving will have 184 calories, 44.5g carbs, and 25g sugars.

DIRECTIONS

Preheat oven to 350 degrees. Spray an 8-inch by 8-inch baking pan with nonstick spray.

Fill a large microwave-safe bowl with ½ inch of water. Add squash and cover. Microwave for about 8 minutes, or until squash is tender enough to mash.

Drain excess water from squash. Thoroughly mash. Stir in soymilk, syrup, sweetener, cinnamon, vanilla extract, and salt.

Stir in egg substitute, and transfer mixture to the baking pan. Bake until mostly firm, 45 to 50 minutes.

Top with marshmallows. Bake until marshmallows begin to brown, about 5 minutes. Mmmmm!

MAKES 8 SERVINGS

CUBING BUTTERNUT SQUASH . . .

You can usually find pre-cubed b-nut squash in the produce section. Wanna cut it up yourself? Here are some tips . . .

* Choose a squash that's mostly long and narrow with a short round section. The round part is hollow and full of seeds; the long section is solid squash and the best part to cube.

* If the squash is too firm to cut, pop it in the microwave for a minute to soften it.

* Slice off the ends and peel squash. Cut in half widthwise, just above the round section. Cut the round piece in half lengthwise and scoop out the seeds.

Cube to your heart's content!

Holy cow . . . have you SEEN the stats for regular egg nog?!
Try these NOGS . . . you just might get a thank-you note from your arteries . . .

NO-NONSENSE NOG

98 calories PER SERVING

You'll Need: blender, pitcher | **Prep:** 5 minutes | **Chill:** 3 hours

⅕th of recipe (about 1 cup):
98 calories, 2g fat, 382mg sodium, 13g carbs, 0.5g fiber, 6g sugars, 6g protein

INGREDIENTS

5 cups light vanilla soymilk

One 4-serving box Jell-O Sugar Free
    Fat Free Vanilla Instant pudding mix

6 no-calorie sweetener packets

1 teaspoon rum extract

½ teaspoon ground nutmeg

Optional toppings: Fat Free Reddi-wip,
    cinnamon

DIRECTIONS

Combine all ingredients in a blender, and blend at high speed until smooth.

Transfer to a pitcher, cover, and refrigerate until thickened, at least 3 hours. Yum time!

MAKES 5 SERVINGS

FUN WITH EGG NOG . . .

✳Spiked!
Nix the rum extract and reduce the soymilk to 4½ cups—then add 5 ounces rum to the recipe. Just tack on an additional 58 calories per serving.

✳In Your Coffee!
A generous splash will add creamy flavor to your cup. Mmmmm!

✳Nogsicles!
If you've got ice-pop molds for making freezy treats at home, fill 'em with nog and freeze until solid. Or just use small plastic cups, cover 'em with foil, and slide a Popsicle stick through the foil to make your pops. Sooo good!

CINN-FULLY GOOD CHOCO-NOG

104 calories
PER SERVING

You'll Need: tall glass, blender, pitcher
Prep: 5 minutes
Chill: 3 hours

⅕th of recipe (about 1 cup): 104 calories, 2g fat, 370mg sodium, 15g carbs, 2g fiber, 6g sugars, 7g protein

INGREDIENTS

1 packet hot cocoa mix with 20 to 25 calories

5 cups light vanilla soymilk

One 4-serving box sugar-free fat-free instant chocolate pudding mix

1 teaspoon rum extract

½ teaspoon cinnamon

¼ teaspoon ground nutmeg

Optional toppings: Fat Free Reddi-wip, additional cinnamon

DIRECTIONS

In a tall glass, combine cocoa mix with ¼ cup hot water and stir to dissolve.

Transfer cocoa mixture to a blender. Add all other ingredients and blend at high speed until smooth.

Transfer to a pitcher, cover, and refrigerate until thickened, at least 3 hours. Enjoy!

MAKES 5 SERVINGS

PUMPKIN-LICIOUS NOG

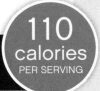

110 calories
PER SERVING

You'll Need: blender, pitcher
Prep: 5 minutes
Chill: 3 hours

⅕th of recipe (about 1 cup): 110 calories, 2g fat, 344mg sodium, 16g carbs, 2g fiber, 6.5g sugars, 6g protein

INGREDIENTS

5 cups light vanilla soymilk

One 4-serving box Jell-O Sugar Free Fat Free Vanilla Instant pudding mix

6 no-calorie sweetener packets

⅔ cup canned pure pumpkin

1 teaspoon rum extract

½ teaspoon ground nutmeg

½ teaspoon pumpkin pie spice

¼ teaspoon cinnamon

Optional topping: additional cinnamon

DIRECTIONS

Combine all ingredients in a blender, and blend at high speed until smooth.

Transfer to a pitcher, cover, and refrigerate until thickened, at least 3 hours. Mmmmm!

MAKES 5 SERVINGS

Hungry for More Holiday Favorites?

The Sweet Stuff chapter has a whole section of holiday desserts, starting on page 418!

CHAPTER 16

SWEET STUFF: FROM BROWNIES & FUDGE TO KRISPYMALLOWS

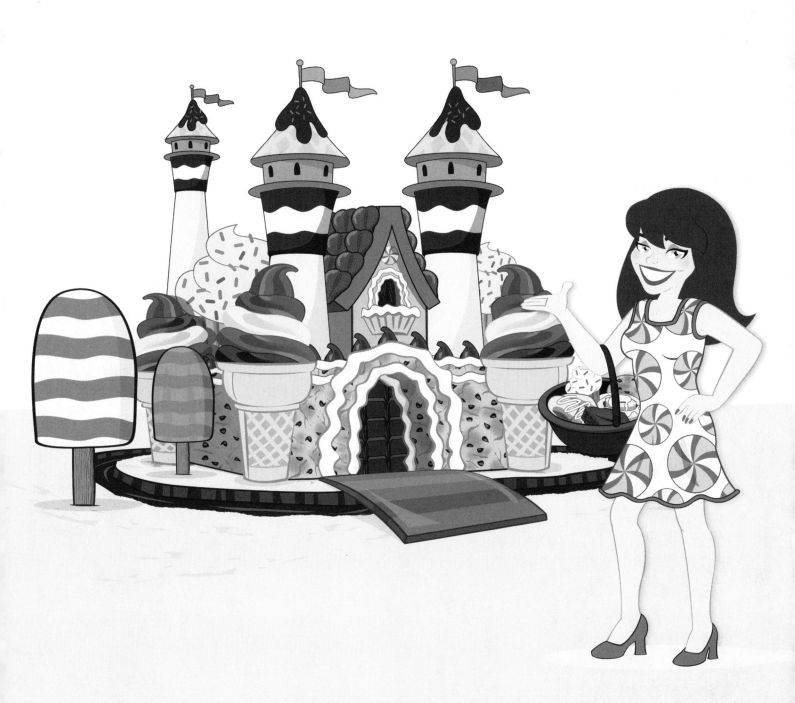

SWEET STUFF: FROM BROWNIES & FUDGE TO KRISPYMALLOWS

Yum Yum Brownie Muffins

Nutty-Good PB Brownies

PB&J Brownies

Death-by-Chocolate Brownies

Swirls-Gone-Wild Cheesecake Brownies

Gooey Caramel Coconut Brownies

Dreamy Chocolate Peanut Butter Fudge

Old Time Rocky Road Fudge

Marshmallow Fudge Mania!

Peppermint-Bark Fudge

Holy Moly Cannoli Cones

Peppermint Cannoli Cones

Eggnog Puddin' Pie

Upside-Down Pumpkin Pie

Candy Corn Custard Parfait

Guilt-Free Dirt & Worms Surprise

Ghosts-with-the-Most Meringues

Candyland Peppermint Pie

Happy Holiday Hot Fruit Crumble

Spice Cake Muffins

Chocolate Chip Pumpkin Muffins

Chippee Chocolate Chip Muffins

Big Fat Blueberry Muffins

Gooey-Good German Chocolate Cupcakes

Chocolate Marshmallow Madness Cupcakes

Red Velvet Insanity Cupcakes

14-Carat Cupcakes

Chocolate PB Pretzel Cupcakes

Expresso Cake in a Mug

Mississippi Mug Pie

Red Hot Apple Pie in a Cup

Diet Soda Cake

Chocolate-on-Chocolate Frosted Cake

Frosty the Vanilla Cake

Apple of My Cake

Upside-Down Pineapple-Applesauce Cake

Best of My Lava Chocolate Cake

Super-Duper Strawberry Shortcake

Ba Na Na Crazy Caramel Shortcakes

Turbo-Tremendous Tiramisu

Blueberry Bliss Cheesecake

Upside-Down Chocolate PB Cheesecake

Too-Good Turtle Cheesecake

PB Cup Cheesecake

Cookies 'n Dream Cheesecake

Bananarama Cream Pie

Gooey-Good Fuji Apple Pie

Crazy-Amazing Coconut Cream Pie

Freezy Downside-Up PB Dream Pie

Awesome Apple Pie Pockets

Blueberry-Apple Pie Pockets

Apple-Cherry Pie Pockets

PB 'n Chocolate Bread Pudding

Scoopable S'mores Bread Pudding

Caramel Bread Pudding for Two

Caramel Apple Bread Pudding

Perfect Pumpkin Bread

Top Banana Bread

Banana Split Bread

Swingin' Cinna-Monkey Bread Singles

Vanilla Almond Fruit Tartlets

Crispy Pecan Pie Bites

BFFs (Black Forest Fillo-Cups)

Double-Chocolate Pretzel Tarts

Caramel Apple Pie Bites

Chocolate-Chippy Cheese Danish

Cheesy Cherry Danish

Cinnamon Apple-Cranberry Danish

Blueberry Cheese Danish

Perfect Peach Dumplings

Crazy-Delicious Apple Dumplings

Bestest Baked Apples

Downtown Apple Betty Brown

Freezy-Cool Whoopie Pie

Freezy-Good Whoopie S'mores

Freezy-Cool Banana Whoopie Pies

Double-Trouble Chocolate Trifle

Ooey-Gooey German Chocolate Trifle

Gooey Cinnamon Rolls with
    Cream Cheese Icing

Strawberry Coconut Cinnamon Buns

Caramel Apple Cinnamon Buns

Nutty Caramel-Coated Sticky Buns

Grab 'n Go Breakfast Cookies

Oatmeal Raisin Softies

Peanut Butter Oatmeal Softies

Pumpkin Softies

Chocolate Chip Oatmeal Softies

Apple Cinnamon Softies

Snickerdoodle Softies

Cranberry White Chocolate Softies

Chocolate-Drizzled PB Chip Softies

Rocky Road Softies

Freezylicious Strawberry Squares

Big Beautiful Baked Alaska

Freezy PB&J Minis

Freezy Movie Night Concession
    Stand-wiches

Too-Cool Key Lime Pie Sandwiches

Creamy Frozen Caramel Crunchcake

Cool 'n Creamy Birthday Cake Sandwich

Chocolate-Coconut Freezies

Freezy-Cool Snickers Stackers

Freezy Candy Cane Snack-wiches

Mini Ice Cream Cakes

Krispymallow Treats

Cocoa Loco Krispymallow Treats

S'mores Krispymallow Treats

PB Chocolate Krispymallow Treats

Candy Corn MegaMallow Treats

HEY! You like dessert? SWEET!

You're in the right place. Dive in . . . face first!

SPLENDA & SUGAR SWAPPIN'!

* Many HG dessert recipes call for Splenda No Calorie Sweetener (granulated) because it has nearly 90 percent fewer calories than sugar. We use real sugar in recipes when only a little bit of sweetener is needed or when the taste of real sugar makes a big difference.

* Since we know some people prefer one or the other across the board, we've provided recipe stats when the alternative is used for every recipe! The few exceptions are recipes in which the nutritional difference is negligible; in those cases, the ingredients are listed interchangeably.

A QUICK GUIDE TO SYMBOLS:

15 Minutes or Less	30 Minutes or Less	Meatless	Single Serving	5 Ingredients or Less	Photos
This symbol lets you know a recipe should take you no more than fifteen minutes from start to finish! That includes prep and cook time.	Just like the 15-minute version, this one points out recipes that take 30 minutes or less to whip up.	You guessed it—no meat here! That includes beef, poultry, and fish. Some recipes give the option of a meatless ingredient. If you want your meal without meat, go with the meatless choice.	Pretty straightforward. These are recipes for one.	Fans of HG know that we like to keep things simple. And these recipes contain just five ingredients or less!	These recipes can be seen in one of the book's photo inserts. The number in the symbol tells you which insert. Find photos of all the recipes at hungry-girl.com/books!

HG BROWNIES call for devil's food cake mix and pumpkin.
Don't question the unique pairing, just enjoy its fudgy allure . . .

YUM YUM BROWNIE MUFFINS

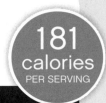
181 calories
PER SERVING

You'll Need: 12-cup muffin pan, foil baking cups or nonstick spray, large bowl
Prep: 5 minutes
Cook: 20 minutes

1/12th of recipe (1 muffin): 181 calories, 3.5g fat, 357mg sodium, 37g carbs, 2g fiber, 20g sugars, 2g protein

INGREDIENTS

1 box moist-style devil's food cake mix (15.25 to 18.25 ounces)
One 15-ounce can pure pumpkin

DIRECTIONS

Preheat oven to 400 degrees. Line a 12-cup muffin pan with foil baking cups, or spray it with nonstick spray.

In a large bowl, mix cake mix with pumpkin until completely smooth and uniform. (Batter will be thick.)

Evenly distribute batter into the cups of the muffin pan. Bake until a toothpick inserted into the center of a muffin comes out mostly clean, about 20 minutes. Enjoy!

MAKES 12 SERVINGS

NUTTY-GOOD PB BROWNIES

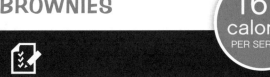
160 calories
PER SERVING

You'll Need: 9-inch by 13-inch baking pan, nonstick spray, large bowl, small bowl
Prep: 10 minutes
Cook: 30 minutes

1/16th of recipe (1 brownie): 160 calories, 4g fat, 293mg sodium, 30g carbs, 2g fiber, 15.5g sugars, 2.5g protein

INGREDIENTS

1 box moist-style devil's food cake mix (15.25 to 18.25 ounces)
One 15-ounce can pure pumpkin
1/4 cup creamy reduced-fat peanut butter, room temperature
1 tablespoon light soymilk

DIRECTIONS

Preheat oven to 400 degrees. Spray a 9-inch by 13-inch baking pan with nonstick spray.

In a large bowl, mix cake mix with pumpkin until completely smooth and uniform. (Batter will be thick.) Spread mixture into the baking pan.

In a small bowl, thoroughly mix peanut butter with soymilk. Swirl the peanut butter mixture over the top of the batter with a knife or spoon handle.

Bake until a toothpick inserted into the center comes out mostly clean, 25 to 30 minutes.

Let brownies cool. Slice and enjoy!

MAKES 16 SERVINGS

HG HEADS-UP:

These brownie recipes call for canned pure pumpkin. Don't confuse pumpkin puree with cans of pumpkin pie mix or filling—those are loaded with too many extra sugary calories!

PB&J BROWNIES

171 calories PER SERVING

You'll Need: 9-inch by 13-inch baking pan, nonstick spray, large bowl
Prep: 10 minutes
Cook: 30 minutes

¹⁄₁₆th of recipe (1 brownie): 171 calories, 3g fat, 270mg sodium, 34g carbs, 1.5g fiber, 20g sugars, 2g protein

INGREDIENTS

1 box moist-style devil's food cake mix (15.25 to 18.25 ounces)

One 15-ounce can pure pumpkin

¾ cup low-sugar strawberry preserves (about half of a 15.5-ounce jar)

¼ cup peanut butter baking chips, finely chopped

DIRECTIONS

Preheat oven to 400 degrees. Spray a 9-inch by 13-inch baking pan with nonstick spray.

In a large bowl, mix cake mix with pumpkin until completely smooth and uniform. (Batter will be thick.) Spread mixture into the baking pan.

Bake until a toothpick inserted into the center comes out mostly clean, 25 to 30 minutes.

Let cool completely.

Spread with preserves and sprinkle with chopped peanut butter chips. Slice and serve!

MAKES 16 SERVINGS

DEATH-BY-CHOCOLATE BROWNIES

174 calories PER SERVING

You'll Need: 9-inch by 13-inch baking pan, nonstick spray, medium bowl, large bowl
Prep: 20 minutes
Cook: 30 minutes
Chill: 15 minutes

¹⁄₁₆th of recipe (1 brownie): 174 calories, 4g fat, 288mg sodium, 33.5g carbs, 1.5g fiber, 19.5g sugars, 2g protein

INGREDIENTS

1 sugar-free chocolate pudding snack with 60 calories or less

⅓ cup chocolate frosting

2 tablespoons light chocolate syrup

1 box moist-style devil's food cake mix (15.25 to 18.25 ounces)

One 15-ounce can pure pumpkin

¼ cup mini semi-sweet chocolate chips

DIRECTIONS

Preheat oven to 400 degrees. Spray a 9-inch by 13-inch baking pan with nonstick spray.

In a medium bowl, mix pudding, frosting, and syrup. Cover and refrigerate.

In a large bowl, thoroughly mix cake mix, pumpkin, and chocolate chips. (Batter will be thick.) Spread mixture into the baking pan.

Bake until a toothpick inserted into the center comes out mostly clean, 25 to 30 minutes.

Let cool completely.

Evenly spread pudding mixture over brownies. Refrigerate until topping is set, about 15 minutes. Slice and enjoy! (Refrigerate leftovers.)

MAKES 16 SERVINGS

CAKE MIX FYI:

Standard boxes of cake mix range from 15.25 to 18.25 ounces, but they yield similar amounts and have similar overall stats. Any box in this size range will work for these recipes, both nutritionally and in terms of recipe results!

SWIRLS-GONE-WILD CHEESECAKE BROWNIES

133 calories PER SERVING

You'll Need: 9-inch by 13-inch baking pan, nonstick spray, large bowl, medium bowl, whisk
Prep: 10 minutes
Cook: 30 minutes

⅟₁₆th of recipe (1 brownie): 133 calories, 1.75g fat, 312mg sodium, 29g carbs, 1.5g fiber, 7.5g sugars, 3g protein

INGREDIENTS

1 box moist-style devil's food cake mix (15.25 to 18.25 ounces)

One 15-ounce can pure pumpkin

1 teaspoon sugar-free French vanilla powdered creamer

¾ths of an 8-ounce tub fat-free cream cheese, room temperature

¼ cup Splenda No Calorie Sweetener (granulated)

¼ teaspoon vanilla extract

DIRECTIONS

Preheat oven to 400 degrees. Spray a 9-inch by 13-inch baking pan with nonstick spray.

In a large bowl, mix cake mix with pumpkin until completely smooth and uniform. (Batter will be thick.) Spread mixture into the baking pan.

In a medium bowl, combine powdered creamer with 2 tablespoons hot water and stir until dissolved. Add cream cheese, Splenda, and vanilla extract. Vigorously whisk until completely blended and smooth.

Spoon cheesy mixture over batter in the pan and use a knife to swirl it in.

Bake until a toothpick inserted into the center comes out mostly clean, 25 to 30 minutes.

Let cool completely. Slice and serve!

MAKES 16 SERVINGS

HG SWEET ALTERNATIVE!

Swap out the Splenda for the same amount of granulated white sugar, and each serving will have 144 calories, 32g carbs, and 10.5g sugars.

GOOEY CARAMEL COCONUT BROWNIES

165 calories PER SERVING

You'll Need: 9-inch by 13-inch baking pan, nonstick spray, large bowl, medium bowl
Prep: 10 minutes
Cook: 30 minutes

⅟₁₆th of recipe (1 brownie): 165 calories, 3.5g fat, 298mg sodium, 32.5g carbs, 2g fiber, 17.5g sugars, 2g protein

INGREDIENTS

1 box moist-style devil's food cake mix (15.25 to 18.25 ounces)

One 15-ounce can pure pumpkin

1 sugar-free caramel pudding snack with 60 calories or less

¼ cup fat-free or light caramel dip

2 tablespoons finely chopped pecans

2 tablespoons shredded sweetened coconut, chopped

DIRECTIONS

Preheat oven to 400 degrees. Spray a 9-inch by 13-inch baking pan with nonstick spray.

In a large bowl, mix cake mix with pumpkin until completely smooth and uniform. (Batter will be thick.) Spread mixture into the baking pan.

Bake until a toothpick inserted into the center comes out mostly clean, 25 to 30 minutes.

Let cool completely. Meanwhile, in a medium bowl, combine pudding, caramel dip, pecans, and coconut. Mix well. Cover and refrigerate.

Evenly spread pudding mixture over brownies. Slice and enjoy!

MAKES 16 SERVINGS

DREAMY CHOCOLATE PEANUT BUTTER FUDGE

65 calories PER SERVING

You'll Need: 8-inch by 8-inch baking pan, nonstick spray, large bowl, aluminum foil
Prep: 10 minutes | **Cook:** 35 minutes | **Chill:** 2 hours

1/36th of recipe (1 square):
65 calories, 1g fat, 57mg sodium, 13.5g carbs, 0.5g fiber, 9g sugars, 0.5g protein

INGREDIENTS

One 18.3-ounce box fudge brownie mix

2 cups canned pure pumpkin

2 tablespoons light chocolate syrup

2 tablespoons reduced-fat
    peanut butter, softened

DIRECTIONS

Preheat oven to 350 degrees. Spray an 8-inch by 8-inch baking pan with nonstick spray.

In a large bowl, mix brownie mix, pumpkin, and chocolate syrup until completely smooth and uniform. (Batter will be thick.) Spread mixture into the baking pan.

Spoon peanut butter over batter in the pan and use a knife to swirl it in.

Bake until edges are slightly firm and top center is dry to the touch, about 35 minutes.

Let fudge cool. Cover the pan with foil and refrigerate until completely chilled, at least 2 hours. Cut into squares and get ready for a fudge frenzy!

MAKES 36 SERVINGS

FUDGE 411
The cooked batter will remain very thick and may look underdone. This is to be expected!

OLD TIME ROCKY ROAD FUDGE

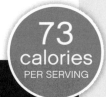

73 calories PER SERVING

You'll Need: 8-inch by 8-inch baking pan, nonstick spray, large bowl
Prep: 10 minutes
Cook: 35 minutes
Chill: 2 hours

⅟₃₆th of recipe (1 square): 73 calories, 1g fat, 52mg sodium, 15.5g carbs, 1g fiber, 10g sugars, 1g protein

INGREDIENTS

One 18.3-ounce box fudge brownie mix
2 cups canned pure pumpkin
2 tablespoons light chocolate syrup
2 cups mini marshmallows
¼ cup slivered almonds, lightly crushed

DIRECTIONS

Preheat oven to 350 degrees. Spray an 8-inch by 8-inch baking pan with nonstick spray.

In a large bowl, mix brownie mix, pumpkin, and chocolate syrup until completely smooth and uniform. (Batter will be thick.) Spread mixture into the baking pan.

Bake for 25 minutes. Leave oven on.

Evenly top with mini marshmallows and sprinkle with crushed almonds. Using a spatula, press down on toppings to help them adhere.

Bake until edges are slightly firm, about 10 minutes.

Let fudge slightly cool. Refrigerate until completely chilled, at least 2 hours. (Do not cover pan.) Cut into squares and serve!

MAKES 36 SERVINGS

MARSHMALLOW FUDGE MANIA!

66 calories PER SERVING

You'll Need: 8-inch by 8-inch baking pan, nonstick spray, large bowl, aluminum foil
Prep: 10 minutes
Cook: 35 minutes
Chill: 2 hours

⅟₃₆th of recipe (1 square): 66 calories, 0.5g fat, 51mg sodium, 14.5g carbs, 0.75g fiber, 9.5g sugars, 0.5g protein

INGREDIENTS

One 18.3-ounce box fudge brownie mix
2 cups canned pure pumpkin
2 tablespoons light chocolate syrup
½ cup Jet-Puffed Marshmallow Creme, room temperature

DIRECTIONS

Preheat oven to 350 degrees. Spray an 8-inch by 8-inch baking pan with nonstick spray.

In a large bowl, mix brownie mix, pumpkin, and chocolate syrup until completely smooth and uniform. (Batter will be thick.)

Spread half of the batter into the baking pan. Spoon ¼ cup marshmallow creme over the batter and use a knife to swirl it in.

Spread remaining batter into the pan. Spoon remaining ¼ cup marshmallow creme over the batter and use a knife to swirl it in.

Bake until edges are slightly firm and top center is dry to the touch, about 35 minutes.

Let fudge cool. Cover the pan with foil and refrigerate until completely chilled, at least 2 hours. Cut into squares and serve it up!

MAKES 36 SERVINGS

PEPPERMINT-BARK FUDGE

 67 calories PER SERVING

You'll Need: 8-inch by 8-inch baking pan, nonstick spray, large bowl, aluminum foil
Prep: 10 minutes
Cook: 35 minutes
Chill: 2 hours

1/36th of recipe (1 square): 67 calories, 1g fat, 50mg sodium, 14g carbs, 0.5g fiber, 9.5g sugars, 0.5g protein

INGREDIENTS

One 18.3-ounce box fudge brownie mix

2 cups canned pure pumpkin

3 tablespoons white chocolate chips, roughly chopped

1 standard-size candy cane *or* 5 mini candy canes, lightly crushed

DIRECTIONS

Preheat oven to 350 degrees. Spray an 8-inch by 8-inch baking pan with nonstick spray.

In a large bowl, mix brownie mix with pumpkin until completely smooth and uniform. (Batter will be thick.) Spread mixture into the baking pan.

Bake until edges are slightly firm and top center is dry to the touch, about 35 minutes.

Sprinkle with chopped chocolate chips and crushed candy cane(s). Using a spatula, press down on toppings to help them adhere.

Let fudge cool. Cover the pan with foil and refrigerate until completely chilled, at least 2 hours. Cut into squares and eat up!

MAKES 36 SERVINGS

HOLY MOLY CANNOLI CONES

 134 calories PER SERVING

You'll Need: medium-large bowl, electric mixer, large plastic bag
Prep: 15 minutes
Chill: 15 minutes

1/6th of recipe (1 cannoli cone): 134 calories, 1.75g fat, 184mg sodium, 21g carbs, 0g fiber, 10.5g sugars, 6g protein

INGREDIENTS

1 tablespoon Jell-O Sugar Free Fat Free Vanilla Instant pudding mix

1 cup plus 2 tablespoons fat-free ricotta cheese

2/3 cup Cool Whip Free (thawed)

2½ tablespoons Splenda No Calorie Sweetener (granulated)

1 tablespoon powdered sugar

2 tablespoons mini semi-sweet chocolate chips

6 sugar cones

DIRECTIONS

In a medium-large bowl, mix pudding mix with 2 tablespoons water until slightly thickened. Add ricotta cheese, Cool Whip, Splenda, and sugar. Mix until smooth with an electric mixer set to high speed.

Stir in 1 tablespoon chocolate chips. Cover and refrigerate until chilled, about 15 minutes.

Transfer mixture to a large plastic bag and squeeze it down toward a bottom corner. Snip off that corner with scissors, creating a hole for piping mixture.

Evenly pipe mixture into the cones. Top with remaining 1 tablespoon chocolate chips. Eat and enjoy!

MAKES 6 SERVINGS

HG SWEET ALTERNATIVE!

Swap out the Splenda for the same amount of granulated white sugar, and each serving will have 152 calories, 26g carbs, and 16g sugars.

PEPPERMINT CANNOLI CONES

143 calories PER SERVING

You'll Need: medium-large bowl, electric mixer, large plastic bag | **Prep:** 15 minutes | **Chill:** 15 minutes

⅙th of recipe (1 cannoli cone):
143 calories, 1.5g fat, 153mg sodium, 24g carbs, <0.5g fiber, 12.5g sugars, 5g protein

INGREDIENTS

1 tablespoon Jell-O Sugar Free Fat Free Vanilla Instant pudding mix

1 cup plus 2 tablespoons fat-free ricotta cheese

⅔ cup Cool Whip Free (thawed)

2½ tablespoons Splenda No Calorie Sweetener (granulated)

1 tablespoon powdered sugar

⅛ teaspoon peppermint extract

2 tablespoons mini semi-sweet chocolate chips

3 hard peppermint candies, crushed

6 sugar cones

HG SWEET ALTERNATIVE!

Swap out the Splenda for the same amount of granulated white sugar, and each serving will have 161 calories, 29g carbs, and 18g sugars.

DIRECTIONS

In a medium-large bowl, mix pudding mix with 2 tablespoons water until slightly thickened. Add ricotta cheese, Cool Whip, Splenda, sugar, and extract. Mix until smooth with an electric mixer set to high speed.

Stir in 1 tablespoon chocolate chips and half of the crushed candies. Cover and refrigerate until chilled, about 15 minutes.

Transfer mixture to a large plastic bag and squeeze it down toward a bottom corner. Snip off that corner with scissors, creating a hole for piping mixture.

Evenly pipe mixture into the cones. Top with remaining 1 tablespoon chocolate chips and crushed candies. Eat and enjoy!

MAKES 6 SERVINGS

EGGNOG PUDDIN' PIE

125
calories
PER SERVING

You'll Need: deep-dish pie pan, nonstick spray, blender or food processor, medium bowl, small microwave-safe bowl, large bowl, whisk | **Prep:** 15 minutes | **Cook:** 10 minutes | **Chill:** 1 hour 35 minutes

⅛th of pie:
125 calories, 3.5g fat, 286mg sodium, 22g carbs, 3.75g fiber, 6.5g sugars, 3g protein

INGREDIENTS

Crust
1 cup Fiber One Original bran cereal

2 sheets (8 crackers) low-fat honey graham crackers, broken into pieces

3 tablespoons Splenda No Calorie Sweetener (granulated)

½ teaspoon cinnamon

¼ cup light whipped butter or light buttery spread

Filling
2 cups fat-free milk

One 4-serving box Jell-O Sugar Free Fat Free Vanilla Instant pudding mix

1 teaspoon rum extract

½ teaspoon vanilla extract

¼ teaspoon ground nutmeg

2 dashes cinnamon

2 cups Cool Whip Free (thawed)

Optional topping: additional cinnamon

DIRECTIONS

Preheat oven to 350 degrees. Spray a deep-dish pie pan with nonstick spray.

In a blender or food processor, grind cereal and graham cracker pieces into crumbs. Transfer to a medium bowl and mix in Splenda and cinnamon.

In a small microwave-safe bowl, microwave butter and 2 tablespoons water for 30 seconds, or until butter has melted. Add to the medium bowl and thoroughly mix.

Evenly distribute mixture along the bottom of the pie pan, using your hands or a flat utensil to firmly press and form the crust. Press it into the edges and up along the sides of the pan.

Bake until firm, about 10 minutes. Let cool.

To make the filling, pour milk into a large bowl. Add pudding mix, rum extract, vanilla extract, nutmeg, and cinnamon. Whisk until smooth, about 2 minutes. Fold in 1 cup Cool Whip. Refrigerate until thickened, at least 5 minutes.

Evenly spread filling into the crust. Spread with remaining 1 cup Cool Whip. Refrigerate until completely chilled and set, at least 1½ hours.

Slice and serve!

MAKES 8 SERVINGS

HG SWEET ALTERNATIVE!
Swap out the Splenda for the same amount of granulated white sugar, and each serving will have 141 calories, 26g carbs, and 11g sugars.

UPSIDE-DOWN PUMPKIN PIE

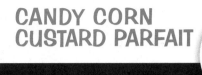 **144 calories** PER SERVING

You'll Need: deep-dish pie pan, nonstick spray, large bowl, whisk
Prep: 15 minutes
Cook: 45 minutes
Chill: 3 hours

⅛th of pie: 144 calories, 0.5g fat, 110mg sodium, 30g carbs, 2g fiber, 26g sugars, 5g protein

INGREDIENTS

One 15-ounce can pure pumpkin (not pumpkin pie filling)
One 12-ounce can evaporated fat-free milk
⅔ cup granulated white sugar
½ cup fat-free liquid egg substitute
2 teaspoons pumpkin pie spice
2 sheets (8 crackers) low-fat cinnamon graham crackers, finely crushed
Optional toppings: Fat Free Reddi-wip, cinnamon

DIRECTIONS

Preheat oven to 350 degrees. Spray a deep-dish pie pan with nonstick spray.

In a large bowl, thoroughly whisk all ingredients *except* graham crackers.

Transfer mixture to the pie pan. Bake until partially firm, about 45 minutes.

Refrigerate until completely chilled and firm, at least 3 hours.

Sprinkle with crushed graham crackers. Enjoy!

MAKES 8 SERVINGS

HG SWEET ALTERNATIVE!

If made with an equal amount of Splenda No Calorie Sweetener (granulated) in place of the sugar, each serving will have 88 calories, 15g carbs, and 9g sugars.

CANDY CORN CUSTARD PARFAIT

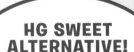

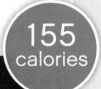 **155 calories**

You'll Need: mid-sized glass
Prep: 5 minutes

Entire recipe: 155 calories, 1g fat, 234mg sodium, 34.5g carbs, 0.5g fiber, 15g sugars, 1.5g protein

INGREDIENTS

1 sugar-free vanilla pudding snack with 60 calories or less
2 drops yellow food coloring
⅓ cup mandarin orange segments packed in juice, drained
¼ cup Cool Whip Free (thawed)
5 pieces candy corn

DIRECTIONS

In a mid-sized glass, thoroughly mix food coloring into pudding.

Top with orange segments, and spread with Cool Whip.

Arrange candy corn prettily on top (or haphazardly—it's your parfait), and dive in!

MAKES 1 SERVING

GUILT-FREE DIRT & WORMS SURPRISE

159 calories PER SERVING

You'll Need: large bowl, whisk, wide serving bowl
Prep: 10 minutes
Chill: 15 minutes

⅛th of recipe (about ⅔ cup):
159 calories, 1g fat, 403mg sodium, 30g carbs, 1g fiber, 15g sugars, 7g protein

INGREDIENTS

2 small (4-serving) boxes sugar-free fat-free instant chocolate pudding mix

4 cups fat-free milk

12 gummy worms, chopped into thirds

4 sheets (16 crackers) chocolate graham crackers, crushed

DIRECTIONS

In a large bowl, whisk pudding mix with milk until thoroughly mixed and thickened, 2 to 4 minutes.

Pour mixture into a wide serving bowl. Cover and refrigerate until set, at least 15 minutes.

Just before serving, top with chopped gummy worms. Sprinkle with crushed graham crackers and enjoy!

MAKES 8 SERVINGS

HG SWEET ALTERNATIVE!

Replace the Splenda with an equal amount of additional granulated white sugar; each serving will have 75 calories, 17.5g carbs, and 16.5g sugars. We don't recommend making this recipe with Splenda only. (It doesn't taste great.)

GHOSTS-WITH-THE-MOST MERINGUES

47 calories PER SERVING

You'll Need: 2 large baking pans, parchment paper, large bowl, electric mixer, large plastic bag
Prep: 15 minutes
Cook: 1 hour 10 minutes
Rest: 1 hour

⅛th of recipe (2 meringues): 47 calories, <0.5g fat, 20mg sodium, 9.5g carbs, 0g fiber, 8.5g sugars, 1g protein

INGREDIENTS

⅓ cup plus 1 tablespoon liquid egg whites (about 3 egg whites)

¼ teaspoon cream of tartar

⅓ cup granulated white sugar

⅓ cup Splenda No Calorie Sweetener (granulated)

½ teaspoon vanilla extract

32 mini semi-sweet chocolate chips

DIRECTIONS

Preheat oven to 200 degrees. Line 2 large baking pans with parchment paper.

In a large bowl, combine egg whites with cream of tartar. With an electric mixer set to high speed, beat until fluffy and slightly stiff, about 3 minutes. Continue to beat while gradually adding sugar, Splenda, and vanilla extract. Beat until thoroughly mixed, about 1 minute.

Transfer mixture to a large plastic bag and squeeze it down toward a bottom corner. Snip off that corner with scissors, creating a hole for piping mixture.

Pipe mixture onto the parchment paper in a 3-inch ghost shape; do the outline first, and then fill it in. Use the tip of the bag to smooth mixture and solidly fill the shape.

Repeat for a total of 16 evenly spaced ghosts. Place 2 mini chips on each ghost for eyes.

Bake for 70 minutes. Do not remove meringues.

Turn off oven and let meringues set in the oven for 1 hour.

Chomp away!

MAKES 8 SERVINGS

CANDYLAND PEPPERMINT PIE

202 calories PER SERVING

You'll Need: pie pan, nonstick spray, blender or food processor, medium bowl, small microwave-safe bowl, large bowl, whisk | **Prep:** 15 minutes | **Cook:** 10 minutes | **Chill:** 1 hour 30 minutes

⅛th of pie:
202 calories, 4.5g fat, 250mg sodium, 37g carbs, 0.25g fiber, 24g sugars, 2.5g protein

INGREDIENTS

Crust
4 sheets (16 crackers) chocolate graham crackers, broken into pieces
2 tablespoons light whipped butter or light buttery spread

Filling
½ cup fat-free sweetened condensed milk
¼ cup fat-free milk
One 4-serving box Jell-O Sugar Free Fat Free Vanilla Instant pudding mix
3 cups Cool Whip Free (thawed)
3 tablespoons mini semi-sweet chocolate chips
2 standard-sized peppermint candy canes *or* 10 mini candy canes, lightly crushed

Optional topping: Fat Free Reddi-wip

DIRECTIONS

Preheat oven to 400 degrees. Spray a pie pan with nonstick spray.

In a blender or food processor, grind graham cracker pieces into crumbs. Transfer to a medium bowl.

In a small microwave-safe bowl, microwave butter for 15 seconds, or until melted. Add to the medium bowl and thoroughly mix.

Evenly distribute mixture along the bottom of the pie pan, using your hands or a flat utensil to firmly press and form the crust. Press it into the edges and up along the sides of the pan.

Bake until firm, about 10 minutes. Let cool.

To make the filling, pour condensed milk into a large bowl. Add milk and pudding mix. Whisk until smooth, about 2 minutes. Fold in Cool Whip. Stir in chocolate chips and ¾ths of the candy cane pieces.

Evenly spread filling into the crust. Refrigerate until completely chilled and set, at least 1½ hours.

Sprinkle with remaining candy cane pieces. Dig in!

MAKES 8 SERVINGS

✳ Flip to the photo inserts to see over 100 recipe pics! And for photos of ALL the recipes, go to **hungry-girl.com/books**.

HAPPY HOLIDAY HOT FRUIT CRUMBLE

123 calories
PER SERVING

You'll Need: 8-inch by 8-inch baking pan, nonstick spray, large bowl, aluminum foil, medium bowl
Prep: 15 minutes | **Cook:** 45 minutes

⅑th of recipe (about ¾ cup):
123 calories, 1.5g fat, 81mg sodium, 30g carbs, 4.5g fiber, 19.5g sugars, 1g protein

INGREDIENTS

Fruit Mixture
3 apples, peeled, cored, and thinly sliced
3 pears, peeled, cored, and thinly sliced
1 tablespoon lemon juice
1 cup cranberries
⅓ cup granulated white sugar
1 tablespoon cornstarch
½ teaspoon cinnamon
Dash salt

Topping
½ cup Fiber One Original bran cereal, lightly crushed
¼ cup old-fashioned oats
2 tablespoons brown sugar (not packed)
2 tablespoons light whipped butter or light buttery spread, room temperature
½ teaspoon cinnamon
⅛ teaspoon salt

DIRECTIONS

Preheat oven to 350 degrees. Spray an 8-inch by 8-inch baking pan with nonstick spray.

In a large bowl, combine sliced apples and pears with lemon juice and toss to coat. Add all remaining ingredients for fruit mixture. Toss until thoroughly mixed.

Transfer mixture to the baking pan, and cover pan with foil.

Bake for 30 minutes, or until fruit has softened. Leave oven on.

Meanwhile, in a medium bowl, combine all ingredients for topping. Stir until well mixed and crumbly.

Remove foil from the pan and mix well. Smooth out surface and sprinkle with topping. Bake uncovered until topping is slightly crisp, about 15 minutes. Dig in!

MAKES 9 SERVINGS

HG SWEET ALTERNATIVE!
If made with an equal amount of Splenda No Calorie Sweetener (granulated) in place of the sugar, each serving will have 98 calories, 23g carbs, and 12g sugars.

SPICE CAKE MUFFINS

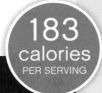

183 calories PER SERVING

You'll Need: 12-cup muffin pan, foil baking cups or nonstick spray, large bowl
Prep: 5 minutes
Cook: 20 minutes

1/12th of recipe (1 muffin): 183 calories, 3.5g fat, 301mg sodium, 37g carbs, 1.25g fiber, 20.5g sugars, 2g protein

INGREDIENTS

1 box moist-style spice cake mix (15.25 to 18.25 ounces)
One 15-ounce can pure pumpkin

DIRECTIONS

Preheat oven to 400 degrees. Line a 12-cup muffin pan with foil baking cups, or spray it with nonstick spray.

In a large bowl, mix cake mix with pumpkin until completely smooth and uniform. (Batter will be thick.)

Evenly distribute batter into the cups of the muffin pan. Bake until a toothpick inserted into the center of a muffin comes out clean, about 20 minutes. Enjoy!

MAKES 12 SERVINGS

CHOCOLATE CHIP PUMPKIN MUFFINS

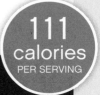

111 calories PER SERVING

You'll Need: 12-cup muffin pan, foil baking cups or nonstick spray, large bowl, whisk, medium bowl
Prep: 20 minutes
Cook: 20 minutes

1/12th of recipe (1 muffin): 111 calories, 2.5g fat, 248mg sodium, 27.5g carbs, 1g fiber, 5g sugars, 2.5g protein

INGREDIENTS

2 cups Bisquick Heart Smart baking mix
1/2 cup Splenda No Calorie Sweetener (granulated)
1 teaspoon baking powder
1 teaspoon pumpkin pie spice
1 teaspoon cinnamon
1/8 teaspoon salt
1 cup canned pure pumpkin
1/4 cup no-sugar-added applesauce
1/4 cup fat-free liquid egg substitute
1 teaspoon vanilla extract
1/4 cup mini semi-sweet chocolate chips

DIRECTIONS

Preheat oven to 350 degrees. Line a 12-cup muffin pan with foil baking cups, or spray it with nonstick spray.

In a large bowl, whisk baking mix, Splenda, baking powder, pumpkin pie spice, cinnamon, and salt.

In a medium bowl, whisk pumpkin, applesauce, egg substitute, and vanilla extract. Add mixture to the large bowl and thoroughly mix. Fold in chocolate chips.

Evenly distribute mixture among cups of the muffin pan. Bake until a toothpick inserted into the center of a muffin comes out clean, about 20 minutes. Enjoy!

MAKES 12 SERVINGS

HG SWEET ALTERNATIVE!

Swap out the Splenda for the same amount of granulated white sugar, and each serving will have 140 calories, 18.5g carbs, and 13.5g sugars.

CHIPPEE CHOCOLATE CHIP MUFFINS

175 calories PER SERVING

You'll Need: 6-cup or 12-cup muffin pan, foil baking cups or nonstick spray, 2 large bowls, whisk
Prep: 15 minutes
Cook: 25 minutes

⅙th of recipe (1 muffin): 175 calories, 5g fat, 299mg sodium, 29g carbs, 3g fiber, 11g sugars, 4.5g protein

INGREDIENTS

1 cup whole-wheat flour
¼ cup Splenda No Calorie Sweetener (granulated)
3 tablespoons brown sugar (not packed)
1½ teaspoons baking powder
¼ teaspoon salt
½ cup light vanilla soymilk
¼ cup sugar-free pancake syrup
¼ cup fat-free liquid egg substitute
2 tablespoons light whipped butter or light buttery spread, room temperature
2 tablespoons no-sugar-added applesauce
½ teaspoon vanilla extract
¼ cup mini semi-sweet chocolate chips

DIRECTIONS

Preheat oven to 400 degrees. Line a 6-cup muffin pan (or 6 cups of a 12-cup muffin pan) with foil baking cups, or spray it with nonstick spray.

In a large bowl, whisk flour, Splenda, brown sugar, baking powder, and salt.

In another large bowl, whisk all other ingredients *except* chocolate chips. Add the flour mixture and stir until smooth. Fold in chocolate chips.

Evenly distribute batter among the 6 lined or sprayed cups of the muffin pan. Bake until a toothpick inserted into the center of a muffin comes out clean, about 22 minutes. Enjoy!

MAKES 6 SERVINGS

HG SWEET ALTERNATIVE!

Swap out the Splenda for the same amount of granulated white sugar, and each muffin will have 203 calories, 36.5g carbs, and 19g sugars.

BIG FAT BLUEBERRY MUFFINS

137 calories PER SERVING

You'll Need: 6-cup or 12-cup muffin pan, foil baking cups or nonstick spray, 2 large bowls, whisk
Prep: 15 minutes
Cook: 25 minutes

⅙th of recipe (1 muffin): 137 calories, 2.25g fat, 269mg sodium, 26.5g carbs, 3g fiber, 7.5g sugars, 4g protein

INGREDIENTS

1 cup whole-wheat flour
¼ cup Splenda No Calorie Sweetener (granulated)
3 tablespoons brown sugar (not packed)
1½ teaspoons baking powder
¼ teaspoon salt
½ cup light vanilla soymilk
¼ cup sugar-free pancake syrup
¼ cup fat-free liquid egg substitute
2 tablespoons light whipped butter or light buttery spread, room temperature
2 tablespoons no-sugar-added applesauce
½ teaspoon vanilla extract
1 cup blueberries

DIRECTIONS

Preheat oven to 400 degrees. Line a 6-cup muffin pan (or 6 cups of a 12-cup muffin pan) with foil baking cups, or spray it with nonstick spray.

In a large bowl, whisk flour, Splenda, brown sugar, baking powder, and salt.

In another large bowl, whisk all other ingredients *except* blueberries. Add the flour mixture and stir until smooth. Fold in blueberries.

Evenly distribute batter among the 6 lined or sprayed cups of the muffin pan. Bake until a toothpick inserted into the center of a muffin comes out clean, about 22 minutes. Enjoy!

MAKES 6 SERVINGS

HG SWEET ALTERNATIVE!

Swap out the Splenda for the same amount of granulated white sugar, and each muffin will have 165 calories, 34g carbs, and 16g sugars.

GOOEY-GOOD GERMAN CHOCOLATE CUPCAKES

138 calories PER SERVING

You'll Need: 12-cup muffin pan, foil baking cups or nonstick spray, small bowl, glass, large bowl, whisk
Prep: 15 minutes | **Cook:** 20 minutes

¹⁄₁₂th of recipe (1 cupcake):
138 calories, 3g fat, 258mg sodium, 25.5g carbs, 1g fiber, 15g sugars, 2.5g protein

INGREDIENTS

¼ cup fat-free or light caramel dip

1 tablespoon finely chopped pecans

2 tablespoons shredded sweetened coconut

Half a sugar-free caramel pudding snack with 60 calories or less

2 tablespoons mini semi-sweet chocolate chips

2 packets hot cocoa mix with 20 to 25 calories each

1 teaspoon granulated white sugar or Splenda No Calorie Sweetener (granulated)

⅛ teaspoon salt

1¾ cups moist-style devil's food cake mix

½ cup fat-free liquid egg substitute

DIRECTIONS

Preheat oven to 350 degrees. Line a 12-cup muffin pan with foil baking cups, or spray it with nonstick spray.

In a small bowl, thoroughly mix caramel dip, pecans, coconut, and pudding. Cover and refrigerate.

In a glass, combine chocolate chips, cocoa mix, sugar or Splenda, and salt. Add ¼ cup very hot water, and stir until ingredients have dissolved.

Transfer mixture to a large bowl and add ¾ cup cold water.

Add cake mix and egg substitute. Whisk until smooth.

Evenly distribute batter among cups of the muffin pan. Bake until a toothpick inserted into the center of a cupcake comes out mostly clean, 15 to 18 minutes.

Let cool completely.

Evenly top with caramel mixture, serve, and enjoy!

MAKES 12 SERVINGS

BATTER UP: CUPCAKES AND MUFFINS!

Before filling the cups, transfer batter to a liquid measuring cup with a spout. (Super-thick batters excluded.) Then pour evenly with ease—no mess!

CHOCOLATE MARSHMALLOW MADNESS CUPCAKES

109 calories
PER SERVING

You'll Need: 12-cup muffin pan, foil baking cups or nonstick spray, glass, large bowl, whisk, small bowl
Prep: 20 minutes | **Cook:** 20 minutes

¹⁄₁₂th of recipe (1 cupcake):
109 calories, 2g fat, 230mg sodium, 21g carbs, 0.75g fiber, 12.5g sugars, 2g protein

INGREDIENTS

1 packet hot cocoa mix with 20 to 25 calories
1¾ cups moist-style devil's food cake mix
½ cup fat-free liquid egg substitute
1 tablespoon Splenda No Calorie Sweetener (granulated)
⅛ teaspoon salt
¼ cup Jet-Puffed Marshmallow Creme
1 teaspoon light soymilk or fat-free milk
1 tablespoon mini semi-sweet chocolate chips
12 mini marshmallows

HG SWEET ALTERNATIVE!
Swap out the Splenda for the same amount of granulated white sugar, and each serving will have 113 calories, 22g carbs, and 13.5g sugars.

DIRECTIONS

Preheat oven to 350 degrees. Line a 12-cup muffin pan with foil baking cups, or spray it with nonstick spray.

In a glass, combine cocoa mix with ¼ cup hot water and stir to dissolve.

Transfer mixture to a large bowl and add ¾ cup cold water. Add cake mix, egg substitute, Splenda, and salt. Whisk until smooth.

Evenly distribute mixture among the cups of the muffin pan. Bake until a toothpick inserted into the center of a cupcake comes out mostly clean, 15 to 18 minutes.

Let cupcakes completely cool.

In a small bowl, thoroughly mix marshmallow creme with soymilk or milk. Drizzle over cupcakes. Top each cupcake with ¼ teaspoon chocolate chips and 1 mini marshmallow. Enjoy!

MAKES 12 SERVINGS

DESSERT TOPPING TIP!

When mixing up a small amount of icing or another topping, use a narrow spoon handle to stir. This is especially helpful with sticky ingredients!

RED VELVET INSANITY CUPCAKES

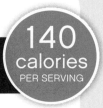

140 calories PER SERVING

You'll Need: 12-cup muffin pan, foil baking cups or nonstick spray, medium bowl, glass, large bowl, whisk
Prep: 15 minutes | **Cook:** 20 minutes

¹⁄₁₂th of recipe (1 cupcake):
140 calories, 3g fat, 262mg sodium, 24.5g carbs, 0.5g fiber, 15g sugars, 3g protein

INGREDIENTS

¼ cup plus 2 tablespoons Jet-Puffed Marshmallow Creme

¼ cup fat-free cream cheese, room temperature

1 tablespoon plus 1 teaspoon Splenda No Calorie Sweetener (granulated)

¼ cup plus 2 tablespoons Cool Whip Free (thawed)

2 packets hot cocoa mix with 20 to 25 calories each

¼ cup mini semi-sweet chocolate chips

1 cup moist-style devil's food cake mix

1 cup moist-style yellow cake mix

½ cup fat-free liquid egg substitute

1 tablespoon red food coloring

⅛ teaspoon salt

HG SWEET ALTERNATIVE!
Swap out the Splenda for the same amount of granulated white sugar, and each serving will have 145 calories, 25.5g carbs, and 16.5g sugars.

DIRECTIONS

Preheat oven to 350 degrees. Line a 12-cup muffin pan with foil baking cups, or spray it with nonstick spray.

In a medium bowl, mix marshmallow creme, cream cheese, and 1 tablespoon Splenda until completely smooth. Fold in Cool Whip. Cover and refrigerate.

In a glass, combine cocoa mix with 2 tablespoons chocolate chips. Add ½ cup very hot water and stir until ingredients have mostly dissolved.

Transfer mixture to a large bowl and add 1 cup cold water. Add cake mixes, egg substitute, food coloring, salt, remaining 2 tablespoons chocolate chips, and remaining 1 teaspoon Splenda. Whisk until smooth.

Evenly distribute batter among cups of the muffin pan. Bake until a toothpick inserted into the center of a cupcake comes out mostly clean, 15 to 20 minutes.

Let cool completely. Top with marshmallow mixture and devour!

MAKES 12 SERVINGS

14-CARAT CUPCAKES

You'll Need: 12-cup muffin pan, foil baking cups or nonstick spray, 2 medium bowls, whisk, large bowl
Prep: 15 minutes | **Cook:** 25 minutes

1/12th of recipe (1 frosted cupcake):
133 calories, 1g fat, 197mg sodium, 26g carbs, 2g fiber, 11.5g sugars, 5g protein

INGREDIENTS

Frosting
Half an 8-ounce tub fat-free cream cheese, room temperature
⅔ cup Splenda No Calorie Sweetener (granulated)
⅓ cup plain fat-free Greek yogurt
½ teaspoon vanilla extract

Cupcakes
¾ cup canned pure pumpkin
⅔ cup fat-free liquid egg substitute
1 cup moist-style yellow cake mix
¾ cup whole-wheat flour
½ cup Splenda No Calorie Sweetener (granulated)
2 tablespoons brown sugar (not packed)
1½ teaspoons pumpkin pie spice
1½ teaspoons cinnamon
1 teaspoon baking powder
1½ cups shredded carrots, roughly chopped if shreds are long
⅔ cup crushed pineapple packed in juice (not drained)
¼ cup raisins (not packed)

DIRECTIONS

Preheat oven to 350 degrees. Line a 12-cup muffin pan with foil baking cups, or spray it with nonstick spray.

In a medium bowl, thoroughly whisk frosting ingredients until smooth. Cover and refrigerate.

In another medium bowl, thoroughly mix pumpkin, egg substitute, and ¼ cup water.

In a large bowl, thoroughly mix cake mix, flour, Splenda, brown sugar, pumpkin pie spice, cinnamon, and baking powder. Add pumpkin mixture and whisk until smooth.

Stir in carrots, pineapple, and raisins. Evenly distribute mixture among cups of the muffin pan.

Bake until a toothpick inserted into the center of a cupcake comes out mostly clean, 23 to 25 minutes.

Let cool completely.

Spread with frosting and refrigerate until set. Enjoy!

MAKES 12 SERVINGS

HG SWEET ALTERNATIVE!

Swap out the Splenda for the same amount of granulated white sugar, and each serving will have 198 calories, 43.5g carbs, and 31g sugars.

CHOCOLATE PB PRETZEL CUPCAKES

135 calories PER SERVING

You'll Need: 12-cup muffin pan, foil baking cups or nonstick spray, large bowl, whisk, 2 small bowls
Prep: 20 minutes
Cook: 25 minutes

1/12th of recipe (1 cupcake): 135 calories, 4g fat, 273mg sodium, 22.5g carbs, 0.5g fiber, 12g sugars, 3g protein

INGREDIENTS

1 ¾ cups moist-style devil's food cake mix
½ cup fat-free liquid egg substitute
¾ teaspoon baking powder
½ cup Cool Whip Free (thawed)
¼ cup reduced-fat peanut butter, room temperature
2 tablespoons light chocolate syrup
1 tablespoon chocolate frosting, room temperature
12 small hard pretzel sticks, broken into small pieces

DIRECTIONS

Preheat oven to 350 degrees. Line a 12-cup muffin pan with foil baking cups, or spray it with nonstick spray.

In a large bowl, whisk cake mix, egg substitute, baking powder, and 1 cup water. Evenly distribute among cups of the muffin pan.

Bake until a toothpick inserted into the center of a cupcake comes out mostly clean, 23 to 25 minutes.

Let cool completely.

In a small bowl, thoroughly mix Cool Whip with peanut butter. In another small bowl, mix syrup with frosting.

Spread cupcakes with peanut butter mixture, drizzle with syrup mixture, and sprinkle with pretzel pieces. Enjoy!

MAKES 12 SERVINGS

EXPRESSO CAKE IN A MUG

147 calories

You'll Need: microwave-safe mug, nonstick spray
Prep: 5 minutes
Cook: 5 minutes

Entire recipe: 147 calories, 3.25g fat, 446mg sodium, 25.5g carbs, 0.5g fiber, 14.5g sugars, 3.5g protein

INGREDIENTS

1 teaspoon instant coffee granules
1 teaspoon mini semi-sweet chocolate chips
3 tablespoons moist-style devil's food cake mix
1 tablespoon fat-free sour cream
1 tablespoon fat-free liquid egg substitute
¼ teaspoon vanilla extract
⅛ teaspoon baking powder
1 no-calorie sweetener packet
Dash salt

DIRECTIONS

Place coffee granules and chocolate chips in a microwave-safe mug sprayed with nonstick spray. Add 2 tablespoons hot water and stir until ingredients have dissolved.

Mix in remaining ingredients. Microwave for 1 minute and 45 seconds, or until set. Enjoy!

MAKES 1 SERVING

MISSISSIPPI MUG PIE

  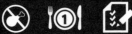

223 calories

You'll Need: large microwave-safe mug, nonstick spray
Prep: 5 minutes
Cook: 5 minutes

Entire recipe: 223 calories, 5g fat, 588mg sodium, 45.5g carbs, 2.75g fiber, 19g sugars, 6.5g protein

INGREDIENTS

3 tablespoons moist-style devil's food cake mix
1 tablespoon fat-free liquid egg substitute
1 packet hot cocoa mix with 20 to 25 calories
1 teaspoon mini semi-sweet chocolate chips
One sugar-free chocolate pudding snack with 60 calories or less

Optional topping: Fat Free Reddi-wip

DIRECTIONS

Spray a large microwave-safe mug with nonstick spray. Add cake mix, egg substitute, cocoa mix, and 2 tablespoons water. Mix well.

Stir in chocolate chips and ⅓rd of the pudding. Microwave for 1 minute.

Fluff with a fork. Gently mix in remaining pudding. Microwave for 1 more minute, or until set. Dig in!

MAKES 1 SERVING

RED HOT APPLE PIE IN A CUP

140 calories

You'll Need: microwave-safe cup or mug
Prep: 5 minutes
Cook: 5 minutes

Entire recipe: 140 calories, 0.5g fat, 44mg sodium, 47g carbs, 3.5g fiber, 24.5g sugars, 0.5g protein

INGREDIENTS

1 medium Fuji apple, cored and cut into ½-inch cubes
12 to 15 pieces Red Hots Cinnamon Flavored Candy
2 low-fat cinnamon graham crackers (½ sheet), crushed
2 tablespoons Fat Free Reddi-wip
Dash cinnamon

DIRECTIONS

Place apple cubes in a microwave-safe cup or mug. Top with Red Hots—the more you use, the hotter the results! Cover and microwave for 2 minutes.

Stir well. Re-cover and microwave for 1 to 2 minutes, until apple cubes are soft.

Mix well. Let cool.

Top with crushed graham crackers, Reddi-wip, and cinnamon. Voilà!

MAKES 1 SERVING

DIET SODA CAKE

171 calories
PER SERVING

You'll Need: 9-inch by 13-inch baking pan, nonstick spray, large bowl, whisk
Prep: 5 minutes
Cook: 40 minutes

1/12th of cake: 171 calories, 3.5g fat, 301mg sodium, 34g carbs, <0.5g fiber, 19g sugars, 1.5g protein

INGREDIENTS

1 box moist-style cake mix (15.25 to 18.25 ounces)
One 12-ounce can diet soda

DIRECTIONS

Preheat oven to 350 degrees. Spray a 9-inch by 13-inch baking pan with nonstick spray.

In a large bowl, whisk cake mix with soda until smooth. Pour into the baking pan.

Bake until a toothpick inserted into the center comes out clean, 35 to 40 minutes.

Slice and enjoy!

**MAKES
12 SERVINGS**

HG FYI:

Yellow cake mix + diet cream soda is the best flavor combo for this recipe! Runners-up include lemon cake mix + diet lemon-lime soda and devil's food cake mix + diet cherry cola.

CHOCOLATE-ON-CHOCOLATE FROSTED CAKE

217 calories
PER SERVING

You'll Need: 9-inch round cake pan, nonstick spray, medium-large bowl, glass, large bowl, whisk, large plate
Prep: 15 minutes
Cook: 30 minutes
Chill: 15 minutes

1/8th of cake: 217 calories, 5.5g fat, 476mg sodium, 40g carbs, 1.5g fiber, 24g sugars, 4g protein

INGREDIENTS

1 sugar-free chocolate pudding snack with 60 calories or less
1/3 cup chocolate frosting
2 tablespoons light chocolate syrup
2 tablespoons mini semi-sweet chocolate chips
2 packets hot cocoa mix with 20 to 25 calories each
1 3/4 cups moist-style devil's food cake mix
1/2 cup fat-free liquid egg substitute
1 teaspoon granulated white sugar or Splenda No Calorie Sweetener (granulated)
1 teaspoon baking powder
1/8 teaspoon salt

DIRECTIONS

Preheat oven to 350 degrees. Spray a 9-inch round cake pan with nonstick spray.

In a medium-large bowl, thoroughly mix pudding, frosting, and syrup. Cover and refrigerate.

In a glass, combine chocolate chips with cocoa mix. Add 1/2 cup very hot water and stir to dissolve.

Transfer mixture to a large bowl and add 3/4 cup cold water. Add all remaining ingredients and whisk until smooth.

Pour batter into the cake pan. Bake until a toothpick inserted into the center comes out mostly clean, about 30 minutes.

Let cake completely cool.

Transfer cake to a large plate and evenly spread with pudding mixture.

Refrigerate until pudding mixture has set, at least 15 minutes.

Slice, serve, and enjoy! (Refrigerate leftovers.)

MAKES 8 SERVINGS

FROSTY THE VANILLA CAKE

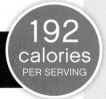

192 calories
PER SERVING

You'll Need: 9-inch round cake pan, nonstick spray, 2 medium bowls, large bowl, whisk, electric mixer, large plate
Prep: 10 minutes | **Cook:** 30 minutes

⅛th of cake:
192 calories, 3g fat, 525mg sodium, 35g carbs, 0g fiber, 17.5g sugars, 6g protein

INGREDIENTS

Topping

3 tablespoons (about ¾ths of a 4-serving box) Jell-O Sugar Free Fat Free Vanilla Instant pudding mix

3 tablespoons Splenda No Calorie Sweetener (granulated)

½ teaspoon vanilla extract

¾ cup fat-free cream cheese, room temperature

1½ cups Cool Whip Free (thawed)

Cake

1¾ cups moist-style white cake mix

¾ teaspoon baking powder

1 cup club soda, room temperature

1 teaspoon vanilla extract

½ cup liquid egg whites (about 4 egg whites)

DIRECTIONS

Preheat oven to 350 degrees. Spray a 9-inch round cake pan with nonstick spray.

To make the topping, in a medium bowl, combine pudding mix, Splenda, and vanilla extract. Add 3 tablespoons cold water and stir vigorously until smooth and slightly thickened. Stir in cream cheese until completely mixed and smooth. Add Cool Whip and mix well. Cover and refrigerate.

To make the cake, in a large bowl, thoroughly mix cake mix with baking powder. Add club soda and vanilla extract, and whisk until completely smooth.

Place egg whites in another medium bowl. With an electric mixer set to medium speed, beat until fluffy, 1 to 2 minutes.

Gently but thoroughly fold egg whites into cake mixture. Pour batter into the cake pan. Bake until a toothpick inserted into the center comes out clean, about 30 minutes.

Once cool, transfer cake to a large plate. Evenly spread with topping. Slice, serve, and enjoy! (Refrigerate leftovers.)

MAKES 8 SERVINGS

HG SWEET ALTERNATIVE!

If made with an equal amount of granulated white sugar in place of Splenda, each serving will have 208 calories, 39g carbs, and 22g sugars.

APPLE OF MY CAKE

153 calories PER SERVING

You'll Need: 9-inch round cake pan, nonstick spray, skillet, large bowl, whisk
Prep: 15 minutes
Cook: 45 minutes

⅛th of cake: 153 calories, 2.75g fat, 260mg sodium, 31g carbs, 0.75g fiber, 18.5g sugars, 1.5g protein

INGREDIENTS

2 sweet apples (like Fuji), peeled, cored, and thinly sliced
1¾ cups moist-style yellow cake mix
1 teaspoon baking powder
½ teaspoon plus 1 dash cinnamon
¼ teaspoon ground nutmeg
⅛ teaspoon ground ginger
½ cup no-sugar-added applesauce
½ cup club soda

DIRECTIONS

Preheat oven to 350 degrees. Spray a 9-inch round cake pan with nonstick spray.

Bring a skillet sprayed with nonstick spray to medium-high heat. Add ¾ths of the apple slices. Cook and stir until softened, 6 to 8 minutes.

In a large bowl, combine cake mix, baking powder, ½ teaspoon cinnamon, nutmeg, and ginger. Add applesauce and soda, and whisk until smooth. Stir in cooked apple slices.

Transfer mixture to the cake pan and smooth out the surface, making sure all the apple slices in the batter are covered.

Top with uncooked apple slices and sprinkle with remaining dash cinnamon. Bake until a toothpick inserted into the center comes out clean, 30 to 35 minutes.

Let cool, slice, and eat!

MAKES 8 SERVINGS

UPSIDE-DOWN PINEAPPLE-APPLESAUCE CAKE

189 calories PER SERVING

You'll Need: 9-inch round cake pan, nonstick spray (butter flavored, if available), small microwave-safe bowl, large bowl, whisk, large plate
Prep: 15 minutes
Cook: 40 minutes

⅛th of cake: 189 calories, 3.5g fat, 298mg sodium, 39g carbs, 0.5g fiber, 26.5g sugars, 1.5g protein

INGREDIENTS

1 tablespoon light whipped butter or light buttery spread
¼ cup brown sugar (not packed)
7 pineapple rings packed in juice, drained and patted dry
7 maraschino cherries, patted dry
1¾ cups moist-style yellow cake mix
1½ teaspoons baking powder
½ cup club soda
¼ cup no-sugar-added applesauce

DIRECTIONS

Preheat oven to 350 degrees. Spray a 9-inch round cake pan with nonstick spray (butter flavored, if available).

In a small microwave-safe bowl, microwave butter for 15 seconds, or until just melted. Add brown sugar and mix well. Spread mixture along the bottom of the cake pan.

Add pineapple rings to the pan in an even layer, and place a cherry in the center of each ring.

In a large bowl, mix cake mix with baking powder. Add club soda and applesauce, and whisk until smooth.

Evenly pour cake batter into the pan. Bake until a toothpick inserted into the center comes out clean, 30 to 35 minutes.

Let cake cool until just slightly warm, 15 to 20 minutes.

Firmly and securely place a large plate over the pan, and carefully flip so the plate is on the bottom. Gently lift pan to release the cake. (If needed, pop just the pan back in the warm oven, right side up, to help release the cake.) Slice and devour!

MAKES 8 SERVINGS

BEST OF MY LAVA CHOCOLATE CAKE

182 calories PER SERVING

You'll Need: four 4-inch baking ramekins (or oven-safe mugs), nonstick spray, microwave-safe bowl, parchment paper, plate, glass, large bowl, whisk | **Prep:** 10 minutes | **Freeze:** 25 minutes | **Cook:** 15 minutes

¼th of recipe (1 lava cake):
182 calories, 4.5g fat, 433mg sodium, 32g carbs, 1.5g fiber, 18g sugars, 4g protein

INGREDIENTS

Filling
½ tablespoon mini semi-sweet chocolate chips
1 teaspoon fat-free liquid creamer
½ teaspoon light whipped butter or light buttery spread
Half of a sugar-free chocolate pudding snack with 60 calories or less

Cake
1 tablespoon mini semi-sweet chocolate chips
1 packet hot cocoa mix with 20 to 25 calories
1 cup moist-style chocolate cake mix
¼ cup fat-free liquid egg substitute
½ teaspoon granulated white sugar or Splenda No Calorie Sweetener (granulated)
2 dashes salt

DIRECTIONS

Preheat oven to 350 degrees. Spray four 4-inch baking ramekins (or oven-safe mugs) with nonstick spray.

To make the filling, place chocolate chips, creamer, and butter in a microwave-safe bowl. Microwave for 20 seconds, or until butter has melted and creamer is hot. Stir until chips have mostly dissolved. Let cool slightly. Stir in pudding.

Spoon mixture into 4 evenly spaced mounds onto a sheet of parchment paper on a plate. Freeze until firm but not frozen solid, about 25 minutes.

To make the cake, combine chocolate chips and cocoa mix in a glass. Add ¼ cup very hot water and stir until ingredients have dissolved. Transfer mixture to a large bowl. Add ½ cup cold water. Add all remaining cake ingredients, and whisk until smooth.

Evenly pour cake batter into the ramekins. Place one mound of filling in the center of each. Bake until top centers are firm, about 15 minutes. Enjoy!

MAKES 4 SERVINGS

Flip to the photo inserts to see over 100 recipe pics! And for photos of ALL the recipes, go to hungry-girl.com/books.

SUPER-DUPER STRAWBERRY SHORTCAKE

191 calories

You'll Need: small bowl
Prep: 5 minutes

Entire recipe: 191 calories, 2g fat, 172mg sodium, 41.5g carbs, 2g fiber, 20.5g sugars, 3.5g protein

INGREDIENTS

1 tablespoon sugar-free strawberry jam/preserves
1 shortcake dessert shell (often found in the produce section)
⅓ cup sliced strawberries
⅓ cup fat-free vanilla ice cream
2 tablespoons Fat Free Reddi-wip

DIRECTIONS

In a small bowl, thoroughly mix jam/preserves with ½ tablespoon hot water.

Layer ingredients on the shortcake shell: ⅓rd of strawberries, ice cream, ⅓rd of strawberries, preserves mixture, Reddi-wip, and remaining strawberries. Dive in!

MAKES 1 SERVING

BA NA NA CRAZY CARAMEL SHORTCAKES

150 calories PER SERVING

You'll Need: 2 baking sheets, nonstick spray, large bowl, rolling pin (optional), microwave-safe bowl
Prep: 10 minutes
Cook: 10 minutes

⅑th of recipe (1 shortcake): 150 calories, 4.25g fat, 250mg sodium, 26.5g carbs, <0.5g fiber, 9g sugars, 1.5g protein

INGREDIENTS

2 cups Cool Whip Free (thawed)
1 sugar-free caramel pudding snack with 60 calories or less
1 large banana, sliced
1 package refrigerated Pillsbury Crescent Recipe Creations Seamless Dough Sheet
¼ cup fat-free or light caramel dip

DIRECTIONS

Preheat oven to 350 degrees. Spray 2 baking sheets with nonstick spray.

In a large bowl, mix Cool Whip and pudding until just blended. Stir in banana slices. Cover and refrigerate.

Unroll dough on a dry surface. Roll or stretch into a large rectangle of even thickness. Cut dough into 18 evenly sized pieces, each about 3 inches by 2 inches.

Place the pieces of dough on the baking sheets, evenly spaced. Bake until lightly browned, about 10 minutes.

Let dough pieces cool.

Just before serving, lay out 9 dough pieces, and evenly distribute Cool Whip mixture among them, about ¼ cup each. Gently top each with another dough piece.

Microwave caramel dip in a microwave-safe bowl for 20 seconds, or until softened and warm. Stir and drizzle over the shortcakes, about ½ tablespoon each. ENJOY!!!

MAKES 9 SERVINGS

TURBO-TREMENDOUS TIRAMISU

275 calories

You'll Need: glass, medium bowl, wide bowl (or plate)
Prep: 10 minutes | **Chill:** 1 hour

Entire recipe:
275 calories, 3g fat, 448mg sodium, 48.5g carbs, 1g fiber, 22g sugars, 9g protein

INGREDIENTS

1 teaspoon instant coffee granules

1 teaspoon sugar-free French vanilla powdered creamer

2 no-calorie sweetener packets

1 tablespoon Jell-O Sugar Free Fat Free Vanilla Instant pudding mix

¼ cup fat-free ricotta cheese

¼ teaspoon vanilla extract

¼ cup Cool Whip Free (thawed)

6 ladyfingers (found in the produce or bakery section)

1 teaspoon unsweetened cocoa powder

DIRECTIONS

In a glass, combine coffee granules, creamer, and 1 sweetener packet. Add ¼ cup hot water and stir until ingredients have dissolved. Add ¼ cup cold water.

Transfer 2 tablespoons of the mixture to a medium bowl. Add pudding mix and stir until mostly smooth. Mix in ricotta cheese, vanilla extract, and remaining sweetener packet. Fold in Cool Whip.

Place 3 ladyfingers side by side in a wide bowl (or on a plate). Drizzle with half of the remaining coffee mixture, about 3 tablespoons. Evenly spread with half of the pudding mixture; sprinkle with ½ teaspoon cocoa powder.

Evenly layer with remaining ingredients: 3 ladyfingers (side by side), coffee mixture, pudding mixture, and ½ teaspoon cocoa powder.

Refrigerate until chilled, at least 1 hour. Enjoy!

MAKES 1 SERVING

BLUEBERRY BLISS CHEESECAKE

168 calories PER SERVING

You'll Need: 9-inch springform cake pan, nonstick spray, large bowl, electric mixer, medium nonstick pot
Prep: 25 minutes | **Cook:** 45 minutes | **Chill:** 1 hour

⅛th of cake:
168 calories, 1g fat, 395mg sodium, 27g carbs, 1g fiber, 22g sugars, 12g protein

INGREDIENTS

Cheesecake
16 ounces fat-free cream cheese, room temperature

½ cup granulated white sugar

1 teaspoon vanilla extract

6 ounces (about ¾ cup) fat-free vanilla Greek yogurt, room temperature

½ cup liquid egg whites (about 4 egg whites), room temperature

2 tablespoons lemon juice, room temperature

2 tablespoons all-purpose flour

¼ teaspoon cinnamon

Topping
2 cups frozen unsweetened blueberries

2 tablespoons granulated white sugar

1 tablespoon cornstarch

¼ teaspoon cinnamon

Dash salt

DIRECTIONS

Preheat oven to 350 degrees. Spray a 9-inch springform cake pan with nonstick spray.

In a large bowl, combine cream cheese, sugar, and vanilla extract. With an electric mixer set to medium speed, beat until smooth, 1 to 2 minutes. Continue to beat while gradually adding yogurt, egg whites, lemon juice, flour, and cinnamon. Beat until thoroughly mixed, about 2 minutes.

Evenly pour mixture into the cake pan. Bake until firm, 40 to 45 minutes.

Let cool completely.

Meanwhile, bring a medium nonstick pot to medium-high heat. Add all topping ingredients. Add ½ cup cold water and mix well. Bring to a boil. Reduce to a simmer. Cook and stir until thick and gooey, 2 to 3 minutes.

Remove from heat and let cool completely.

Evenly pour blueberry topping over the cheesecake in the pan. Refrigerate until fully chilled, at least 1 hour. Once ready to serve, release and remove the springform. Slice and dig in!

MAKES 8 SERVINGS

HG SWEET ALTERNATIVE!

If made with an equal amount of Splenda No Calorie Sweetener (granulated) in place of the sugar, each serving will have 116 calories, 13g carbs, and 6g sugars.

HG TIP:

The topping may run down the edges of the cake once the springform is removed. To catch all of that deliciousness, place the pan on a larger plate before removing the springform.

UPSIDE-DOWN CHOCOLATE PB CHEESECAKE

143 calories PER SERVING

You'll Need: glass, 2 medium bowls, electric mixer, deep-dish pie pan, whisk | **Prep:** 10 minutes | **Chill:** 2 hours

⅛th of recipe (about ½ cup):
143 calories, 3.5g fat, 320mg sodium, 19.5g carbs, 1g fiber, 6g sugars, 6.5g protein

INGREDIENTS

1 packet hot cocoa mix with 20 to 25 calories

One 8-ounce tub fat-free cream cheese, room temperature

2 sugar-free chocolate pudding snacks with 60 calories or less each

⅓ cup Splenda No Calorie Sweetener (granulated)

2 teaspoons vanilla extract

2 cups Cool Whip Free (thawed)

3 tablespoons reduced-fat peanut butter, room temperature

2 packs Nabisco 100 Cal Oreo Thin Crisps cookies *or* 3 sheets (12 crackers) chocolate graham crackers, finely crushed

Optional topping: Fat Free Reddi-wip

HG SWEET ALTERNATIVE!
Swap out the Splenda for the same amount of granulated white sugar, and each serving will have 171 calories, 27g carbs, and 14.5g sugars.

DIRECTIONS

In a glass, combine cocoa mix with 2 tablespoons hot water and stir to dissolve.

Transfer to a medium bowl. Add cream cheese, pudding, Splenda, and vanilla extract. With an electric mixer set to medium speed, beat until smooth.

Fold in ½ cup Cool Whip. Transfer mixture to a deep-dish pie pan.

In another medium bowl, combine peanut butter with remaining 1½ cups Cool Whip. Whisk until smooth. Spread mixture over cheesecake layer.

Cover and refrigerate until chilled and slightly firm, about 2 hours.

Top pie with crushed crisps or graham crackers. Enjoy with a spoon!

MAKES 8 SERVINGS

QUICK Q&A WITH HG:

Why do some cheesecake ingredients need to be at room temperature?
To prevent large cracks in your cheesecake.

What if I forgot to bring them to room temperature in advance?
Microwave them individually at 50 percent power in 15-second intervals, stirring between intervals, until they just reach room temp. Do NOT overheat them.

TOO-GOOD TURTLE CHEESECAKE

213 calories PER SERVING

You'll Need: 9-inch springform cake pan, nonstick spray, large bowl, electric mixer
Prep: 25 minutes | **Cook:** 45 minutes | **Chill:** 1 hour

⅛th of cake:
213 calories, 4.5g fat, 420mg sodium, 32g carbs, 0.5g fiber, 24g sugars, 12g protein

INGREDIENTS

Cheesecake
16 ounces fat-free cream cheese, room temperature
½ cup granulated white sugar
1 teaspoon vanilla extract
6 ounces (about ¾ cup) fat-free vanilla Greek yogurt, room temperature
½ cup liquid egg whites (about 4 egg whites), room temperature
2 tablespoons lemon juice, room temperature
2 tablespoons all-purpose flour
2 tablespoons mini semi-sweet chocolate chips

Topping
1 sheet (4 crackers) chocolate graham crackers, crushed
¼ cup fat-free or light caramel dip
¼ cup chopped pecans

DIRECTIONS

Preheat oven to 350 degrees. Spray a 9-inch springform cake pan with nonstick spray.

Combine cream cheese, sugar, and vanilla extract in a large bowl. With an electric mixer set to medium speed, beat until smooth, 1 to 2 minutes. Continue to beat while gradually adding yogurt, egg whites, lemon juice, and flour. Beat until thoroughly mixed, about 2 minutes.

Evenly pour mixture into the cake pan. Sprinkle with chocolate chips. Bake until firm, 40 to 45 minutes.

Let cool completely.

Evenly top with crushed graham crackers. Drizzle with caramel dip and sprinkle with pecans.

Refrigerate until chilled, at least 1 hour. Release springform, slice, and dig in!

MAKES 8 SERVINGS

HG SWEET ALTERNATIVE!
If made with an equal amount of Splenda No Calorie Sweetener (granulated) in place of the sugar, each serving will have 170 calories, 20g carbs, and 12g sugars.

For more recipes, tips & tricks, sign up for FREE daily emails at hungry-girl.com!

PB CUP CHEESECAKE

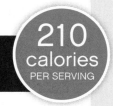

210 calories PER SERVING

You'll Need: 9-inch springform cake pan, nonstick spray, medium bowl, large bowl, electric mixer
Prep: 25 minutes | **Cook:** 45 minutes | **Chill:** 1 hour

⅛th of cake:
210 calories, 4g fat, 458mg sodium, 29g carbs, 0.5g fiber, 24g sugars, 13.5g protein

INGREDIENTS

6 ounces (about ¾ cup) fat-free vanilla Greek yogurt, room temperature

3 packets hot cocoa mix with 20 to 25 calories each

16 ounces fat-free cream cheese, room temperature

½ cup granulated white sugar

1 teaspoon vanilla extract

½ cup liquid egg whites (about 4 egg whites), room temperature

2 tablespoons all-purpose flour

¼ cup peanut butter baking chips, chopped

One 1.53-ounce bag (about 3 tablespoons) Reese's Pieces candies, chopped

HG SWEET ALTERNATIVE!

If made with an equal amount of Splenda No Calorie Sweetener (granulated) in place of the sugar, each serving will have 168 calories, 18g carbs, and 12g sugars.

DIRECTIONS

Preheat oven to 350 degrees. Spray a 9-inch springform cake pan with nonstick spray.

In a medium bowl, stir cocoa mix into yogurt until smooth.

In a large bowl, combine cream cheese, sugar, and vanilla extract. Beat until smooth with an electric mixer set to medium speed, 1 to 2 minutes.

Continue to beat the mixture while gradually adding cocoa-yogurt mixture, egg whites, and flour. Beat until thoroughly mixed, about 2 minutes.

Fold in chopped peanut butter chips. Evenly pour mixture into the cake pan. Bake until firm, 40 to 45 minutes.

Sprinkle with chopped candies. Let cool completely.

Refrigerate until chilled, at least 1 hour. Release springform, slice, and enjoy!

MAKES 8 SERVINGS

COOKIES 'N DREAM CHEESECAKE

173 calories
PER SERVING

You'll Need: 9-inch springform cake pan, nonstick spray, large bowl, electric mixer
Prep: 25 minutes | **Cook:** 45 minutes | **Chill:** 1 hour

⅛th of cake:
173 calories, 1.5g fat, 435mg sodium, 27.5g carbs, 0.5g fiber, 20.5g sugars, 11.5g protein

INGREDIENTS

16 ounces fat-free cream cheese, room temperature

½ cup granulated white sugar

1 teaspoon vanilla extract

6 ounces (about ¾ cup) fat-free vanilla Greek yogurt, room temperature

½ cup liquid egg whites (about 4 egg whites), room temperature

2 tablespoons all-purpose flour

3 packs Nabisco 100 Cal Oreo Thin Crisps cookies, roughly crushed

DIRECTIONS

Preheat oven to 350 degrees. Spray a 9-inch springform cake pan with nonstick spray.

Combine cream cheese, sugar, and vanilla extract in a large bowl. Beat until smooth with an electric mixer set to medium speed, 1 to 2 minutes.

Continue to beat the mixture while gradually adding yogurt, egg whites, and flour. Beat until thoroughly mixed, about 2 minutes.

Fold in crushed cookies. Evenly pour mixture into the cake pan. Bake until firm, 40 to 45 minutes.

Let cool completely.

Refrigerate until chilled, at least 1 hour. Release springform, slice, and serve!

MAKES 8 SERVINGS

HG SWEET ALTERNATIVE!

If made with an equal amount of Splenda No Calorie Sweetener (granulated) in place of the sugar, each serving will have 131 calories, 16g carbs, and 8g sugars.

SUPER-HELPFUL CHEESECAKE TIP:

Set out *all* measured ingredients before assembling. You'll want 'em all within reach so you can easily add 'em gradually while whisking.

BANANARAMA CREAM PIE

163
calories
PER SERVING

You'll Need: 9-inch pie pan, nonstick spray, blender or food processor, medium bowl, small microwave-safe bowl, medium nonstick pot, whisk | **Prep:** 10 minutes | **Cook:** 25 minutes | **Chill:** 2 hours

⅛th of cake:
163 calories, 4.5g fat, 216mg sodium, 31.5g carbs, 4.5g fiber, 13g sugars, 2g protein

INGREDIENTS

Crust
1 cup Fiber One Original bran cereal
2 sheets (8 crackers) low-fat honey graham crackers, broken into pieces
3 tablespoons Splenda No Calorie Sweetener (granulated)
¼ teaspoon cinnamon
¼ cup light whipped butter or light buttery spread

Filling
2 medium bananas
¼ cup granulated white sugar
¼ cup Splenda No Calorie Sweetener (granulated)
¼ cup cornstarch
¼ teaspoon salt
2 cups light plain soymilk
1½ tablespoons light whipped butter or light buttery spread
1 teaspoon vanilla extract
1 cup Cool Whip Free (thawed)

DIRECTIONS

Preheat oven to 350 degrees. Spray a 9-inch pie pan with nonstick spray.

In a blender or food processor, grind cereal and graham cracker pieces into crumbs. Transfer to a medium bowl and mix in Splenda and cinnamon.

In a small microwave-safe bowl, microwave butter and 2 tablespoons water for 30 seconds, or until butter has melted. Add to the medium bowl and thoroughly mix.

Evenly distribute mixture along the bottom of the pie pan, using your hands or a flat utensil to firmly press and form the crust. Press it into the edges and up along the sides of the pan.

Bake until firm, about 10 minutes. Let crust cool.

Slice 1 banana into coins, and evenly place half of the coins in the crust in a single layer.

In a medium nonstick pot, combine sugar, Splenda, cornstarch, and salt. Set temperature to medium-high heat and slowly add soymilk. Stirring constantly with a whisk, bring to a boil. (Don't raise heat to high.) Cook until thickened, whisking constantly, about 4 minutes.

Remove pot from heat, and stir in butter and vanilla extract.

Pour half of the filling mixture over the banana coins in the crust, and smooth out the surface. Layer with remaining banana coins, followed by remaining filling mixture, and smooth out the surface.

Refrigerate until chilled and set, at least 2 hours. Just before serving, evenly top pie with Cool Whip. Slice the remaining banana into coins and evenly layer over the Cool Whip. Slice pie and serve! (P.S. Refrigerate leftovers!)

MAKES 8 SERVINGS

HG SWEET ALTERNATIVES!

Swap the Splenda (in the crust and filling) for equal amounts of additional granulated white sugar; each serving will have 200 calories, 41g carbs, and 23.5g sugars. Or skip the sugar and use an equal amount of additional Splenda; then each serving will have 142 calories, 26g carbs, and 6.5g sugars. Yay for options!

GOOEY-GOOD FUJI APPLE PIE

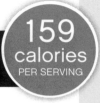
159
calories
PER SERVING

You'll Need: deep-dish pie pan, nonstick spray, blender or food processor, medium bowl, small microwave-safe bowl, large nonstick pot | **Prep:** 20 minutes | **Cook:** 50 minutes

⅛th of pie:
159 calories, 3g fat, 167mg sodium, 37g carbs, 5.5g fiber, 23g sugars, 1g protein

INGREDIENTS

Crust
1 cup Fiber One Original bran cereal

2 sheets (8 crackers) low-fat honey graham crackers, broken into pieces

3 tablespoons granulated white sugar

¼ teaspoon cinnamon

¼ cup light whipped butter or light buttery spread

Filling
6 to 8 Fuji apples (enough to yield 8 cups once sliced)

¼ cup brown sugar (not packed)

2 tablespoons cornstarch

1 tablespoon plus 1 teaspoon granulated white sugar

2 teaspoons cinnamon

2 teaspoons lemon juice

½ teaspoon vanilla extract

¼ teaspoon salt

Optional topping: Fat Free Reddi-wip

DIRECTIONS

Preheat oven to 350 degrees. Spray a deep-dish pie pan with nonstick spray.

In a blender or food processor, grind cereal and graham cracker pieces into crumbs. Transfer to a medium bowl and mix in white sugar and cinnamon.

In a small microwave-safe bowl, microwave butter and 2 tablespoons water for 30 seconds, or until butter has melted. Add to the medium bowl and thoroughly mix.

Evenly distribute mixture along the bottom of the pie pan, using your hands or a flat utensil to firmly press and form the crust. Press it into the edges and up along the sides of the pan.

Bake until firm, about 10 minutes. Let cool.

Set oven to 375 degrees. Peel, core, and thinly slice 8 cups' worth of apples.

In a large nonstick pot, combine all filling ingredients *except* apples. Add 1½ cups cold water and mix until ingredients have dissolved. Add sliced apples and stir.

Bring pot to medium-high heat. Stirring frequently, cook until liquid has thickened and apples have softened, 12 to 15 minutes.

Transfer filling to the pie pan and smooth out the surface. Bake until apples are very tender, 20 to 25 minutes.

Let pie completely cool and set. Slice and enjoy!

MAKES 8 SERVINGS

HG SWEET ALTERNATIVE!

Want to save even more calories? Use granulated Splenda No Calorie Sweetener instead of granulated white sugar. Just swap equal amounts! Each slice will then have 138 calories, 31.5g carbs, and 17.5g sugars. Hooray for options!

CRAZY-AMAZING COCONUT CREAM PIE

143 calories
PER SERVING

You'll Need: deep-dish pie pan, nonstick spray, blender or food processor, medium bowl, small microwave-safe bowl, large bowl, whisk, skillet (optional) | **Prep:** 10 minutes | **Cook:** 15 minutes | **Chill:** 1 hour

⅛th of pie:
143 calories, 4.5g fat, 365mg sodium, 24.5g carbs, 3.75g fiber, 7.5g sugars, 2.5g protein

INGREDIENTS

Crust
1 cup Fiber One Original bran cereal

2 sheets (8 crackers) low-fat honey graham crackers, broken into pieces

3 tablespoons Splenda No Calorie Sweetener (granulated)

¼ cup light whipped butter or light buttery spread

Filling and Topping
1½ cups fat-free milk

½ teaspoon coconut extract

One 6-serving box Jell-O Sugar Free Fat Free Vanilla Instant pudding mix

2 cups Cool Whip Free (thawed)

¼ cup plus 2 tablespoons shredded sweetened coconut

HG SWEET ALTERNATIVE!
Swap out the Splenda for the same amount of granulated white sugar, and each serving will have 159 calories, 29g carbs, and 12g sugars.

DIRECTIONS

Preheat oven to 350 degrees. Spray a deep-dish pie pan with nonstick spray.

In a blender or food processor, grind cereal and graham cracker pieces into crumbs. Transfer to a medium bowl and mix in Splenda.

In a small microwave-safe bowl, microwave butter and 2 tablespoons water for 30 seconds, or until butter has melted. Add to the medium bowl and thoroughly mix.

Evenly distribute mixture along the bottom of the pie pan, using your hands or a flat utensil to firmly press and form the crust. Press it into the edges and up along the sides of the pan.

Bake until firm, about 10 minutes. Let cool.

Pour milk into a large bowl. Add coconut extract and pudding mix and whisk until smooth, about 2 minutes. Fold in 1 cup Cool Whip. Stir in ¼ cup shredded coconut.

Evenly spread filling into the crust. Spread remaining 1 cup Cool Whip over the filling. Refrigerate until completely chilled and set, at least 1 hour.

For a toasted coconut topping (optional), bring a skillet to medium heat. Cook and stir remaining 2 tablespoons shredded coconut until lightly browned, about 4 minutes. Let cool.

Just before serving, sprinkle toasted or un-toasted shredded coconut over the pie. Slice and enjoy!

MAKES 8 SERVINGS

FREEZY DOWNSIDE-UP PB DREAM PIE

159 calories PER SERVING

You'll Need: large bowl, electric mixer, pie pan | **Prep:** 15 minutes | **Freeze:** 2 hours

⅛th of pie:
159 calories, 6.5g fat, 235mg sodium, 18g carbs, 1g fiber, 8.5g sugars, 7g protein

INGREDIENTS

½ cup reduced-fat creamy peanut butter, room temperature
Half an 8-ounce tub fat-free cream cheese, room temperature
¼ cup powdered sugar
½ cup light vanilla soymilk
1 cup Cool Whip Free (thawed)
2 sheets (8 crackers) low-fat honey graham crackers, crushed

Optional topping: Fat Free Reddi-wip

DIRECTIONS

In a large bowl, combine peanut butter with cream cheese. With an electric mixer set to medium speed, beat until smooth and uniform.

Set mixer to low speed. Continue to beat while gradually adding powdered sugar, followed by soymilk.

Fold in Cool Whip. Transfer filling to a pie pan. Top with crushed graham crackers. Cover and freeze until firm, at least 2 hours.

Slice and enjoy!

MAKES 8 SERVINGS

HG TIP:
If frozen until solid, let pie sit at room temperature for 10 to 15 minutes before cutting and serving.

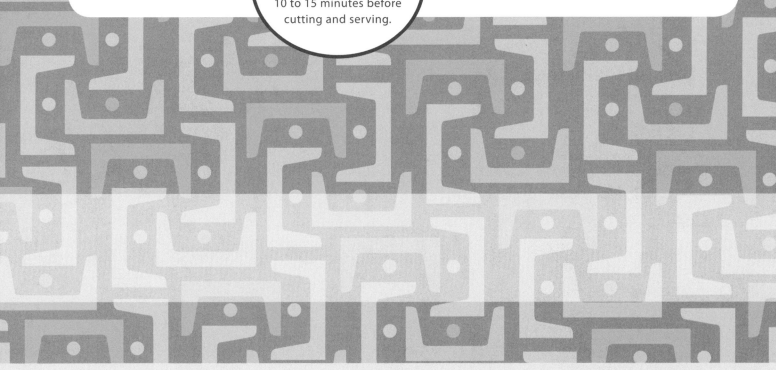

AWESOME APPLE PIE POCKETS

You'll Need: baking sheet, nonstick spray, medium nonstick pot, medium bowl
Prep: 25 minutes | **Cook:** 35 minutes

⅙th of recipe (1 pie pocket):
110 calories, 0.5g fat, 156mg sodium, 25g carbs, 1.25g fiber, 10.5g sugars, 2g protein

INGREDIENTS

2 tablespoons granulated white sugar

2 teaspoons cornstarch

1 teaspoon cinnamon

¼ teaspoon vanilla extract

⅛ teaspoon salt

3 cups peeled and chopped Fuji apples

6 large square egg roll wrappers

18 sprays I Can't Believe It's Not Butter! Spray

Optional toppings: Fat Free Reddi-wip or
    Cool Whip Free, additional cinnamon

HG SWEET ALTERNATIVE!

If made with an equal amount
of Splenda No Calorie Sweetener
(granulated) in place of the
sugar, each serving will have
96 calories, 21g carbs,
and 6.5g sugars.

DIRECTIONS

Preheat oven to 350 degrees. Spray a baking sheet with nonstick spray.

In a medium nonstick pot, combine sugar, cornstarch, cinnamon, vanilla extract, and salt. Add ½ cup cold water and stir until ingredients have dissolved. Add apples and stir. Bring to medium-high heat and, stirring frequently, cook until apples have softened, 7 to 10 minutes.

Reduce heat to low. Stirring often, cook until thick and gooey, 1 to 2 minutes. Transfer to a medium bowl and let cool.

Lay an egg roll wrapper flat on a dry surface. Moisten all four edges with water. Evenly distribute ⅙th of apple mixture (about ⅓ cup) on the bottom half of the wrapper. Fold the top half over the mixture so the top edge meets the bottom. Dab the edges with water and press firmly with the prongs of a fork to seal.

Repeat to make 5 more pie pockets. Transfer to the baking sheet. Spray the top of each pie pocket with 3 sprays butter spray.

Bake until edges begin to brown, 15 to 18 minutes. Dig in!

MAKES 6 SERVINGS

BLUEBERRY-APPLE PIE POCKETS

113 calories PER SERVING

You'll Need: baking sheet, nonstick spray, medium bowl, small bowl
Prep: 25 minutes
Cook: 20 minutes

¼th of recipe (1 pie pocket):
113 calories, 0.5g fat, 197mg sodium, 25.5g carbs, 1.5g fiber, 10g sugars, 2g protein

INGREDIENTS

⅔ cup peeled and chopped Fuji apple
⅔ cup frozen blueberries, thawed and patted dry
½ tablespoon lemon juice
2 drops almond extract
2 tablespoons granulated white sugar
½ tablespoon cornstarch
¼ teaspoon cinnamon
⅛ teaspoon salt
4 large square egg roll wrappers
12 sprays I Can't Believe It's Not Butter! Spray

DIRECTIONS

Preheat oven to 350 degrees. Spray a baking sheet with nonstick spray.

In a medium bowl, mix apple, blueberries, lemon juice, and almond extract.

In a small bowl, mix sugar, cornstarch, cinnamon, and salt. Add to the medium bowl and stir.

Lay an egg roll wrapper flat on a dry surface. Moisten all four edges with water. Evenly distribute ¼th of fruit mixture (about ⅓ cup) on the bottom half of the wrapper. Fold the top half over the mixture so the top edge meets the bottom. Dab the edges with water and press firmly with the prongs of a fork to seal.

Repeat to make 3 more pie pockets. Transfer to the baking sheet and spray the top of each pocket with 3 sprays butter spray.

Bake until edges begin to brown, 15 to 18 minutes. Mmmmm!

MAKES 4 SERVINGS

HG SWEET ALTERNATIVE!

If made with an equal amount of Splenda No Calorie Sweetener (granulated) in place of the sugar, each serving will have 93 calories, 20g carbs, and 4.5g sugars.

APPLE-CHERRY PIE POCKETS

126 calories PER SERVING

You'll Need: baking sheet, nonstick spray, medium bowl, small bowl
Prep: 25 minutes
Cook: 20 minutes

¼th of recipe (1 pie pocket): 126 calories, 0.5g fat, 183mg sodium, 28.5g carbs, 1.5g fiber, 14g sugars, 2.5g protein

INGREDIENTS

1 cup peeled and chopped Fuji apple
1 cup pitted dark sweet cherries, fresh or thawed from frozen
½ tablespoon lemon juice
2 drops almond extract
2 tablespoons granulated white sugar
½ tablespoon cornstarch
¼ teaspoon cinnamon
⅛ teaspoon ground nutmeg
⅛ teaspoon salt
4 large square egg roll wrappers
16 sprays I Can't Believe It's Not Butter! Spray

HG SWEET ALTERNATIVE!

If made with an equal amount of Splenda No Calorie Sweetener (granulated) in place of the sugar, each serving will have 106 calories, 23.5g carbs, and 8g sugars.

DIRECTIONS

Preheat oven to 350 degrees. Spray a baking sheet with nonstick spray.

In a medium bowl, mix apple, cherries, lemon juice, and almond extract.

In a small bowl, mix sugar, cornstarch, cinnamon, nutmeg, and salt. Add to the medium bowl and stir.

Lay an egg roll wrapper flat on a dry surface. Moisten all four edges with water. Evenly distribute ¼th of fruit mixture on the bottom half of the wrapper. Fold the top half over the mixture so the top edge meets the bottom. Dab the edges with water and press firmly with the prongs of a fork to seal.

Repeat to make 3 more pie pockets. Transfer to the baking sheet. Spray the top of each pie pocket with 4 sprays butter spray.

Bake until edges begin to brown, 15 to 18 minutes. Yum time!

MAKES 4 SERVINGS

PB 'N CHOCOLATE BREAD PUDDING

225 calories PER SERVING

You'll Need: loaf pan, nonstick spray, blender
Prep: 10 minutes
Cook: 50 minutes

¼th of bread pudding (1 heaping cup):
225 calories, 8.5g fat, 294mg sodium, 30g carbs, 4g fiber, 15.5g sugars, 10g protein

INGREDIENTS

4 slices light bread
3 tablespoons semi-sweet mini
    chocolate chips
1⅓ cups light vanilla soymilk
⅓ cup fat-free liquid egg substitute
3 tablespoons reduced-fat peanut butter
2½ tablespoons brown sugar (not packed)
Dash salt

Optional topping: Cool Whip Free or
    Fat Free Reddi-wip

DIRECTIONS

Preheat oven to 350 degrees. Spray a loaf pan with nonstick spray.

Lightly toast bread. Cut into ½-inch cubes, place in the pan, and sprinkle with chocolate chips.

In a blender, combine soymilk, egg substitute, peanut butter, brown sugar, and salt. Blend at medium speed until smooth.

Pour mixture into the loaf pan, completely covering the bread cubes. Let stand for 5 minutes.

Bake until pudding is firm, 45 to 50 minutes. Enjoy!

MAKES 4 SERVINGS

SCOOPABLE S'MORES BREAD PUDDING

170 calories PER SERVING

You'll Need: 8-inch by 8-inch baking pan, nonstick spray, large bowl, whisk
Prep: 10 minutes
Cook: 55 minutes

⅛th of bread pudding (about ⅔ cups):
170 calories, 4g fat, 245mg sodium, 29g carbs, 3g fiber, 16g sugars, 7g protein

INGREDIENTS

8 slices light bread
¼ cup plus 2 tablespoons mini semi-sweet
    chocolate chips
2 sheets (8 crackers) low-fat honey graham crackers,
    broken into bite-sized pieces
2½ cups light vanilla soymilk
⅔ cup fat-free liquid egg substitute
¼ cup brown sugar (not packed)
⅛ teaspoon salt
½ cup mini marshmallows

Optional topping: Cool Whip Free or Fat Free Reddi-wip

DIRECTIONS

Preheat oven to 350 degrees. Spray an 8-inch by 8-inch baking pan with nonstick spray.

Lightly toast bread. Cut into ½-inch cubes, and place in the pan. Sprinkle with chocolate chips and graham cracker pieces.

In a large bowl, thoroughly whisk soymilk, egg substitute, brown sugar, and salt.

Pour mixture into the baking pan, completely covering the bread cubes. Let stand for 5 minutes.

Bake until firm, 45 to 50 minutes.

Set oven to broil.

Evenly top bread pudding with marshmallows. Broil until marshmallows have lightly browned, 1 to 2 minutes. Enjoy!

MAKES 8 SERVINGS

CARAMEL BREAD PUDDING FOR TWO

190 calories PER SERVING

You'll Need: 2 microwave-safe mugs, nonstick spray, small bowl
Prep: 5 minutes
Cook: 5 minutes

½ of recipe (1 mug): 190 calories, 2g fat, 388mg sodium, 40.5g carbs, 5g fiber, 11.5g sugars, 8.5g protein

INGREDIENTS

4 slices light bread
1 sugar-free vanilla pudding snack with 60 calories or less
¼ cup fat-free liquid egg substitute
½ teaspoon vanilla extract
2 tablespoons fat-free or light caramel dip
¼ cup Fat Free Reddi-wip
¼ teaspoon cinnamon

DIRECTIONS

Lightly toast bread. Let slightly cool.

Spray 2 microwave-safe mugs with nonstick spray. Tear bread into bite-sized pieces, and divide the pieces between the mugs.

In a small bowl, mix pudding, egg substitute, and vanilla extract. Divide mixture between the mugs, about ¼ cup each, and gently stir to coat the bread.

Place both mugs in the microwave and cook for 2 minutes, or until mostly set.

Add 1 tablespoon caramel dip to each mug and gently stir to evenly distribute. Microwave for 1 minute, or until set.

Once slightly cool, top each mug with 2 tablespoons Reddi-wip. Sprinkle with cinnamon and dig in!

MAKES 2 SERVINGS

CARAMEL APPLE BREAD PUDDING

143 calories PER SERVING

You'll Need: loaf pan, nonstick spray, small nonstick pot with a lid, large bowl, whisk
Prep: 10 minutes
Cook: 1 hour

¼th of bread pudding: 143 calories, 1g fat, 274mg sodium, 28.5g carbs, 3.5g fiber, 16.5g sugars, 6.5g protein

INGREDIENTS

½ teaspoon cornstarch
¼ teaspoon cinnamon
3 tablespoons brown sugar (not packed)
2 dashes salt
1 cup diced Fuji apple
4 slices light bread
1 cup light vanilla soymilk
⅓ cup fat-free liquid egg substitute
2 tablespoons fat-free or light caramel dip

Optional topping: Cool Whip Free or Fat Free Reddi-wip

DIRECTIONS

Preheat oven to 350 degrees. Spray a loaf pan with nonstick spray.

In a small nonstick pot, combine cornstarch, cinnamon, ½ tablespoon brown sugar, and 1 dash salt. Add ¼ cup cold water and stir to dissolve. Stir in apple and bring to medium heat. Cover and cook until apple has softened and liquid has thickened, about 6 minutes, uncovering often to stir.

Remove from heat and let cool. Meanwhile, lightly toast bread and cut into ½-inch cubes.

In a large bowl, thoroughly whisk soymilk, egg substitute, remaining 2½ tablespoons brown sugar, and remaining dash salt. Mix in bread cubes and apple mixture. Transfer to the loaf pan.

Bake until set, 45 to 50 minutes.

Drizzle with caramel dip and enjoy!

MAKES 4 SERVINGS

PERFECT PUMPKIN BREAD

143 calories PER SERVING

You'll Need: loaf pan, nonstick spray, 2 large bowls, whisk | **Prep:** 15 minutes | **Cook:** 50 minutes

⅛th of loaf:
143 calories, 0.5g fat, 281mg sodium, 31g carbs, 4.5g fiber, 9g sugars, 5g protein

INGREDIENTS

1 ¼ cups whole-wheat flour
¼ cup all-purpose flour
½ cup Splenda No Calorie Sweetener (granulated)
¼ cup brown sugar (not packed)
2 ¼ teaspoons baking powder
1 ½ teaspoons cinnamon
½ teaspoon salt
⅓ teaspoon pumpkin pie spice
One 15-ounce can pure pumpkin
½ cup fat-free liquid egg substitute
1 teaspoon vanilla extract
¼ cup sweetened dried cranberries or
    raisins (not packed), chopped

DIRECTIONS

Preheat oven to 350 degrees. Spray a loaf pan with nonstick spray.

In a large bowl, mix both types of flour, Splenda, brown sugar, baking powder, cinnamon, salt, and pumpkin pie spice.

In another large bowl, whisk pumpkin, egg substitute, and vanilla extract. Add this mixture to the large bowl and stir until just blended.

Stir in chopped cranberries or raisins. Transfer batter to the loaf pan and smooth out the surface. Bake until a toothpick inserted into the center comes out clean, about 50 minutes.

MAKES 8 SERVINGS

HG SWEET ALTERNATIVE!

Swap out the Splenda for the same amount of granulated white sugar, and each serving will have 185 calories, 42.5g carbs, and 21.5g sugars.

BATTER UP: BROWNIES AND BREADS!

To smooth out the surface, try spraying a spatula or the back of a spoon with a little nonstick spray. No stickiness while you spread . . .

TOP BANANA BREAD

140 calories
PER SERVING

You'll Need: loaf pan, nonstick spray, 2 large bowls | **Prep:** 10 minutes | **Cook:** 50 minutes

⅛th of loaf:
140 calories, 0.5g fat, 267mg sodium, 31g carbs, 3.75g fiber, 7g sugars, 5g protein

INGREDIENTS

1¼ cups whole-wheat flour
¼ cup all-purpose flour
¾ cup Splenda No Calorie Sweetener (granulated)
2 teaspoons baking powder
½ teaspoon cinnamon
½ teaspoon salt
1½ cups mashed extra-ripe bananas
½ cup fat-free liquid egg substitute
½ cup no-sugar-added applesauce
1 teaspoon vanilla extract

DIRECTIONS

Preheat oven to 350 degrees. Spray a loaf pan with nonstick spray.

In a large bowl, mix both types of flour, Splenda, baking powder, cinnamon, and salt.

In another large bowl, thoroughly mix bananas, egg substitute, applesauce, and vanilla extract. Add to the flour mixture and stir until just blended.

Transfer batter to the loaf pan and smooth out the surface. Bake until a toothpick inserted into the center comes out clean, about 50 minutes. Slice and chew!

MAKES 8 SERVINGS

HG SWEET ALTERNATIVE!

Swap out the Splenda for the same amount of granulated white sugar, and each serving will have 203 calories, 48g carbs, and 26g sugars.

BANANA SPLIT BREAD

169 calories PER SERVING

You'll Need: loaf pan, nonstick spray, 2 large bowls, small microwave-safe bowl
Prep: 20 minutes | **Cook:** 50 minutes

⅛th of loaf:
169 calories, 1.5g fat, 267mg sodium, 35.5g carbs, 3.75g fiber, 13g sugars, 5g protein

INGREDIENTS

1 ¼ cups whole-wheat flour
¼ cup all-purpose flour
½ cup Splenda No Calorie Sweetener (granulated)
2 teaspoons baking powder
½ teaspoon salt
1 ½ cups mashed extra-ripe bananas
½ cup fat-free liquid egg substitute
½ cup no-sugar-added applesauce
1 teaspoon vanilla extract
2 tablespoons mini semi-sweet chocolate chips
¼ cup low-sugar strawberry preserves

Optional topping: Fat Free Reddi-wip

HG SWEET ALTERNATIVE!

Swap out the Splenda for the same amount of granulated white sugar, and each serving will have 211 calories, 47g carbs, and 25.5g sugars.

DIRECTIONS

Preheat oven to 350 degrees. Spray a loaf pan with nonstick spray.

In a large bowl, mix both types of flour, Splenda, baking powder, and salt.

In another large bowl, thoroughly mix bananas, egg substitute, applesauce, and vanilla extract. Add to the flour mixture and stir until just blended.

Stir in chocolate chips. Transfer half of the batter into the loaf pan.

Microwave preserves in a microwave-safe bowl for 20 seconds, or until softened. Stir until smooth.

Drizzle preserves over batter in the pan. Evenly top with remaining batter.

Bake until a toothpick inserted into the center comes out clean, about 50 minutes. Slice, serve, and enjoy!

MAKES 8 SERVINGS

SWINGIN' CINNA-MONKEY BREAD SINGLES

154 calories PER SERVING

You'll Need: 12-cup muffin pan, nonstick spray, large bowl, small nonstick pot
Prep: 20 minutes
Cook: 25 minutes

⅙th of recipe: 154 calories, 7.5g fat, 369mg sodium, 21g carbs, 0.5g fiber, 6.5g sugars, 2g protein

INGREDIENTS

3 tablespoons Splenda No Calorie Sweetener (granulated)
2 teaspoons cinnamon
1 package refrigerated Pillsbury Crescent Recipe Creations Seamless Dough Sheet
½ teaspoon baking powder
2 tablespoons light whipped butter or light buttery spread
2 tablespoons sugar-free pancake syrup
2 tablespoons brown sugar (not packed)

DIRECTIONS

Preheat oven to 350 degrees. Spray 6 cups of a 12-cup muffin pan with nonstick spray.

In a large bowl, mix 1 tablespoon Splenda and 1 teaspoon cinnamon.

Lay dough sheet on a dry surface and sprinkle with baking powder. Gently press baking powder into the sheet.

Cut dough sheet widthwise into six even strips. Cut each strip into four squares. Roll each square into a ball, for a total of 24 dough balls.

Place 12 dough balls in the bowl with the Splenda-cinnamon mixture. Lightly toss to coat. Gently place 4 coated dough balls in each of 3 sprayed cups of the muffin pan. Repeat with remaining dough balls and sprayed cups.

In a small nonstick pot, combine butter, syrup, brown sugar, remaining 2 tablespoons Splenda, and remaining 1 teaspoon cinnamon. Bring to medium heat. Stirring frequently, cook just until butter has melted and contents are well mixed, about 2 minutes.

Evenly spoon butter mixture over the dough balls. Bake until puffy and firm, 15 to 20 minutes. Enjoy!

MAKES 6 SERVINGS

VANILLA ALMOND FRUIT TARTLETS

71 calories PER SERVING

You'll Need: baking sheet, medium bowl
Prep: 10 minutes
Cook: 5 minutes

⅕th of recipe (3 tartlets): 71 calories, 3g fat, 55mg sodium, 10.5g carbs, 0.5g fiber, 1.5g sugars, 2g protein

INGREDIENTS

15 frozen mini fillo shells
1 sugar-free vanilla pudding snack with 60 calories or less
½ cup chopped strawberries
2 tablespoons sliced almonds, lightly crushed
15 blueberries

DIRECTIONS

Preheat oven to 350 degrees.

Place shells on a baking sheet and bake until lightly browned and crispy, 3 to 5 minutes.

In a medium bowl, mix pudding, strawberries, and crushed almonds. Evenly distribute mixture among the shells. Top each shell with a blueberry. Serve it up!

MAKES 5 SERVINGS

HG SWEET ALTERNATIVE!

Swap out the Splenda for the same amount of granulated white sugar, and each serving will have 175 calories, 26.5g carbs, and 13g sugars.

CRISPY PECAN PIE BITES

106 calories PER SERVING

You'll Need: baking sheet, medium bowl
Prep: 10 minutes
Cook: 20 minutes

⅕th of recipe (3 pieces): 106 calories, 6g fat, 87mg sodium, 12g carbs, 0.5g fiber, 5.5g sugars, 3g protein

INGREDIENTS

15 frozen mini fillo shells
¼ cup fat-free liquid egg substitute
3 tablespoons brown sugar (not packed)
½ tablespoon light whipped butter or light buttery spread, room temperature
1 drop vanilla extract
Dash salt
¼ cup roughly chopped pecans

Optional topping: Fat Free Reddi-wip

DIRECTIONS

Preheat oven to 375 degrees. Place shells on a baking sheet.

In a medium bowl, thoroughly mix egg substitute, brown sugar, butter, vanilla extract, and salt. Stir in 2 tablespoons chopped pecans. Evenly distribute mixture among the fillo shells.

Evenly distribute remaining 2 tablespoons chopped pecans among the shells, about ½ teaspoon each.

Bake until edges are crisp, 15 to 18 minutes. Enjoy!

MAKES 5 SERVINGS

BFFS (BLACK FOREST FILLO-CUPS)

80 calories PER SERVING

You'll Need: baking sheet
Prep: 10 minutes
Cook: 5 minutes

⅕th of recipe (3 BFFs): 80 calories, 3.5g fat, 70mg sodium, 12.5g carbs, 0.5g fiber, 3g sugars, 0.5g protein

INGREDIENTS

15 frozen mini fillo shells
1 sugar-free chocolate pudding snack with 60 calories or less
5 tablespoons Fat Free Reddi-wip
15 pitted dark sweet cherries, fresh or thawed from frozen

DIRECTIONS

Preheat oven to 350 degrees.

Place shells on a baking sheet and bake until lightly browned and crispy, 3 to 5 minutes.

Let cool slightly. Evenly distribute pudding among shells, and top each with a 1-teaspoon squirt of Reddi-wip. Add a cherry to each cup, and prepare for some quality time with your new BFFs!

MAKES 5 SERVINGS

DOUBLE-CHOCOLATE PRETZEL TARTS

70 calories PER SERVING

You'll Need: baking sheet, nonstick spray, medium bowl | **Prep:** 10 minutes | **Cook:** 5 minutes

⅕th of recipe (3 tarts):
70 calories, 2.5g fat, 85mg sodium, 12g carbs, <0.5g fiber, 1.5g sugars, 2g protein

INGREDIENTS

15 frozen mini fillo shells

1 sugar-free chocolate pudding snack with 60 calories or less

15 small hard pretzel sticks, broken into small pieces

1 tablespoon mini semi-sweet chocolate chips

DIRECTIONS

Preheat oven to 350 degrees.

Place shells on a baking sheet and bake until lightly browned and crispy, 3 to 5 minutes.

In a medium bowl, mix pudding, pretzel stick pieces, and chocolate chips. Evenly distribute mixture among the shells. Yum time!

MAKES 5 SERVINGS

CARAMEL APPLE PIE BITES

66 calories PER SERVING

You'll Need: baking sheet, medium bowl | **Prep:** 10 minutes | **Cook:** 15 minutes

⅕th of recipe (3 pieces):
66 calories, 1.5g fat, 46mg sodium, 13g carbs, <0.5g fiber, 4.5g sugars, 1.5g protein

INGREDIENTS

15 frozen mini fillo shells

½ cup diced Fuji apple

Dash cinnamon

2 tablespoons fat-free or light caramel dip

DIRECTIONS

Preheat oven to 350 degrees. Place shells on a baking sheet.

In a medium bowl, sprinkle apple with cinnamon. Add caramel dip and stir to coat. Evenly divide among shells.

Bake until shells are lightly browned and crispy and filling is hot, about 12 minutes. Eat up!

MAKES 5 SERVINGS

CHOCOLATE-CHIPPY CHEESE DANISH

141 calories PER SERVING

You'll Need: baking sheet, nonstick spray, small microwave-safe bowl, medium bowl, rolling pin (optional)
Prep: 20 minutes | **Cook:** 20 minutes

⅛th of Danish:
141 calories, 6g fat, 313mg sodium, 18.5g carbs, 0.5g fiber, 6g sugars, 4g protein

INGREDIENTS

Icing
1½ teaspoons Splenda No Calorie Sweetener (granulated)
1 teaspoon powdered sugar
1 teaspoon cornstarch
1 drop vanilla extract
1 tablespoon Jet-Puffed Marshmallow Creme
1 tablespoon Cool Whip Free (thawed)

Danish
Half an 8-ounce tub fat-free cream cheese, room temperature
2 tablespoons Splenda No Calorie Sweetener (granulated)
1 tablespoon light vanilla soymilk
½ teaspoon vanilla extract
¼ teaspoon cinnamon
¼ cup old-fashioned oats
2 tablespoons mini semi-sweet chocolate chips
1 package refrigerated Pillsbury Crescent Recipe Creations Seamless Dough Sheet

DIRECTIONS

Preheat oven to 350 degrees. Spray a baking sheet with nonstick spray.

To make the icing, mix Splenda, sugar, and cornstarch in a small microwave-safe bowl. Add vanilla extract and 1½ teaspoons cold water, and stir until ingredients have dissolved.

Add marshmallow creme and microwave for 5 seconds, or until creme is soft. Stir until smooth. Stir in Cool Whip, cover, and refrigerate.

In a medium bowl, thoroughly mix cream cheese, Splenda, soymilk, vanilla extract, and cinnamon. Stir in oats and chocolate chips.

On the baking sheet, roll or stretch out dough into a large rectangle of even thickness. Arrange sheet with the short sides on the left and right. Spoon cream cheese filling lengthwise across the middle third of the dough, leaving ½-inch borders on the sides.

Make vertical cuts about 1 inch apart along the top section of the dough, stopping about ½ inch above the filling, to create 1-inch-wide strips of dough. Repeat with the bottom section of the dough.

Alternate folding the top and bottom strips over the filling, covering it completely and creating a "braided" criss-cross. Cross the last few strips toward the middle of the Danish. Fold the sides of the dough in and firmly pat to seal.

Bake until crispy and golden brown, 15 to 20 minutes.

Let cool completely.

Stir icing and drizzle over Danish. Slice and enjoy!

MAKES 8 SERVINGS

HG SWEET ALTERNATIVE!

If made with an equal amount of granulated white sugar in place of Splenda, each serving will have 154 calories, 22g carbs, and 10g sugars.

CHEESY CHERRY DANISH

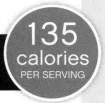
135 calories
PER SERVING

You'll Need: baking sheet, nonstick spray, small microwave-safe bowl, medium bowl, rolling pin (optional)
Prep: 20 minutes | **Cook:** 20 minutes

⅛th of Danish:
135 calories, 4.75g fat, 312mg sodium, 19.5g carbs, 0.5g fiber, 6g sugars, 4g protein

INGREDIENTS

Icing

1½ teaspoons Splenda No Calorie Sweetener (granulated)

1 teaspoon powdered sugar

1 teaspoon cornstarch

1 drop vanilla extract

1 tablespoon Jet-Puffed Marshmallow Creme

1 tablespoon Cool Whip Free (thawed)

Danish

Half an 8-ounce tub fat-free cream cheese, room temperature

2 tablespoons Splenda No Calorie Sweetener (granulated)

1 tablespoon light vanilla soymilk

¼ teaspoon almond extract

1 cup frozen unsweetened pitted dark sweet cherries, thawed

¼ cup old-fashioned oats

1 package refrigerated Pillsbury Crescent Recipe Creations Seamless Dough Sheet

DIRECTIONS

Preheat oven to 350 degrees. Spray a baking sheet with nonstick spray.

To make the icing, mix Splenda, sugar, and cornstarch in a small microwave-safe bowl. Add vanilla extract and 1½ teaspoons cold water, and stir until ingredients have dissolved.

Add marshmallow creme and microwave for 5 seconds, or until creme is soft. Stir until smooth. Stir in Cool Whip, cover, and refrigerate.

In a medium bowl, thoroughly mix cream cheese, Splenda, soymilk, and almond extract. Stir in cherries and oats.

On the baking sheet, roll or stretch out dough into a large rectangle of even thickness. Arrange sheet with the short sides on the left and right. Spoon cherry filling lengthwise across the middle third of the dough, leaving ½-inch borders on the sides.

Make vertical cuts about 1 inch apart along the top section of the dough, stopping about ½ inch above the filling, to create 1-inch-wide strips of dough. Repeat with the bottom section of the dough.

Alternate folding the top and bottom strips over the filling, covering it completely and creating a "braided" criss-cross. Cross the last few strips toward the middle of the Danish. Fold the sides of the dough in and firmly pat to seal.

Bake until crispy and golden brown, 15 to 20 minutes.

Let cool completely.

Stir icing and drizzle over Danish. Slice and eat!

MAKES 8 SERVINGS

HG SWEET ALTERNATIVE!

If made with an equal amount of granulated white sugar in place of Splenda, each serving will have 148 calories, 23g carbs, and 10g sugars.

HG ALTERNATIVE!

When a recipe calls for a very small amount of soymilk, feel free to use your milk or milk swap of choice. It'll barely affect the taste or nutritionals. Hooray for options!

CINNAMON APPLE-CRANBERRY DANISH

152 calories
PER SERVING

You'll Need: baking sheet, nonstick spray, medium nonstick pot, rolling pin (optional), small bowl
Prep: 20 minutes | **Cook:** 35 minutes

⅛th of Danish:
152 calories, 4g fat, 316mg sodium, 25g carbs, 0.5g fiber, 13g sugars, 3.5g protein

INGREDIENTS

2 tablespoons granulated white sugar

1 tablespoon brown sugar (not packed)

½ tablespoon cornstarch

1 teaspoon cinnamon

¼ teaspoon plus 1 drop vanilla extract

2 cups peeled and chopped Fuji apples

2 tablespoons sweetened dried cranberries, chopped

Half an 8-ounce tub fat-free cream cheese

1 package refrigerated Pillsbury Crescent Recipe Creations Seamless Dough Sheet

2 tablespoons powdered sugar

HG SWEET ALTERNATIVE!

If made with an equal amount of Splenda No Calorie Sweetener (granulated) in place of the sugar, each serving will have 142 calories, 22g carbs, and 10g sugars.

DIRECTIONS

Preheat oven to 350 degrees. Spray a baking sheet with nonstick spray.

Combine white sugar, brown sugar, cornstarch, and cinnamon in a medium nonstick pot. Add ¼ teaspoon vanilla extract and ½ cup cold water, and stir until ingredients dissolve. Add apples and cranberries and stir well. Bring to medium-high heat. Stirring frequently, cook until sauce has thickened and apples have partially softened, 10 to 12 minutes.

Remove pot from heat and let cool slightly. Add cream cheese and mix thoroughly. Let cool completely.

On the baking sheet, roll or stretch out dough into a large rectangle of even thickness. Arrange sheet with the short sides on the left and right. Spoon fruit filling lengthwise across the middle third of the dough, leaving ½-inch borders on the sides.

Make vertical cuts about 1 inch apart along the top section of the dough, stopping about ½ inch above the filling, to create 1-inch-wide strips of dough. Repeat with the bottom section of the dough.

Alternate folding the top and bottom strips over the filling, covering it completely and creating a "braided" criss-cross. Cross the last few strips toward the middle of the Danish. Fold the sides of the dough in and firmly pat to seal.

Bake until crispy and golden brown, 15 to 20 minutes.

Let cool completely.

Just before serving, in a small bowl, combine powdered sugar, remaining drop vanilla extract, and 1 teaspoon cold water. Stir until smooth, and drizzle over the Danish. Slice and indulge!

MAKES 8 SERVINGS

BLUEBERRY CHEESE DANISH

134
calories
PER SERVING

You'll Need: baking sheet, nonstick spray, small microwave-safe bowl, medium bowl, rolling pin (optional)
Prep: 20 minutes | **Cook:** 20 minutes

⅛th of Danish:
134 calories, 4g fat, 317mg sodium, 19g carbs, 1g fiber, 5.5g sugars, 4g protein

INGREDIENTS

Icing

1½ teaspoons Splenda No Calorie Sweetener (granulated)

1 teaspoon powdered sugar

1 teaspoon cornstarch

1 drop vanilla extract

1 tablespoon Jet-Puffed Marshmallow Creme

1 tablespoon Cool Whip Free (thawed)

Danish

Half an 8-ounce tub fat-free cream cheese, room temperature

2 tablespoons Splenda No Calorie Sweetener (granulated)

1 tablespoon light vanilla soymilk

¼ teaspoon almond extract

1 cup frozen unsweetened blueberries, thawed

¼ cup old-fashioned oats

1 package refrigerated Pillsbury Crescent Recipe Creations Seamless Dough Sheet

DIRECTIONS

Preheat oven to 350 degrees. Spray a baking sheet with nonstick spray.

To make the icing, mix Splenda, sugar, and cornstarch in a small microwave-safe bowl. Add vanilla extract and 1½ teaspoons cold water, and stir until ingredients have dissolved.

Add marshmallow creme and microwave for 5 seconds, or until creme is soft. Stir until smooth. Stir in Cool Whip, cover, and refrigerate.

In a medium bowl, thoroughly mix cream cheese, Splenda, soymilk, and almond extract. Stir in blueberries and oats.

On the baking sheet, roll or stretch out dough into a large rectangle of even thickness. Arrange sheet with the short sides on the left and right. Spoon blueberry filling lengthwise across the middle third of the dough, leaving ½-inch borders on the sides.

Make vertical cuts about 1 inch apart along the top section of the dough, stopping about ½ inch above the filling, to create 1-inch-wide strips of dough. Repeat with the bottom section of the dough.

Alternate folding the top and bottom strips over the filling, covering it completely and creating a "braided" criss-cross. Cross the last few strips toward the middle of the Danish. Fold the sides of the dough in and firmly pat to seal.

Bake until crispy and golden brown, 15 to 20 minutes.

Let cool completely.

Stir icing and drizzle over Danish. Slice and enjoy!

MAKES 8 SERVINGS

HG SWEET ALTERNATIVE!

Swap out the Splenda for the same amount of granulated white sugar, and each serving will have 145 calories, 22.5g carbs, and 10g sugars.

PERFECT PEACH DUMPLINGS

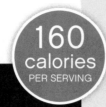

You'll Need: 9-inch by 13-inch baking pan, nonstick spray, rolling pin (optional), aluminum foil
Prep: 20 minutes
Cook: 40 minutes

⅙th of recipe (1 dumpling):
160 calories, 5g fat, 301mg sodium, 26g carbs, 1.5g fiber, 11.5g sugars, 2.5g protein

INGREDIENTS

1 package refrigerated Pillsbury Crescent Recipe Creations Seamless Dough Sheet

3 cups chopped peaches

1 tablespoon brown sugar (not packed)

1 teaspoon cinnamon

DIRECTIONS

Preheat oven to 375 degrees. Spray a 9-inch by 13-inch baking pan with nonstick spray.

Lay dough sheet on a dry surface with the shorter sides on the left and right. Horizontally cut into 2 even strips. Vertically cut each strip into 3 even pieces. Slightly stretch or roll out each piece into larger squares.

Evenly distribute peaches among dough squares, ½ cup each.

Sprinkle with brown sugar and cinnamon. One dough square at a time, gently bring all four corners up around the filling to overlap at the top and pinch edges to seal, enclosing the filling. Place in the baking pan.

Cover pan with foil and bake for 40 minutes, or until dough has lightly browned and peaches are tender. Enjoy!

MAKES 6 SERVINGS

CRAZY-DELICIOUS APPLE DUMPLINGS

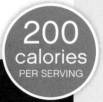

You'll Need: 9-inch by 13-inch baking pan, nonstick spray, aluminum foil, rolling pin (optional)
Prep: 20 minutes
Cook: 50 minutes

⅙th of recipe (1 dumpling): 200 calories, 6.5g fat, 308mg sodium, 36g carbs, 2.5g fiber, 19g sugars, 2.5g protein

INGREDIENTS

1 package refrigerated Pillsbury Crescent Recipe Creations Seamless Dough Sheet

6 small baking apples (preferably Fuji), peeled and cored

2 tablespoons sweetened dried cranberries

½ tablespoon brown sugar (not packed)

½ tablespoon light whipped butter or light buttery spread

1 teaspoon cinnamon

¼ teaspoon ground nutmeg

DIRECTIONS

Preheat oven to 375 degrees. Spray a 9-inch by 13-inch baking pan with nonstick spray.

Lay dough sheet on a dry surface with the shorter sides on the left and right. Horizontally cut into 2 even strips. Vertically cut each strip into 3 even pieces. Slightly stretch or roll out each piece into larger squares.

Place an apple in the center of each dough square. Evenly distribute cranberries among the openings of the apples, 1 teaspoon each. Evenly distribute brown sugar and butter among the openings, about ¼ teaspoon of each per apple. Sprinkle with cinnamon and nutmeg.

One dough square at a time, gently bring all four corners up around the apple to overlap at the top and pinch edges to seal, enclosing the apple. Place in the baking pan, evenly spaced.

Cover the pan with enough foil to secure at the sides without resting on top of the apples. Bake for 45 to 50 minutes, until dough is browned and apples are tender. Dive in!

MAKES 6 SERVINGS

BESTEST BAKED APPLES

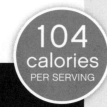

104 calories PER SERVING

You'll Need: 8-inch by 8-inch baking pan
Prep: 10 minutes
Cook: 45 minutes

¼th of recipe (1 apple): 104 calories, <0.5g fat, 10mg sodium, 27g carbs, 4g fiber, 21g sugars, 0.5g protein

INGREDIENTS

4 medium Rome or Braeburn apples
One 12-ounce can diet black cherry soda
1 teaspoon granulated white sugar or
    Splenda No Calorie Sweetener (granulated)
¼ teaspoon cinnamon
½ cup Fat Free Reddi-wip

Optional topping: additional cinnamon

DIRECTIONS

Preheat oven to 375 degrees.

Core apples and place in an 8-inch by 8-inch baking pan. Pour the entire can of soda over the apples. Sprinkle with sugar or Splenda and cinnamon.

Bake until apples are tender, about 45 minutes.

Top each apple with 2 tablespoons of the Reddi-wip. Enjoy!

MAKES 4 SERVINGS

DOWNTOWN APPLE BETTY BROWN

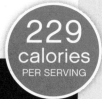

229 calories PER SERVING

You'll Need: 9-inch by 13-inch baking pan, nonstick spray, 2 large bowls, blender or food processor, medium bowl
Prep: 20 minutes
Cook: 40 minutes

⅙th of recipe: 229 calories, 4.5g fat, 387mg sodium, 48g carbs, 12g fiber, 22g sugars, 7.5g protein

INGREDIENTS

8 slices light bread
5 Fuji apples, cored and thinly sliced
1 tablespoon lemon juice
¼ teaspoon salt
3 tablespoons brown sugar (not packed)
2 teaspoons cinnamon
1 cup Fiber One Original bran cereal
¼ cup light whipped butter or light buttery spread
¾ cup fat-free liquid egg substitute
½ cup light vanilla soymilk
1 teaspoon vanilla extract

Optional topping: Cool Whip Free

DIRECTIONS

Preheat oven to 350 degrees. Spray a 9-inch by 13-inch baking pan with nonstick spray.

Lightly toast bread and tear into bite-sized pieces.

Place apple slices in a large bowl, top with lemon juice, and toss to coat. Sprinkle with salt, 2 tablespoons brown sugar, and 1 teaspoon cinnamon. Mix well.

In a blender or food processor, grind cereal into crumbs. Transfer to a medium bowl and mix in remaining 1 tablespoon brown sugar and ½ teaspoon cinnamon. Mix in butter until evenly dispersed; mixture will be crumbly.

In another large bowl, thoroughly mix egg substitute, soymilk, vanilla extract, and remaining ½ teaspoon cinnamon. Add bread pieces and stir to coat. Transfer mixture to bowl of apple slices and thoroughly mix.

Evenly spoon apple-bread mixture into the baking pan and top with crumb mixture. Bake until firm and lightly browned, 35 to 40 minutes. Enjoy!

MAKES 6 SERVINGS

FREEZY-COOL WHOOPIE PIE

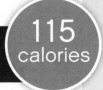

115 calories

You'll Need: plate | **Prep:** 5 minutes | **Freeze:** 1 hour

Entire recipe:
115 calories, 1.5g fat, 145mg sodium, 24g carbs, 6g fiber, 10g sugars, 3g protein

INGREDIENTS

1 Vitalicious Deep Chocolate VitaTop
  (partially thawed)

2 tablespoons Cool Whip Free (thawed)

DIRECTIONS

Carefully slice VitaTop in half lengthwise (like you would a hamburger bun), so that you are left with 2 thin round "slices."

Spread Cool Whip on one slice and top with the other slice. Place on a plate and freeze until solid, about 1 hour. Enjoy!

MAKES 1 SERVING

QUICK Q&A WITH HG:

What are VitaTops, and where can I find 'em?

They're high-fiber, low-fat muffin tops with just 100 calories (or less) per Top! You can find the Deep Chocolate and a few other flavors at select markets (in the freezer aisle). You can also order online at **Vitalicious.com**.

FREEZY-GOOD WHOOPIE S'MORES

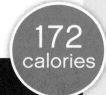 **172 calories**

You'll Need: small bowl, 2 small plates
Prep: 5 minutes
Freeze: 1 hour

Entire recipe: 172 calories, 2.5g fat, 175mg sodium, 40.5g carbs, 9g fiber, 19g sugars, 4.5g protein

INGREDIENTS

1 Vitalicious Deep Chocolate VitaTop (partially thawed)
3 tablespoons Cool Whip Free (thawed)
10 mini marshmallows
½ teaspoon mini semi-sweet chocolate chips
1 low-fat graham cracker (¼ sheet), crushed

DIRECTIONS

Carefully slice VitaTop in half lengthwise (like you would a hamburger bun), so that you are left with 2 thin round "slices."

Place Cool Whip in a small bowl. Stir in marshmallows and chocolate chips.

Place crushed graham cracker on a small plate.

Evenly spoon Cool Whip mixture over the bottom Vita slice. Top with the other Vita slice to form a sandwich. Gently press the sides of the sandwich into the crushed graham cracker, covering the exposed filling with crumbs.

Place on another small plate and freeze until solid, about 1 hour. Tada!

MAKES 1 SERVING

FREEZY-COOL BANANA WHOOPIE PIES

 150 calories PER SERVING

You'll Need: large plate
Prep: 5 minutes
Freeze: 1 hour

¼th of recipe (1 whoopie pie):
150 calories, 2g fat, 155mg sodium, 34g carbs, 9g fiber, 18.5g sugars, 4g protein

INGREDIENTS

4 Vitalicious Deep Chocolate VitaTops (partially thawed)
¾ cup Cool Whip Free (thawed)
1 medium banana, thinly sliced

DIRECTIONS

Carefully slice one VitaTop in half lengthwise (like you would a hamburger bun), so that you are left with 2 thin round "slices." Place ¼th of the Cool Whip on the bottom Vita slice; then top with ¼th of the banana slices, followed by the top Vita slice.

Repeat with remaining ingredients for a total of 4 whoopie pies. Place on a large plate and freeze until solid, about 1 hour. So good!

MAKES 4 SERVINGS

DOUBLE-TROUBLE CHOCOLATE TRIFLE

193 calories PER SERVING

You'll Need: 2 medium bowls, whisk, blender, medium serving bowl
Prep: 10 minutes
Chill: 5 minutes

¼th of trifle: 193 calories, 1.5g fat, 346mg sodium, 39.5g carbs, 6.5g fiber, 15g sugars, 5.5g protein

INGREDIENTS

1 cup fat-free milk
2 tablespoons sugar-free fat-free chocolate instant pudding mix
1⅔ cups Cool Whip Free (thawed)
1½ tablespoons sugar-free chocolate syrup
4 Vitalicious Deep Chocolate VitaTops (thawed)

DIRECTIONS

In a medium bowl, combine milk with pudding mix. Whisk until thickened and smooth, about 2 minutes. Refrigerate for at least 5 minutes.

In another medium bowl, mix syrup into 1 cup Cool Whip. Refrigerate for at least 5 minutes.

Break VitaTops into pieces and place in a blender. Pulse into crumbs.

Layer ingredients in a medium serving bowl: ¼th of Vita crumbs, half of the pudding, remaining ⅔ cup Cool Whip, ¼th of Vita crumbs, and remaining pudding.

Top with the chocolate Cool Whip mixture and sprinkle with remaining Vita crumbs. Dig in!

MAKES 4 SERVINGS

OOEY-GOOEY GERMAN CHOCOLATE TRIFLE

216 calories PER SERVING

You'll Need: medium bowl, whisk, blender, small microwave-safe bowl, medium serving bowl
Prep: 10 minutes
Chill: 10 minutes
Cook: 5 minutes

⅕th of trifle (about ⅔ cup): 216 calories, 4.5g fat, 330mg sodium, 41g carbs, 6g fiber, 20g sugars, 5.5g protein

INGREDIENTS

1 cup plus 2 tablespoons fat-free milk
2 tablespoons sugar-free fat-free chocolate instant pudding mix
1 cup Cool Whip Free (thawed)
4 Vitalicious Deep Chocolate VitaTops (thawed)
¼ cup fat-free or light caramel dip
2 tablespoons chopped pecans
2 tablespoons shredded sweetened coconut

DIRECTIONS

In a medium bowl, combine 1 cup milk with pudding mix. Whisk until thickened and smooth, about 2 minutes. Refrigerate for 5 minutes.

Fold in Cool Whip and refrigerate for at least 5 more minutes.

Break VitaTops into pieces and place in a blender. Pulse into crumbs.

In a small microwave-safe bowl, combine caramel dip with remaining 2 tablespoons milk. Microwave for 45 seconds, or until softened. Mix well. Stir in pecans and coconut.

Place ⅓rd of the Vita crumbs in a medium serving bowl. Top with half of the pudding mixture, and drizzle with half of the caramel mixture.

Repeat layering with half of the remaining Vita crumbs, the remaining pudding mixture, the remaining Vita crumbs, and the remaining caramel mixture. Serve with 5 spoons!

MAKES 5 SERVINGS

GOOEY CINNAMON ROLLS WITH CREAM CHEESE ICING

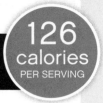

126 calories PER SERVING

You'll Need: baking sheet, nonstick spray, small bowl, medium bowl, rolling pin (optional)
Prep: 15 minutes | **Cook:** 15 minutes

⅛th of recipe (1 iced roll):
126 calories, 5g fat, 308mg sodium, 18.5g carbs, <0.5g fiber, 6.5g sugars, 3g protein

INGREDIENTS

Icing
¼ cup Cool Whip Free (thawed)
3 tablespoons fat-free cream cheese, room temperature
1 tablespoon Splenda No Calorie Sweetener (granulated)

Filling
¼ cup dark brown sugar (not packed)
¼ cup Splenda No Calorie Sweetener (granulated)
½ tablespoon light whipped butter or light buttery spread, room temperature
1½ teaspoons cinnamon
⅛ teaspoon salt

Rolls
1 package refrigerated Pillsbury Crescent Recipe Creations Seamless Dough Sheet
16 sprays I Can't Believe It's Not Butter! Spray

DIRECTIONS

Preheat oven to 350 degrees. Spray a baking sheet with nonstick spray.

In a small bowl, thoroughly mix all icing ingredients. Cover and refrigerate.

In a medium bowl, thoroughly mix all filling ingredients.

Unroll dough on a dry surface with the long sides on the left and right. Roll or stretch into a large rectangle of even thickness. Evenly spray with butter.

Evenly spread filling onto dough, leaving a 1-inch border. Tightly roll up dough into a log. Pinch the long seam to seal.

Turn log so the seam side is down. Cut widthwise into 8 equally sized rolls, and lay rolls on the baking sheet, swirl sides up.

Bake until golden brown, 12 to 15 minutes.

Drizzle icing over rolls and enjoy!

MAKES 8 SERVINGS

HG SWEET ALTERNATIVE!

Swap out the Splenda for the same amount of granulated white sugar, and each serving will have 152 calories, 25.5g carbs, and 14.5g sugars.

STRAWBERRY COCONUT CINNAMON BUNS

125 calories PER SERVING

You'll Need: baking sheet, nonstick spray, blender or food processor, small nonstick pot, rolling pin (optional), small bowl | **Prep:** 20 minutes | **Cook:** 20 minutes

⅛th of recipe (1 bun):
125 calories, 4.5g fat, 256mg sodium, 18g carbs, 1g fiber, 6.5g sugars, 1.5g protein

INGREDIENTS

Filling

1 cup frozen unsweetened strawberries, partially thawed

2 tablespoons Splenda No Calorie Sweetener (granulated)

1½ teaspoons cornstarch

3 drops coconut extract

Dash cinnamon

Dash salt

Buns

1 package refrigerated Pillsbury Crescent Recipe Creations Seamless Dough Sheet

Topping

2 tablespoons powdered sugar

1 drop coconut extract

¼ cup shredded sweetened coconut, chopped

DIRECTIONS

Preheat oven to 350 degrees. Spray a baking sheet with nonstick spray.

Puree strawberries in a blender or food processor with ¼ cup water. Transfer to a small nonstick pot and stir in all other filling ingredients. Set heat to high and bring to a boil.

Reduce to a simmer. Cook and stir until thick and gooey, 2 to 3 minutes. Remove from heat and let cool.

Unroll dough on a dry surface with the long sides on the left and right. Roll or stretch into a large rectangle of even thickness. Evenly spread filling onto dough, leaving a 1-inch border. Tightly roll up dough into a log. Pinch the long seam to seal.

Turn log so the seam side is down. Cut widthwise into 8 equally sized buns, and lay buns on the baking sheet, swirl sides up.

Bake until golden brown, 12 to 15 minutes.

In a small bowl, thoroughly mix powdered sugar, remaining drop coconut extract, and 1 teaspoon cold water. Drizzle over buns, sprinkle with coconut, and enjoy!

MAKES 8 SERVINGS

HG SWEET ALTERNATIVE!

Swap out the Splenda for the same amount of granulated white sugar, and each serving will have 136 calories, 21g carbs, and 9.5g sugars.

CARAMEL APPLE CINNAMON BUNS

137 calories
PER SERVING

You'll Need: baking sheet, nonstick spray, microwave-safe bowl, rolling pin (optional), small bowl
Prep: 20 minutes | **Cook:** 15 minutes

⅛th of recipe (1 bun):
137 calories, 4g fat, 280mg sodium, 24g carbs, 0.5g fiber, 10.5g sugars, 1.5g protein

INGREDIENTS

Filling
1 cup finely chopped Granny Smith apple
¼ cup fat-free or light caramel dip
1 teaspoon cinnamon
Dash salt

Buns
1 package refrigerated Pillsbury Crescent Recipe Creations Seamless Dough Sheet

Icing
2 tablespoons powdered sugar
2 teaspoons fat-free or light caramel dip

DIRECTIONS

Preheat oven to 350 degrees. Spray a baking sheet with nonstick spray.

In a microwave-safe bowl, microwave apple for 1 minute, or until slightly softened. Add remaining filling ingredients and thoroughly stir.

Unroll dough on a dry surface with the long sides on the left and right. Roll or stretch into a large rectangle of even thickness. Evenly spread filling onto dough, leaving a 1-inch border. Tightly roll up dough into a log. Pinch the long seam to seal.

Turn log so the seam side is down. Cut widthwise into 8 equally sized buns, and lay buns on the baking sheet, swirl sides up.

Bake until golden brown, 12 to 15 minutes.

In a small bowl, mix powdered sugar with 1 teaspoon cold water until dissolved. Thoroughly mix in caramel dip. Drizzle over buns and enjoy!

MAKES 8 SERVINGS

CARAMEL DIP TIP:

If your dip is extra thick 'n sticky, stir it before measuring it out. If it's still tough to work with, microwave it in a microwave-safe bowl until just softened.

NUTTY CARAMEL-COATED STICKY BUNS

169 calories PER SERVING

You'll Need: 12-cup muffin pan, nonstick spray, small microwave-safe bowl, rolling pin (optional), medium microwave-safe bowl   **Prep:** 20 minutes | **Cook:** 15 minutes

⅛th of recipe (1 bun):
169 calories, 7.5g fat, 323mg sodium, 23.5g carbs, 0.5g fiber, 10.5g sugars, 2g protein

INGREDIENTS

Filling
¼ cup brown sugar (not packed)
1 tablespoon light whipped butter or light buttery spread
1½ teaspoons cinnamon
⅛ teaspoon salt

Buns
1 package refrigerated Pillsbury Crescent Recipe
    Creations Seamless Dough Sheet

Topping
3 tablespoons fat-free or light caramel dip
2 tablespoons light whipped butter or light buttery spread
2 tablespoons sugar-free pancake syrup
1 tablespoon brown sugar (not packed)
3 tablespoons chopped pecans

DIRECTIONS

Preheat oven to 350 degrees. Spray 8 cups of a 12-cup muffin pan with nonstick spray.

To make filling, combine brown sugar with butter in a small microwave-safe bowl. Microwave for 10 seconds, or until butter has mostly melted. Mix in cinnamon and salt.

Unroll dough on a dry surface with the long sides on the left and right. Roll or stretch into a large rectangle of even thickness. Evenly spread filling onto dough, leaving a 1-inch border. Tightly roll up dough into a log. Pinch the long seam to seal.

Turn log so the seam side is down. Cut widthwise into 8 equally sized buns. Place a bun in each of the 8 sprayed muffin cups, spiral side up.

In a medium microwave-safe bowl, combine all topping ingredients *except* pecans. Microwave for 30 to 45 seconds, until butter has mostly melted. Add pecans and mix well. Evenly distribute topping among buns, about 1 tablespoon each.

Bake until golden brown, 12 to 15 minutes.

Gently remove buns from pan while still warm. Enjoy!

MAKES 8 SERVINGS

GRAB 'N GO BREAKFAST COOKIES

154 calories
PER SERVING

You'll Need: baking sheet, nonstick spray, large bowl, whisk | **Prep:** 20 minutes | **Cook:** 15 minutes

¼th of recipe (1 cookie):
154 calories, 1.5g fat, 166mg sodium, 32.5g carbs, 5g fiber, 10.5g sugars, 5g protein

INGREDIENTS

⅓ cup pureed peaches (like the kinds found in the baby food aisle)

¼ cup Splenda No Calorie Sweetener (granulated)

¼ cup canned pure pumpkin

¼ cup fat-free liquid egg substitute

2 tablespoons brown sugar (not packed)

¼ cup plus 2 tablespoons whole-wheat flour

¼ cup Fiber One Original bran cereal, finely crushed

2 teaspoons sugar-free French vanilla powdered creamer

½ teaspoon baking powder

½ teaspoon cinnamon

⅛ teaspoon salt

½ cup old-fashioned oats

1 tablespoon golden raisins, chopped

1 tablespoon dried sweetened cranberries, chopped

DIRECTIONS

Preheat oven to 375 degrees. Spray a baking sheet with nonstick spray.

In a large bowl, thoroughly whisk peaches, Splenda, pumpkin, egg substitute, and brown sugar.

Add flour, crushed cereal, creamer, baking powder, cinnamon, and salt. Stir until smooth. Fold in oats, chopped raisins, and chopped cranberries.

Spoon batter onto the sheet in 4 evenly spaced mounds. Use the back of a spoon to spread and flatten into 3-inch circles.

Bake until a toothpick inserted into the center of a cookie comes out clean, 12 to 14 minutes. Grab 'n go!

MAKES 4 SERVINGS

HG SWEET ALTERNATIVE!

Swap out the Splenda for the same amount of granulated white sugar, and each serving will have 196 calories, 44g carbs, and 23g sugars.

✳ Flip to the photo inserts to see over 100 recipe pics! And for photos of ALL the recipes, go to **hungry-girl.com/books**.

OATMEAL RAISIN SOFTIES

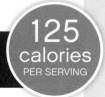

125 calories PER SERVING

You'll Need: baking sheet, nonstick spray, medium bowl, whisk | **Prep:** 10 minutes | **Cook:** 10 minutes

⅙th of recipe (1 softie):
125 calories, 2.5g fat, 120mg sodium, 23.5g carbs, 2g fiber, 10g sugars, 3g protein

INGREDIENTS

¼ cup brown sugar (not packed)

2 tablespoons Splenda No Calorie Sweetener (granulated)

2 tablespoons light whipped butter or light buttery spread, room temperature

2 tablespoons no-sugar-added applesauce

2 tablespoons fat-free liquid egg substitute

¼ teaspoon vanilla extract

⅓ cup whole-wheat flour

¼ teaspoon baking powder

¼ teaspoon cinnamon

Dash salt

¾ cup old-fashioned oats

¼ cup raisins (not packed), chopped

DIRECTIONS

Preheat oven to 350 degrees. Spray a baking sheet with nonstick spray.

In a medium bowl, thoroughly whisk brown sugar, Splenda, butter, applesauce, egg substitute, and vanilla extract.

Add flour, baking powder, cinnamon, and salt, and stir until smooth. Fold in oats and chopped raisins.

Spoon batter onto the sheet in 6 evenly spaced mounds. Use the back of a spoon to spread and flatten into 3-inch circles.

Bake until a toothpick inserted into the center of a softie comes out clean, about 10 minutes. Enjoy!

MAKES 6 SERVINGS

HG SWEET ALTERNATIVE!

Swap out the Splenda for the same amount of granulated white sugar, and each serving will have 139 calories, 27.5g carbs, and 14g sugars.

SAVE THOSE SOFTIES!
Refrigerate leftovers . . . They'll last longer.

PEANUT BUTTER OATMEAL SOFTIES

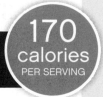
170 calories
PER SERVING

You'll Need: baking sheet, nonstick spray, medium bowl, whisk | **Prep:** 10 minutes | **Cook:** 10 minutes

⅙th of recipe (1 softie):
170 calories, 6.25g fat, 169mg sodium, 23.5g carbs, 2.5g fiber, 7.5g sugars, 5.5g protein

INGREDIENTS

¼ cup reduced-fat peanut butter, room temperature

¼ cup brown sugar (not packed)

2 tablespoons Splenda No Calorie Sweetener (granulated)

2 tablespoons light whipped butter or light buttery spread, room temperature

2 tablespoons no-sugar-added applesauce

2 tablespoons fat-free liquid egg substitute

¼ teaspoon vanilla extract

⅓ cup whole-wheat flour

½ teaspoon baking powder

Dash salt

¾ cup old-fashioned oats

DIRECTIONS

Preheat oven to 350 degrees. Spray a baking sheet with nonstick spray.

In a medium bowl, thoroughly whisk peanut butter, brown sugar, Splenda, butter, applesauce, egg substitute, and vanilla extract.

Add flour, baking powder, and salt, and stir until smooth. Fold in oats.

Spoon batter onto the sheet in 6 evenly spaced mounds. Use the back of a spoon to spread and flatten into 3-inch circles.

Bake until a toothpick inserted into the center of a softie comes out clean, about 10 minutes.

Let cool completely. Enjoy!

MAKES 6 SERVINGS

HG SWEET ALTERNATIVE!

Swap out the Splenda for the same amount of granulated white sugar, and each serving will have 184 calories, 27.5g carbs, and 11.5g sugars.

HG ALTERNATIVE!

If you can find Better'n Peanut Butter, use it. If you do, each softie will have 140 calories, 3.25g fat, and 2g fiber. Woohoo!

PUMPKIN SOFTIES

116 calories PER SERVING

You'll Need: baking sheet, nonstick spray, medium bowl, whisk | **Prep:** 10 minutes | **Cook:** 15 minutes

⅛th of recipe (1 softie):
116 calories, 2g fat, 93mg sodium, 22.5g carbs, 3g fiber, 8g sugars, 3g protein

INGREDIENTS

1 cup canned pure pumpkin
¼ cup brown sugar (not packed)
2 tablespoons Splenda No Calorie Sweetener (granulated)
2 tablespoons light whipped butter or light buttery spread
2 tablespoons fat-free liquid egg substitute
¼ teaspoon vanilla extract
¾ cup whole-wheat flour
1 teaspoon pumpkin pie spice
1 teaspoon cinnamon
½ teaspoon baking powder
⅛ teaspoon salt
½ cup old-fashioned oats
¼ cup raisins (not packed), chopped

DIRECTIONS

Preheat oven to 350 degrees. Spray a baking sheet with nonstick spray.

In a medium bowl, thoroughly whisk pumpkin, brown sugar, Splenda, butter, egg substitute, and vanilla extract.

Add flour, pumpkin pie spice, cinnamon, baking powder, and salt, and stir until smooth. Fold in oats and chopped raisins.

Spoon batter onto the sheet in 8 evenly spaced mounds. Use the back of a spoon to spread and flatten into 3-inch circles.

Bake until a toothpick inserted into the center of a softie comes out clean, 12 to 15 minutes. Enjoy!

MAKES 8 SERVINGS

HG SWEET ALTERNATIVE!

Swap out the Splenda for the same amount of granulated white sugar, and each serving will have 126 calories, 25.5g carbs, and 11g sugars.

CHOCOLATE CHIP OATMEAL SOFTIES

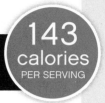
143 calories
PER SERVING

You'll Need: baking sheet, nonstick spray, medium bowl, whisk | **Prep:** 10 minutes | **Cook:** 10 minutes

⅙th of recipe (1 softie):
143 calories, 4.5g fat, 111mg sodium, 23g carbs, 2.5g fiber, 10.5g sugars, 3g protein

INGREDIENTS

¼ cup brown sugar (not packed)

2 tablespoons Splenda No Calorie Sweetener (granulated)

2 tablespoons light whipped butter or light buttery spread, room temperature

2 tablespoons no-sugar-added applesauce

2 tablespoons fat-free liquid egg substitute

½ teaspoon vanilla extract

⅓ cup whole-wheat flour

¼ teaspoon baking powder

⅛ teaspoon salt

¾ cup old-fashioned oats

3 tablespoons mini semi-sweet chocolate chips

DIRECTIONS

Preheat oven to 350 degrees. Spray a baking sheet with nonstick spray.

In a medium bowl, thoroughly whisk brown sugar, Splenda, butter, applesauce, egg substitute, and vanilla extract.

Add flour, baking powder, and salt, and stir until smooth. Fold in oats and chocolate chips.

Spoon batter onto the sheet in 6 evenly spaced mounds. Use the back of a spoon to spread and flatten into 3-inch circles.

Bake until a toothpick inserted into the center of a softie comes out clean, about 10 minutes. Enjoy!

MAKES 6 SERVINGS

HG SWEET ALTERNATIVE!
Swap out the Splenda for the same amount of granulated white sugar, and each serving will have 157 calories, 27g carbs, and 14.5g sugars.

APPLE CINNAMON SOFTIES

123 calories PER SERVING

You'll Need: baking sheet, nonstick spray, microwave-safe bowl, medium bowl, whisk
Prep: 10 minutes | **Cook:** 15 minutes

⅙th of recipe (1 softie):
123 calories, 2.5g fat, 111mg sodium, 22.5g carbs, 2g fiber, 10g sugars, 2.5g protein

INGREDIENTS

1 cup peeled and finely chopped apple
¼ cup plus ½ tablespoon brown sugar (not packed)
1¼ teaspoons cinnamon
2 tablespoons Splenda No Calorie Sweetener (granulated)
2 tablespoons light whipped butter or light buttery spread, room temperature
2 tablespoons no-sugar-added applesauce
2 tablespoons fat-free liquid egg substitute
¼ teaspoon vanilla extract
⅓ cup whole-wheat flour
¼ teaspoon baking powder
⅛ teaspoon salt
¾ cup old-fashioned oats

DIRECTIONS

Preheat oven to 350 degrees. Spray a baking sheet with nonstick spray.

In a microwave-safe bowl, sprinkle apple with ½ tablespoon brown sugar and ¼ teaspoon cinnamon and stir to coat. Microwave for 2 minutes, or until slightly softened. Mix well.

In a medium bowl, thoroughly whisk Splenda, remaining ¼ cup brown sugar, butter, applesauce, egg substitute, and vanilla extract.

Add flour, baking powder, salt, and remaining 1 teaspoon cinnamon, and stir until smooth. Fold in oats and apple mixture.

Spoon batter onto the sheet in 6 evenly spaced mounds. Use the back of a spoon to spread and flatten into 3-inch circles.

Bake until a toothpick inserted into the center of a softie comes out clean, about 10 minutes.

Let cool slightly and enjoy!

MAKES 6 SERVINGS

HG SWEET ALTERNATIVE!

Swap out the Splenda for the same amount of granulated white sugar, and each serving will have 137 calories, 26.5g carbs, and 14g sugars.

SNICKERDOODLE SOFTIES

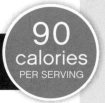

You'll Need: baking sheet, nonstick spray, medium bowl, whisk, small bowl
Prep: 10 minutes | **Cook:** 10 minutes

⅙th of recipe (1 softie):
90 calories, 1.5g fat, 110mg sodium, 16g carbs, 1g fiber, 6.5g sugars, 2g protein

INGREDIENTS

¼ cup brown sugar (not packed)

2 tablespoons plus 2 teaspoons Splenda No Calorie Sweetener (granulated)

2 tablespoons light whipped butter or light buttery spread, room temperature

2 tablespoons no-sugar-added applesauce

2 tablespoons fat-free liquid egg substitute

¼ teaspoon vanilla extract

⅓ cup whole-wheat flour

¼ cup all-purpose flour

¼ teaspoon baking powder

¾ teaspoon cinnamon

⅛ teaspoon salt

DIRECTIONS

Preheat oven to 350 degrees. Spray a baking sheet with nonstick spray.

In a medium bowl, thoroughly whisk brown sugar, 2 tablespoons Splenda, butter, applesauce, egg substitute, and vanilla extract.

Add whole-wheat flour, all-purpose flour, baking powder, ¼ teaspoon cinnamon, and salt. Stir until smooth.

Spoon batter onto the sheet in 6 evenly spaced mounds. Use the back of a spoon to spread and flatten into 2-inch circles.

In a small bowl, mix remaining 2 teaspoons Splenda with remaining ½ teaspoon cinnamon. Sprinkle over batter.

Bake until a toothpick inserted into the center of a softie comes out clean, about 10 minutes. Enjoy!

MAKES 6 SERVINGS

HG SWEET ALTERNATIVE!

Swap out the Splenda for the same amount of granulated white sugar, and each serving will have 109 calories, 21g carbs, and 12g sugars.

✳ Flip to the photo inserts to see over 100 recipe pics! And for photos of ALL the recipes, go to **hungry-girl.com/books**.

CRANBERRY WHITE CHOCOLATE SOFTIES

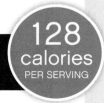

128 calories PER SERVING

You'll Need: baking sheet, nonstick spray, medium bowl, whisk | **Prep:** 10 minutes | **Cook:** 10 minutes

⅙th of recipe (1 softie):
128 calories, 3.5g fat, 115mg sodium, 21.5g carbs, 1.5g fiber, 11g sugars, 2.5g protein

INGREDIENTS

¼ cup brown sugar (not packed)

2 tablespoons Splenda No Calorie Sweetener (granulated)

2 tablespoons light whipped butter or light buttery spread, room temperature

2 tablespoons no-sugar-added applesauce

2 tablespoons fat-free liquid egg substitute

¼ teaspoon vanilla extract

⅓ cup whole-wheat flour

¼ teaspoon baking powder

⅛ teaspoon salt

½ cup old-fashioned oats

2 tablespoons sweetened dried cranberries, chopped

2 tablespoons white chocolate chips, finely chopped

HG SWEET ALTERNATIVE!

Swap out the Splenda for the same amount of granulated white sugar, and each serving will have 142 calories, 25.5g carbs, and 15g sugars.

DIRECTIONS

Preheat oven to 350 degrees. Spray a baking sheet with nonstick spray.

In a medium bowl, thoroughly whisk brown sugar, Splenda, butter, applesauce, egg substitute, and vanilla extract.

Add flour, baking powder, and salt, and stir until smooth. Fold in oats and chopped cranberries.

Spoon batter onto the sheet in 6 evenly spaced mounds. Use the back of a spoon to spread and flatten into 3-inch circles. Sprinkle with chopped chocolate chips.

Bake until a toothpick inserted into the center of a softie comes out clean, about 10 minutes. Enjoy!

MAKES 6 SERVINGS

CHOCOLATE-DRIZZLED PB CHIP SOFTIES

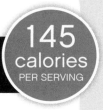

145 calories
PER SERVING

You'll Need: baking sheet, nonstick spray, medium bowl, whisk, very small microwave-safe bowl
Prep: 10 minutes | **Cook:** 15 minutes

⅙th of recipe (1 softie):
145 calories, 5g fat, 124mg sodium, 22g carbs, 2g fiber, 11g sugars, 3g protein

INGREDIENTS

¼ cup brown sugar (not packed)

2 tablespoons Splenda No Calorie Sweetener (granulated)

2 tablespoons light whipped butter or light buttery spread, room temperature

2 tablespoons no-sugar-added applesauce

2 tablespoons fat-free liquid egg substitute

¼ teaspoon vanilla extract

⅓ cup whole-wheat flour

¼ teaspoon baking powder

⅛ teaspoon salt

½ cup old-fashioned oats

2 tablespoons peanut butter baking chips, finely chopped

2 tablespoons mini semi-sweet chocolate chips

DIRECTIONS

Preheat oven to 350 degrees. Spray a baking sheet with nonstick spray.

In a medium bowl, thoroughly whisk brown sugar, Splenda, butter, applesauce, egg substitute, and vanilla extract.

Add flour, baking powder, and salt, and stir until smooth. Fold in oats.

Spoon batter onto the sheet in 6 evenly spaced mounds. Use the back of a spoon to spread and flatten into 3-inch circles. Sprinkle with chopped peanut butter chips.

Bake until a toothpick inserted into the center of a softie comes out clean, about 10 minutes.

In a very small microwave-safe bowl, microwave chocolate chips at 50 percent power for 1 minute. Stir and microwave at 50 percent power for 30 seconds; repeat, as needed, until melted.

Stir melted chocolate and drizzle over softies. Enjoy immediately or refrigerate until chocolate drizzle is firm. Yum!

MAKES 6 SERVINGS

HG SWEET ALTERNATIVE!

Swap out the Splenda for the same amount of granulated white sugar, and each serving will have 159 calories, 26g carbs, and 15g sugars.

ROCKY ROAD SOFTIES

You'll Need: baking sheet, nonstick spray, medium bowl, whisk | **Prep:** 10 minutes | **Cook:** 15 minutes

⅙th of recipe (1 softie):
144 calories, 4.5g fat, 160mg sodium, 23g carbs, 2g fiber, 11.5g sugars, 3g protein

INGREDIENTS

¼ cup brown sugar (not packed)
2 tablespoons Splenda No Calorie Sweetener (granulated)
2 tablespoons light whipped butter or light buttery spread, room temperature
2 tablespoons no-sugar-added applesauce
2 tablespoons fat-free liquid egg substitute
¼ teaspoon vanilla extract
⅓ cup whole-wheat flour
2 packets hot cocoa mix with 20 to 25 calories each
¼ teaspoon baking powder
⅛ teaspoon salt
½ cup old-fashioned oats
2 tablespoons mini semi-sweet chocolate chips
2 tablespoons sliced almonds, roughly chopped
24 mini marshmallows (about ¼ cup)

DIRECTIONS

Preheat oven to 350 degrees. Spray a baking sheet with nonstick spray.

In a medium bowl, thoroughly whisk brown sugar, Splenda, butter, applesauce, egg substitute, and vanilla extract.

Add flour, cocoa mix, baking powder, and salt, and stir until smooth. Fold in oats, chocolate chips, and chopped almonds.

Spoon batter onto the sheet in 6 evenly spaced mounds. Use the back of a spoon to spread and flatten into 3-inch circles.

Bake until a toothpick inserted into the center of a softie comes out mostly clean, about 9 minutes. Leave oven on.

Meanwhile, cut each marshmallow into 2 coin-shaped halves.

Top each softie with 8 marshmallow halves, cut sides down. Bake until marshmallows just begin to melt, 1 to 2 minutes. (Do not overbake, as marshmallows will completely melt.) Enjoy!

MAKES 6 SERVINGS

HG SWEET ALTERNATIVE!

Swap out the Splenda for the same amount of granulated white sugar, and each serving will have 158 calories, 26.5g carbs, and 15.5g sugars.

HG HEADS-UP:

If refrigerating leftovers, let cool completely first.

FREEZYLICIOUS STRAWBERRY SQUARES

173 calories PER SERVING

You'll Need: 8-inch by 8-inch baking pan, nonstick spray, blender or food processor, medium bowl, small microwave-safe bowl | **Prep:** 15 minutes | **Cook:** 10 minutes | **Freeze:** 6 hours

⅑th of recipe (1 square):
173 calories, 2.75g fat, 142mg sodium, 35g carbs, 5g fiber, 21.5g sugars, 4g protein

INGREDIENTS

Crust
1 cup Fiber One Original bran cereal

1 cup Fiber One Caramel Delight cereal

3 tablespoons Splenda No Calorie Sweetener (granulated)

1 teaspoon cinnamon

¼ cup light whipped butter or light buttery spread

Filling
Half of a 14-ounce can (½ cup plus 2 tablespoons) fat-free sweetened condensed milk

2 cups frozen unsweetened strawberries, partially thawed

2 cups fat-free strawberry yogurt

1 cup Cool Whip Free (thawed)

1 teaspoon vanilla extract

HG SWEET ALTERNATIVE!
Swap out the Splenda for the same amount of granulated white sugar, and each serving will have 187 calories, 39g carbs, and 25.5g sugars.

DIRECTIONS

Preheat oven to 350 degrees. Spray an 8-inch by 8-inch baking pan with nonstick spray.

In a blender or food processor, grind both cereals into crumbs. Transfer to a medium bowl and mix in Splenda and cinnamon.

In a small microwave-safe bowl, microwave butter and 2 tablespoons water for 30 seconds, or until butter has melted. Add to the medium bowl and thoroughly mix.

Evenly distribute mixture along the bottom of the baking pan, using your hands or a flat utensil to firmly press and form the crust. Press it into the edges, but not up the sides.

Bake until firm, about 10 minutes. Let cool.

Clean blender, and add all filling ingredients. Blend at high speed until smooth. Pour mixture over the crust in the pan.

Cover and freeze until firm, about 6 hours.

Let thaw for 5 to 10 minutes before serving. Cut into squares and enjoy!

MAKES 9 SERVINGS

For more recipes, tips & tricks, sign up for FREE daily emails at **hungry-girl.com!**

BIG BEAUTIFUL BAKED ALASKA

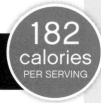

182 calories
PER SERVING

You'll Need: medium-large bowl with an 8-inch diameter at the top (with a capacity of at least 1½ quarts), plastic wrap, large bowl, electric mixer, 9-inch pie pan, baking sheet
Prep: 15 minutes | **Freeze:** 8 hours | **Cook:** 5 minutes

⅛th of dessert:
182 calories, 2g fat, 109mg sodium, 37g carbs, 0.5g fiber, 23.5g sugars, 4.5g protein

INGREDIENTS

3 cups fat-free vanilla ice cream, softened
2 cups light strawberry ice cream, softened
16 Reduced Fat Nilla Wafers
½ cup liquid egg whites (about 4 egg whites)
⅛ teaspoon cream of tartar
¼ cup granulated white sugar
¼ cup Splenda No Calorie Sweetener (granulated)
¼ teaspoon vanilla extract

HG SWEET ALTERNATIVES!

Skip the Splenda in this recipe and double the granulated white sugar; each serving will have 203 calories, 42g carbs, and 29g sugars. Or double the Splenda and leave out the sugar; then each serving will have 161 calories, 31.5g carbs, and 17.5g sugars. Score!

DIRECTIONS

Begin with a medium-large bowl with an 8-inch diameter at the top (with a capacity of at least 1½ quarts). Line the bowl with plastic wrap, draping excess wrap over the sides.

Evenly and firmly pack vanilla ice cream into the bowl. Smooth out the surface, and repeat with strawberry ice cream, yielding two packed layers with a flat surface. Place wafers, rounded side down, in a single layer over the strawberry ice cream. Cover with plastic wrap and freeze until completely firm, at least 8 hours.

Preheat oven to 500 degrees. Set out all remaining measured ingredients.

To make the meringue, combine egg whites with cream of tartar in a large bowl. With an electric mixer set to high speed, beat until fluffy and slightly stiff, about 3 minutes. Continue to beat while gradually adding sugar, Splenda, and vanilla extract. Beat until fully blended and stiff peaks form, 2 to 3 minutes.

Remove bowl from the freezer and uncover. Place a 9-inch pie pan firmly over the bowl, upside down, and carefully flip so the pie pan is on the bottom. Gently tug on the plastic wrap to release the ice cream from the bowl, leaving the ice cream in the pie pan. Remove the plastic wrap.

Quickly and evenly spread meringue over the ice cream mound. Place pie pan on a baking sheet.

Bake until meringue is cooked through and lightly browned, about 3 minutes. Slice and enjoy! (Freeze the leftovers and eat 'em frozen.)

MAKES 8 SERVINGS

These **FREEZY FAUX ICE CREAM SANDWICHES** are not made with actual ice cream . . . but they're packed with freezy-cool creamy goodness!

FREEZY PB&J MINIS

110 calories
PER SERVING

You'll Need: small bowl, plate | **Prep:** 5 minutes | **Freeze:** 1 hour

¼th of recipe (4 mini sandwiches):
110 calories, 1.5g fat, 187mg sodium, 21g carbs, <0.5g fiber, 7.5g sugars, 2g protein

INGREDIENTS

1 tablespoon low-sugar strawberry preserves

1 tablespoon reduced-fat creamy peanut butter, room temperature

½ cup Cool Whip Free (thawed)

32 caramel-flavored mini rice cakes

DIRECTIONS

In a small bowl, mix preserves with peanut butter until smooth. Stir in Cool Whip until just mixed.

Lay 16 mini rice cakes on a plate, and evenly distribute Cool Whip mixture among them.

Lightly place another rice cake over each mixture-topped cake to form 16 sandwiches. Freeze until filling is firm, at least 1 hour. Yum!

MAKES 4 SERVINGS

FREEZY MOVIE NIGHT CONCESSION STAND-WICHES

158 calories PER SERVING

You'll Need: medium-large bowl, 2 plates or baking sheet
Prep: 15 minutes
Freeze: 1 hour 30 minutes

⅐th of recipe (1 sandwich): 158 calories, 2g fat, 128mg sodium, 32g carbs, <0.5g fiber, 7g sugars, 2.5g protein

INGREDIENTS

One 8-ounce container Cool Whip Free (thawed)
3 pieces Twizzlers Strawberry Twists, finely chopped
1 tablespoon mini semi-sweet chocolate chips
1 tablespoon chopped peanuts
14 full-sized butter-flavored rice cakes

DIRECTIONS

Place Cool Whip in a medium-large bowl. Gently stir in chopped Twizzlers, chocolate chips, and chopped peanuts.

Evenly distribute Cool Whip mixture among 7 rice cakes, a heaping ¼ cup each.

Lightly place another rice cake over each filling-topped cake to form 7 sandwiches.

Place sandwiches in an even layer on 2 plates or a baking sheet and freeze until filling is firm, at least 1½ hours. Eat up!

MAKES 7 SERVINGS

TOO-COOL KEY LIME PIE SANDWICHES

128 calories PER SERVING

You'll Need: medium bowl, plate
Prep: 10 minutes
Freeze: 1 hour 30 minutes

½ of recipe (1 sandwich): 128 calories, 1g fat, 105mg sodium, 24g carbs, 0.5g fiber, 16g sugars, 7g protein

INGREDIENTS

½ cup fat-free plain Greek yogurt
1½ tablespoons granulated white sugar
1 tablespoon lime juice (key lime, if available)
2 sheets (8 crackers) low-fat cinnamon graham crackers, broken into 4 squares

DIRECTIONS

In a medium bowl, thoroughly mix yogurt, sugar, and lime juice. Cover and freeze until very thick but soft enough to stir, 25 to 30 minutes.

Place two graham cracker squares on a plate, cinnamon sides down. Stir yogurt mixture and divide between the two squares, about ¼ cup each. Gently top each with another graham cracker square, cinnamon sides up.

Freeze until filling is firm, at least 1 hour. Enjoy!

MAKES 2 SERVINGS

HG SWEET ALTERNATIVE!

If made with an equal amount of Splenda No Calorie Sweetener (granulated) in place of the sugar, each serving will have 97 calories, 15.5g carbs, and 6.5g sugars.

CREAMY FROZEN CARAMEL CRUNCHCAKE

130 calories

You'll Need: small bowl | **Prep:** 5 minutes | **Freeze:** 1 hour 30 minutes

Entire recipe:
130 calories, 0.5g fat, 70mg sodium, 28g carbs, 0g fiber, 8g sugars, 2g protein

INGREDIENTS

¼ cup Cool Whip Free (thawed)

Dash cinnamon, or more to taste

2 full-sized caramel-flavored rice cakes

DIRECTIONS

In a small bowl, stir cinnamon into Cool Whip. Spoon mixture over 1 rice cake. Gently top with the other rice cake.

Freeze until filling is firm, at least 1 ½ hours. Enjoy!

MAKES 1 SERVING

COOL 'N CREAMY BIRTHDAY CAKE SANDWICH

192 calories

You'll Need: small bowl | **Prep:** 5 minutes | **Freeze:** 1 hour 30 minutes

Entire recipe:
192 calories, 2.5g fat, 75mg sodium, 37g carbs, <0.5g fiber, 16.5g sugars, 2g protein

INGREDIENTS

¼ cup Cool Whip Free (thawed)

1 drop vanilla extract

2 teaspoons rainbow sprinkles

1 teaspoon mini semi-sweet chocolate chips

2 full-sized caramel-flavored rice cakes

DIRECTIONS

In a small bowl, mix Cool Whip with vanilla extract. Stir in sprinkles and chocolate chips. Evenly spoon mixture onto 1 rice cake. Lightly top with the other rice cake to form a sandwich.

Freeze until filling is firm, at least 1½ hours. Enjoy!

MAKES 1 SERVING

CHOCOLATE-COCONUT FREEZIES

102 calories PER SERVING

You'll Need: small bowl, plate
Prep: 5 minutes
Freeze: 1 hour

¼th of recipe (4 mini sandwiches):
102 calories, 2g fat, 63mg sodium, 20g carbs,
0.5g fiber, 7g sugars, 1g protein

INGREDIENTS

½ cup Cool Whip Free (thawed)
2 teaspoons mini semi-sweet chocolate chips
1 teaspoon shredded sweetened coconut
⅛ teaspoon coconut extract
32 chocolate-flavored mini rice cakes

DIRECTIONS

In a small bowl, mix Cool Whip, chocolate chips,
shredded coconut, and coconut extract. Lay
16 mini rice cakes on a plate, and evenly distribute
mixture among them.

Lightly place another rice cake over each
mixture-topped cake to form 16 sandwiches.
Freeze until filling is firm, at least 1 hour. Yum!

MAKES 4 SERVINGS

FREEZY-COOL SNICKERS STACKERS

186 calories PER SERVING

You'll Need: medium bowl
Prep: 5 minutes
Freeze: 1½ hours

½ of recipe (1 sandwich): 186 calories,
3g fat, 178mg sodium, 30.5g carbs,
2g fiber, 7.5g sugars, 4g protein

INGREDIENTS

½ cup Cool Whip Free (thawed)
1 tablespoon chopped peanuts
1 sugar-free chocolate pudding snack
    with 60 calories or less
4 full-sized caramel-flavored rice cakes

DIRECTIONS

In a medium bowl, stir peanuts into Cool
Whip. Gently swirl in the pudding.

Evenly distribute mixture between
2 rice cakes. Lightly top each with another
rice cake to form 2 sandwiches.

Freeze until filling is firm, at least 1½ hours.
Enjoy!

MAKES 2 SERVINGS

FREEZY CANDY CANE SNACK-WICHES

93 calories PER SERVING

You'll Need: medium bowl, large plate | **Prep:** 5 minutes | **Freeze:** 1 hour

¼th of recipe (4 mini sandwiches):
93 calories, 1g fat, 60mg sodium, 20.5g carbs, 0g fiber, 7g sugars, 1g protein

INGREDIENTS

½ cup Cool Whip Free (thawed)

3 mini candy canes *or* ½ standard-sized candy cane, lightly crushed

32 chocolate-flavored mini rice cakes

DIRECTIONS

In a medium bowl, gently stir crushed candy cane(s) into Cool Whip. Lay 16 mini rice cakes on a large plate, and evenly distribute filling among them.

Lightly place another rice cake over each mixture-topped cake to form 16 sandwiches. Freeze until filling is firm, at least 1 hour. Mmmm!

MAKES 4 SERVINGS

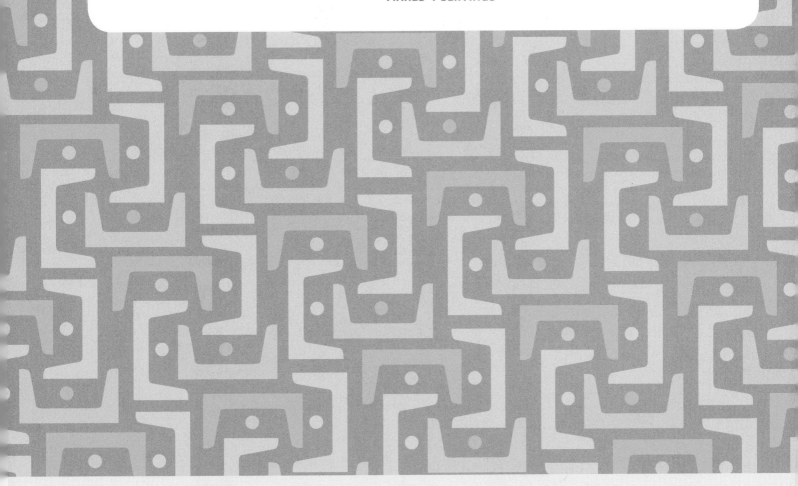

MINI ICE CREAM CAKES

136 calories PER SERVING

You'll Need: 12-cup muffin pan, foil baking cups, large bowl, whisk, large platter (optional)
Prep: 20 minutes | **Cook:** 25 minutes | **Freeze:** 1 hour 30 minutes

¹⁄₁₂th of recipe (1 mini ice cream cake):
136 calories, 3.5g fat, 131mg sodium, 22.5g carbs, <0.5g fiber, 14g sugars, 2.5g protein

INGREDIENTS

1 cup moist-style devil's food cake mix
¼ cup fat-free liquid egg substitute
1 tablespoon mini semi-sweet chocolate chips
3 cups light chocolate chip ice cream (vanilla with chocolate chips)
1½ cups Cool Whip Free (thawed)
2 tablespoons sprinkles

DIRECTIONS

Preheat oven to 350 degrees. Line a 12-cup muffin pan with foil baking cups.

In a large bowl, whisk cake mix, egg substitute, and ½ cup water. Stir in chocolate chips. Evenly distribute among the cups of the muffin pan. (Cups will be about ⅓rd full.)

Bake until a toothpick inserted into the center of a cupcake comes out mostly clean, 20 to 22 minutes.

Let cool completely.

Remove cupcakes from the pan. Evenly top with ice cream, ¼ cup per cupcake. Evenly top ice cream layers with remaining ingredients: 2 tablespoons Cool Whip and ½ teaspoon sprinkles each.

Transfer cupcakes to a large platter that will fit in your freezer or place them back in the cooled muffin pan.

Freeze until ice cream is firm and Cool Whip is frozen, at least 1½ hours. Eat!

MAKES 12 SERVINGS

HG TIP:
If frozen for longer than 1½ hours, allow cupcakes to slightly thaw before eating, about 5 minutes.

Flip to the photo inserts to see over 100 recipe pics! And for photos of ALL the recipes, go to **hungry-girl.com/books**.

Unconventional, RICE KRISPIE-LESS, CEREAL SNACK fun for humans of all ages . . .

KRISPYMALLOW TREATS

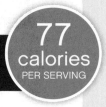

77 calories PER SERVING

You'll Need: 9-inch by 13-inch baking pan, nonstick spray, large nonstick pot
Prep: 5 minutes | **Cook:** 15 minutes

⅟₁₅th of recipe (1 treat):
77 calories, 1.5g fat, 54mg sodium, 18.5g carbs, 4g fiber, 6.5g sugars, 1.5g protein

INGREDIENTS

3 tablespoons light whipped butter or light buttery spread

3 cups miniature marshmallows

5 cups puffed wheat cereal

2 cups Fiber One Original bran cereal

DIRECTIONS

Spray a 9-inch by 13-inch baking pan with nonstick spray.

Place butter in a large nonstick pot and bring to low heat. Once butter has melted, add marshmallows. Cook and stir until melted, about 10 minutes.

Remove pot from heat. Add both cereals and gently stir until coated.

Using a spatula sprayed with nonstick spray, evenly press mixture into the baking pan.

Let cool completely. Cut and devour!

MAKES 15 SERVINGS

HG HISTORY:

Have you noticed our Krispymallows have gotten LARGER over the years? The stats were so impressive we increased the serving sizes. Yay!

KRISPYMALLOW TREAT MOLDING TRICK!

Lay a sheet of wax paper or parchment paper over the mixture in the pan . . . then just press to smooth. SO EASY.

COCOA LOCO KRISPYMALLOW TREATS

122 calories PER SERVING

You'll Need: 9-inch by 13-inch baking pan, nonstick spray, large nonstick pot
Prep: 5 minutes
Cook: 15 minutes

⅕th of recipe (1 treat): 122 calories, 2.75g fat, 99mg sodium, 25.5g carbs, 3.5g fiber, 12g sugars, 1.5g protein

INGREDIENTS

3 tablespoons light whipped butter or light buttery spread

3 cups mini marshmallows

3 cups Chocolate Cheerios cereal

3 cups puffed wheat cereal

1½ cups Fiber One Original bran cereal

One 1.53-ounce package Reese's Pieces candy, lightly crushed

One 1.69-ounce package Milk Chocolate M&M's candy, lightly crushed

DIRECTIONS

Spray a 9-inch by 13-inch baking pan with nonstick spray.

Place butter in a large nonstick pot and bring to low heat. Once butter has melted, add marshmallows. Cook and stir until melted, about 10 minutes.

Remove pot from heat. Add all three cereals and gently stir until coated.

Using a spatula sprayed with nonstick spray, evenly press mixture into the baking pan.

Sprinkle both types of crushed candy evenly over the treats and press down with the spatula to help them adhere.

Let cool completely. Cut it up and eat it up!

MAKES 15 SERVINGS

S'MORES KRISPYMALLOW TREATS

95 calories PER SERVING

You'll Need: 9-inch by 13-inch baking pan, nonstick spray, large nonstick pot
Prep: 5 minutes
Cook: 15 minutes

⅕th of recipe (1 treat): 95 calories, 1.5g fat, 87mg sodium, 20g carbs, 2.5g fiber, 8.5g sugars, 0.5g protein

INGREDIENTS

3 tablespoons light whipped butter or light buttery spread

3 cups mini marshmallows

4 cups puffed wheat cereal

2 cups Golden Grahams cereal

1 cup Fiber One Original bran cereal

5 teaspoons mini semi-sweet chocolate chips

DIRECTIONS

Spray a 9-inch by 13-inch baking pan with nonstick spray.

Place butter in a large nonstick pot and bring to low heat. Once butter has melted, add marshmallows. Cook and stir until melted, about 10 minutes.

Remove pot from heat. Add all three cereals and gently stir until coated.

Using a spatula sprayed with nonstick spray, evenly press mixture into the baking pan.

Sprinkle with chocolate chips, and press down with the spatula to help them adhere.

Let cool completely. Slice and enjoy!

MAKES 15 SERVINGS

PB CHOCOLATE KRISPYMALLOW TREATS

127 calories PER SERVING

You'll Need: 9-inch by 13-inch baking pan, nonstick spray, large nonstick pot, small microwave-safe bowl
Prep: 5 minutes
Cook: 15 minutes

¹⁄₁₅th of recipe (1 treat): 127 calories, 3.5g fat, 89mg sodium, 25g carbs, 3.5g fiber, 11g sugars, 2g protein

INGREDIENTS

3 tablespoons light whipped butter or light buttery spread
3 cups mini marshmallows
3 cups puffed wheat cereal
3 cups Peanut Butter Multi Grain Cheerios cereal
1½ cups Fiber One Original bran cereal
¼ cup mini semi-sweet chocolate chips
3 tablespoons peanut butter baking chips, roughly chopped

DIRECTIONS

Spray a 9-inch by 13-inch baking pan with nonstick spray.

Place butter in a large nonstick pot and bring to low heat. Once butter has melted, add marshmallows. Cook and stir until melted, about 10 minutes.

Remove pot from heat. Add all three cereals and gently stir until coated.

Using a spatula sprayed with nonstick spray, evenly press mixture into the baking pan.

Let cool completely.

In a small microwave-safe bowl, microwave chocolate chips at 50 percent power for 1 minute. Stir and microwave at 50 percent power for 30 seconds; repeat, as needed, until melted.

Stir and drizzle melted chocolate over the treats and sprinkle with chopped peanut butter chips.

Once chocolate drizzle is firm, cut and eat up!

MAKES 15 SERVINGS

CANDY CORN MEGAMALLOW TREATS

132 calories PER SERVING

You'll Need: 9-inch by 13-inch baking pan, nonstick spray, large nonstick pot
Prep: 5 minutes
Cook: 15 minutes

¹⁄₁₂th of recipe (1 treat): 132 calories, 1.5g fat, 167mg sodium, 33g carbs, 4.5g fiber, 14.5g sugars, 1.5g protein

INGREDIENTS

3 tablespoons light whipped butter or light buttery spread
3 cups mini marshmallows
4 cups (about one 3.5-ounce bag) mini caramel-flavored rice cakes, lightly crushed
2 cups Fiber One Original bran cereal
1 cup puffed wheat cereal
3 ounces (about ½ cup) candy corn, chopped

DIRECTIONS

Spray a 9-inch by 13-inch baking pan with nonstick spray.

Place butter in a large nonstick pot and bring to low heat. Once butter has melted, add marshmallows. Cook and stir until melted, about 10 minutes.

Remove pot from heat. Add crushed rice cakes and both cereals and stir to coat.

Using a spatula sprayed with nonstick spray, evenly press mixture into the baking pan.

Evenly sprinkle with chopped candy corn and press firmly into the mixture.

Let cool completely. Cut and EAT!

MAKES 12 SERVINGS

RECIPES THAT TAKE 15 MINUTES OR LESS

⏱ RECIPES THAT TAKE 15 MINUTES OR LESS

RECIPES THAT TAKE 15 MINUTES OR LESS

Super-Sour Lemon Drop
Kickin' Cranberry Cosmo
Apple Cinnamon Cosmo
Night & Day Nog-tinis
ChocoMint Martinis

Candy Corn Custard Parfait
Expresso Cake in a Mug
Mississippi Mug Pie
Red Hot Apple Pie in a Cup
Super-Duper Strawberry Shortcake
Caramel Bread Pudding for Two
Vanilla Almond Fruit Tartlets
BFFs (Black Forest Fillo-Cups)
Double-Chocolate Pretzel Tarts
Double-Trouble Chocolate Trifle

⏱ RECIPES THAT TAKE 30 MINUTES OR LESS

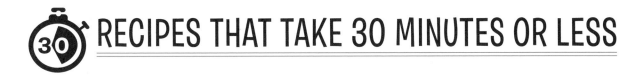

RECIPES THAT TAKE 30 MINUTES OR LESS

Creamy Salmon Girlfredo
Beef Strogataki
Clam-tastic Shirataki Pasta
Chicken Carbonara a la Hungry Girl
Spicy Southern Shrimp Fettuccine
Vodka Impasta
Super-Delicious Shrimp Scampi
Chicken Florentine
Slaw and Order
Funkadelic Chili Mac

PIZZA 220

Crispy White Pizza
Thin-Crust Enchilada Pizza
Garlic Chicken Pizza
Best BBQ Chicken Pizza
The Great Greek Pizza
American Buffalo Chicken Pizza
Mediterranean Pizza
Veggie & Ricotta Pizza
Sloppy Joe Pizza
Garlic-Bread White Pizza
Salad-Topped Pita Pizza
Sausage-Topped Pizza Swap
Meat Lover's Breakfast Pizza
Perfect Pepperoni Pizzas
Chicken Girlfredo Pizza
Pizza Luau
Purple Pizza Eaters
Pesto Pizzas
Pizza-bellas
White Pizza-bellas
Sausage-Loaded Pizza-bellas
Greek Pizza-bellas

MEXICAN 244

Shrimp Cocktail Tacos
Crunchy BBQ Chicken Tacos
iHungry Spaghetti Tacos
Saucy-Q Chicken Soft Tacos
Peach-BBQ Soft Fish Tacos
Amazing Ate-Layer Tostada
Chicken Fajita Burrito
Caramelized Onion Cheese Quesadilla
Clubhouse Chicken Quesadilla
Cheeseburger Quesadilla
Cheesy Pizza Quesadilla
Lean 'n Green Shrimp-chilada
Cheesy Chicken Enchiladas
Lean Bean 'n Cheese Enchiladas
Pizza-ladas
Spinach Enchiladas
Surprise, It's Pumpkin! Enchiladas
Buffalo Chicken Taquitos
Jalapeño Cheese Taquitos
'Bella Asada Fajitas

BURGERS & FRIES 268

Island Insanity Burger
Philly-licious Cheesesteak Burger
Spinach Arti-Cheeseburger
Portabella Guac Burger
HG's 100-Calorie Beef Patties
Bacon Cheeseburger Patty
Outside-In Cheeseburger Patty
OMG! Onion Mushroom Goodness Burgers
Thanksgiving Burgers
Mamma Mia! Patties
Tremendous Top-Shelf Turkey Burger
Red Hot & Blue Burger
Unique Greek Turkey Burgers
Cheesed-Up Taco Turkey Burgers

⏱ RECIPES THAT TAKE 30 MINUTES OR LESS

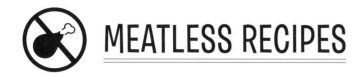

MEATLESS RECIPES

EGG MUGS AND EGG BAKES   8

The Egg Mug Classic
Bean 'n Cheesy Soft Taco in an Egg Mug
California Love Mug
Crunchy Beefy Taco Egg Mug
Say Cheese! Egg Mug
Mexi-licious Egg Mug
It's All Greek to Me Egg Mug
Egg Mug Burger-rama
All-American Egg Mug
Egg Mug Florentine
Chili Cheese Egg Mug
Veggie Eggs-plosion Mug
Cheesy Jalapeño Egg Mug
The Original Ginormous Egg Bake
Egg Bake Olé
El Ginormo Southwest Egg Bake
Cheesy-Onion Egg Bake
Cheesy Sausage 'n Hash Egg Bake
Caramelized Onion 'n Spinach Egg Bake
Sweet Treat a la Soufflé

GROWING OATMEAL BOWLS   34

Banana Split Oatmeal
Happy Trail Mix Oatmeal
PB&J Oatmeal Heaven
S'mores Oatmeal
Large & In Charge Neapolitan Oatmeal
Strawberry Shortcake Oatmeal
Caramel Apple Oatmeal
Choco-Monkey Oatmeal
Cinna-Raisin Oatmeal
Skinny Elvis Oatmeal
Piña Colada Oatmeal
Pumpkin Chocolate Chip Oatmeal
Complete & Utter Oatmeal Insanity
Major Mocha Cappuccino Oatmeal

Chocolate Caramel Coconut Oatmeal
Apple Pie Oatmeal Bonanza
PB & Chocolate Oatmeal Blitz
Cranberry-Walnut Maple Oatmeal

PARFAITS   48

Magical Maui Oatmeal Parfait
Peaches 'n Cream Oatmeal Parfait
Blueberry Pie Oatmeal Parfait
Bananas Foster Oatmeal Parfait
Pumpkin Pie Oatmeal Parfait
Super-Sized Berry-nana Oatmeal Parfait
PB&J Oatmeal Parfait
Cinn-a-nilla Apple Oatmeal Parfait
Bananas Foster Puddin' Parfait
Peachy Maple–Caramel Crunch Parfait
Creamy Crunchy Freeze-Dried Frenzy
PB&J Yogurt Parfait
Big Black-and-White Berry Parfait
Carnival Parfait
Dessert Island Parfait
Bananas for Brownies Parfait
Pumpkin Pudding Parfait
Very Berry Dreamboat Parfaits
Crunchy Caramel Chocolate Parfaits
Caramel Apple Parfait
Strawberry Shortcake Parfait
Piña Colada Parfait Surprise
Very Berry Vanilla Parfait
Banana Split Yogurt Parfait
Sun-Up Waffle Parfait
Coconut Cream Pie Parfait
Sausage McMuffin Parfait
Cheeseburger Mashed Potato Parfaits

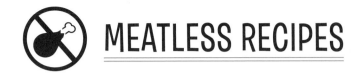

MEATLESS RECIPES

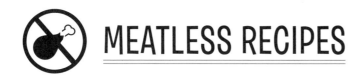

MEATLESS RECIPES

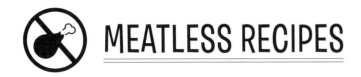

MEATLESS RECIPES

SINGLE-SERVING RECIPES

① SINGLE-SERVING RECIPES

SINGLE-SERVING RECIPES

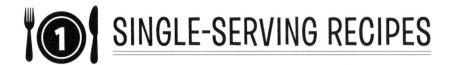

SINGLE-SERVING RECIPES

RECIPES WITH 5 INGREDIENTS OR LESS

RECIPES WITH 5 INGREDIENTS OR LESS

RECIPES WITH 5 INGREDIENTS OR LESS

Guilt-Free Dirt & Worms Surprise

Spice Cake Muffins

Mississippi Mug Pie

Red Hot Apple Pie in a Cup

Diet Soda Cake

Super-Duper Strawberry Shortcake

Ba Na Na Crazy Caramel Shortcakes

Vanilla Almond Fruit Tartlets

BFFs (Black Forest Fillo-Cups)

Double-Chocolate Pretzel Tarts

Caramel Apple Pie Bites

Perfect Peach Dumplings

Bestest Baked Apples

Freezy-Cool Whoopie Pie

Freezy-Good Whoopie S'mores

Freezy-Cool Banana Whoopie Pies

Double-Trouble Chocolate Trifle

Freezy PB&J Minis

Freezy Movie Night Concession Stand-wiches

Too-Cool Key Lime Pie Sandwiches

Creamy Frozen Caramel Crunchcake

Cool 'n Creamy Birthday Cake Sandwich

Chocolate-Coconut Freezies

Freezy-Cool Snickers Stackers

Freezy Candy Cane Snack-wiches

Krispymallow Treats

📷 RECIPES IN PHOTO INSERT ONE

RECIPES IN PHOTO INSERT TWO

There you go! A whopping 650 GUILT-FREE RECIPES for your chewing (and sipping) pleasure! I hope you LOVE them as much as we do here at the HG HQ. (I've got a feeling you will!) Have questions, comments, or just want to say hi? Email me at ask@hungry-girl.com. And for all the latest guilt-free food news, product finds, and brand-new recipes, sign up for FREE daily emails at hungry-girl.com.

Now, who's hungry?

Lisa :)

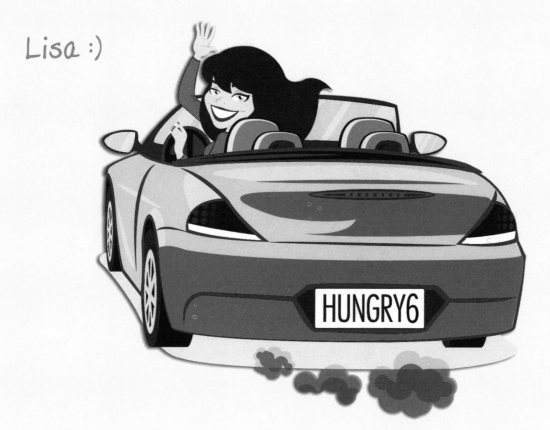

INDEX

Greenwood Public Library
PO Box 839 Mill St.
Greenwood, DE 19950

DISCARD